RESEARCH EXAMPLES

1–1. Role Conflict—A Challenge to Reality Shock 27

2–1. Autocratic, Democratic, and Laissez-Faire Leadership 35

2–2. Leadership Style and Nursing Staff Job Satisfaction 39

2–3. The Famous Hawthorne Studies 43

2–4. Which Approach do Successful Managers Use? 48

3–1. The Effect of Leader Competence 65

4–1. Tasks of First-Line Nurse Managers 88

10–1. Being Sane in Insane Places 191

11–1. How Often Should Patient Classification Ratings Be Done? 224

12–1. Interruptions in Nursing Managers' Schedules 244

14–1. Nurses' Purposes Versus Management's Perceptions in Collective
Bargaining 265

14–2. Hospital Employee's Opinions About Their Work 275

15–1. A Simulated Negotiation 306

18–1. A Case Study of Participative Decision Making 381

19–1. Successful Planned Changes 417

NURSING LEADERSHIP AND MANAGEMENT:
Concepts and Practice

Second Edition

NURSING LEADERSHIP AND MANAGEMENT:
Concepts and Practice

Second Edition

RUTH M. TAPPEN, R.N., Ed.D.
Professor, School of Nursing
University of Miami
Coral Gables, Florida

F.A. DAVIS COMPANY • Philadelphia

Printed in the United States of America

Last digit indicates print number: 10 9 8 7 6 5 4 3

Library of Congress Cataloging-in-Publication Data

Tappen, Ruth M.
  Nursing leadership and management.
  Rev. ed. of: Nursing leadership. c1983.
  Includes bibliographies and index.
  1. Nursing services — Administration.
2. Leadership.   I. Tappen, Ruth M.   Nursing leadership.
II. Title.   [DNLM: 1. Leadership — nurses' instruction.
2. Nursing, Supervisory.   WY 105 T175n]
RT89.T36   1989   362.1'73'068   88-33504
ISBN 0-8036-8335-9

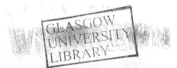

PREFACE TO THE SECOND EDITION

In the six years since the first edition of this book was published, a great deal has happened in the nursing profession. We have seen changes in the supply and demand for nurses, more public debate about these changes, widespread computerization, greater sophistication in nursing practice and research, the movement of highly technical care into the home, and many others too numerous to mention. There is no reason to believe that the amount of change will decrease soon or even that the rate of change might slow down in the next few years. It is an exciting time in nursing, and the study of leadership and management can help us take advantage of the opportunities that such changes present.

Just as the profession is experiencing change, this textbook has undergone some changes in preparation for the second edition. The leadership content in the first edition has been tightened up, redundancy reduced, and the order somewhat rearranged, but little information has actually been deleted. On the other hand, much has been added, most of it management-oriented content. This includes new chapters on "The Components of Effective Management" (Chapter 4), "The Context: A Changing Environment" (Chapter 5), "Project Planning" (Chapter 8), "Time Management" (Chapter 12), and "Computer Applications" (Chapter 13). A number of chapters have also been substantially expanded. They include: "Leadership and Management Theories" (Chapter 2), "Financial Management" (Chapter 9), "Organizing Care" (Chapter 11), "Collective Bargaining" (Chapter 14), "Formal and Informal Evaluation Procedures" (Chapter 21), "Accountability and Quality Assurance" (Chapter 22), and "Staff Development" (Chapter 23). These additions were in response to requests from readers and reviewers, and they are reflected in the new title, *Nursing Leadership and Management: Concepts and Practice.*

From another viewpoint, the book may be seen as containing both basic and advanced concepts of leadership and management. *The most fundamental material is found in Chapters:* 1 ("Conceptual Base for Leadership and Management"), 3 ("The Components of Effective Leadership"), 4 ("The Components of Effective Management"), 5 ("The Context: A Changing Environment"), 6 ("Critical Thinking"), 7 ("Problem Solving and Goal Setting"), 15 ("Communication"), 16 ("Understanding Groups"), and 17 ("Leading Meetings and Conferences"). *Material of moderate difficulty and complexity is in Chapters:* 2 ("Leadership and Management Theories"), 10 ("Health Care Organizations"), 11 ("Organizing Care"), 12 ("Time Management"), 13

("Computer Applications"), 18 ("Teamwork and Motivation"), 19 ("Strategies for Planned Change"), 20 ("Leadership in the Community"), 21 ("Formal and Informal Evaluation Procedures"), 22 ("Accountability and Quality Assurance"), and 24 ("Leading Information Conferences"). *Material of considerable complexity is found in Chapters:* 8 ("Project Planning"), 9 ("Financial Management"), 14 ("Collective Bargaining"), and 23 (Staff Development").

The philosophy underlying the first edition has not changed. The viewpoint remains holistic within an open system framework. I have continued to advocate a participative style of leadership and management that recognizes and respects as much as possible the rights and needs of all people in a leadership-management situation. Knowledge and skill in leadership are considered essential to every practicing professional. Management knowledge and skills are built upon the fundamentals of essential leadership.

As I wrote in the Preface to the first edition, the observation and study of people's behavior is continually fascinating to me. The practice of leadership and management has been a stimulating and constantly challenging experience, and I hope that the reader will share this interest and enthusiasm for the subject as he or she progresses through the pages of this newly expanded second edition.

R.M.T.

PREFACE TO THE FIRST EDITION

When this book was first proposed, there was a limited choice of nursing leadership and management texts available. Since then, many more have appeared but some gaps in content continue to exist. For example, the stages of group development and group roles are not even touched upon in most texts. Teamwork has also been a neglected area and yet most nurses work as part of a team, often as parts of several different teams. The same is true for the more complex subjects of organizations and political action in the community.

An exclusive focus on the hospital setting ignores the variety of settings in which nurses at all levels are practicing today. Leadership has generally been treated as if it were a subject entirely separate from the rest of nursing practice although there are actually many concepts in common between the two. For example, good communication skills are helpful no matter with whom you are using them. Maslow's hierarchy of needs applies to both patient and coworker and sociocultural factors influence the behavior of both. In much the same way, effective leadership is needed equally (and probably more) when teaching a group of patients as when teaching a group of coworkers; therefore, this book contains examples of working with clients or patients as well as examples of working with colleagues.

The purpose of this book, then, is to provide a more comprehensive and readable text, one that contains all the leadership information needed by the practicing professional nurse and ample illustrations of the application of this information in practice. This book is written for the student or nurse who desires a strong basic foundation in leadership and management. Even the individual who is suddenly thrust into a supervisory or administrative role will find that, aside from learning the specific routines of the organization, these basic leadership concepts and skills are the most essential tools for effective functioning in these positions.

For me, the observation and study of people's behavior has always been a source of great fascination but the greatest rewards of studying leadership come from the opportunity to practice it. This is the real purpose of studying leadership and I hope that the reader will agree that it is a stimulating and constantly challenging experience.

R.M.T.

ACKNOWLEDGMENTS

CONTRIBUTORS

Patricia Z. Lund, R.N., Ed.D.
Assistant Professor
Columbia University School of
    Nursing
New York, New York

Phyllis M. George, R.N., M.A.
Director of Public Health Nursing
Dutchess County Health Department
Poughkeepsie, New York

Cynthia Daubman, R.N., M.S.
Poughkeepsie, New York

REVIEWERS

Marilyn Schluterman Bauer, R.N.,
    B.S.N., M.Ed.
Level Coordinator
St. John's Hospital School of Nursing
Springfield, Missouri

Evelyn N. Behanna, R.N., M.S.N.,
    Col. (Ret.)
Clinical Coordinator
Graduate Health System
Rancocas Division
Willingboro, New Jersey

Kathaleen C. Bloom, R.N., M.S.
Assistant Professor
University of North Florida
Jacksonville, Florida

Gloria Goldman, R.N., B.S.N.,
    M.Ed., M.S.
Professor
Sinclair Community College
Dayton, Ohio

*Elaine Graveley, R.N., M.A.
Assistant Professor
University of Texas Health Science
    Center
School of Nursing
San Antonio, Texas

Margaret C. Jopp, R.N., Ed.D.
Instructor
Delaware Technical and
    Community College
Dover, Delaware

Jean A. Massey, R.N., Ph.D.
Associate Professor
University of South Carolina
College of Nursing
Columbia, South Carolina

Elaine McIlwain Reimels, R.N., M.S.
Assistant Clinical Professor
University of South Carolina
College of Nursing
Columbia, South Carolina

Marian Costopoulos Slater, R.N.,
    M.N.
Assistant Professor of Nursing
Widener University
School of Nursing
Chester, Pennsylvania

*F.A. Davis offers a special acknowledgment to Elaine Graveley, who shared her expertise and time.

Cecilia Volden, R.N., M.S.
Associate Professor
University of North Dakota
College of Nursing
Grand Forks, North Dakota

Rebekah F. Wood, R.N., M.S.N.
Director
St. John's Hospital School of Nursing
Springfield, Missouri

CONTENTS

INTRODUCTION . . . .   *xv*

Unit I FRAMEWORK FOR LEADERSHIP AND MANAGEMENT. .   **1**

Chapter 1
CONCEPTUAL BASE FOR LEADERSHIP
AND MANAGEMENT. **2**

Chapter 2
LEADERSHIP AND MANAGEMENT THEORIES. **30**

Chapter 3
THE COMPONENTS OF EFFECTIVE LEADERSHIP **56**

Chapter 4
THE COMPONENTS OF EFFECTIVE MANAGEMENT **84**

Chapter 5
THE CONTEXT: A CHANGING ENVIRONMENT **105**
Patricia Lund, R.N., Ed.D. and
Ruth M. Tappen, R.N., Ed.D.

UNIT I LEARNING ACTIVITIES **121**

Unit II PLANNING AND DECISION MAKING **123**

Chapter 6
CRITICAL THINKING **124**

Chapter 7
PROBLEM SOLVING AND GOAL SETTING **134**

Chapter 8
PROJECT PLANNING **147**

Chapter 9
FINANCIAL MANAGEMENT **169**

UNIT II LEARNING ACTIVITIES **184**

Unit III ORGANIZING.................................... 185

Chapter 10
HEALTH CARE ORGANIZATIONS........................... 186

Chapter 11
ORGANIZING CARE..................................... 215
Phyllis George, R.N., M.A. and
Ruth M. Tappen, R.N., Ed.D.

Chapter 12
TIME MANAGEMENT.................................... 231

Chapter 13
COMPUTER APPLICATIONS.............................. 247

Chapter 14
COLLECTIVE BARGAINING.............................. 262

UNIT III LEARNING ACTIVITIES.......................... 281

Unit IV LEADERSHIP AND MOTIVATION................... 283

Chapter 15
COMMUNICATION...................................... 284

Chapter 16
UNDERSTANDING GROUPS.............................. 310

Chapter 17
LEADING MEETINGS AND CONFERENCES.................. 339
Ruth M. Tappen, R.N., Ed.D. and
Cynthia Daubman, R.N., M.S.

Chapter 18
TEAMWORK AND MOTIVATION.......................... 368

Chapter 19
STRATEGIES FOR PLANNED CHANGE..................... 393

Chapter 20
LEADERSHIP IN THE COMMUNITY....................... 434

UNIT IV LEARNING ACTIVITIES.......................... 454

UNIT V EVALUATION AND PROFESSIONAL DEVELOPMENT.... 455

Chapter 21
FORMAL AND INFORMAL EVALUATION PROCEDURES........ 456
Ruth M. Tappen, R.N., Ed.D. and
Phyllis George, R.N., M.A.

Chapter 22
ACCOUNTABILITY AND QUALITY ASSURANCE   474
Ruth M. Tappen, R.N., Ed.D. and
Phyllis George, R.N., M.A.

Chapter 23
STAFF DEVELOPMENT   489

Chapter 24
LEADING INFORMATION CONFERENCES   503

UNIT V LEARNING ACTIVITIES   519

INDEX   521

■ *INTRODUCTION*

LEADERSHIP ──────────────────────────────

Acquiring leadership knowledge and skill is an essential part of the health care professional's preparation for practice. In fact, experienced professional people often say that most of the major problems, conflicts, and challenges that they face in their work are not technical problems but people problems. These are the kind of problems that leadership knowledge and skill can help you resolve.

The primary purpose for studying leadership is to learn how to work with people, as individuals or as members of groups, teams, organizations, and even whole communities. The acquisition and appropriate use of the leadership concepts and skills can give you a feeling of greater understanding and control of events in a work situation. It can provide you with a sense of personal power and self-direction in situations that would otherwise be bewildering, frustrating, discouraging, or a combination of these.

The study of leadership encompasses many facets of human behavior. It includes the study of motivation, the effects of social roles and norms, leadership theories, group development, teamwork, organizational dynamics, and community structure. It also includes learning effective communication skills such as confrontation and negotiation, critical thinking, problem solving, conducting meetings and conferences, providing evaluation feedback, and implementing changes on both a small and grand scale. All of this is discussed in this book because leaders need to know why the people with whom they work act the way they do and how the leader can influence that behavior.

Leadership is often defined as *the process of influencing others* (Tannenbaum, Weschler, & Massarik, 1974). A somewhat more complex but challenging definition of leadership is *the ability to translate intention into reality and to sustain it* (Bennis & Nanus, 1985). It is purposive (goal-oriented) behavior involving an exchange with other people. Although the emphasis in this book is on work situations, leadership behavior can also occur in social situations.

An act of leadership is an attempt to influence others. Therefore, whenever you attempt to influence people, you are exercising leadership. The attempt defines the leadership action — it does not always have to be successful. It is also not necessary to be designated the leader. Any member of a group can act as its leader. You do not have to be called a team leader, manager, or supervisor in order to be a leader, although people in these positions do need to use leadership concepts and skills. The following example may help to clarify this point:

A student is observing a hospital team attempting to resuscitate a patient. A nurse is ready to administer electroshock but others are still leaning against the patient's metal bed. The student calls out "Everybody off the bed!" and they quickly move back. Here, the student has exercised leadership in spite of being a junior member of this team.

If the student had thought, "Hmm, I don't think they ought to be leaning on the bed like that" but had not said anything, the student would not have shown any leadership at all despite having had the right idea.

In order to be a leader, you have to implement your plans and ideas in some way. This reflects that more complex definition of leadership. Leaders put good ideas, plans, and suggestions into practice. Doing so requires skill, knowledge, energy, and action, things that we will talk more about in a later chapter. To be a leader you must make a decision to act.

A leadership action always involves some kind of exchange with other people, an exchange in which there is some attempt to influence them, either directly or indirectly. The "other people" referred to may be a single coworker or client, the team to which you belong, the organization in which you are employed, or a whole community with which you are working to improve health care. The correct use of leadership concepts and skills can help you to improve your effectiveness in all of these different exchanges and relationships.

MANAGEMENT

This book also includes a substantial amount of information about basic nursing management. Actually, leadership and management are closely related, sometimes intertwined, concepts. Leadership, as it was defined earlier, is the process of influencing others with a specific goal in mind. Management, too, is a process of influencing others *with the specific intention that they perform effectively and contribute to meeting the organization's goals* (Drucker, 1967). This is done by obtaining and correctly utilizing the people, money, and other resources needed to get the work done (Longenecker & Pringle, 1981). You can see why management is often called the process of getting work done through other people.

A manager is formally and officially responsible for the work of a given group, for ensuring that the right kind and amount of work is done and that it is done well. To fulfill this responsibility, the manager may be expected to hire and fire people; formally evaluate staff members; recommend raises and promotions; prepare and adhere to a budget; approve expenses and purchases; review the work done by staff members; assign and schedule the work of staff members; handle work and personnel problems; contribute technically; and plan the current and future activities of the department.

The study of management also encompasses a broad range of knowledge and skills. It includes such things as financial management, the principles and techniques of formal appraisal procedures, staff development, project planning, and collective bargaining. It also includes an understanding of management theories, of the different ways in which organizations have developed their hierarchies and structured their work groups, and of both the internal and external factors that affect the organization and its ability to survive and grow. Finally, the study of management includes an understanding of all of the facets of effective leadership.

Many nurses move quickly into beginning managerial or quasi-managerial positions, such as assistant head nurse, assistant supervisor, coordinator or project director, in which they are expected to already be cognizant of the basic concepts of management. Without this preparation, you could feel quite lost, unable to understand or carry out the expectations of your new position.

What is the difference between management and leadership? First, management is a formal, specifically designated position within the organization. Each work group, unit, or department has a manager. Leadership, on the other hand, is an unofficial, achieved position. A group may have more than one leader and should have many members who assume leadership functions. You could say that management is an assigned role, while leadership is an attained role. Second, to be a good manager, it is absolutely essential to be an effective leader. In fact, some use the term *leader-manager* to emphasize the importance of the leadership aspects of management and to combine (synthesize) the concepts from both into the role of the leader-manager (Williamson, 1986). The opposite is not true, however. You do not have to be a manager to be an effective leader; anyone within a group can exert leadership.

It is every health care professional's responsibility to assume some leadership within the profession. Not every professional can or needs to be a manager, but it is helpful for all professionals to have a good understanding of the basics of management, especially when some aspects of the manager's tasks and functions are delegated to other members of the group and staff members are increasingly being asked to have input into managerial decisions.

SOME ADDITIONAL COMMENTS ───────────────────

Although the usual approach has been to concentrate on leadership and management in institutional settings, especially in hospitals, community and long term care situations are also included in this book in order to better represent the whole spectrum of settings in which health care is given and leadership and management can be practiced. Much of what you will read in this book is also applicable to working with clients, again as individuals, groups, or communities. The examples used in this book reflect this diversity and the potential for broad application of the concepts and skills it contains.

One additional comment on the practice of leadership and management. As a leader or manager, you are in a responsible position which requires that you maintain the confidence and trust of the people with whom you work. Many of these skills and strategies are quite powerful in their effect. Instead of being used to help people and improve working relationships, they can, and have been, turned around and used to increase stress and to manipulate people. The health care professional who takes advantage of opportunities to use these skills and strategies also assumes the responsibility to use them constructively.

REFERENCES

Bennis, W. & Nanus, B. (1985). *Leaders: The strategies for taking charge*. New York: Harper and Row.

Drucker, P.F. (1967). *The effective executive*. New York: Harper and Row.

Longenecker, J.G. & Pringle, C.D. (1981). *Management*. (Fifth Edition). Columbus, Ohio: Charles E. Merrill.

Tannenbaum, R., Weschler, I.R. & Massarik, F. (1974). *Leadership: A frame of reference*. In Cathcart, R.S. & Samopvar, L.A. (eds): *Small group communication: A reader*. Dubuque: William C. Brown.

Williamson, J.N. (1986). *The leader-manager*. New York: John Wiley.

Unit I

FRAMEWORK FOR LEADERSHIP AND MANAGEMENT

Chapter 1.   Conceptual Base for Leadership and Management
Chapter 2.   Leadership and Management Theories
Chapter 3.   Components of Effective Leadership
Chapter 4.   Components of Effective Management
Chapter 5.   The Context: A Changing Environment
Unit I Learning Activities

Chapter 1

OUTLINE

Theory
   Uses of Theory
     Organization
     Perspective
     Explanation
     Prediction
     Application
   Theory Selection

Open Systems: The Interaction of People With Their Environment
   Systems Defined
   System Characteristics
     Hierarchy of Systems
     Wholeness
     Openness
     Energy Fields
     Growth
     Patterns
     Individuality
     Sentience
   Multiple Factors Influencing Behavior

Individual Factors Affecting Human Behavior
   Assumptions About Human Behavior

Coping Behavior Patterns
   Reflex Actions
   Nondeliberative Mechanisms
   Deliberative Mechanisms
Motivation and Human Needs: Maslow's Hierarchy
   Human Needs
   Physiologic Needs
   Safety and Security
   Love and Belonging
   Esteem
   Self-Actualization

Sociocultural Influences
   Culture
     Cultural Differences in Shared Meaning
     Working With Cultural Differences
   The Influence of Roles
     Sources of Role Stress
     Role Stress Reduction

Summary

LEARNING OBJECTIVES

Upon completion of this chapter, the reader will be able to:

▷ Use an open systems framework when analyzing leadership and management situations.

▷ Explain the concept that all human behavior has meaning.

▷ Apply Maslow's need hierarchy to leadership and management situations.

▷ Identify cultural influences on people's behavior at work.

▷ Identify the effect of role stresses and conflicts on people's behavior.

CONCEPTUAL BASE FOR LEADERSHIP AND MANAGEMENT

T his chapter and the four that follow provide the theoretical foundation on which the rest of this book is based. Chapter 1 presents the more general theories and concepts that are used to explain human behavior. These are important because a leader needs to understand human behavior in order to be able to influence it. Chapter 2 surveys the major theories of leadership and management which attempt to explain what leadership and management are and how one can influence others in the work setting. Chapters 3 and 4 are more specific in their application; they describe the components of effective leadership and management that can be applied directly to practice. Chapter 5 considers current trends and issues that affect the practice of leadership and management.

Why do people behave the way they do? In this chapter we will look at several very important theories that explain human behavior. Some will be familiar from other contexts. Maslow's hierarchy, for example, is often used to explain patient needs and behaviors but can be applied to nonpatients and to leadership and management situations. Our particular interest here is to consider how these theories can be of use to us in leadership and management. The chapter begins with a brief explanation of how theory is of use to us and then looks at several important theories that serve as background to the rest of this book. The first is the very general open systems theory, followed by some explanations of individual behavior and, finally, explanations of the broader social and cultural influences on people's behavior.

THEORY

Uses of Theory ›

Why have a theoretical framework? A brief explanation of the ways in which theory can be used will help you see the purpose of a theoretical framework.

ORGANIZATION. A theory provides a framework in which you can organize your ideas and experiences. Like a desk organizer that has many compartments to tuck things into, a theory has components or categories into which you can group your thoughts and observations. Like an organizer, a theory helps you to detect similarities, differences, and other patterns in data and to provide explanations for these patterns.

PERSPECTIVE. A theory also provides a perspective, or a certain way of looking at things. The particular theory you use influences how you interpret what you see. The following is an example:

A woman is hurling angry words at a male companion. A traditional Freudian analyst could see this woman as "suffering from penis envy." In contrast, a follower of Thomas Harris and Eric Berne would describe this as an "I'm OK, You're not OK" situation. To someone using communications theory, the situation represents "a failure to communicate." To a sociologist, it may be an example of "women's liberation" or someone being "aggressive rather than assertive."

Each person in the example above was looking at the same event from a different theoretical perspective. One perspective focuses on physical differences between the sexes, another emphasizes feelings about self and others, a third is concerned with the prevailing social climate, and so forth. In fact, the Freudian analyst, the sociologist, and the communications theorist could actually have difficulty talking to each other about this situation. Each one might also choose a different intervention if the angry woman were a client.

EXPLANATION. Theories not only organize information, they also provide explanations of events (Duldt & Giffin, 1985). Theories are general statements that help us understand *why* certain things do or do not happen. Why, for example, does Nurse A work harder than Nurse B? One management theory will say that it is because Nurse A receives a larger salary than Nurse B. Another theory will say that it is because Nurse B is not interested in the type of work that has been assigned to her. A third will say that both factors are operating: Nurse A has interesting, stimulating work and is paid more than Nurse B who is dissatisfied with her work in several ways.

PREDICTION. A theory should also help you to predict what is likely to happen in a given situation. For example, developmental theory predicts that certain crises will occur during adolescence, including conflicts between parents and teenagers. Familiarity with this theory enables a nurse to provide anticipatory guidance to a family with children entering adolescence. The ability to predict people's behavior enables a leader to anticipate what will happen given a certain set of circumstances. You could, for example, expect a more experienced nurse who has achieved some degree of success in the profession to be more interested in being a mentor than a nurse who is still relatively inexperienced.

APPLICATION. A theory that predicts what is likely to happen in a given situation can provide some direction regarding what action is to be taken. This is particularly important in a practice profession such as nursing. The example above shows how theory can guide practice. Leadership and management theories also serve as guides to selecting the most effective action to take.

Theory Selection

There is no single theory to explain all human behavior. Some of the theories conflict with each other but others are complementary and together explain more than any one theory alone does. This was the basis on which the theories discussed in this chapter were selected.

A thorough and scholarly evaluation of a particular theory is a complex process beyond the scope of this book. However, there are several questions (Fawcett, 1984) you can ask about any theory to help you decide whether or not it is as helpful to you in the practice of leadership and management.

Is the theory internally consistent? Are the different parts of the theory congruent with each other or is there some inconsistency in the way human behavior is explained or predicted? An inconsistent management theory might claim that people try to avoid work and then suggest that the manager allows staff members to work as independently as possible.

Does the theory provide useful guidelines for practice? Our primary purpose for studying theories that explain human behavior is to apply them to practice. Some theories are so broad, however, that it is difficult to apply them to specific situations. Open systems theory, for example, provides little specific advice on how to respond to a particular problem. On the other hand, it provides us with a valuable perspective, an understanding of the complexity of most situations that will help us avoid trying simplistic solutions for complex situations.

Has empirical testing yielded evidence in support of the theory? Some theories have a natural appeal that tempts us to accept them without sufficient evaluation. The purpose of subjecting theories to empirical (research) testing is to provide us with some objective evidence about the theory's ability to explain and predict human behavior. The research examples in this book can help you begin this process of evaluation.

Is the theory congruent with your values and your philosophy of nursing? A management theory that supports the growth and development of the individual employee implies a very different set of values from one that supports immediate termination when the employee's skills are no longer needed.

Why were the particular theories discussed in this chapter selected? Open systems theory is part of the theoretical framework because it encompasses the complex interrelationships that health care professionals continually deal with. From the complexity of the human being to the organization that dispenses health care services. Maslow's Hierarchy of Needs provides a way to bridge the gap between physical, social, and emotional needs. Attention is also given to culture, role theory, and to coping behaviors because they provide more detailed information about the way in which people interact with their environment.

OPEN SYSTEMS: THE INTERACTION OF PEOPLE WITH THEIR ENVIRONMENT

System Defined

An ameba, a heart, a dog, a person, a group, and a community are all systems. They are systems because you can define them as whole entities having some kind of identifiable parts and a definable boundary. A more formal definition of a system is: *a system is a set of objects together with relationships between the objects and between their attributes* (Hall, 1968).

System Characteristics

To fully understand a system, it is necessary to look at three aspects: its components, its attributes as a whole, and the relationships within the system and with the environment. The *objects* spoken of in the formal definition are the parts or components of the system. They can be almost anything: molecules, cells, organs, people, or groups of people. *Attributes* are the characteristics of the system such as color, temperature, speed, maturity, personality, and energy level. The *relationships* are what tie the system together, the processes that occur between parts. The possibilities for relationships are innumerable: ionization, metabolism, circulation, communication, and negotiation, for example.

Open systems exhibit a number of other important characteristics including a hierarchical nature, wholeness, openness, energy, growth, patterns, individuality, and sentience.

HIERARCHY OF SYSTEMS. There are multiple levels of systems within systems. This is called the hierarchical order of systems (Laszlo, 1972). The smaller systems within systems are called *subsystems*. Larger systems may also be parts of an even more inclusive *suprasystem*. Whatever is outside of the suprasystem, is referred to as the *environment*. Figure 1–1 gives some examples of subsystems, systems, and suprasystems. You can see that they are named in order of increasing size and complexity, the basis for the ordering of systems within a hierarchy.

You may have noticed the vast difference in size between the systems in the two examples. The choice of what level to begin with depends on your purpose in defining a hierarchy of systems and on what level is of most interest to you (Ashby, 1968; Bell, 1968). In leadership these are usually the individual, the group, the organization, and the community.

WHOLENESS. Wholeness means that the system is an integrated set of components (parts) with its *own* attributes and relationships that are different from those of its parts. The system as a whole has characteristics that are different from and greater than the sum of its parts (Von Bertalanffy, 1976; Rogers, 1970). An individual, for example, is not just a collection of bones, skin, heart, lungs, and intestines, but something quite different: a living, breathing, self-aware organism.

A group as a whole also has its own characteristics and relationships that cannot be predicted from the properties of the individual members (Glisson, 1986). The following are examples:

> An audit committee can be dynamic and productive even if it has one member who sleeps through most of the meetings.
> Another group can consist of dynamic, high energy individuals but get nothing done because each member is caught up in competing with the others.
> Even though it is made up of mature individuals, a newly formed group will be immature as a whole in terms of its working relationships until its members develop ways to work together.

The parts or subsystems of a whole system do influence the larger system, although they do not define it. For instance, in the last example given, the fact that the group's members are mature individuals will proba-

SUBSYSTEM:	CELL	INDIVIDUAL	LOCAL GROUP
SYSTEM:	ORGAN	TEAM	STATE ORGANIZATION
SUPRASYSTEM:	INDIVIDUAL	AGENCY	NATIONAL ORGANIZATION

Figure 1–1. Examples of the hierarchy of systems.

bly speed the process of developing ways to work together. Their individual maturity, however, does not make the group mature when it first forms. The same is true for other large systems.

The concept of wholeness has many implications. In nursing practice, for example, its use emphasizes how important it is to assess the client as a whole who has feelings that affect bodily functions and vice versa. This is the basis for many complaints about the medical model which not only concentrates on illness rather than health, but also treats lungs, stomachs, and uteri instead of people. The problem inherent in this model has been well documented.

The concept of wholeness also has implications for leadership. Some communities as a whole are friendly; others are hostile, especially to strangers. Organizations actually take on personalities in a sense. It makes a real difference whether you work for a progressive, growth-oriented organization that encourages innovation or for a schizophrenic one that tells you to do one thing and expects you to do another. You also cannot predict the behavior of a group as a whole by getting to know its members individually —you need to study the behavior of the entire group.

OPENNESS. A system is open if it exchanges matter, energy, or information with its environment (Hall, 1968). There is some disagreement on whether or not a truly closed system (which would *not* exchange any matter, energy, or information with its environment) can exist (Fawcett, 1984). It is difficult to imagine a system that is totally impervious to its environment. Even an object as inanimate as a stone is affected if, for example, its environment became warmer or colder. If you put a cold stone in hot water the water would become cooler and the stone warmer. This is clearly an exchange of energy.

It will be assumed in this book, that no matter how little exchange there may be between some systems and environments, there are no living or natural systems that are completely closed off from their environments. The term "closed" is often used to mean that the system has relatively impermeable boundaries or that it resists input and change. Family theorists, for example, often refer to "closed family systems." In leadership, certain types of organizations or institutions may be called "closed." These systems may be less open to their environments than others but they are not completely closed.

The exchange of matter, information, and energy between a human system and its environment is an active relationship. A human being is active, not passive or just reactive, in relationship to the environment. At the same time that the living system is being influenced by its environment, it is also influencing that environment.

An act of leadership involves a particular kind of interpersonal exchange in which there is an attempt to influence. Whenever this exchange between people occurs, there are at least three elements or systems involved: the leader, the person or groups to be influenced (the co-actors) (Scheflen, 1982), and the environment (surroundings) in which the attempt to influence takes place (Fig. 1–2). These can be broken down into many more elements but the leader, co-actor(s), and the environment are the essential elements that need to be considered whenever you analyze a leadership event.

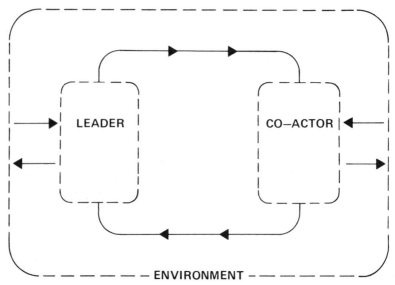

Figure 1–2. Elements of a leadership event.

A *feedback loop* has been used to illustrate this dynamic interplay (Kantor, 1976) between the leader, co-actor(s), and the environment. This loop is meant to represent a simultaneous interaction between the three elements, not a linear model of interaction in which the leader acts and the person or group merely reacts (it is not a stimulus-response model).

The leader and co-acting system continually influence each other even when there is no apparent action or reaction. The following example shows how people can influence each other without any overt action:

> The team leader enters the conference room to distribute assignments for the team. The rest of the team sit silently as the leader enters. The team is usually noisy and talkative in the conference room, so the leader wonders why they are silent today. Is this silence a respectful hush so that the leader can begin talking or is it a hostile refusal to make the leader feel welcome? In either case, the silence has definitely affected the leader.

ENERGY FIELDS.   Every living system requires energy in order to grow and to maintain itself (Hanchett, 1979). The energy may be in the form of matter, including food and oxygen or it may be an exchange of information, such as how to carry out a procedure. Economic energy in the form of money available to spend is an important source of energy for most organizations. Other types include measurable ones in such as light, heat, or sound and the less measurable forces of love, hate, fear, caring, or healing.

Energy can flow or be exchanged in different amounts and directions. There can be very small, hard-to-detect amounts or enormously explosive amounts of energy exchanged. Energy can be unused and can accumulate to the point where there is intensive pressure to release it. A balance of positive energies flowing in and out of a system is usually a sign of a healthy system.

When you study a system, you need to look at how that system exchanges energy with its environment. You may ask, for example, whether or not your nursing unit effectively exchanges information with other departments such as pharmacy, dietary, and social services. You may also ask whether or not the organization as a whole provides sufficient economic energy (budgeted funds) to support its nursing services and to provide adequate salaries for the nurses employed there.

GROWTH.   The process of growth proceeds *unidirectionally*; it does not reverse itself or regress back in time (Boulding, 1968). People do not go back to being like they were last week, last year, or when they were children. Aging, for example, is not a regression but a progression to new conditions and behaviors. (You may wonder about those elderly people who are described as having "regressed". They have not gone back to being children which is obvious from their physical size among other things. Instead, they continue to change but in a negative or pathologic manner). The same is true for older coworkers: they continue to have the need to grow and develop despite their older age and years of experience.

Human growth and development reflect an increasing complexity of pattern and organization (Rogers, 1970). To successfully traverse the adult years, an individual must continue to learn and grow developmentally. Many opportunities are found in the work setting. They range from learning new technical skills to improving one's ability to work as part of an interdisciplinary team. Work can also contribute to the accomplishment of such developmental tasks as developing a sense of identity or guiding the next generation.

A leader-manager who is aware of these needs can organize the work of a group of caregivers in such a way that it can contribute substantially to each staff member's learning and growth. The following is an example of how a nurse manager can do this:

> A staff nurse has worked in the same position long enough to know the job very well. In fact, the nurse knows it so well that it is beginning to get boring. The nurse, however, will not be eligible for a promotion into a more challenging position until finished with school.
>
> The nurse manager recognized this problem and assigned the staff nurse to orient new nurses to the team. The staff nurse has gotten a great deal of satisfaction out of this opportunity to share his expertise with others and to gain some recognition for his experience. The nurse also had to learn new leadership skills by effectively carrying out this new assignment.

It is not only individuals who show evidence of growth and change over time. Teams, groups, organizations, and communities are also open systems that change and evolve over time, either positively or negatively. The positive growth and development of a group or organization could include such things as successful innovations or improved working relationships.

These larger systems can also be thought of as having life cycles in which they begin as immature systems with poorly defined behavior patterns and gradually develop into mature systems with well-defined highly functional behavior patterns. Like other living systems, their existence also has an ending at some point in time.

PATTERNS.   Any action or relationship that recurs at regular intervals can be called a pattern of that system. Many patterns can be observed by the leader but some are more subtle and can only be detected by careful measurement (Laszlo, 1972; Luce, 1971).

Some patterns vary over short periods of time and others extend beyond the life span of an individual. The unidirectional and predictable stages of the life cycle are long-interval patterns. There are seasonal patterns to the occurrence of certain illnesses and to some kinds of behavior, such as suicide. Seasonal variations affect hospital admissions and agency workloads. The patterns of our clients' daily lives also affect service delivery. For example, some community health agencies have extended services into evening and weekend hours to better meet working people's needs.

Patterns with shorter intervals can also be significant to leadership and management. Many biorhythms, for example, are disrupted by rotating shifts, leaving people fatigued and irritable. Although the effects are often subtle, they influence the way a person feels and behaves at work.

Interpersonal relationships have a rhythmic nature that most people are not aware of, but which affects the way they feel about the relationship. People with the same or complementary communication patterns get along better than those whose patterns are asynchronous. Some people are quite flexible and can adjust to another's rhythms, while others can do this only within a narrow range (Chapple, 1979).

There are also patterns in the interpersonal relations within larger systems. Groups may have free-flowing patterns of communication or stilted patterns that discourage spontaneity. Every work group, from a small team to an entire organization, develops patterns of behavior, commonly called routines.

If there were no patterns, we would have chaos. The patterns of a system allow us to predict the behavior of that system with some degree of accuracy. The leader who knows the common patterns of the relevant human systems and who has observed the actual patterns of a particular system can not only better predict its behavior, but also have an influence on its patterns.

INDIVIDUALITY.   Each system has a unique pattern, organization, and behavior unlike any other system. Do you remember having learned in elementary school that no two snowflakes are alike? In the same way, no two people, no two groups, and no two organizations or communities are alike.

While systems have many commonalities, each one has a unique configuration within these commonalities. For example, every person has a need for food and shelter. Just think, however, of the infinite variety of ways in which these common needs have been met. In leadership we study the common attributes and responses of certain systems, but it is important to stay alert to the uniqueness of each system as well. For example:

> When something threatens the integrity of an open system (for example, a person, group, organization, or community), you can expect that system to react to the threat. But without an intimate knowledge of the particular system's attributes, you cannot predict whether the reaction will be to withdraw, to resist the threat, or to attack the source of the threat.

SENTIENCE.   People have the capacity for thought, abstraction, and feeling. This capacity is called sentience. Sentience brings into play the uniquely human importance of emotions, values, and personal and culture-bound meanings. People are not simply aware of the world around them—they are actively involved in trying to make sense out of it and in trying to organize or influence their environment (Boulding, 1968).

The capacity for sentience affects behavior and shows how complex people are. People respond to events as totalities (wholes). A focus on just one aspect, such as a person's culture, does not adequately explain human behavior. Although sometimes difficult, it is necessary to recognize the full complexity of a system as a whole in order to really understand it.

In a sense, larger human systems (such as groups) also possess this capacity to think, feel, reflect, and make choices. Evidence of sentience in these larger systems can be seen in comments such as:

"Our group views this situation as a very serious threat to our new program."

"The community is incensed over the new health department regulation."

"This agency is proud of its record in delivering the highest quality care to its clients."

Multiple Factors Influencing Behavior

Although it may sometimes seem that a person's or group's action was caused by a single stimulus, in fact, there are always multiple factors affecting that response. For an individual, these include past experiences with similar stimuli, the present condition of the individual, and the environment in which this interaction takes place. Other factors include the person's cultural background, personal and social values, and social roles. The following example shows how these multiple factors can influence a single action:

Ms. T., a home health aide, walked up the path to a client's home. The aide stopped suddenly when she found a dog blocking the path.

Her behavior was influenced by many factors, including the size of the dog, the "Beware of the Dog" sign on the lawn, her dislike of dogs, and the way the dog approached. Also, in Ms. T.'s homeland, dogs are used to guard property and are rarely kept as housepets. As a small child, Ms. T. was badly bitten by a guard dog when she put her hand through a fence to feed it. The appearance of the dog threatened Ms. T.'s feelings of safety and security. At the same time, her startled response excited the dog, who began barking and ran after her.

Ms. T. returned to the agency and refused to go back to that home. The supervisor did not explore the factors that had influenced Ms. T.'s refusal and fired her for insubordination.

Responses of groups, teams, organizations, and communities are also affected by multiple factors. A simplistic approach to understanding their responses fails to appreciate this complexity and is likely to result in inadequate understanding of human behavior.

INDIVIDUAL FACTORS AFFECTING HUMAN BEHAVIOR

Assumptions About Human Behavior

Before discussing specific behaviors, it may be helpful to consider two important assumptions about human behavior. The first of these assumptions is that *all human behavior has some kind of meaning* (Brown & Fowler, 1971). Simple observation is often sufficient to reveal the meaning of that behavior (Das, 1988). While the meaning of a particular action may be obscure or unintelligible to the observer, it is still assumed to have some purpose for that person. This purpose may be to meet a need for security, to express a feeling, or to cope with a perceived threat.

People are not always aware of the purpose of their behavior. In fact, they may not be any more aware of the purpose than the observer is although they have the potential for developing this awareness.

It is also assumed that the *present state of the individual in relation to the current state of the environment* determines current behavior. For example, a person whose energy level is very low may make a much weaker response to a problem than would seem justified by the seriousness of the problem, while another person who has been storing up a great deal of tension may seem to overreact to a problem. Every behavior reflects the person as a whole—one's physical state as well as one's emotional state.

Coping Behavior Patterns

Actions taken for the purpose of reducing tension or dealing with a perceived threat may be divided into three categories: reflex actions, nondeliberative mechanisms, and deliberative mechanisms. Their importance is difficult to overstate. In fact, it has been said that many illnesses are a response to inadequate or inappropriate coping efforts (Garland & Bush, 1982). These illnesses are not confined to our patients. They affect us and our colleagues as well.

REFLEX ACTIONS. Reflex actions are automatic responses. They occur rapidly, without any conscious effort, but are nevertheless purposeful. The purpose is usually protective in some way. People are born with many reflexes and can acquire others during their lives. Reacting automatically to a sudden loud noise and pulling away from a source of pain are examples of reflex actions.

NONDELIBERATIVE MECHANISMS. The term nondeliberative is used to indicate that these particular coping mechanisms seem to operate primarily below the full awareness of the individual. Since they are below awareness, their connection to the perceived threat or problem is not always apparent. Recalling these mechanisms helps the leader-manager to explain the often puzzling and seemingly inexplicable behavior of others.

The description of these nondeliberative mechanisms originated with the work of Freud (Schwartz & Schwartz, 1972), but they have been used to explain behavior even by those who do not employ other elements of Freudian psychology. While their purpose is generally self-protective, inappropriate or excessive use is considered harmful.

Compensation. When people believe they lack a particular ability they may try to compensate for this lack by excelling in another area. For example, a person who has difficulty with technical skills may make up for this deficit by concentrating on developing social skills and becoming popular at work.

Repression. Repression is the complete blocking of certain feelings or thoughts from awareness because they are unacceptable or intolerable in some way. A caregiver may repress anger toward a particular patient because anger is a completely unacceptable response. The result is that the caregiver is not aware of these angry feelings except perhaps as a vague sense of tension or unease when interacting with this patient.

Denial.   Denial is a blocking of something occurring in the environment while repression refers to blocking something within the individual. A common example is the denial of a life-threatening illness. People can also deny problems at work and seem, for example, to believe that everything is going well when they are actually on the verge of being fired.

Suppression.   Suppression is a more deliberate form of repression. It is a temporary putting aside of disturbing feelings or thoughts until they can be handled. For example, you may see a nurse suppress emotions and act calmly in an emergency but have shaking hands afterward.

Displacement.   Displacement occurs when a person holds back or suppresses feelings and then later unleashes these feelings in another situation or toward a different person. For example, you might be angry at your boss but afraid to express this feeling directly. Later you displace the anger and yell at your friends for leaving their shoes in the living room.

Projection.   Projection is another way to deal with painful or unacceptable feelings by attributing them to other people. For example, supervisors who feel anxious about the institution of a new evaluation procedure may say (and actually believe) that they oppose it because the people they supervise are threatened by it. Another kind of projection that can cause first-line managers some serious problems is when staff members blame others for their own failures.

Withdrawal.   Withdrawal and avoidance of threatening situations is sometimes the only solution available to a person facing a problem.

Rationalization.   Rationalization is a logical and reasonable explanation of, but not the real reason for, that behavior. For example, a supervisor may deny a promotion to an eligible employee whom the supervisor dislikes intensely. The supervisor rationalizes this explaining that this was done "because the employee isn't ready to move into that position yet and will be better off staying at the present level for at least another year."

Substitution.   Socially acceptable energy outlets are often substituted for a less acceptable but desirable outlet. For example, the urge to retaliate against an agency that has drawn clients away from a person's own agency can be replaced by a drive to improve their own agency. The substitution chosen is not always constructive. For example, some people substitute excessive eating or drinking for desired but unattainable outlets.

Identification.   Identification involves experiencing the same feelings as another person or behaving the same way. It is often a means of filling some deficit in self-confidence or identity. People frequently identify with people they especially admire or with whom they have something in common. For example, new nurses may identify with a head nurse they admire and model their behavior after that head nurse.

DELIBERATIVE MECHANISMS.   The deliberative coping mechanisms that people use more consciously to avoid discomfort, reduce tension, and solve problems are even more varied and individualistic than the nondeliberative mechanisms. Most of these mechanisms are usually helpful but they also can be misused. They are more straightforward and self-explanatory behaviors as you will see in the examples below (Ardell, 1986; Menninger, 1963; Feuerstein, Labbe & Kuczmierczyk, 1986). A few of the deliberative mechanisms people use include:

Seeking Comfort and Reassurance.   Touch, hugging, and comforting words can soothe and calm people who are distressed.

Using Sound and Rhythm. Dancing, listening to music, and other rhythmic activities are a means for expressing feelings and releasing tension.

Ventilating Feelings. Crying, swearing, and laughing, to name only a few, are ways to relieve tensions and share feelings with others.

Eating. Eating can relieve tension and substitute for the satisfaction of other needs. When done in the company of others, it can become a time of sharing and support that contributes to well-being.

Smoking and Stimulants. Although not healthful, these are often used to ease tension and reduce feelings of fatigue.

Relaxation Techniques and Exercise. These are nondrug methods that are often effective in reducing tension, although they do not solve underlying problems.

Discussing a Problem. Simply talking about a problem with a person who is a good listener often makes the problem seem smaller and more manageable.

Drawing on Past Experience. Having successfully managed a similar experience in the past not only provides clues to action—but also confidence in your ability to cope adequately the next time.

Taking One Thing at a Time. A seemingly unmanageable problem or demand may seem less impossible to deal with if it is broken down into manageable parts that are considered and resolved one at a time. This is a kind of "tunnel vision" that may help a person get through a time of crisis.

Becoming Passive, Rigid, or Vague. These behaviors conserve energy temporarily but do not relieve the stress. People using this mechanism tend to internalize their stress.

Aggression. This discharges energy but often exacerbates the problem. Assertiveness is a more positive response.

Taking Stock of Your Resources. This mechanism has both a calming and strengthening effect.

Sleeping. This is a means of temporary escape but also restores energy reserves.

Repetitive Activity. Seemingly purposeless, repetitive actions, such as pacing, rocking, grinding teeth, drumming fingers on a table, or swinging a leg while sitting, discharge excess energy. These behaviors are evident at meetings or at nurses stations where there are few other outlets available.

People often engage in these activities at times when other behaviors would seem more appropriate to the observer who is not aware of their need to reduce tension or resolve a problem. The leader who is aware of the meaning of such behaviors can avoid misinterpretations and can sometimes help the individual resolve the problem that led to the need for these coping mechanisms.

Motivation and Human Needs: Maslow's Hierarchy

Maslow (1970) developed a theory of motivation based on the idea that some human needs are more basic, or prepotent, than others. These more basic needs must be at least partially filled before a person has sufficient energy and motivation to work toward gratifying the higher, less prepotent

	Individual Need	**Management Example**
Highest Level	Self Actualization	Developing a new nursing diagnosis category
	Esteem	Receiving recognition for one's accomplishments
	Love and Belonging	Working with a friendly cohesive group
	Safety and Security	Protection from communicable disease spread
Lowest Level	Physiologic	Adequate time for meal breaks

Figure 1–3. Maslow's hierarchy of human needs applied to leadership and management.

(less powerful or influential) needs. These human needs form a hierarchy beginning with the lowest and most basic physiologic needs, working up through the safety and security needs, love and belonging needs, esteem needs, and up to the highest level of self-actualization needs (Fig. 1–3).

HUMAN NEEDS.   The needs dealt with in Maslow's theory of motivation may be loosely termed *intrinsic* factors because they originate primarily from within the individual. You will see, though, that gratification of these needs is certainly influenced by the environment. Hunger and thirst, for example, are influenced by the availability of food and water. The social and cultural factors discussed later may be thought of as *extrinsic* because they originate primarily within the environment.

Each of the levels of needs from the most basic or prepotent physiologic needs up to the self-actualization needs are discussed here with emphasis on their application to leadership. Within these categories, specific needs are discussed in what is believed to be their general order of prepotency (Campbell, 1978). These needs do not explain *all* behavior but they do provide another very useful explanation of the intrinsic motivating forces behind people's actions.

PHYSIOLOGIC NEEDS.   Some physiologic needs are constant and immediate. Any situation in which they are not met would be life-threatening —a person can live only a few minutes without adequate oxygen and blood circulation, for example.

Because of their immediacy, when one of these needs is not sufficiently met, a person is motivated to act on meeting this need and nothing else. The person will think of nothing but this need and will focus all attention and energy on satisfying the need. The following is an example of this focusing:

> If you began to choke on a piece of steak in a restaurant, you would immediately stop whatever you were doing and try to dislodge that piece of meat. Although ordinarily not considered polite, you might put your fingers in your mouth to pull the meat out.

If this didn't work, you would probably try to get someone's attention to help you with other maneuvers.

During such an emergency, would you care about disturbing other people? Would you care about the approval of others, your dignity, or your need for independence? Not at all. This also happens during emergencies on nursing units. Although you might care at a later time, belonging, esteem, or even other basic physiologic needs become less important.

Other needs that are not of such an immediate nature but still necessary to maintain health include a normal temperature, adequate sleep, adequate activity and stimulation, freedom from pain, and sexual gratification. These are important to you as a leader because people will direct their attention and energy toward meeting these needs and will not be very interested in working toward higher level needs until the basic needs are at least partially met. The following are some examples:

Temperature. If you hold a meeting in a hot, stuffy room, the people at the meeting will concentrate more on staying cool rather than on the purpose of the meeting.

Sleep. People whose sleep patterns are interrupted because they often have to work overtime or irregular hours will be tired and irritable at work.

Activity and Stimulation. Sitting at a desk in the nursing station or in a classroom all day can make a person feel dull and listless. Alternating active and quiet work and allowing time to walk around provides some stimulation.

Pain. A person who is ill or injured will have difficulty concentrating on work.

Sex. Opportunities to meet people may be provided in a work setting.

The leader who acts to assure that these very basic human needs are met (as much as is possible in the work setting) will be helping people to free their energies for work on higher-level needs and, therefore, perform their jobs more effectively. This is also true for the next level of needs, safety and security.

SAFETY AND SECURITY. Both actual safety and the feeling of being safe are included in this second level of needs. Physical safety is the most prepotent of these needs, followed by perceived security, stability, and dependency.

Safety. While work in health care settings is not generally considered physically dangerous, there are still some threats to safety which should be eliminated, or at least reduced, by the alert leader. These threats to safety include exposure to infection, radiation, electric shock, and potentially violent individuals, as well as the risk of back injuries. Many nurses also work in high-crime areas. The effective leader-manager takes action to identify and minimize these and other potential threats to the safety of one's self and coworkers.

Security. Providing a feeling of security is an important and challenging leadership function. People who do not feel secure in their work setting focus most of their energy on attempts to reduce the threats in order to increase their feeling of security.

Fostering security and trust is a complex task because there are so many potentially threatening situations in a work setting and also because people differ in their reactions to threats. What one person sees as a minor threat may be seen by another as a major threat demanding a total response. The following are examples of situations that may be perceived by a person as a threat:

▷ Assignment to a task one does not feel able to do correctly.
▷ Joining a new group.
▷ Hearing rumors that the new boss is planning to bring in new people and eliminate current staff.
▷ Evaluation procedures, especially those that are new, inconsistent, or subjective.

▷ Being asked to lead a conference or give a presentation.
▷ The hiring of a more skilled person who could easily do the present employee's job.

Virtually any situation could be perceived by some as a threat so the leader-manager needs to be alert to individual reactions as well as to responses of the group as a whole.

Stability. People also need some constancy in their lives. While change is stimulating and too much stability is deadening, too much change at one time can threaten the integrity of a system. It can also create a situation that is so chaotic that people cannot deal with it.

People need some regularity or pattern in the rhythms of their daily lives—in their sleep, meals, work, and play. Some predictability is needed at work. This does not mean that people need or want a rigid routine which is stultifying and probably impossible in a profession such as nursing that deals with human behavior and unexpected emergencies. The following are some ways to provide stability in a work setting:

▷ Regular work hours and meal times.
▷ Predictability of job expectations.
▷ Clear standards for quality care.
▷ Regular opportunities to give and receive feedback.
▷ Preparation in advance for handling emergencies.
▷ Continuity in patient or client assignments.

There are many things you can do to increase stability in the work setting and to free people's energies to address higher level needs.

Dependency. According to Maslow, people also have a need for dependency. This means that people need to be able to ask for help. Of course, healthy adults have fewer dependency needs than young children or sick people but there are still times when they need assistance from another person such as:

▷ Learning a new job.
▷ Grieving after a serious loss.
▷ Lifting a heavy object.
▷ Solving a difficult problem.
▷ Carrying out a complex task that requires more than two hands.

The leader's function is to ensure that adequate assistance and support are available to people at work and to assure people that it is acceptable for an adult to seek help. Asking for help when it is needed is a sign of maturity, not immaturity.

LOVE AND BELONGING. People also need love and affection. They need to feel accepted, to give and receive approval, and to be part of a group (such as a family, neighborhood, gang, team, club) in which they can give and receive affection. They need opportunities for communication and satisfying contact with people. A person whose love and belonging needs are not met will feel lonely, friendless, rejected, or alienated.

The work setting can be an important source of gratification of these needs. For some people, the opportunity to be part of a congenial work group and to have the acceptance and approval of this group are their major sources of satisfaction from their jobs. This is particularly true when the work itself is monotonous or unsatisfying in some way.

Unfortunately, not every work group is warm and accepting of its members and interpersonal conflict is a prime source of difficulty in many work settings. As a leader-manager you probably will find that much of your energy is directed toward resolution of interpersonal conflicts and the development of warmth, acceptance, and group feeling among coworkers.

Some people may question the appropriateness of meeting belonging needs at work. Isn't time wasted when there's too much socializing? Shouldn't the leader concentrate on getting the work done? Some leadership theorists raise these same questions and conclude that attention to these needs is not important. They believe that people are motivated to work hard in order to avoid punishment such as being reprimanded or fired.

But many more theorists, including Maslow, point out that people cannot concentrate their efforts on getting their work done unless their basic needs, including belonging, are met. People put more effort into their work when they are given opportunities to grow and develop on the job. Interpersonal conflicts can paralyze a team to the point where it is nonfunctional. The effective leader will take action to reduce the conflicts so that the team can resume its function. Purely social activities are beneficial but need to be kept within limits so that they enhance rather than interfere with the major goal of carrying out professional health care functions.

ESTEEM. People need to think well of themselves (self-esteem) and to be well thought of by others (esteem from others). When the other, more basic needs are satisfactorily met, then these esteem needs will emerge and become primary motivators of behavior. The work setting can provide many opportunities for filling esteem needs. Along with the next level of needs (self-actualization needs), esteem needs are frequently important sources of motivation for people.

Self-Esteem. People need to feel good about themselves. They need to feel that they have an intrinsic worth. This feeling of self-worth is related to a sense of being useful, adequate, competent, independent, and autonomous. The alert reader may note that dependency was listed as one of the safety and security needs while independence and autonomy are listed here as esteem needs. A person can be independent most of the time and yet occasionally need to ask for help. The healthy adult has some dependency needs but, overall, is far more independent than dependent.

Maslow says that a healthier and firmer sense of worth is developed when it is based on what a person really is rather than on a façade or on a role into which a person has forced himself or herself. A person's need for self-esteem is better satisfied when worth is based on what the person is rather than on what that person could be or pretends to be. The leader needs to take this into consideration when developing ways to help staff increase their sense of worth and meet their esteem needs.

The work setting can provide many opportunities for increasing self-esteem. People feel competent when they are able to use their talents and abilities in their work and when they can do a job well. They feel useful and necessary when they are able to help others. They feel autonomous when they can make their own decisions. These are just a few ways in which self-esteem needs can be met at work and all of them can be influenced by the actions of an effective leader-manager.

Esteem from Others.   Respect and recognition from others is another source of esteem. This respect and recognition from others is more satisfying if it is based on a true appreciation of the real person rather than on a facade or on the opinion of others that is not based on fact. The implication for leadership is that unearned praise is not as effective a motivation as praise that has been earned. Unearned praise may even be counterproductive because it implies that the person is not sufficiently competent to earn it.

People want others to pay attention to them. They want their uniqueness recognized and their need for dignity respected. They need to feel important, to feel that they have some kind of status within their social groups, and to feel that they are able to influence others. Learning and practicing leadership skills is one way to increase esteem.

Any expression of recognition or genuine appreciation helps to build esteem. Some more specific ways in which a nurse manager can provide opportunities to meet these needs and thereby increase staff motivation are by:

▷ Letters of commendation.
▷ Merit raises and promotions.
▷ Positive and frequent evaluative feedback.
▷ Individualized assignments that suit staff members' abilities.
▷ Mentioning a person's positive qualities and accomplishments to that person and to others.

Several of the actions listed (raises, promotions, assignments) are dependent on your having the authority to grant them or the ability to influence the decisions to grant these things.

SELF-ACTUALIZATION.   Self-actualization is the next and highest level in the hierarchy of needs. Self-actualization is the growth and development to an individual's fullest potential. Maslow uses many terms to describe his ideal of the fully self-actualized person: perceptive, accepting, spontaneous, natural, autonomous, secure, unselfish, philosophic, creative, flexible, and satisfied.

These terms offer an image of a truly mature and highly functional human being. But self-actualized people are not perfect—they can be lazy, thoughtless, or bad tempered at times. They are not always happy, either. In other words, while self-actualized people are highly functional, they are not perfect.

If every human being is unique, then what constitutes a person's fullest potential is also unique. Some people have more potential capability than others. Some find expression of their fullest development in artistic ways, others in work with people, and others in work with ideas or material things. The definition of self-actualization may also be influenced by the cultural background of the person (Szapocznik, 1978).

If you are to be an effective leader, you will seek ways to promote your own self-actualization as well as that of your coworkers. You need to know a great deal about yourself or others before you can effectively promote self-actualization. Also, the lower-level needs must be at least partially filled before people are motivated to use their time and energy working toward self-actualization.

Because of the individuality of self-actualization needs, it is difficult to describe exactly what actions will promote it. (It would be easier to say what will *not* promote self-actualization.) The following are some suggestions:

▷ Encourage innovation.
▷ Include staff members in planning processes.
▷ Provide opportunities for enhancing current skills.
▷ Allow the testing of new ideas in practice.
▷ Include staff in decisions about assignments.
▷ Encourage people to write their job descriptions and to set their own goals or objectives.
▷ Encourage staff to develop and implement new projects and programs.
▷ Provide resources for continued learning.
▷ Offer challenging work.

SOCIOCULTURAL INFLUENCES

Culture

There are also a number of social forces within the environment that have an influence on the way a person behaves. The broad concept of culture, the more specific concept of roles, and the way in which they influence attitudes and behavior are discussed in this section.

The culture of the group or society within which people live and work determines the language they speak and influences their behavior patterns —the kind of food they eat, the way they dress, how they relate to others, their values, their aspirations, and their view of the world. Behavior patterns are also affected by the particular roles people play and how those roles are defined. While these sociocultural factors are not the sole determinants of behavior, they are a pervasive and often subtle influence that needs to be considered when trying to understand why people behave the way they do.

Culture includes all of the beliefs, values, and behavior patterns common to a particular group of people (Leininger, 1986). These patterns are shared by the whole group, but there are usually differences in the degree to which the patterns are evident in the attitudes and behavior of a particular individual.

Because these patterns are learned, not intrinsic, they can differ widely from one group to another. These differences are of some concern to leaders because they may lead to misunderstandings and conflicts between people from different cultures.

CULTURAL DIFFERENCES IN SHARED MEANING.   One of the classic ways of describing how cultures differ in beliefs, values and behavior patterns is the model developed by Kluckhohn (1976). According to this model, there are five fundamental areas in which every culture develops a set of shared meanings.

Innate Goodness or Evil.   Are people thought to be basically good, evil, or neither? The Puritan ancestors of some Americans believed that people were inherently evil but that it was possible to overcome this evil nature. This point of view leads to an emphasis on the need for a great deal of discipline and control. An alternative view that people have the potential to be either good or bad is probably more common today. You can also find humanists who believe that people are inherently good and their badness is due to environmental influences. You will see this difference in the motivational theories of leadership in the next chapter.

Relationship With Nature.   Do people dominate natural forces or are they dominated by them? Those who believe that people dominate nature are likely to put a great deal of energy into altering their environment, while those who believe that nature dominates them tend to accept their environment as it is. For example, one group would accept a harsh work environment as a given, while another group would protest its harshness and try to change it. A third view point is to see man as part of the environment, affecting it and being affected by it, which is closer to the open system approach.

Time Orientation.   Are people most concerned with the past, present, or future? Some groups have a great deal of respect for tradition and are likely to see change as a threat to their traditions. Others are oriented primarily to the present and consider the future too unpredictable to do any planning for it. An orientation to the future leads to an emphasis on planning ahead. People with a future orientation are more likely to see their present job as a stepping stone to better positions and to be more interested in career planning.

Another way in which time orientations can differ is the definition of being "on time". For some groups, a two o'clock appointment means that they will expect to enter your office at precisely two o'clock or, even better, a minute or two early. For people from other cultures, however, a two o'clock appointment means that they can expect to see you at two forty-five or so, depending on what else is happening at the time. They would not expect you to be upset with them unless they arrived well past three o'clock.

Being, Becoming, or Doing.   Which aspect is given the most attention —what a person is, what that person can be, or what that person does? People of cultures with a being orientation focus primarily on a person's present characteristics while those with a becoming orientation focus on development of the self as a whole (for example, becoming more knowledgeable, aware, or creative). The third orientation focuses on action and accomplishment. In terms of work and leadership, people with this third orientation (doing) would emphasize an individual's contribution to productivity and profit as measures of success. Those with a becoming orientation would look at the individual, what that individual is learning or how the person is developing, and how this contributes to the purposes of the group or organization.

Relationships With Others.   In some societies, the vertical or lineal relationships, that is, who a person's ancestors and parents were, are of great importance. In others, the emphasis is on lateral relationships, that is, the members of the groups to which a person belongs including the extended family, usually with an accompanying concern for others and mutual dependency on others. For people with this lateral orientation, group goals take priority over individual goals. A third orientation, commonly found in American business, has an emphasis on the independence and autonomy of the individual. For people with this orientation, dependence has negative connotations and individual goals take priority over group goals. People with this individualistic orientation are likely to have more difficulty working as members of a group or team than those with a lateral orientation. They are also more likely to be competitive rather than cooperative.

Other Differences. In addition to the fundamental areas described, there are a number of other general differences among cultures that are significant for leadership. These include differences in (1) relationship to people in authority, (2) spatial relationships, (3) the use of eye contact, (4) expressiveness, (5) language, and (6) modes of thinking (Hall & Whyte, 1976; Sue, 1981).

1. *Relationship to people in authority.* People in some cultural groups, Asian Americans for example, show their respect for people in authority by remaining silent. They expect communications with people in authority, such as supervisors, to be primarily one way, that is, from the supervisor to the employee. This respectful silence can be misinterpreted as rudeness or lack of intelligence by people from cultural groups in which an employee is expected to relate to the supervisor on an equal or near equal basis and to engage in two-way communication.

2. *Spatial relationships.* There are significant measurable differences between cultural groups in regard to the amount of space that feels comfortable between people in conversation. Anglo-Americans prefer to keep at least two feet between people during a conversation with a colleague, but Latin-Americans and Black Americans generally consider this amount of space between people too distant and often try to move closer, which makes the Anglo-American feel uncomfortable. The person moving away may be thought of as cold, distant, and indifferent while the person moving closer may be thought of as pushy or inappropriately intimate.

3. *Eye contact.* Generally speaking, Anglo-Americans use eye contact to indicate that they are listening but look away frequently when they are speaking. Black Americans make greater eye contact when they are speaking and this nonverbal communication can be misinterpreted by Anglo-Americans as glaring. In contrast, Mexican Americans and Japanese Americans may avoid eye contact to show respect.

4. *Expressiveness.* People from traditional Chinese, Japanese, and American Indian cultural groups value restraint in the expression of strong feelings or discussion of personal matters, while people from the Middle East are more likely to be loud and exuberant in expressing their feelings. Somewhere in between is the Northern American who values a calm, logical approach but also values expressing feelings more openly.

5. *Language.* When people speak different languages, the communication problem is obvious. However, when they speak the same language, they may not be aware that they speak different versions of that language. For example, the use of non-standard English and regional differences in the use of certain words or expressions can lead to misinterpretations and misunderstandings. In health care organizations, the frequent use of abbreviations and shortened words can be mystifying to clients or new employees who thought they spoke the same language.

6. *Modes of thinking.* There are differences in modes of thinking among

cultural groups. Some emphasize the intuitive and creative approach to knowing, others emphasize the objective, logical, and scientific method. Some groups make a clear distinction between physical and mental health (a distinction that is evident in the structure of our health care system), others do not. Some are familiar with abstract thought (such as the use of theories and principles) and comfortable with ambiguity while others prefer a concrete, structured mode that uses examples and offers specific directions. Each of these differences affects exchange between people from different cultures.

A number of crosscultural and crossnational research studies have identified differences in leadership and management approaches and preferences across cultures. Mexican managers, for example, perceive participative management as a threat to their managerial image and have been described as "anti-delegation" in comparison to American managers (Negandhi, 1985).

Most managers across cultures seem to be relatively practical and pragmatic in their outlook. But some emphasize competition more than others. Regard for the scientific method has also been found to be higher in developed countries. Developing countries in general allow more subjective (intuitive, emotional) factors in decision making. These differences may cause difficulty in adaptation for people who are new to the U.S., a significant concern in a health care system which employs people of many different cultural backgrounds.

These cultural differences should not be overemphasized because one can find almost as many differences within a culture as among cultures (Negandhi, 1985). They are generalizations, meant to stimulate your awareness of these differences and the ways in which they can affect behavior and also to increase your sensitivity to often overlooked potential for misunderstanding among people from different cultures. Many of these differences are subtle and easily overlooked by the leader who is not alert to them.

WORKING WITH CULTURAL DIFFERENCES. Work in the health care field attracts people from many different cultures. You may work with people from your own culture or with people from a culture that is entirely unfamiliar to you. You may find yourself a part of the majority, or, in other situations, a part of the minority culture. This is generally a more uncomfortable position.

When you are a part of the majority culture it will be especially important for you to show respect and consideration for people from different cultural groups. If you are in the minority, you may have to demand this respect and consideration from others. In either case, knowledge of both your own cultural patterns and those of other cultures is an essential first step in developing effective working relationships among people of different cultures.

There is no shortcut to cultural awareness and effectiveness in working with people of different cultures. This process requires some insight into your own responses to difference as well as time to learn about these differences and develop your ability to recognize them. The following is a set of guidelines that can help you move in this direction:

1. *Learn more about culture beliefs, values, and practices.* Knowledge comes before understanding. Learning about your own culture may actually be more difficult than learning about another culture. This is true because it is so much a part of you that it is below awareness until you begin studying your own culture or until you are exposed to other cultures.
2. *Resist seeing everyone in a particular culture as being alike.* If you read about your own culture, you will probably find that some of the descriptions fit you personally but others do not. The same is true for people from other cultures.
3. *Interpret behavior on the basis of its meaning to the other person and that person's culture.* Try not to interpret the behavior of people from a different culture on the basis of your own culture. The difference in use of direct eye contact is an example. For some cultural groups it communicates interest and openness, for others, it communicates rudeness and insubordination.
4. *Observe different cultural patterns in behavior.* If you watch the ways in which people from different cultural groups interact, you can begin to get a feeling for the customary distance they maintain between one another, the degree of expressiveness and eye contact considered appropriate, and so forth. This both increases your awareness and helps you to feel more comfortable with different patterns of behavior.
5. *Adjust your own patterns somewhat to reduce the difference between your own and other people's patterns.* This does not mean that you must give up your culture and become the same as the people with whom you work. It does mean that you can make some accommodations, such as speaking a little softer or louder, moving a little closer or farther away, or using more abstract or concrete expressions, in order to facilitate communication and comfortable working relationships.
6. *Distinguish between behavior that needs to be changed and behavior that can be accommodated.* This is especially important. In some jobs, for example, it is necessary for an employee to arrive at exactly the agreed upon time so that people on the previous shift can leave their patients and go home. It is also necessary to learn enough of your clients' language to be able to communicate with them, especially if you counsel them. On the other hand, a wide variation in differences such as preferred personal distance, expressiveness, and responses to people in authority can be tolerated in most work situations. In fact, we can learn to appreciate and value diversity (Sargent, 1987).

The Influence of Roles

Roles are social prescriptions for behavior. They specify what kind of behavior is appropriate for a person who has a specific position within a group. Role can also be defined as the actual (rather than prescribed) behavior of a person occupying a specific position within a group. This is the definition we will use later in talking about group roles.

Like cultural patterns, role behavior is learned through interactions with people in a process called socialization. Learning a role involves acquiring certain skills, attitudes, and patterns of behavior. However, cultural patterns are more general than role prescriptions and a person usually fills many different roles but has one or a limited number of different cultural patterns (Biddle & Thomas, 1966), (Hardy & Conway, 1978).

Socialization into a particular role includes changes in attitudes and behavior and an acceptance of the expectations of that role. People can become deeply committed to their roles, can get a great deal of satisfaction from them, and can suffer anger or sorrow at the loss of a role. The roles that an individual plays can affect that individual's identity and self-esteem. The roles can also help or thwart their attempts to meet their basic needs. For example, the role of nursing assistant carries little status or prestige and can fail to meet a person's need for recognition although it can help to meet a person's needs for security or belonging.

People occupy different roles in different situations and within different groups. A single individual can occupy the roles of caregiver, colleague, friend, parent, spouse, sibling, cousin, partner, and many more. You may find yourself in the role of leader in one situation and in the role of someone responding to leadership in another situation. Both a person's understanding of a particular role and a person's unique characteristics as an individual affect the way a role is carried out. In other words, you will find variations in the way a role is enacted. For example, although there is a great deal of similarity in the way all critical care nurses in a particular hospital function, no two nurses will behave exactly the same way in that role despite the fact that they are filling the same role within the parameters set by the hospital and by society.

The existence of different roles and the fact that they influence behavior by describing the kind of behavior that is expected helps to explain why people can be observed to act somewhat differently at various times and in various places. The person as a whole has not changed but different aspects of the self become more evident in different roles.

SOURCES OF ROLE STRESS. There are a number of ways in which stress can arise within a role or between roles.

Role Conflict. Conflicts can occur within a particular role or between two or more roles. For example, nurses may be expected to make independent decisions and to be accountable for their own practice and yet be expected to follow a physician's directions without question.

The differences *between* roles can also be a source of conflict. For example, some people may be expected to be nurturing and supportive parents within their families but dominant and controlling in their particular positions at work. This conflict of expectations can be a source of stress to people who cannot easily switch from home to work roles and back again.

Ambiguity. Some roles are vague and inadequately defined. Without adequate guidelines you cannot be sure that you are fulfilling the role according to expectations. For example, imagine being assigned to a newly formed drug treatment team. You may find that the nurse's role is ambiguous. You may not know whether you are expected to monitor drug intake, counsel individuals, be responsible for the client's physical well being, or all of these.

Incongruity. Some role expectations are not congruent with a person's usual patterns of behavior. For example, an experienced nurse who is asked to be a preceptor for a nursing student may find it difficult to step back and let the student give the nursing care when the nurse is accustomed to doing it. Another common example of incongruity occurs when a person who enjoys working with highly technical equipment is suddenly promoted to a managerial position, and expected to enjoy dealing with people problems.

Overload.   Some roles demand too much of the individual. For example, a nurse is expected to be an expert clinician, teacher, counselor, researcher, and leader. For some who enter nursing, these demands constitute an overload of expectations that they cannot meet.

Incompetence.   People sometimes find that they do not have the knowledge or skills a roll demands. The highly skilled technician, in the earlier example, finds that the skills needed to fulfill a manager's role are not the same as those previously needed.

Overqualification.   This is the opposite of role incompetence. People sometimes find themselves in a role that does not utilize all of their abilities. In the drug treatment team example mentioned previously, if you find that the only expectation of you as a nurse is to monitor drug intake, much of your knowledge and skill will be unused.

Research Example 1–1 examines the frequency with which some of the different types of role conflicts are encountered by caregivers in hospitals.

The sources of stress just described are a matter of concern to the leader because of their potential negative effect on job satisfaction and productivity. They can be a problem for both the leader and the people with whom the leader works.

ROLE STRESS REDUCTION.   A number of ways to reduce role stress have been suggested by Hardy (1978). Not all of the suggestions are suitable for every situation or type of stress. The suggestions are as follows:

1. *Problem solving.* This is usually the first step to take when trying to resolve a dilemma. The problem-solving process includes identifying the problem and then seeking alternative actions that will solve the problem. For example, if the problem is role ambiguity, it may be possible to better define the role yourself or to request clarification from the people with whom you work.
2. *Role bargaining.* When role stress cannot be reduced by clarification or another simple solution, then direct or indirect role bargaining can be used. In *direct bargaining,* the individual communicates the role problem to those who have established the role expectations and then negotiates a change in those expectations. For example, if you joined the drug treatment team and found that your only expected duty was to monitor drug intake, you could discuss the problem of role overqualification with team members or with the person in authority. Then you could negotiate an expansion of the nurse's role.

   Indirect bargaining involves the same kind of role alteration but it is done solely by the dissatisfied individual. Instead of discussing it first with others, the individual simply begins to alter the role in the hope that a gradual change will be accepted by the people involved. For example, you could begin to gradually add to your functions on the drug treatment team without discussing the change with the team members. Although not always appropriate, indirect bargaining is sometimes an effective way

---

RESEARCH EXAMPLE 1–1. Role Conflict—A Challenge to Reality Shock

How much role conflict do nurses experience? What types of conflicts? Are these conflicts related to job dissatisfaction and turnover? Rosse and Rosse (1981) questioned registered nurses, practical nurses, and aides about the types of conflicts they experienced, how satisfied they were with their jobs and the likelihood of leaving their jobs in the next six to nine months.

The role conflicts measured were role ambiguity, role overload, intersender conflict (incompatible demands from different people such as physicians and administrators), inter-role conflict (demands of multiple roles) and person-role conflict (conflict between values or beliefs and actions required by the role). For example, coworkers were asked if they ever had to work under incompatible policies, do things that were against their better judgment, or if they had conflicts with their families. The coworkers were also asked to choose one of seven faces from a scowl to a broad smile to represent their feelings about work. Altogether, 220 RNs, 188 LPNs, 78 nursing aides, and 17 nursing supervisors representing all three shifts at five different hospitals in Illinois completed the questionnaire. Their median length of employment at the hospitals was 3.5 years.

Although a high level of conflict was expected for all types listed, only intersender (incompatible demands) and role overload had means about the midpoint of the scale used. The researchers expected that role overload would be higher for those who worked in intensive and coronary care units and that intersender conflicts would be higher for RNs (especially those with higher degrees) than for LPNs or aides, but they found no significant differences on any of these variables. They did find, however, that role conflicts were related to work stress but did not find as strong a relationship to job satisfaction or to intentions to resign as had been expected.

Increased conflicts were found in nurses who had been in their positions for a greater length of time. This contradicts the concept of reality shock, the role stress phenomenon occurring when a new, unexperienced nurse first enters the job market. Head nurses and supervisors had higher levels of both role overload and intersender conflicts (incompatible demands), probably because of their roles as mediator between nursing staff, physicians, and administrators, as well as with patients.

The results of this study raise many questions about the role conflicts experienced by nursing personnel. They seem to indicate that many factors commonly believed to be the sources of role conflict—working in intensive care units, holding a bachelor's or higher degree, and being a new graduate—are not as influential as many have assumed. The researchers conclude that many of our beliefs about the sources of role conflict have not been sufficiently researched.

---

to bring about subtle role changes without provoking resistance to the change.

3. **Nonconformity.** Nonconformity is the refusal to meet unrealistic or conflicting role expectations. It is similar to indirect role bargaining in that dissatisfied individuals proceed to carry out the role the way they want it to be. However, indirect bargaining is an attempt to gain the support of the other people involved while nonconformity is used in spite of resistance. Nonconforming actions involve a higher risk than indirect bargaining does.

4. **Withdrawal.** Withdrawal from the problematic role may be partial or complete. Some roles are essentially voluntary ones from which it is easy

to withdraw completely. But other roles have a more central position and cannot be easily abandoned. It would, for example, be much harder to withdraw from the role of nurse than it would be to withdraw from the role of student in an evening recreational class.

A partial withdrawal is accomplished by limiting the amount of time, energy, attention, and other forms of commitment devoted to the role. For example, some people who are dissatisfied with their jobs but for some reason feel that they cannot leave them will put minimal energy into their jobs—just enough to get by—and put the rest of their energy into roles outside of work. This kind of withdrawal could seriously affect a person's performance at work.

Withdrawal is usually a last resort action taken to eliminate the stress when other actions have failed. However, it is sometimes a necessary and constructive action.

SUMMARY

Theories provide us with an organizing framework, particular perspective, explanations, predictions, and guides to application in practice. According to open system theory, an open system is different from and greater than the sum of its parts (subsystems). The open system (which may be an individual, group, organization, or community) interacts mutually and simultaneously with its environment, exchanging energy, matter, and information with its environment. It is characterized by its patterns including growth; by its individuality; and by the capacity to think and feel, known as sentience.

Human behavior is postulated to have meaning and to reflect the present state of the individual as a whole in relation to the environment. Automatic reflex actions, nondeliberative coping mechanisms (compensation, expression, denial, suppression, displacement, projection, withdrawal, rationalization, substitution, and identification), and a large number of deliberative mechanisms are used by people to cope with the everyday challenges and stresses of living and working.

Maslow developed a hierarchy of needs that begins with the most basic physiologic needs followed by safety and security, love and belonging, esteem, and self-actualization needs. The more basic or prepotent need must be at least partially met before a person is motivated to seek gratification of the next higher needs. The leader can help people meet these basic needs in order to free their energy to work on higher level needs.

Culture includes the learned patterns of beliefs, values and behaviors common to a group or society. Cultures vary in many ways including their beliefs about the nature of people, their time orientation, and their relationships to nature and to other people. Variations of particular interest to leadership include relationships to people in authority, spatial relationships, use of eye contact, expressiveness, language, modes of thinking and preferred leadership and management styles.

Roles are more specific, socially prescribed patterns of behavior. Role stresses such as role conflict, ambiguity, incongruity, overload, and inappropriate preparation for the role can be dealt with by problem solving, role bargaining, nonconformity, or withdrawal.

REFERENCES*

*Ardell, D.B. (1986). *High level wellness.* Berkeley, California: Ten Speed Press.

Ashby, W.R. (1968). *Principles of the self-organizing system.* In Weckley, W. *Modern systems research for the behavioral scientist.* Chicago: Aldine Publishing.

Bell, N.W. & Vogel, E.F. (1968). *A modern introduction to the family.* New York: The Free Press.

Biddle, B. & Thomas, E. (1966). *Role theory: perspectives for health professionals.* New York: John Wiley & Sons.

Boulding, K.E. (1968). *General system theory—the skeleton of science.* In Buckley, W. *Modern systems research for the behavioral scientist.* Chicago: Aldine Publishing.

Brown, M.M. & Fowler, G.R. (1971). *Psychodynamic nursing: a biosocial orientation.* Philadelphia: W.B. Saunders.

Campbell, C. (1978). *Nursing diagnosis and intervention in nursing practice.* New York: John Wiley & Sons.

Chapple, E.D. (1979). *The biological foundations of individuality and culture.* Huntington, New York: Robert Krieger.

Das, H. (1988). Relevance of symbolic interactionist approach in understanding power: A preliminary analysis. *Journal of Management Studies,* 25, 251–267.

Duldt, B.W. & Griffin, K. (1985). *Theoretical perspectives for nursing.* Boston: Little, Brown.

Fawcett, J. (1975). The family as an open living system: an emerging conceptual framework for nursing. *Journal of International Nursing Review,* 22, 113.

*Fawcett, J. (1984). *Analysis and evaluation of conceptual models of nursing.* Philadelphia: F.A. Davis.

Feuerstein, M., Labbe, E.E. & Kuczmierczyk, A.R. (1986). *Health psychology: a psychological perspective.* New York: Plenum Press.

*Garland, L.M. & Bush, C.T. (1982). *Coping behaviors and nursing.* Reston, Va.: Reston Publishing.

Glisson, C. (1986). The group versus the individual as the unit of analysis in small group research. *Social Work with Groups,* 9,(3), 15–39.

*Hall, A.D. & Fagen, R.E. (1968). *Definition of system.* In Buckley, W. *Modern systems research for the behavioral scientist.* Chicago: Aldine Publishing.

Hall, E.T. & Whyte, W.F. (1976). *Intercultural communication: a guide to men of action.* In Brink, P.J. *Transcultural nursing: a book of readings.* Englewood Cliffs, N.J.: Prentice Hall.

Hanchett, E.S. (1979). *Community health assessment: a conceptual tool kit.* New York: John Wiley & Sons.

Hardy, M.E. (1978). Role stress and role strain. In Hardy, M.E. and Conway, M.E. *Role theory: perspectives for health professionals.* New York: Appleton-Century-Crofts.

Hardy, M.E. & Conway, M.E. (1978). *Role theory: perspectives for health professionals.* New York: Appleton-Century-Crofts.

Jones, K.L., Shainberg, L.W. & Byer, C.O. (1975). *Emotional Health.* ed. 2. San Francisco: Canfield Press.

Joynt, P. & Warner, M. (1985). *Managing in different cultures.* Oslo: Universitetsforlaget AS.

Kantor, D. & Lehr, W. (1976). *Inside the family: toward a theory of family process.* New York: Harper Calophon Books.

*Kluckhohn, F.R. (1976). *Dominant and variant value orientations.* In Brink, P.J. *Transcultural nursing: a book of readings.* Englewood Cliffs, N.J.: Prentice-Hall.

*Laszlo, E. (1972). *The systems view of the world.* New York: George Braziller.

Leininger, M. (1986). *Transcultural nursing: concepts, theories and practices.* New York: John Wiley & Sons.

*Luce, G.G. (1971). *Body time.* New York: Pantheon Books.

*Maslow, A.H. (1970). *Motivation and personality.* ed. 2. New York: Harper & Row.

Menninger, K. (1963). *The vital balance: the life process in mental health and illness.* New York: The Viking Press.

Negandhi, A.R. (1985). *Management in the third world.* In Joynt, P. & Warner, M. *Managing in different cultures.* Oslo: Universitetsforlaget AS.

Rogers, M.E. (1970). *An introduction to the theoretical basis of nursing.* Philadelphia: FA Davis.

Rosse, J.G. & Rosse, P.H. (1981). Role conflict and ambiguity: an empirical investigation of nursing personnel. *Evaluation and the health professionals,* 4, 385.

Sargent, A.G. (1987). Building a multicultural work environment, *Nursing Management,* 18, (u), 45–51.

Scheflen, A.E. (1982). *Comments on the significance of interaction rhythms.* In Dairs, M. *Interaction rhythms: periodicity in communicative behavior.* New York: Human Sciences Press.

Schwartz, L.H. & Schwartz, J.L. (1972). *The psychodynamics of patient care.* Englewood Cliffs, N.J.: Prentice Hall.

*Sue, D.W. (1981). *Counseling the culturally different: theory and practice.* New York: John Wiley & Sons.

Szapocznik, J. et al. (1978). Cuban value structure: treatment implications. *Consult Clinical Psychology,* 46, 961.

Von Bertalanffy, L. (1976). *Introduction.* In Werley, H. et al. *Health research: the systems approach.* New York: Springer Publishing.

---

*References marked with an asterisk are suggested for further reading.

Chapter 2 ▬▬▬▬▬

OUTLINE

Early Leadership Theories
Trait Theories
  Great Man Theory
  Individual Characteristics
  Trait Studies
Behavioral Theories
  Authoritarian-Democratic-Laissez Faire
    Styles (Lewin, Lippitt, & White)
  Leader Behavior Descriptions (Hemphill;
    Halpin & Winer)
  Task vs. Relationship Orientation (Blake
    & Mouton)

Early Management Theories
Scientific Management (Taylor et al)
Human Relations (Mayo et al)

**Contemporary Leader-Manager
Theories**
Motivational Theories
  Theories X and Y (McGregor)

Hygiene and Motivation Factors
  (Herzberg)
Theory Z (Ouchi)
Behavioral Management (Miller)

Situational Theories
Contingency Theory (Fiedler)
Path-Goal Theory (House)
Situational Determinants
Interactional Theories
  Complex Man and Open Systems
    (Schein)
  Elements of a Leader Situation
    (Hollander)
  Leader-Group Interaction (Schreisheim,
    Howday, & Stodgill)
  The Work-Unit Culture (Lashbrook)
Discussion

Summary

LEARNING OBJECTIVES ▬▬▬▬▬

Upon completion of this chapter, the reader will be able to:

▷ Trace the evolution of early leadership and management theories into the contemporary leader-manager theories.

▷ Distinguish a simplistic leadership or management theory from a comprehensive theory.

▷ Critique the major theories in terms of the degree to which they include the four basic elements of a leadership-management situation.

▷ Compare and contrast the democratic style with the authoritarian and laissez-faire styles; Theory X to Theories Y and Z; task orientation to relationship orientation; and the humanistic approach to the behavioral management approach.

▷ Discuss the effect of one's choice of leader-manager theories on the practice of leadership and management.

LEADERSHIP AND MANAGEMENT THEORIES

T he first chapter dealt with attempts to explain human behavior. This second chapter focuses on theories and concepts specific to leadership and management. They have been developed over the years to explain how people influence each other's behavior in work situations.

You will see that some of the earlier approaches tried to explain leadership in terms of a single characteristic or single aspect of a leadership situation. Some are so limited that they hardly deserve to be called theories. Although only partial explanations of how leaders influence people, they do have some value and are used more often than you might expect.

Early management theories were also somewhat limited in scope. They focused primarily on methods to increase a worker's productivity but did not consider all of the factors that might affect the worker's development, motivation, and productivity. Their primary concern was the factory worker, someone whose output could be measured in terms of the number of welds completed or objects assembled. The output of many workers today, including those in the health care system with whom we are primarily concerned, is not so concrete or easy to measure and the factors which affect the output are not at all clearcut.

The later theories are more complex but they also explain more. They are far more successful in avoiding the problem of being too simplistic than are the earlier theories.

The first section of this chapter deals with the earlier leadership theories and the second section considers the earlier management theories. The last section discusses some of the more recent approaches, most of which acknowledge the need for a more complex, open systems perspective to provide an adequate explanation for leadership and management (Heimann, 1976; Lee, 1980; Maloney, 1979; Stogdill, 1974; Williamson, 1986; Deaux & Wrightsman, 1983). Figure 2–1 is a diagram of these different categories. It may help you to refer back to this diagram or to the outline at the beginning of the chapter from time to time as you read about these theories.

EARLY LEADERSHIP THEORIES

Trait Theories

If you have ever heard the statement that "leaders are born, not made," then you have heard someone expressing the fundamental belief underlying the trait theories of leadership. Trait theories assume that a person must

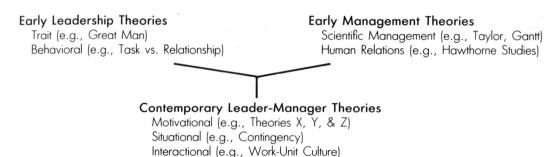

Figure 2–1. Diagrammatic representation of the evolution of leader-manager theories.

have certain innate abilities, personality traits, or other characteristics in order to be a leader. If true, it would mean that some people are naturally better leaders than others.

Since trait theories emphasize given ability over the effects of learning, they lead to the popular conclusion that some people cannot be leaders, no matter how hard they try. This approach also leads to efforts to identify people who have the characteristics of a leader rather than to the development of leaders.

The desire to distinguish leaders who have these innate characteristics from nonleaders who do not led to a search for a single trait or cluster of traits. Trait theorists have studied the biographies of historic leaders and the characteristics of people in positions that require leadership ability. The study of biographies was the basis of the Great Man theory of leadership.

GREAT MAN THEORY. According to the Great Man theory of leadership, the tremendous influence of some well-known people has actually determined or changed the course of history. These people are said to have possessed innate characteristics that made them great leaders. The opposite, deterministic viewpoint would be that they happened to be in the right place at the right time and that it was the events of their time that made them great.

Important historical figures, such as Caesar, Alexander the Great, and Hitler, have been studied to find the characteristics that made them outstanding leaders of their time. Royalty was also of interest to trait theorists. For example, when the characteristics of the rulers of 14 European countries over 500 years were studied, it was found that the countries were strong when they had a strong ruler but that the conditions in these countries were bad when they had a weak ruler (Gemmill, 1986; Woods, 1913). The Great Man Theory assumed that the condition of the country was due to the influence of the abilities with which the ruler was born, ignoring the fact that the condition of the country could have affected the success of the ruler.

INDIVIDUAL CHARACTERISTICS. The search for traits that determine whether or not a person will be an effective leader has been the focus of many studies. So far, however, no single trait or characteristic has been found in all leaders. In spite of this limitation, the trait approach is often used to choose people for leadership positions.

Many people believe in and try to implement a number of different—and even contradictory—versions of the trait theory. Certain physical characteristics are often thought to augment leadership ability. For example, it is commonly believed that tall individuals are better leader material than short individuals because they seem stronger and more dominating. A tall person can literally look down on other people and can be physically imposing. A contradictory but also popular belief is that a person who was always smaller than his or her peers has had to learn how to defend himself or herself and is, therefore, a tougher fighter and a potentially stronger leader than taller people.

There are also personality traits and talents commonly associated with leadership ability. For example, the most outspoken person in a group is often assumed to be the leader even when other evidence does not support this assumption. The most intelligent or skilled person in a group is often designated the leader because other group members admire this person. Manipulative people (sometimes called "smooth operators," "wheeler-dealers," or "trouble-makers") and people who are especially courageous are also thought of as good leader material.

Despite their limitations and contradictions, these popular versions are often used as the basis for leadership decisions. The most physically imposing or most highly skilled nurse in a group may be chosen for a supervisory position solely on the basis of this supposed leadership trait.

TRAIT STUDIES. The beliefs about leadership mentioned above are very subjective, but even the more objective research studies have not really succeeded in finding any one set of traits that distinguish leaders from nonleaders. The results have been inconsistent. Dozens of different traits have been identified but, so far, none can repeatedly predict who will be an effective leader and who will not.

There are some characteristics, however, that were found repeatedly in a large proportion of these studies. They are intelligence and skill, initiative, assertiveness and persistence, ability to relate to other people, a strong sense of self, ability to tolerate stress and take the consequences of a decision, originality (creativity), and status within the group. Intelligence and initiative are the two most often cited.

By themselves, the trait theories are too limited because they focus on the leader and ignore the other elements of a leadership-management situation (co-actor and the environment). Also, they focus on the capacities a leader brings to a situation rather than on what the leader actually does in a situation. They do contribute to our understanding of leadership by indicating those characteristics, especially intelligence and initiative, that are more likely to be found in leaders than nonleaders. Many of these traits associated with leadership may actually be indicators of motivation or desire to lead rather than the innate capacities of an individual to lead.

Behavioral Theories

The behavioral theories, sometimes called the functional theories of leadership, still focus on the leader. The primary difference between the trait and behavioral theories is that the behavioral theories are concerned with what a leader *does* rather than who the leader *is*. They are still limited primarily to the leader element in a situation but are far more action oriented and do give some consideration to the co-actor. We will consider one theory based upon the description of leader functions and two different approaches to describing leadership styles.

AUTHORITARIAN, DEMOCRATIC, LAISSEZ-FAIRE STYLES (LEWIN, LIPPITT, & WHITE). A major breakthrough in the development of leadership theories came in the late 1930s. The classic research done by Lewin, Lippitt and White (1960) on the interaction between leaders and group members indicated that the behavior of the leader could substantially influence the climate and outcomes of the group. The leader behaviors were divided into three distinct patterns called leadership styles: authoritarian, democratic, and laissez-faire. More details about their study can be found in the Research Example 2–1. These styles can be thought of as a continuum from a highly controlling and directive type of leadership to a very passive, inactive style as illustrated in Figure 2–2.

The *authoritarian* leader maintains strong control over the people in the group. This control may be benevolent and considerate (paternalistic leadership) or it may be dictatorial with complete disregard for group members.

Authoritarian leaders give orders often and expect group members to obey these orders. Directions are given as commands, not suggestions. Criticism is more common from the authoritarian leader, although not necessarily a constant occurrence. Many authoritarian leaders are also quite punitive.

Decision making is done by the leader alone, not by the group. Some will try to make decisions congruent with the group's goals but the less benevolent leaders often make decisions that are directly opposed to the group's needs or goals.

Authoritarian leadership emphasizes differences in status. The autocratic leader clearly dominates the group, making the status of the leader separate from, and higher than, the status of group members. This reduces the degree of trust and openness between leader and group members, particularly if the leader tends to be punitive as well.

Procedures and group actions are well defined and usually predictable. This reduces frustration and increases group members' feelings of security. Productivity is high but creativity, autonomy, and self-motivation are stifled. Dependency needs are usually met but growth and autonomy needs often are not.

Authoritarian leadership is particularly suitable in crisis situations when clear directions are the highest priority. It is also appropriate when the entire focus is on getting the job done or when it is difficult to share decision making for some reason. It is often referred to today as a directive or controlling style of leadership.

Democratic leadership is based on the following principles:

1. Every group member should participate in decision making.
2. Freedom of belief and action is allowed within reasonable bounds that are set by society and by the group.
3. Each individual is responsible for himself or herself and for the welfare of the group.
4. There should be concern and consideration for each group member as a unique individual.

STUDY DESIGN

A classic study of the effects of different leadership styles on groups was done by Lewin, Lippitt and White in 1938. Twenty 11-year old boys (described as middle class, from the Midwest, and well-adjusted) were assigned to groups with either autocratic, democratic or laissez-faire leaders.

The groups met once a week in after-school clubs in which the boys made masks, plaster molds, and other craft items. Each group was exposed to three different leaders and at least two different styles of leadership. Each leader played at least two different styles of leadership in order to control the effects of differences in skills and personal style of the individual leaders.

The autocratic leaders made all the decisions and expected the boys to obey them. When the groups had democratic leaders, the boys participated in making decisions. The laissez-faire leader avoided making any decisions and allowed the group to work or play without any supervision or direction.

The original plan was to test only the autocratic and democratic styles, but it was observed that one of the four leaders in the first series of club meetings was more anarchic than democratic and that this was having a substantial effect on his group. This leader was then encouraged to assume the laissez-faire style for that series of six meetings and another leader did the same in the second series of meetings in order to study the effects of laissez-faire leadership.

At each club meeting, an observer sat unobtrusively in the corner of the room to record the behavior of both the leader and group members for later analysis. Raw scores and percentages were reported for the behavior observed such as the number and proportion of friendly, aggressive, or dependent statements made by the boys. The differences were found to be statistically significant at the 0.05 level of confidence or better.

RESULTS

The researchers found that the groups behaved very differently under different leadership styles. When the groups had laissez-faire leaders they were less organized, less efficient, and less satisfying for their members. Laissez-faire groups got less work done, spent more time horsing around, and their work was done poorly. When the boys were interviewed later by a neutral party, all of them (100 percent) preferred the democratic leader over the laissez-faire leader.

Autocratic leadership was found to result in much more hostility (in a ratio of 30 to 1), more demands for attention, more dependence on the leaders, and other more subtle kinds of discontent in the groups. In fact, all four boys who dropped out of the clubs did so when their groups were led by autocratic leaders. It is interesting to note that groups with autocratic leaders were found to be either quite aggressive or quite submissive. The observers thought that less individuality was allowed in the autocratic groups. Motivation to work was clearly lower than in the democratic groups: when the autocratic leader left the room, the work stopped. However, the overall quantity of work done was greatest under the autocratic leaders.

Democratic groups were more cohesive. They were described as being friendlier and more group-minded. Although they produced somewhat less work than the autocratic groups, both motivation and originality were found to be higher. Nineteen out of a total of twenty boys expressed a preference for the leader who used the democratic style of leadership.

	AUTHORITARIAN	DEMOCRATIC	LAISSEZ-FAIRE
Degree of Freedom	Little freedom	Moderate freedom	Much freedom
Degree of Control	High control	Moderate control	No control
Decision Making	By the leader	Leader and group together	By the group or by no one
Leader Activity Level	High	High	Minimal
Assumption of responsibility	Primarily the leader	Shared	Abdicated
Output of the Group	High quantity, good quality	Creative, high quality	Variable, may be poor quality
Efficiency	Very efficient	Less efficient than authoritarian	Inefficient

Figure 2–2. Comparison of authoritarian, democratic, and laissez-faire leadership styles.

Democratic leadership is much more participative and far less control-ling than authoritarian leadership. Democratic leadership is not passive, however. The democratic leader actively stimulates and guides the group toward fulfillment of the principles above and toward achievement of its goals.

Rather than issuing commands, democratic leaders offer information, ask stimulating questions and make suggestions to guide the work of the group. They are catalysts rather than controllers, more likely to say "we" than "I" and "you" when talking about the group. They set limits, enforce rules, and encourage productivity. Criticism is constructive rather than punitive.

Control is shared with group members who are expected to participate to the best of their abilities and experience. The democratic style demands a strong faith in the ability of group members to solve problems and to ultimately make wise choices when setting group goals and deciding how to accomplish these goals. Not every leader finds this easy.

Because group members participate actively in decision making and have more responsibility for the outcomes of those decisions, dependence on the leader is minimized and independence and originality are encouraged. Participation in goal setting increases the group's commitment to those goals and motivation to get the work done comes from the entire group rather than through pressure from the leader. Group members are usually more satisfied with democratic leadership than with authoritarian or laissez-faire leadership.

Most studies indicate that democratic leadership is not as efficient quantitatively as authoritarian leadership. While the work done by a demo-cratic group is more creative and the group is more self-motivated, the democratic style is also more cumbersome. First, it takes more time to ensure that everyone in the group has participated in making a decision and this can be very frustrating to people who want to get a job done as fast as possible. Second, disagreements are more likely to arise and must be resolved, which can also require a great deal of effort.

Democratic leadership is particularly appropriate for groups of people who will work together for an extended period of time, when interpersonal relationships can substantially affect the work of the group. It is also appropriate when a great deal of cooperation and coordination between group members is needed, or when the nature of the work makes close and detailed supervision difficult or impossible. This is often true of health care.

Democratic leadership is often called supportive or participative leadership. There are variations in the degree to which decision making is shared with the group, with styles midway between democratic and autocratic. For example, a leader may encourage input from group members and take their views into consideration but makes the final decision.

The *laissez-faire* leader is generally inactive, passive and nondirective. The laissez-faire leader leaves virtually all of the control and decision making to the group and provides little or no direction, guidance or encouragement.

Laissez-faire leaders offer very little to the group: few commands, questions, suggestions or criticism. They are permissive, set almost no limits, and allow almost any behavior. However, many are inconsistent and will occasionally become very directive and command group members to take a particular action. When this happens, group members often ignore the command or react negatively to this attempt to exert leadership.

Some laissez-faire leaders are quite supportive of individual group members and will provide information or suggestions when asked. The more extreme laissez-faire leader, however, will direct an individual back to the group. When the laissez-faire style of leadership becomes extreme, no leadership is evident.

In a laissez-faire group, members act independently of each other and often at cross purposes because there is little cooperation or coordination. In some groups, disinterest and apathy set in, in others the activity becomes chaotic and the frustration level rises. In either case, goals are unclear and procedures are often confusing or totally lacking. Neither the task nor the relationship concerns of group members are dealt with in a satisfactory manner.

When all group members are highly self-directed, motivated, and able to coordinate their own activities with others, laissez-faire leadership can give them the freedom they need to be highly creative and productive. In most situations, however, laissez-faire leadership is unproductive, inefficient and unsatisfactory. Laissez-faire leadership is also called permissive or nondirective leadership.

LEADER BEHAVIOR DESCRIPTIONS (HEMPHILL; HALPIN & WINER). When attention turned from the qualities of the person to the kinds of behavior exhibited by leaders, it became apparent that leadership could be a shared function. For example, on a health care team each member of the team may be knowledgeable about some aspect of patient care and have some influence on patient care decisions made by the team.

Beginning in the 1940s and 1950s, a large number of research studies were done to define these leader functions (Stogdill & Coons, 1957). The purpose of these studies was to describe and categorize the behaviors of actual leaders. Unlike the subjects of the earlier trait theorists, however, these leaders were not political or historic figures. Instead, they were supervisors or leaders of a diverse array of teams including Air Force crews, school personnel, and, more recently, nurses.

Over 1800 different behaviors were identified in these studies. The behaviors were then organized into nine categories:

1. Integration (increasing cooperation)
2. Communication
3. Production emphasis
4. Representation (speaking for the group)
5. Fraternization
6. Organization
7. Evaluation
8. Initiation
9. Domination

These categories were later modified, tested, and finally reduced to two major categories that are still widely used. The first of these categories, called *initiating structure*, includes task-related functions such as:

▷ Assigns members to particular tasks.
▷ Criticizes poor work.

Initiating structure also includes behaviors that clarify roles, organize work, define procedures and move the group toward its goals.

The second category, *consideration*, includes relationship-oriented functions such as:

▷ Finds time to listen to team members.
▷ Does personal favors for team members. (Halpin & Winer in Stogdill & Coons, 1957).

Consideration also includes behaviors that build trust and show respect for the individual group members.

These categories have been used in many research studies and in evaluations of leaders by both superiors and subordinates (see Research Example 2–2 for an example from nursing). Both seem to have a significant effect on leader effectiveness. For example, when leaders are rated high on both initiating structure and consideration, their groups are more cohesive and harmonious. High consideration behavior results in increased satisfaction, lower absenteeism, fewer grievances, and lower employee turnover. High initiating structure seems to improve group productivity.

Leaders who are low in both initiating structure and consideration are usually rated ineffective by both their supervisors and the members of the group. The most effective leader is high on both initiating structure and consideration.

TASK VS. RELATIONSHIP ORIENTATION (BLAKE & MOUTON). The task and relationship orientations are closely related to the initiating structure and consideration categories. The task-oriented leader is concerned

RESEARCH EXAMPLE 2–2. Leadership Style and Nursing Staff Job Satisfaction

Does leadership style affect the behavior and attitudes of subordinates? In a study of 238 nurses working in 14 neonatal intensive care units, Duxbury and associates (1984) looked at the relationship between job satisfaction, staff burnout, and head nurse leadership style. The sample was drawn from a larger national random sample.

The head nurses' leadership styles were separated into four categories: high structure-high consideration; low structure-low consideration; high structure-low consideration; and low structure-high consideration. The researchers found a fairly strong relationship ($r = 0.55$) between staff nurse job satisfaction and high consideration and less relationship to staff burnout ($r = 0.29$). There was little relationship between structure and job satisfaction or burnout except that staff burnout was highest when the head nurse's style was one of high structure and low consideration.

The researchers point out that the work environment should also be considered in analyzing these results. The head nurse's style could be a reaction to different work environments. In other words, head nurses can also suffer burnout and may, as a result, have a high structure, low consideration style of leadership. It was concluded that neonatal intensive care head nurses can increase satisfaction and reduce burnout by displaying a high consideration style of leadership.

with getting the work done and focuses on activities that encourage group productivity. The relationship oriented leader, on the other hand, is especially concerned with interpersonal relationships and focuses on activities that meet group member's needs.

Unlike the single continuum of authoritarian, democratic and laissez-faire leadership styles, the task and relationship orientations are bipolar (Fig. 2–3). This means that a leader can be high on one scale and low on the other or vice versa. Blake and Mouton (Blake & Mouton, 1964; Blake, Mouton & Tapper, 1981) have developed what they call a Managerial Grid to show the various combinations of high and low (relationship and task orientation). The leader with a 1,1 score is low on both task and relationship concerns, while a leader with a 9,9 score is high on both and considered to have the most effective style of leadership.

The 1,1 leader can be described as an inactive and uninvolved leader who does little planning, shows little concern for team members and rarely takes the initiative to make changes. This is similar to the style of the laissez-faire leader. The high task, low relationship (9,1) leader can be described as a controlling, directive leader who closely supervises team members and does most of the planning. Team members are expected to do what they are told and those who do not may be punished. On the other hand, the low task, high relationship leader (1,9) can be described as an accepting, considerate leader who encourages team members and emphasizes good feelings between people but does little planning and allows team members to make many of their own decisions.

The high task, high relationship (9,9) leader can be described as an active leader who promotes open communication and team members' participation in setting goals. Leaders using this style also provide constructive

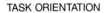

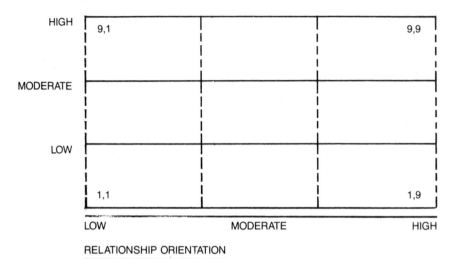

Figure 2–3. Bipolar leader orientation to task and relationships. [Adapted from Blake, Mouton, and Tapper (1981).]

(not destructive) criticism, intervene when a conflict arises, and introduce changes after discussing them with team members. This leader has been found to be the most effective, as was the case with high initiating structure and consideration leaders.

EARLY MANAGEMENT THEORIES

In contrast to the early leadership theories which described the person who was the leader, the early management theories began with a concern about getting as much work as possible out of each employee. Most attention was given at first to blue collar workers (assembly lines, construction gangs and similar workers). There are two particularly important branches of the early management theories: the forerunners of present management science with its emphasis on cost and productivity, and the behavioral approach to getting the best out of an employee.

Scientific Management (Taylor et al)

Almost every management book mentions Frederick Taylor as the founder of management science. Taylor had an engineering background and was experienced as a machine shop foreman. You can see the influence of his machine shop and engineering background in the management principles that he developed in the 1890s and 1900s (Lee, 1980; Locke, 1982).

Taylor and his associates' principles center on ways to increase the efficiency or productivity of each worker. He concentrated on the amount of time an employee took to do a certain task, ways to make the task easier, and ways to get it done in the least amount of time possible so that more work could be done in a day. To do this, the elements of the task were analyzed for useless movements that could be eliminated; workers who seemed to have found the fastest way to do the job were identified and their methods examined; designs for work aids (such as devices for moving heavy objects) to get the task done faster were developed; and the amount of rest needed to keep workers from becoming too exhausted to work was determined.

One incentive Taylor used was that of paying by the piece, that is, to pay for each item completed rather than by the day or by the hour. The focus was on getting more work out of the individual employee and calculating exactly how many employees were needed to do how much work. This, by the way, occasionally prompted vigorous protests from workers and their unions (Lee, 1980).

> There is a famous story about Taylor and how he convinced a worker named "Schmidt" to quadruple his output by providing the right incentives. The average worker loaded 12 tons of iron a day and was paid $1.15 per day at a cost of 9 cents per ton to the company. Under Taylor's incentive plan, the legendary Schmidt increased his output to 45 tons when offered a raise to $1.85 per day, reducing the company's cost to 4 cents per ton. Unfortunately, the veracity of Taylor's accounts of his success with Schmidt and other workers has been questioned, particularly in regard to whether or not Taylor himself actually conducted these experiments and in regard to the fact that he told many different versions of the same stories (Lee, 1980).

Despite these questions about the foundations of his principles, the suggestions of Taylor and associates (such as Gantt, whose famous charts [see Chapter 8] are still used today) were the forerunners of many current business techniques such as inventory control, cost volume analysis, and other quantitative approaches.

A summary of the basic components of early scientific management includes:

1. Analysis and synthesis of the elements of operation.
2. Scientific selection of the worker.
3. Training of the worker.
4. Proper tools and equipment.
5. Proper incentive. (Kendall, 1914, p. 123).

Some characteristics a management science follower would look for in a first-line manager include:

1. Someone who knows the work that is being done in the department very well.
2. A good disciplinarian.
3. Able to get work through and out of the department quickly.
4. Cautious and accurate.
5. Able to keep track of innumerable details.

Human Relations (Mayo et al)

The human relations group called for a new mix of managerial skills: understanding human behavior, counseling, motivating, leading, and communicating with workers. The Hawthorne studies of Mayo and his associates may be the most famous set of research studies in leadership and management literature. In fact, people often use the term "Hawthorne Effect" to describe how other people's behavior improves when you give them some kind of extra attention. The studies themselves are summarized in Research Example 2–3 and help to clarify what the real "Hawthorne Effect" is.

Actually, these researchers started out to test some of the concepts of scientific management:

> It is interesting to note that the Hawthorne studies began with the idea that changing simple physical conditions such as the amount of lighting in the work area or the number of breaks during the day could directly affect the workers' output. They were particularly interested in the relationship of working conditions to the degree of fatigue and boredom experienced by the employees. But they soon found that changing physical conditions alone did not explain workers' responses and productivity. There were other important factors that had been previously neglected, especially the interpersonal aspects of the situation (Landsberger, 1958).

The employees' attitudes, hopes, fears, personal problems, sensitivity to differences in status within the plant, and ideas about fair treatment had a strong influence on their responses to management. This led to the concept that the employee should be viewed as a whole, not just a worker. (Critics have said this was not genuinely holistic because it only views the worker as a producing unit.) The employee's perception of a situation affects his or her response and should be considered, particularly when implementing change.

Another important aspect that had been previously neglected was the effect of informal groupings of workers. These are important because they provide employees with the support needed to resist unwelcome pressure from supervisors (to increase output or change routines, for example).

The function of the manager and supervisor, then, is to obtain the cooperation of the workers in working toward the goals of the organization. Recognizing their needs and concerns is necessary to gain their acceptance and cooperation. Some critics of the human relations approach point out that conflicts between administration and labor do exist and that simply being nice is not sufficient. They have called its proponents the "happiness boys." Manager effectiveness comes also from the ability to protect the workers from higher administration's imposition of unwelcome pressure and changes (Wren, 1972).

CONTEMPORARY LEADER-MANAGER THEORIES _____

Motivational Theories

The motivational theories expand upon the attention given to the co-actor element (staff member or follower) which began with the behavioral theories. People's needs and motivations become the central focus and the distinction between leader and manager begins to blur.

Motivational theorists and researchers have concentrated on identifying the factors that stimulate satisfaction and productivity and on eliminating those factors that inhibit them. The most effective leader or manager is the one who creates an environment in which people are highly motivated and, therefore, highly productive.

RESEARCH EXAMPLE 2–3. The Famous Hawthorne Studies

A series of evolving research studies was conducted over many years at the Hawthorne plant of the Western Electric Company, a division of American Telephone and Telegraph, by an interdisciplinary team including people from Harvard University and from Western Electric. (Landsberger, 1958; Lee, 1980: Roethlisberger & Dickson, 1939). The major studies were done between 1927 and 1932 but the whole series extends both before and after this time.

ILLUMINATION STUDIES. The preliminary studies, begun in 1924, attempted to determine the effects of increasing and decreasing the level of illumination in several departments. The experimental groups, who were given more lighting, did produce more than they had previously but, surprisingly, so did those whose lighting level was kept the same or even decreased (until it became extremely low).

THE RELAY ASSEMBLY TEST ROOM. In the next series, the researchers tried to better control the many variables that would affect the workers' output. To do this, they selected six women from the relay assembly room and placed them in a separate room where various factors thought to affect output could be tested. The various changes that they tried were as follows:

Phase I.   The weekly output of the women was measured for two weeks before they were transferred.
Phase II.   The women spent five weeks in the test room without any other changes.
Phase III.   A separate incentive system for these women was implemented (eight weeks).
Phase IV.   Two five-minute breaks were added.
Phase V.   The breaks were increased to ten minutes.
Phase VI.   Six shorter (five minute) breaks were allowed.
Phase VII.   Snacks were provided during the midmorning and midafternoon breaks.
Phase VIII.   The workday was shortened by a half hour.
Phase IX.   The work day was shortened by another half hour.
Phase X.   Same as Phase VII.
Phase XI.   Saturday work was eliminated.
Phase XII.   Returned to Phase I through III conditions for twelve weeks.
Phase XIII.   Returned to Phases VII and X.

The result was an *almost uninterrupted increase* in hourly and weekly productivity, especially when they entered Phase VII, even though some phases were repeated and the work day returned to its original length in Phase XII. The comments of the women seemed to indicate that they had become a "special" group envied by the other workers and pleased by the way in which they were treated and supervised, especially with being consulted about the changes being made.

SECOND RELAY ASSEMBLY TESTS. These women stayed in their departments but were put on a similar special incentive program. This single change also resulted in increased output but only a 13% increase compared with the 30% increase in the first series. Both rivalry with the first group and the jealousy of other assemblers may have affected these results.

THE MICA SPLITTING TESTS. This series was set up in the same fashion as the first Relay Assembly tests except these workers were already being paid for their individual output and were already working overtime. Each of the five longer phases in this series represented an improvement over previous phases. This group never developed a special identity and their output increased at first but actually declined in the fourth phase, perhaps due to the worsening employment conditions at the plant (these studies took place over the time of the 1929 Stock Market Crash and the ensuing Depression).

The researchers' conclusions were that the human factors which had been largely neglected before, especially workers' attitudes, were a very important influence on worker output. They did not suggest, as many have quoted them as saying, that the human relations factors were the only ones that influenced productivity.

Many of these theories are based on a humanistic approach and you will see the influence of Maslow's theory of motivation, especially self actualization, in them. The emphasis on small groups and teams changes to an emphasis on the organizations in which people work. McGregor's Theory X and Theory Y, two approaches that developed from Theory X and Y, and one using an opposing stimulus-response approach are discussed.

THEORIES X AND Y (MCGREGOR). In his 1960 book entitled *The Human Side of Enterprise,* McGregor compared two different sets of beliefs about human nature, describing how these led to two very different approaches to leadership and management. The first, more conventional, approach he called Theory X. The second, more humanistic, approach was termed Theory Y (Bennis & Schein, 1966).

Theory X is based on a common view of human nature: the ordinary person is lazy, unmotivated, unresponsible, and not too intelligent; most people do not really like to work. They do not care about meeting the team's or organization's goals and will work only as hard as they must to keep their jobs. Most avoid taking on any additional responsibility and prefer to be directed rather than to act independently. Without specific rules and the threat of punishment, most workers would come in late, goof off most of the day, and produce sloppy, careless work.

Based on this view, leaders must direct and control people in order to ensure that the work is done properly. Detailed rules and regulations need to be set and strictly enforced. People need to be told exactly what to do, and how to do it. Close supervision is necessary to catch mistakes and to make sure employees keep working and that rules (such as 30 minutes for lunch) are obeyed.

Motivation is supplied by a system of rewards and punishments. Those who do not obey the rules are reprimanded, fined, or fired. Those who do obey the rules are rewarded with time off, pay raises and continued employment.

According to Theory Y, the behavior described in Theory X is not inherent but a result of leadership that emphasizes control, direction, reward, and punishment. The passivity, lack of motivation, and avoidance of responsibility are symptoms of poor leadership and indicate that people's needs for belonging, recognition and self-actualization have not been met.

Drawing on Maslow's theory of motivation, Theory Y proposes that the work itself can be motivating and rewarding. People can become enthusiastic about their work and will support the team's and organization's goals when these goals also meet their needs. They can be trusted to put forth adequate effort and to complete their work without constant supervision if they are committed to these goals. Under the right conditions, the ordinary person can be imaginative, creative, and productive.

Given the Theory Y beliefs, the major function of the leader-manager would be to provide such opportunities and an environment in which needs can be met at work. Theory Y leaders remove obstacles, provide guidance, and encourage growth. The extensive external controls of Theory X are not necessary because people can exert self-control and self-direction under Theory Y leadership.

HYGIENE AND MOTIVATION FACTORS (HERZBERG). Herzberg enlarged on Theory Y by dividing the needs that affect a person's motivation to work into two sets of factors that affect dissatisfaction and satisfaction (Herzberg, 1959, 1966; House & Wigdor, 1967). The first set, called *hygiene factors*, meet a person's need to avoid pain, insecurity, and discomfort. If not met, the employee is dissatisfied. The second set, called *motivation factors*, meet needs to grow psychologically. When met, the employee feels satisfied. These sets are distinct and independent sets of factors, according to Herzberg. Meeting hygiene needs will not increase satisfaction and meeting motivation needs will not reduce dissatisfaction.

These two sets of factors were derived from yet another set of research studies. Employees such as engineers and accountants were asked to describe incidents at work that made them feel especially good or especially bad. The lists of influential hygiene and motivation factors were derived from their descriptions of these critical incidents.

The hygiene factors include:

1. Adequate salary
2. Appropriate supervision
3. Good interpersonal relationships
4. Safe and tolerable working conditions (including reasonable policies and procedures).

The motivation factors include:

1. Satisfying, meaningful work
2. Opportunities for advancement and achievement
3. Appropriate responsibility
4. Adequate recognition.

The leader-manager's function is to ensure that both sets of needs are met, some directly and others by providing opportunities for them to be met in a conducive work environment.

THEORY Z (OUCHI).   Ouchi more recently (1981) expanded and enlarged upon Theory Y and the democratic approach to leadership to create what he calls Theory Z. Like Theory Y, Theory Z has a humanistic viewpoint and focuses on developing better ways to motivate people, assuming that this will lead to increased satisfaction and productivity.

Theory Z was developed in part from a study of the most successful and best managed Japanese organizations. It was adapted to the American culture, which is different in some ways but similar in its productivity goals and advanced technology. A number of American organizations that are known for being well-managed, good places to work use elements of Theory Z. These are collective decision making, long term employment, slower promotions, indirect supervision, and a holistic concern for employees.

Collective Decision Making.   A democratic, participative mode of decision making is an essential element of Theory Z. This participation is extensive, involving every one who is affected by a decision. For example, if a decision to provide a new service would affect 70 people in an agency, a small team would be assigned to talk with *each one* of these 70 people to reach a true consensus about offering the new service. If a major change in the plan is made at some point, the team would go back and speak with everyone again. This is a slow way to get things done.

Everyday problems are also dealt with in a participative manner through problem solving groups called quality circles in which all members of a team or department are encouraged to identify and resolve problems faced by the group or organization. The emphasis is on keeping everyone fully informed, encouraging active participation, and gaining their commitment to the final decision rather than on the speed or efficiency with which a decision can be made. Some critics think that Theory Z is faddish; others believe that it slows decision making and stifles innovation (Strader, 1987).

Long Term Employment. Movement *within* the organization rather than *between* organizations is encouraged. Many Japanese workers have been employed by only one organization for their entire career—quite different from the job switching done by many Americans.

There are some Theory Z organizations in the United States in which long term employment is the norm. Employees move around within the organization, taking on different functions and working in different departments. The advantage is that they are better able to understand how other departments work, and what their problems and capabilities are. This results in better communication and coordination between departments and an integration of separate units impossible to achieve otherwise. Many employees also become less specialized but more valuable to the Z organization which is consequently more willing to invest in training its employees and encouraging their growth. Fair treatment also becomes more important when the organization needs to cultivate the commitment and loyalty of this long term employee.

Slower Promotions. Slower promotions may seem to be a disadvantage but there are long term benefits. Rapid promotions can be illusory: if everyone is promoted rapidly, your relative position in the organization does not really change. It also means that close working relationships within groups do not have time to develop, nor is there any incentive to develop them. Slower promotions allow time to thoroughly evaluate the individual's long term contribution to the organization, and discourage the kind of game playing that occurs when people try to make themselves look good by undermining others.

Indirect Supervision. Supervision of employees is subtle and indirect rather than direct. Workers become a part of the culture of the organization and are intimately familiar with its working philosophy, values, and goals. In fact, the goals belong to the workers because they are involved in setting them. Decisions are made partly on the basis of what fits the culture of the organization. A person who is well acquainted with the organization does not need to be told what to do as often as a new, unassimilated employee does.

A similar source of indirect supervision is the influence of the groups in which the employee works. Employees' desire for peer approval motivates group members and supports productive behavior in Theory Z organizations.

Holistic Concern. Trust, fair treatment, commitment, and loyalty are all characteristics of the Theory Z organization. These characteristics are part of the overall consideration for each employee as a whole, including concern for the employee's health and well-being, as well as his or her performance as a worker.

BEHAVIORAL MANAGEMENT (MILLER). Although a number of organizations have successfully adapted the humanistic Theory Y and Theory Z, there are many more people who believe that these approaches are soft-hearted and unproven. Miller's (1978) behavioral management approach is an example of this opposing viewpoint.

Behavioral management is based upon the stimulus-response explanation of human behavior and uses rewards to influence and control employee behavior. For example, if an employee took too long to complete daily reports, the behavioral management approach to this problem would be to remove any distractions, set goals for gradual reduction of the time taken to write one report, and reinforce improvement by giving rewards such as intermittent praise, salary increases, free lunches, and gift items.

Proponents of this approach believe that it is more suitable in a work setting than are the humanistic approaches. The following are some reasons:

1. Maslow's hierarchy of needs simply means that people are motivated to get what they do not have.
2. Theory Y approaches demand too much of the manager whose main function is to meet production goals, not to satisfy human needs.
3. An employer should be interested only in the employee's work performance. Interest in any other aspect of the employee's life is an invasion of privacy and abuse of power. (Drucker, 1973 in Miller, 1978).
4. There is little evidence that training to improve self-awareness or sensitivity to others actually improves leader effectiveness.
5. Many organizations using Theory X have prospered, so McGregor's analysis of its deficiencies was wrong.

The studies done by Hall and Donell (1980) in Research Example 2–4 provide an interesting response to these criticisms.

It is possible that both approaches to motivation are significant and that their effects are additive rather than opposite (Mitchell, 1982). One approach may work better in some situations and the other approach in different situations, a concept that is the essence of the situational theories that are discussed in the next section.

Situational Theories

The motivational theories were a significant advance over the earlier theories because they include consideration of group or staff members (the co-actors) as well as the leader. However, the third element, the environment, is barely acknowledged. Leadership and management do not occur in a vacuum. We need to consider the context in which they take place (McElroy, 1986).

Recognition of the importance of this missing element has led to several leader-manager theories called situational theories. The contingency and path-goal theories are discussed separately, and other aspects of the environment that have been found to have a considerable influence upon employees are listed.

CONTINGENCY THEORY (FIEDLER). Participative leadership is not necessarily effective in every situation according to situational theorists. Fiedler (1974), for example, found that factors such as the nature of the task to be done, the power of the leader, and the favorableness of the situation

RESEARCH EXAMPLE 2–4. Which Approach Do Successful Managers Use?

Do successful managers actually use the humanistic theories in their work? A series of five studies known as the Achieving Manager Research Project was done by Hall and Donnell (1982) comparing a manager's personal success and use of the humanistic behavioral and motivational theories of leadership and management. Altogether, 12,000 male managers in more than 50 organizations ranging from drug companies to government and nonprofit agencies were studied. Managers were divided into low, average, and high achieving groups on the basis of their rate of progress toward the top ranks of the organization.

Study I compared the managers' success with their belief in McGregor's Theory X or Theory Y. Hall and Donnell found a significant ($p < 0.03$) negative relationship between belief in Theory X and managerial achievement: low and average achievers had a much stronger belief in Theory X than did the high achievers.

Study II compared the managers' preferred work incentives, that is, primary motivating factors derived from Maslow, Herzberg, and others, with their success. Low achievers were found to stress the hygiene and maintenance factors, especially safety and security, and virtually ignored the motivation factors of actualization, belonging, or ego status. These factors were emphasized by the high achievers. This emphasis on hygiene factors accounted for 77 percent of the variance between the low achievers and the others. Low achievers were also found to be more self-centered while high achievers were more other-centered.

Study III focused on the use of the participative management approach. The degree to which managers used the participative style was measured by administering a questionnaire to people who worked for them (not by asking the managers themselves). The difference in use of participative management was dramatic: as a group, the high achievers scored five times higher in participative management than did the low achievers. The average achieving group was not much higher than the low group. Managers with low and average success offered their workers few opportunities to participate and used practices that repressed and frustrated the people in their groups. High achievers used the participative style to a much greater extent with accompanying higher levels of satisfaction in their groups.

Study IV measured the extent to which the managers disclosed or shared personal, intellectual and emotional data about themselves and encouraged others to do the same—called interpersonal competence by the researchers. Subordinates, peers, supervisors, and the managers themselves were asked to rate these behaviors. Both self-rating and subordinates' ratings indicated that the high achieving managers were significantly ($p < 0.001$) higher in interpersonal competence measured as disclosure.

Study V measured the task and relationship orientations of the managers. Eighteen hundred seventy-eight managers and their subordinates were given a management style inventory to determine the manager's position on the Blake and Mouton managerial grid. High achievers were found to use a collaborative, participative, high task, high relationship style. Average achievers tended to emphasize task over relationship and low achievers showed a preference for a low risk, defensive style. The managers' styles seemed to be an overall summary of the individual leader's beliefs, attitudes, and practices.

The studies indicate that successful managers apply humanistic theories to their practice. The researchers concluded that, when taken together, the results of the five studies suggest that the use of the humanistic behavioral and motivational approaches to leadership has implications for career growth. They also hypothesize that, although the data cannot be generalized to women, the same leadership practices would distinguish female high and low achievers in management positions.

help to determine the type of leadership that works best. The effectiveness of a certain style of leadership is *contingent* on these other factors.

Fiedler's contingency theory is less straightforward than most discussed so far. The leader's style is reflected in the rating that the leader gives to the least preferred coworker (LPC). On the basis of this rating, leaders are categorized as either high or low LPC. It is not clear exactly what this LPC rating measures. It may be measuring the leader's tolerance for incompetent workers or differences in types of least preferred coworkers. Usually, the high LPC leader is considered predominantly relationship oriented and the low LPC leader is considered primarily task oriented.

On the basis of extensive research since the 1950s, the low LPC leader has been found to be most effective in both very favorable situations, when the leader has a great deal of power and an excellent relationship with group members, and in very unfavorable situations in which the leader has very little power and poor relationships. The low LPC leader is also more effective when the tasks are clear and structured.

The high LPC leader is most effective in moderately favorable situations when the leader's power and authority are weak, the task is not clearly defined, and relationships are good. Fiedler's research indicates that the most effective leaders can adapt their styles to the needs of a particular situation.

PATH-GOAL THEORY (HOUSE).   A different set of situational factors is considered in the path-goal theory developed in the 1970's by House (1971) from earlier work done by Georgopoulas and Vroom. These factors include the scope of the task to be done, role ambiguity, the employee's expectations and perceptions of the task, and ways in which the leader can influence these expectations.

The motivation to perform a certain task is based on a person's expectation that doing this work will result in a desired outcome and that personal satisfaction or reward will be achieved as a result of this outcome. In other words, people estimate their ability to carry out the task, any obstacles in doing the job, and the amount of support they can expect. They also estimate what kind of reward (such as recognition from the group or leader or a sense of satisfaction) they can get from completing the task.

The leader who can recognize and anticipate these expectations can take such actions as providing support, removing obstacles to completing the task, and pointing out the connection between doing the work and receiving the rewards. The name of this theory comes from this last action: the leader clarifies the relationship between the path the employees take and the goal they want to reach.

House found that when a person has a wide variety of tasks to perform, leader consideration is not as great an influence on satisfaction because the work itself is satisfying. However, he also found that all employees need recognition and other forms of consideration from their leaders. The characteristics of the employees and the number of environmental demands they have to deal with to complete their work also affect the kinds of leadership needed to increase motivation.

SITUATIONAL DETERMINANTS.   Both the contingency and path-goal theories indicated that the characteristics of the tasks to be done are an important situational determinant (as did the early work of Frederick Taylor) but did not agree on what the other situational determinants are. There are many other determinants that have been identified in leadership and management research (Stogdill, 1974; Fiedler in Hunt & Larson, 1979; Ford, 1981; Oldham & Hackman, 1981). The following are a sampling of these determinants:

Group Size.   Large groups need more coordination than small groups. Some research also indicates that large groups need leaders who are more task oriented than do small groups.

Position in Group.   Studies of space and territoriality indicate that the leader tends to occupy the head position at a table and that this position reinforces the leader's status. Group members tend to sit opposite the leader rather than next to the leader.

Communication Networks.   A central position for controlling the sending and receiving of information increases the probability of that person emerging as the leader of the group.

Social Status.   People with higher social status usually have more influence on group decisions. (The effect of status may be related to ability and experience.)

Interpersonal Stress.   The existence of stress and tension between an employee and supervisor reduces the employee's ability to think and problem solve creatively. The stress of having a difficult job to do does not seem to affect thinking in the same way.

Designation of Leadership.   Formal designation of a person as a leader by someone in authority outside the group reinforces that person's position as leader of the group.

Organizational Structure.   Organizational structure can affect employees' satisfaction by affecting the characteristics of their jobs. The more formal, hierarchical organization tends to allow less autonomy, identity, feedback, and variety in jobs. In organizations with less emphasis on hierarchy, employees tend to feel more self-confident, more receptive to change, more committed to their work and less powerless. Organizational structure also affects leader behavior. For example, the amount of leader consideration has been found to be negatively related to the size of the organization.

Interactional Theories

Although situational theories contribute some needed complexity, they have a tendency to treat the situation as if it were separate from the leader. Each one also identifies different situational determinants. No theory has yet managed to pull together all the influential factors from each of the four elements of a leader-manager situation (the leader-manager, co-actors, the work, and the environment) into one coherent, integrated theory of leadership and management.

Many earlier theorists were aware of the need to consider other variables but ignored them when proposing their approaches. Theory Z, for example, is more comprehensive than some of the earlier theories and yet it neglects some apparently influential situational factors such as the nature of the work to be done. It also assumes that all group members will respond positively to the same approach.

Some theories have moved in the direction of clarifying and predicting the interaction between the elements of a leader-manager situation. Four examples are (1) complex man and open systems, (2) elements of a leader situation, (3) leader-group interaction, and (4) the work-unit culture and the leader-manager.

COMPLEX MAN AND OPEN SYSTEMS (SCHEIN). After reviewing other viewpoints on human nature, Schein (1970; and in Deaux & Wrightsman, 1983) concluded that they were all overgeneralized and oversimplified. In their place, he proposed a model of complex man based on the following assumptions:

1. People are complex and highly variable. They have multiple motives for doing things, which vary from one person to another. For example, a pay raise can mean security to one person, recognition to another, and both to a third person.
2. People can develop new motives and their motives can change over time.
3. Goals can differ in different situations. For example, in a formal group the goal may be to get the work done. In an informal group the goal may be to socialize, and whether the work gets done or not is not important to its members.
4. The nature of the task affects people's performance and productivity. Ability, experience and motivation also affect productivity.
5. Different leadership actions are needed in different situations. No single strategy will be effective in every situation.

Schein's assumptions synthesize elements of the theories reviewed so far. Use of an open systems framework is implied in these assumptions. Needs, motives, abilities, the nature of the task, the work setting, the type of group, the organizational structure, and the person's past experience and patterns of relating to others all affect the leadership situation. The leader must be able to diagnose the situation and select the appropriate strategy from a large repertoire of skills in order to be effective.

ELEMENTS OF A LEADER SITUATION (HOLLANDER). Hollander (1978) identified three basic elements in a leadership exchange as:

1. The leader, including the leader's personality, perceptions, and abilities.
2. The followers, with their personalities, perceptions, and abilities.
3. The situation within which the leader and followers function, including its norms, size, density, and other characteristics.

Leadership is a dynamic, two-way process of influence. Leader and follower are interdependent. This model also recognizes that both the leader and followers have other roles outside the leadership situation and that they may both be influenced by environmental factors.

According to Hollander, leadership effectiveness requires the use of the problem solving process, maintenance of group cohesiveness, communication skills, leader fairness, competence, dependability, creativity, and identification with the group.

LEADER-GROUP INTERACTION (SCHREISHEIM, MOWDAY & STOGDILL). The leader is not solely responsible for the outcome of an exchange with co-actors (Gemmill, 1986). More attention should be paid to the interdependence between the leader and the group, according to Schreisheim, Mowday and Stogdill (1977). Many interrelated factors influence this relationship. Group cohesiveness, for example, is affected not only by leader behavior but also by group size, stress, relationships between group members, the nature of the task, and external pressures. Leader behaviors are dynamically interrelated with the group behavior, cohesiveness, and motivation. The productivity of the group, then, is not due to the leader alone.

In this model, both task-oriented and relationship-oriented leader behaviors are positively related to group motivation and cohesiveness. In turn, group motivation and cohesiveness (as well as the nature of the task and the group's goal) affect productivity and satisfaction, turnover and absenteeism. The relationships in this model are complex, yet many others could have been added to it.

THE WORK-UNIT CULTURE (LASHBROOK). The context in which the interaction between the manager and staff take place is the central focus of Lashbrook's (1986) conceptualization of the work-unit culture. The interaction between the manager and staff members can lead to a positive, productive work environment or to a negative, unproductive environment. Lashbrook distinguishes between the effect of the organization as a whole and the effect of the smaller work unit influenced by the manager. The objective is to create a positive work-unit culture by attending to five areas: mission, goals, feedback, rewards, and support.

Mission. People need to feel important. Both the manager and staff need a clear idea of the mission or overall purpose of the group and the organization within which it functions. A sense of mission goes beyond the everyday routine to look at the ultimate purpose for doing the work. It gives meaning to the work that people are doing. Creating this sense of mission should not be difficult in a health care system in which most jobs contribute either directly or indirectly to preventing illness, saving lives, or easing distress. Building a sense of purpose answers the employee's question, "Why am I here?"

Goals. People need to feel that they make a specific contribution to the work being done. Goals are more specific than the overall purpose. They provide the reason for everyday work, clarify the manager's expectations, and define the outcomes. Working together on a set of clearly defined goals can be a powerfully unifying force for the group. Clearly defining the goals answers the question, "Where am I going?"

Feedback. People need to know how well they are doing. The manager is responsible for providing this information to members of the group but it may come from coworkers or the employee as well. The feedback should be relevant, accurate, consistent, and constructive. Providing feedback answers the question, "How am I doing?"

Rewards. Rewards provide reinforcement for positive behavior and should be clearly connected to those behaviors. The manager needs to carefully consider what rewards he or she can give to a staff member: a smile, a word of praise, a positive evaluation, or a raise in pay. High performing staff members need as much reinforcement as do low performers. It is important that rewards be given in such a way that they reinforce a positive work-unit culture. Giving rewards answers the question. "What's in it for me?"

Support. In a positive work-unit culture, people feel free to seek help on a regular basis and should be willing to offer constructive support to each other. Lashbrook describes two particularly *unhelpful* ways to respond to a request for help:

Here's how I used to do it.

Let me do it for you. (p. 130)

Both of these are potential threats to the autonomy and self-confidence of the individual employee. In contrast, providing assistance and information that increases the employee's knowledge and skill is far more constructive and helpful in the long run. Giving this type of support contributes to a positive work-unit culture and answers the question, "What happens if I need help?"

The work-unit culture model recognizes the influence of external factors such as an employee's personal problems or the limitations of the organization's resources but does not suggest ways in which to deal with these important factors in the environment. It does, however, provide a helpful definition of the leader-manager's role (and limitations) in increasing the productivity of employees.

DISCUSSION. These interactional approaches have some common themes. They all recognize the multiplicity of factors affecting a leadership situation and attempt, to differing degrees, to synthesize the findings of the preceding theories. Either implicitly or explicitly, they point to the need to consider the leader, co-actors, work, and environment and the reciprocal interactions among them when analyzing a leadership situation. Indirectly, they all indicate the usefulness of an open systems perspective in accounting for all of the factors that influence a leadership situation, the effectiveness of the leader-manager and the productivity of the staff members. However, a common set of assumptions about human nature and how people work best or a complete model that can explain and predict what happens in a leadership-management situation has not yet been developed.

SUMMARY

A number of important theories and models have been developed over time to describe and predict what makes a person an effective leader-manager. The discussion began with the earlier, simpler theories and progressed to more complex interactional models and theories.

Innate capacity for leadership is the focus of the trait theories. According to the Great Man theory, important figures who influenced the course of history had innate characteristics that distinguished them from ordinary people. Popular versions of the trait theory see such characteristics as size, courage, intelligence, or dominance as indicators that a person will be an effective leader. Research also shows that traits such as intelligence and initiative are associated with leadership but that the trait theories are too limited to determine effective leadership alone.

Behavioral theories focus on the behavior or functions of the leader. The authoritarian leader is highly controlling and directive in comparison with the democratic leader who encourages participation in goal setting and planning. The laissez-faire leader is passive and nondirective.

Early management theories took two different paths. The first, characterized by the work of Taylor, emphasized the importance of analyzing the details of a particular task in order to determine how to increase speed and efficiency. He also sought to identify incentives (such as money or rest breaks) that would get more work out of the individual employee. The second path, characterized by the work of Mayo and associates, focused primarily on understanding human behavior and improving communication as a way to increase worker satisfaction and productivity.

There are also two kinds of motivational theories: those that take a humanistic view and those that oppose it, claiming that people will avoid additional work or responsibility if possible and need close supervision and control. McGregor called this opposing view Theory X and proposed a more humanistic Theory Y based on the implementation of Maslow's hierarchy of needs. Herzberg expanded this concept into two independent sets of influential factors, the hygiene and motivational factors. Theory Z extended this further, calling for collective decision making, long term employment, slower promotions, indirect supervision, and holistic concern for people in well-managed organizations.

A major element of a leadership-management situation, the environment, was missing from the preceding theories. A large number of situational determinants have been identified. The contingency theory identified the leader's power, relationship with the group, and clarity of the task as determinants of the most effective leadership style. The path-goal theory also identified the scope of the task, the individual's expectations about the difficulties of completing the task, and resulting rewards as determinants of motivation. Other factors affecting leader effectiveness directly or indirectly include group size, leader status and position in the group, position in the communication network, social status, interpersonal stress, formal designation as leader and organizational structure.

None of the preceding theories could account for all of the factors involved in the complex and dynamic interactions of a leader-manager situation. The complexity and variability of people and of the work that they do, the use of an open systems framework, inclusion of all four elements of a leader-manager situation, and the interrelationships between these elements were all suggested as the basis for a more complete and integrated interactional theory of effective leadership and management.

REFERENCES*

Blake, R.R. & Mouton, J.S. (1964). *The managerial grid.* Houston: Gulf Publishing.

Blake, R.R., Mouton, J.S., & Tapper, M. (1981). *Grid approaches for managerial leadership in nursing.* St. Louis: C.V. Mosby.

Bennis, W.G. & Schein, E.H. (with the collaboration of C. McGregor). (1966). *Leadership and motivation: Essays of Douglas McGregor.* Cambridge, Mass: MIT Press.

Deaux, K. & Wrightsman, L.C. (1983). *Social Psychology in the Eighties.* Monterey, Calif: Brooks/Cole.

Drucker, P. (1973). Management: Tasks, responsibilities and practices. In Miller, L.M. *Behavior management: The new science of managing people at work.* New York: Harper & Row, p. 424.

Duxbury, M.C., Armstrong, G.D., Drew, D.J. & Henley, S.J. (1984). Head nurse leadership style with staff

nurse burnout and job satisfaction in neonatal intensive care units. *Nursing Research, 33,* (2), 97–101.

Fiedler, F.E. (1979). Organizational determinants of managerial incompetence. In Hunt, J.G. & Larson, L.L. (eds). *Crosscurrents in leadership.* Carbondale: Southern Illinois University Press.

Fiedler, F.E. & Chemers, M.M. (1974). *Leadership and effective management.* Glenview, Ill.: Scott, Foresman.

Ford, J. (1981). Departmental context and formal structure as constraints on leader behavior. *Academy of Management Journal. 24,* (4), 274.

Gemmill, G. (1986). The mythology of the leader role in small groups. *Small Group Behavior, 17,* (1), 41–50.

Hall, J. & Donnell, S.M. (1980). *Managerial achievement: The personal side of behavior theory.* In Katz,

D., Kahn, R.L. & Adams, J.S. (eds.) *The study of organizations.* San Francisco: Jossey-Bass.

Heimann, C.G. (1976). Four theories of leadership. *Journal of Nursing Administration.* 6, (6), 18.

Herzberg, F. (1966). *Work and the nature of man.* Cleveland: World Publishing.

Herzberg, F., Mausner, B. & Snyderman, B. (1959). *The motivation to work.* (2nd ed.). New York: John Wiley.

*Hollander, E.P. (1978). *Leadership dynamics: A practical guide to effective relationships.* New York: The Free Press.

House, R.J. (1971). A path goal theory of leader effectiveness. *Administrative Science Quarterly.* 16 (3) 321.

House, R.J. & Wigdor, L.A. (1967). Herzberg's dual-factor theory of job satisfaction and motivation: A review of the evidence and a criticism. *Personnel Psychology.* 20 (4), 369.

Kendall, H.P. (1914). *Unsystematized, systematized, and scientific management.* In Thompson, C.B. *Scientific Management: A collection of the more significant articles describing the Taylor system of management.* Cambridge: Harvard University Press.

Landsberger, H.A. (1958). *Hawthorne revisited: Management and the worker, its critics and developments in human relations in industry.* Ithaca, New York: Cornell University Press.

Lashbrook, L.B. (1986). *Management as a performance system.* In Williamson, J.N. *The leader-manager.* New York: John Wiley.

*Lee, J.A. (1980). *The gold and the garbage in management theories and prescriptions.* Athens, Ohio: Ohio University Press.

Locke, E.A. (1982). The ideas of Frederick W. Taylor: An evaluation. *Academy of Management Review.* 7 (1), 14.

Maloney, M.M. (1979). *Leadership in nursing: Theory, strategies, action.* St. Louis: C.V. Mosby.

McElroy, J.C. (1986). Attribution theories of leadership and network analysis. *Journal of Management,* 12, 351–362.

McFarland, D.E. (1986). *The managerial imperative: The age of macromanagement.* Cambridge, Mass.: Ballinger.

*McGregor, D. (1960). *The human side of enterprise.* New York: McGraw-Hill.

*Miller, L.M. (1978). *Behavior management: The new science of managing people at work.* New York: John Wiley.

Mitchell, T.R. (1982). Motivation: New directions for theory, research and practice. *Academy of Management Review.* 7 (1), 80.

Oldham, G.R. & Hackman, J.R. (1981). Relationships between organizational structure and employee reaction: Comparing alternative frameworks *Administrative Science Quarterly.* 26 (1), 66.

*Ouchi, W.G. (1981). *Theory Z: How American business can meet the Japanese challenge.* Reading, Mass: Addison-Wesley.

Peterson, P.B. (1986). Correspondence from Henry L. Gantt to an old friend reveals new information about Gantt. *Journal of Management,* 12, (3), 339–350.

Roethlisberger, F.J. & Dickson, W.J. (1939). *Management and the worker.* From Landsberger, H.A. (1958) *Hawthorne revisited: Management and the worker: its critics and developments in human relations in industry.*

Schein, E.H. (1970). *Organizational psychology.* (2nd ed.) Englewood Cliffs: Prentice-Hall.

Schreisheim, C.A., Mowday, R.T. & Stogdill, R.M. (1977). Crucial dimensions of leader-group interaction. In Hunt, J.G. & Larson, L.L. (eds). *Crosscurrents in leadership.* Carbondale, Ill.: Southern Illinois University Press.

Strader, M.K. (1987). Adapting Theory Z to nursing management. *Nursing Management,* 18, (4), 61–64.

Stogdill, R.M. (1974). *Handbook of leadership: A survey of theory and research.* New York: The Free Press.

Stogdill, R.M. & Coons, A.E. (eds) (1957). *Leader behavior: Its description and measurement. Research monograph 88.* Columbus, Ohio: The Ohio State University, College of Administrative Science.

Thompson, C.B. (1914). *Scientific management: A collection of the more significant articles describing the Taylor system of management.* Ithaca, New York: Cornell University Press.

White, R.K. & Lippitt, R. (1960). *Autocracy and democracy: An experimental inquiry.* New York: Harper and Row. (Published after Lewin's death).

*Williamson, J.N. (1986). *The leader-manager.* New York: John Wiley.

Woods, F.A. (1913). *The influence of monarchs.* New York: Macmillan.

*Wren, D.A. (1972). *The evolution of management thought.* New York: Ronald Press.

*References marked with an asterisk are recommended for further reading.

Chapter 3 ███████████

OUTLINE

Effective Leadership

Goals
Goal Levels
Congruent, Meaningful Goals
Clear Goals

Knowledge and Skills
Leadership Knowledge
Leadership Skills
Nursing Knowledge and Skills
Critical Thinking

Self Awareness
Openness to Self
Importance of Self Awareness
Increasing Self Awareness
Stages of Self Awareness

Communication
Active Listening
Encouraging a Flow of Information

Directness and Assertiveness
Checking Perceptions
Providing Feedback
Linking
Networking

Energy
Neural and Emotional Energy
Energy and Leadership Effectiveness
Energy Flow and Reserves
An Energy Inventory

Action
Initiating Action
Working with Others
Critical Thinking and Problem Solving
Professional Activities
Deciding to Act

The Leadership Effectiveness Checklist

Summary

LEARNING OBJECTIVES

Upon completion of this chapter, the reader will be able to:

▷ Name and describe the components of effective leadership.

▷ Assess the degree of congruence between goal levels within a group.

▷ Discuss the purpose of a variety of constructive leader actions.

▷ Evaluate his or her own leadership effectiveness in terms of the components of effective leadership.

THE COMPONENTS OF EFFECTIVE LEADERSHIP

Many related concepts have been pulled together here into two simple conceptual frameworks for leadership (Chapter 3) and management (Chapter 4). These include the most essential elements of leadership and management in professional practice and represent a synthesis of philosophy, theory, research, and experience in leadership and management.

What makes a person an effective leader? The answer is found in the components of effective leadership: goals, knowledge and skill, self awareness, communication, energy, and action (Fig. 3–1).

Each of these components is described and explained in this chapter. Together they summarize the most fundamental concepts of leadership. The details are discussed in later chapters.

EFFECTIVE LEADERSHIP

An effective leader is one who is successful in attempts to influence others to work together in a productive and satisfying manner. Occasional failures are inevitable but an effective leader selects the best possible means for influencing others in order to improve the likelihood of success well beyond what would happen by chance.

Before discussing the components in detail, an outline of the components of effective leadership is provided. An effective leader:

1. Sets *goals* that are clear, congruent, and meaningful to the group.
2. Has adequate *knowledge and skill* in leadership and in his or her professional field.
3. Possesses *self awareness* and uses this understanding to recognize both personal needs and the needs of other people.
4. *Communicates* clearly and effectively.
5. Mobilizes adequate *energy* for leadership activities.
6. Takes *action.*

Each of the six components of the framework—goals, knowledge and skill, self awareness, communication, energy, and action—contributes to the effectiveness of a leader.

The components can also be used to test yourself against the ideal of an effective leader. You can ask yourself to what extent you have developed your leadership potential in regard to each of these components.

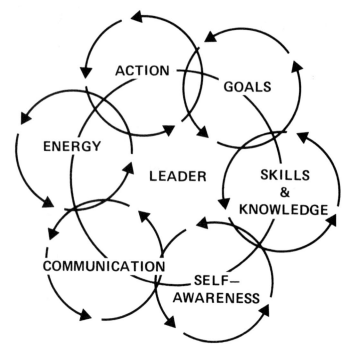

Figure 3–1. Components of effective leadership.

GOALS

All acts of leadership have a goal or objective. The goal is the end result desired, the reason for a particular behavior. Just as all human behavior is believed to have some meaning, it is also assumed that every attempt to influence others has some purpose or intention (Bennis & Nanus, 1985).

Goal Levels

It is unusual to find an individual who has a single goal in mind. It is even rarer to find a group with a single, clearly stated goal with which everyone agrees.

There are three levels of goals that a leader needs to be aware of: the individual level, the group level, and the environmental level, which includes the organization's goals (Tannenbaum, Weschler & Massarik, 1974). Figure 3–2 illustrates these different goal levels.

The individual goals, also called personal goals, are those of one particular person. There are usually several reasons why a person does or does not want something done. The following is an example:

You have invited several other nurses to a conference about a patient whose depression seems to be increasing. Your primary goal is to come up with new ways to intervene with this patient.

GOAL LEVELS	EXAMPLES
Environmental Goals	Organization Wants to Please Accrediting Agency
Group Goals	Have A Coffee Break
Individual Goals	
Personal Goals of Members	Contribute
	Show Conferences Are a Waste of Time
Personal Goals of Leader	Help Patient
	Demonstrate Leadership Ability

Figure 3–2. Levels of goals within a group.

> There are probably other reasons why you are organizing this conference. You may also be hoping to interest the other nurses in holding regular conferences about patients and to show them how well you can lead one of these conferences.

All of the goals described in this example would be your individual goals as leader of the group.

Every person in a group will also have individual goals. Some of these may be quite different and even conflict with your personal goals. For example:

> Some of the nurses invited to the conference want to contribute, but others believe that they have more important work to do and therefore want to hurry through the conference. Some do not want to come at all. One group member, for example, believes that conferences are a waste of time and has the goal of seeing to it that your conference turns out exactly the way this nurse predicted—a complete waste of time.

The goals mentioned in these examples are only a few of the many possible individual goals that members of the group could have.

The next level of goals involves the group as a whole. As you may recall from Chapter 1, the characteristics of the group as a whole, including its goals, are different from those of its individual members.

> When you get the group together for the conference at 10 a.m. it is time for a coffee break. The group, as a whole, is more interested in relaxing and in idle conversation than in discussing the depressed patient.

If it is true that the group prefers a break to a serious discussion, then the goal for the group as a whole conflicts with your goal as the group leader.

There is one more level of goals that needs to be considered, the environmental level. The environment is defined in terms of your particular situation. The most influential part of the environment may be the climate of a particular department or team, the economic health of the organization, or the attitude of the entire community. Referring back to the conference example:

> In this particular case, the environmental setting of concern to you is the organization within which you and the rest of the group work. Your employing organization may be antici-

pating the visit of a national accrediting agency and so be very interested in demonstrating that patient conferences are encouraged.

This example shows that the environmental level may reach as far as the national or even international level.

Goals within and between the different levels can be numerous, different, and conflicting. It is important that the leader recognize this and try to identify the varying goals at the three different levels.

Congruent, Meaningful Goals

In order for your leadership actions to be most effective, the goals at the different levels need to be congruent and meaningful to the group. This means that there should be sufficient agreement about goals so that the entire group, including the leader, can move in the same direction. Looking back at Figure 3–2, you can see that the leader's personal goals and the organizational goals both favor the idea of a conference although the goals themselves are not identical. The group goal and the goals of some individual members, however, are in serious conflict with the leader's goals. If the leader cannot change this situation, the conference will not succeed.

You will be a more effective leader if the group sees you as someone who identifies with them and has their best interests in mind (Hollander, 1974). For example, if the group senses that your main interest in holding a conference is your own personal goal of demonstrating your leadership ability rather than the group goal of helping the patient, their response to the conference is likely to be resistant and resentful. A leader who can identify with the group will be a more effective leader of that group. Another way of saying this is that the leader must "begin where the group is," just as in the helping relationship you begin where your client is and work from there.

How do you increase goal congruence? Suppose you do not agree with the group's goals, or you believe that their goals are unrealistic?

When the problem is a lack of information or understanding, supplying the correct information may be sufficient to change the group's goals. When there is a difference of opinion, remember that you can be accepting of people without accepting their beliefs or opinions. You can also show an interest in another point of view without agreeing with it. Your interest and acceptance will encourage open discussion that leads to finding some area of agreement with which the group may be willing to begin.

How willing you are to compromise your goals is going to depend on you, the gravity of the situation, and the kind of compromise you would need to make. If compromising your goals is going to mean violating your own personal set of values, then you must ask yourself what you will gain by doing it. While showing some flexibility is usually productive, yielding too much is ineffective.

When the actions mentioned (supplying information, expressing an interest in the other point of view, seeking a common ground among diverse goals, and occasionally making some compromises) do not reduce the differences enough, you will need to apply change strategies (Chapter 19) to bring them into congruence. Without congruent goals, group members will work at cross-purposes and are not likely to accomplish anything. But when the goals are congruent, you and your group have a starting point from which you can proceed to work together.

Clear Goals

You cannot be sure that the goals are congruent until they have been clearly stated. People often assume that everyone agrees without really checking out the validity of their assumption. For example, you often hear a comment such as "Everyone knows why we're here, let's get on with the job", at the beginning of a meeting (Beal, Bohlen & Raudabaugh, 1962, p. 130). Talking about a group's goals seems like a waste of time to many; however, people may have not only their own personal goals but also individual goals and very different perceptions of what the group's goals are.

Group members can honestly believe that they share a common goal and yet actually have diverse goals. The following is an example:

> A group called the "Committee to Improve Patient Care" might seem to have an obvious and self-explanatory goal. However, one member, a physician, thinks the committee's goal is to increase the hospital's medical staff. The Administrator expects the committee to endorse the building program that the Administrator proposed. The third member, the Nursing Director, expects more nurses to be hired as a result of the committee's recommendations.

A patient on the committee may not agree with any of these opinions. Every committee member interpreted the committee's goal in their own way, from their own perspectives and particular needs.

A precise statement of the group's goals or objectives is necessary to ensure agreement. A complete statement of each of the group's goals would include:

1. **Who:** The people who will be involved or who "own" the goal.
2. **What:** The target of the goal, which may be people or objects.
3. **Why:** The outcome or end result desired, stated in observable terms (Mager & Beach, 1975).

It is important to state the end result in observable terms so that everyone can see whether or not each goal has been met. Use an action verb to begin the goal statement or objective and state each goal as specifically as possible. This statement should *not* include how you are going to achieve the results—the means should be developed after the goal is chosen. Using the committee example:

> It could take a lot of discussion to make the goal of the Committee to Improve Patient Care more specific. Fulfilling the first criterion is easy in this case. The people who "own" the goal will be the three committee members, the physician, the administrator, the nursing director, and perhaps the group each one represents: the medical staff, the administration, and the nursing department.
>
> Although the overall target population for the committee was *all* patients who received care in their institution, once the committee selected its specific objectives, the target population could be stated more specifically as well. The target populations would be the outpatients using the emergency room, patients receiving radiation therapy, and patients anticipating discharge. In a self-help group, the group itself could be the target population.
>
> In order to please all three members, the committee might finally decide on three specific outcomes to work toward simultaneously. These outcomes include:
>
> Provide 24-hour coverage for the emergency room.
> Renovate the radiation therapy building.
> Supplement the work of the present home care coordinator.
>
> In order to be sure that everyone agrees on the goals, the agreed upon objectives

should be as specific as possible. For example, the committee will need to determine such things as how many patients the home care program should accommodate.

After the goals are clearly stated and acceptable to all concerned, the group can then proceed to discuss how they will achieve these goals or objectives. It is often difficult to separate decisions about goals and the means by which to achieve them.

Now the committee can proceed to a discussion of how they will go about achieving their goals. They may decide to hire more community health nurses to supplement the work of the present home care coordinator. They may decide to hire more physicians to provide 24-hour medical coverage in the emergency room.

The feelings that arise as a group forms and evolves have not yet been discussed, but they will also affect the dynamics of selecting and defining goals in a group.

KNOWLEDGE AND SKILLS

Knowledge and skill in leadership, knowledge and skill in nursing and the ability to think critically are basic requirements for leadership. Knowledge comes before practice: once you have learned basic leadership concepts, you can apply them to specific situations. When you consciously apply them you achieve more consistent results than by using the trial and error approach.

You will find, for example, that when a coworker is not doing the job, you will know some specific steps you can take to remedy the problem. After you have studied group dynamics, you can quickly assess what is happening in a group that seems to be stuck on a particular issue and then select a strategy for helping to motivate the group.

Leadership Knowledge

What does a person need to know in order to be an effective leader? To answer this question, it is necessary to go back to the three basic elements of a leadership event from the first chapter: the leader, co-actor(s), and environment (shown in Fig. 1–2).

As a leader you must know about human needs and motivation and how they affect behavior. You also need to relate this knowledge to your own behavior. This is the *leader* element. Although leadership events can be one-to-one interactions, many of them involve far more people (a health care team or a client population, for example) so a leader needs to know how people act as a group and even as a community as well as how they act individually. This is the *co-actor* element.

Every leadership event takes place within an *environment*, the third basic element. For example, the emotional climate in which an interaction takes place can have a tremendous impact on its outcome. Two frantically busy people are unlikely to arrange a complicated staffing schedule as well as two calm people working without interruption. The time and the arrangement of the space in which an event takes place can also influence its outcome.

There is also the larger system of which the group is a part, another aspect of the environment to consider. For example, the event can take place in an organization that encourages growth and development of its individual members or in an organization with rigid job descriptions. An attempt to bring about a change in nursing roles would proceed very differently in these two environments. In fact, you would approach the change itself very differently in these two environments.

Some people appear to be natural leaders. You may wonder why they would need to learn leadership theory. The theories and concepts of leadership will enhance their natural ability and help them select actions more specific to a particular situation. Also, some of the most seemingly natural leaders actually think and plan very carefully before acting; it's their flexibility in response to a unique situation that makes them seem so natural.

An emphasis on knowledge does not deny the value of intuition. In fact, knowledge, feelings, and intuition can work together synergistically and result in creative solutions to leadership problems. If you let your knowledge and intuition work together, you will be drawing upon more of your inner resources as a leader.

Leadership Skills

You also need to learn some specific leadership skills as well as the situations in which it is appropriate to use them. Once you have analyzed the situation in terms of the basic elements of a leadership event, you are ready to select a strategy. For example, there are several different ways to confront a person or to bring about change. There are political tactics particularly appropriate for the underdog. There are paradoxical methods for change that may appeal to your sense of humor as well as help you become an effective leader.

Nursing Knowledge and Skills

Knowledge and skill in nursing practice are important to the leader. Planning and organizing patient care are leadership responsibilities of the professional nurse. They require accurate assessments and diagnoses based on adequate knowledge. Your peers expect you to share your expertise with them; your patients count on you to give skillful nursing care; and your assistants look to you for guidance.

It takes time to develop this expertise and you can never really be finished learning and improving your skills. Having adequate knowledge and skill gives you confidence and the security needed to try new things and to assert yourself at work. Concern about your skills can result in your focusing most of your attention on them, diverting your energy from more productive activities.

What can you do to increase your knowledge and skill? First, take responsibility for your own education. Your basic education provides you with the knowledge and skill needed to begin practicing nursing. If you feel uncertain about your knowledge or skill, look for extra learning experiences wherever possible. You can study on your own, attend workshops and seminars, ask for extra practice time in laboratory or clinical areas, seek out instructors and supervisors for guidance, and let other staff members know you are interested in observing and learning—most of them will welcome your interest.

If you really have adequate knowledge and skill, but lack self-confidence, focus your attention on this area instead. An assessment of your strengths is a good starting point. You must then follow-up with a real effort to build on these strengths. Assertiveness training is helpful for many people, even for those who feel uncertain behind their aggressive fronts. Leadership skills are surprisingly helpful in building self-esteem because they can provide a genuine sense of personal power to the individual who uses them correctly.

Surprisingly, the leader who has too much knowledge or skill may not be the most effective in leading a group. This seems at first to contradict the previous discussion. The more effective leader, however, is one who identifies with the group. If you know far more than the group and if you are not willing to go back to where the group is in terms of knowledge, you will not appear to be identifying with the group and will not communicate on the same level as the rest of the group.

The leader who is too far ahead of the group can lose them as quickly as the leader who is not as knowledgeable as the group. A leader who is not *too* far ahead of the group seems to be the most effective leader (Beal, Bohlen & Raudabaugh, 1962). It is important to adjust your expectations and choice of terminology to the level of the individual or group:

> You would not tell a brand new aide that a child has "acute pharyngitis." Instead, you would say the child has a sore throat and, if the aide is not overwhelmed by new responsibilities, explain the technical term for future reference.

The importance of leader knowledge and skill was tested in a series of studies, two of which are described in Research Example 3–1.

Critical Thinking

Simply accumulating knowledge and skill is not enough. The leader is an active rather than a passive participant in the learning process. You can make choices regarding what you have learned; you can choose to accept or reject the knowledge offered to you.

A leader needs to maintain an open-minded and questioning attitude. Caregivers frequently fail to question the validity of common practices and often accept the statements of authorities, particularly authorities outside of nursing, without critically evaluating their validity and usefulness in nursing. Although we laugh now at the use of leeches or the old belief that too much learning endangered a woman's health, some of our current practices may seem just as irrational 100 years from now. Many of our current nursing practices are still influenced more by ritual and tradition than by the rationale of theory and the substantiation of research.

Many nursing routines may be customary habits that need critical evaluation. Routines increase efficiency but they can also become too comfortable. You can become mechanical and unthinking about providing nursing care (especially "routine" care) and lose sight of the uniqueness of the individual you are caring for. It is too easy to fall into repetitive ways of thinking and acting without being aware that you are doing it.

RESEARCH EXAMPLE 3–1. The Effect of Leader Competence

Is a leader's perceived competence related to the leader's acceptance and influence in a group? In a series of studies, Hollander and Julian (1978) tested the idea that the leader who helps the group achieve its goals acquires increased influence and esteem from the group. Two of these studies are described here.

EXPERIMENT #1: QUESTIONNAIRE

Six hundred thirty-three undergraduate students in a psychology course were asked to imagine a leader of the same sex who was described as either a good or poor performer of group activities, elected or designated, and interested or not interested in group members. The students rated their willingness (on a scale of 1 to 6) to have this imagined person continue as the leader, serve as the group spokesperson, be a member of the group, or be a close friend.

The greatest difference in ratings was found between the leader described as performing well (5.28) and the leader described as performing poorly (3.19) at the task of the group. A leader's high interest in group activities could raise the leader's level of acceptance when the leader was a poor performer.

The researchers also found that the respondents were more willing to accept the imagined leader as a group member or friend than as a spokesperson. The elected leaders did get a higher rating than the designated leaders but the difference was not statistically significant at the 0.01 level. The researchers concluded that the leader's perceived competence had a significant positive impact on group members' responses to the leader but that they seemed to be wary of granting someone the right to be their spokesperson as it gives the leader a position of authority (parenthetically, a manager is usually expected to have this authority).

EXPERIMENT #2: IN THE LABORATORY

Eighty male undergraduate students were divided into 20 small groups. Ten of these groups held elections to determine the leader. The results of the elections were contrived by the experimenters. The other 10 groups had a leader arbitrarily designated for them.

Group members were then given the task of judging which of three lights on the wall would go off first. Their success in making these judgments was manipulated by the experimenters. Group members were given points for correct guesses.

Again, those leaders seen as competent had significantly more influence over their group's judgments and members of groups in which the leader had been "elected" were more willing to admit that they had been influenced by the leader. Not surprisingly, the leader who distributed points on an equal basis among group members was rated significantly more fair and received a higher evaluation from the group than did the leaders who gave themselves more points. The researchers concluded that the results of this experiment supported the results of the first one in which the leader who was perceived to be competent had more influence on group members.

Holt says that if we do not maintain a questioning attitude, there is a danger that we will "go stupid" (Holt, 1964; Greene, 1973 pp. 5, 80). Experienced staff can be excellent resources but some of them have "gone stupid" and succumbed to the numbing of routine. An alert leader will find many examples of this in everyday practice. The following is one example:

> A nursing assistant developed a time-saving routine for toileting patients in the morning and planned to share this routine with fellow nursing assistants. She systematically worked her way up and down the hall placing each patient, some of them frail and at great risk for developing decubiti, on a bedpan and leaving them for as long as an hour until returning. The routine had become her main concern; the assistant had made the routine more efficient but, unthinkingly, also made it potentially harmful.

SELF AWARENESS

Self awareness is one of the means by which you can increase your effectiveness as a leader. Self awareness or insight is knowing yourself as a thinking, feeling being interacting with an ever-changing world. Its focus is "getting in touch with your feelings" or being "open to experience". These phrases may seem old and trite after being used so frequently and often so casually. But it is difficult to find better words to describe this state of increased sensitivity to the inner self and to your relationship with the world around you, how you respond to people and what effect you have on them.

Self awareness alone is not a solution to leadership problems but it is a heightened sensitivity that will act as a clarifier of peoples' problems, their responses to you, and your responses to them. As Wicks (1977, p. 147) said rather pointedly, "Self-awareness is not an end in itself. The presence of 'enlightened alcoholics' and 'aware neurotics' in the community attests to this fact."

Openness to Self

Self-insight includes being alert to the signals that your body sends you when you are anxious or pushing yourself too hard. As a nurse, you know that these signals can be ignored only at your eventual peril. Self-insight also includes allowing yourself the emotions that well up, including sorrow, jealousy, anger, contentment, love, and joy. Self awareness is acknowledging and expressing the full range of emotions. You probably know the symptoms of anxiety, but can you recognize them in yourself when they arise? If you do recognize the symptoms, how do you cope with them? Are you satisfied with your current coping methods? Can you recognize and constructively express anger or resentment? Can you express feelings of warmth and positive regard for other people?

It may not have occurred to you before, but it seems that there are also people who do not fully recognize their thinking side. On the whole, our society has emphasized the cognitive aspect of a person and rewarded cool, clear thinking rather than emotional responses. Yet, some people also suppress this thinking aspect of themselves. This is especially true of women. If you experience a shiver of fear when you hear the word "research" or are in the habit of saying "I was never good at math," then you might be suppressing your thinking side along with or instead of your feeling side.

Importance of Self Awareness

People who are not self aware tend to define themselves as others see them (Rogers, 1961). They live out their lives in response to other people's demands, including peer and parental pressures, instead of being genuinely themselves. They waste a lot of time and energy trying to be what they are not instead of recognizing and experiencing all that they are (including experiencing the full range of emotions). This lack of awareness tends to make a person defensive and unable to get close to others.

You cannot effectively guide and influence others if you do not feel free to share yourself with others. Rogers believes that everyone really wants to know themselves better. Once you have experienced your genuine and unique self (the mean and nasty side as well as the good and loving side), you become more flexible and more autonomous. This means that you are less dependent on others for approval and are able to act in ways that most satisfy your own needs. It does not mean that you would always be satisfied with yourself. People are forever changing and growing, whether constructively or destructively, and it is natural to experience some discomfort and even distress related to the changes you go through and the decisions you make.

When you can accept yourself as you really are, you will like yourself better. This seems to become a self-fulfilling prophecy: people who like themselves are more likable. On the other hand, people who feel worthless tend to get themselves in situations that will prove them worthless (Egan, 1976). For example, if you are afraid that the people in a certain group will not like you, you will avoid contact with them. As a result, no one pays attention to you and you can say, "See, they don't like me." This self-fulfilling prophecy can be turned around and used to your advantage: if you think of yourself as a leader, you are more likely to be one.

Self awareness also helps you to evaluate your abilities realistically. Being objective about your abilities enables you to identify the areas in which you need to improve and to recognize and build on your strengths. Here is an example:

> If you are afraid to speak in front of a large group, you would not plan to address the PTA about the school health program. Instead, you could involve students in putting on a health fair for their parents. Still, you also need to work on reducing your fear of talking to large groups because, next time, that may be your most effective strategy. (For one way to work on such a fear, see paradoxical change in Chapter 19).

Building up a large repertoire of skills increases your choices and your range of effectiveness.

Being self aware can help you develop more effective interpersonal relationships. If you are not aware of your thoughts and feelings, then you cannot communicate them to others. Also, if you do not see how your actions affect others, you can be badly misled in your interpretations of their behavior and in your choice of leadership strategies. Self awareness also helps you to understand the kinds of motivations that are influencing your behavior. Are you, for example, confronting your colleagues about excuses to avoid doing care plans so that they will improve their work? Or, are you doing it to even a score with them for pointing out something you forgot to do the week before?

Self-insight helps you to develop empathy. Although some psychologists suggest that you try to "get into the other person's skin" to develop empathy, you cannot actually experience or feel exactly what another person is feeling. But you can relate their experiences to your own in order to develop some understanding of what they are feeling. People always mediate what the other person says or feels through their own experience (Laing, 1969). This is one reason why it is important to respond to the other person's messages and to check out your perceptions of what the other person is saying and doing, a basic communication skill discussed later.

Increasing Self Awareness

One way to increase awareness is to develop your understanding of human behavior, especially the role of the emotions, human needs, motivations, and coping behaviors.

Observation of people's reactions to your behavior can give you many clues as to your effect on others. One of the most important ways to do this, and one that you can do every day, is to seek feedback from others. This can be done directly and formally by asking colleagues to evaluate your performance or informally by asking their opinion of how you are doing. It is also worthwhile to ask your patients if you've been of any help to them and, if so, to ask them to tell you in what ways—you may be surprised at some of the responses.

Many people underrate themselves. They dwell on their negative characteristics and downplay their real strengths. If you are one of these people, you may be in for a pleasant surprise when you seek feedback from other people.

Tape recordings and videotapes are good sources of objective feedback. We do not hear our voices the same way others do and the tape recorder can supply another set of ears as well as a record of what you have said. Videotape is even better because a lot of nonverbal communication is apparent on the video screen. Both of these can be played back several times to allow you to think and analyze your behavior and your effect on others. They can also be reviewed in private, which is more comfortable for some people.

Joining a group can be a valuable experience for a developing leader. There are so many kinds of groups that you will have to evaluate both your own needs and the purpose of a group before joining one. Some groups are formed explicitly for the purpose of increasing self awareness. In other groups, however, this goal is secondary or implied. You can learn something from almost any group (even if it is how *not* to conduct a group), but a group that has an open, accepting climate in which you can feel comfortable and free to be yourself is one that would be most productive.

Stages of Self Awareness

Some people do not progress beyond a limited self awareness which enables them to function, but not to the full extent of their ability. When you first begin paying serious attention to yourself, you can become acutely self-conscious. You may find yourself reflecting on just about every response you make to a patient or to a coworker. ("What am I *really* saying?" "Why did I do that?") You can find yourself trying to pick up more of the feeling messages in other people's responses to you ("Why did he do that?" "What are they really trying to say?" But as you become more accustomed to being open to yourself, there seems to be less self-conscious about it. Fully experiencing your thinking, feeling, responding and acting self becomes easier and more natural. It can contribute immeasurably to your effectiveness in relating to other people (Rogers, 1977).

COMMUNICATION

Communication is at the very heart of leadership. It is the essential means through which leadership is accomplished, whether the communication is a spoken word of praise, a written set of instructions, a frown of displeasure or an encouraging squeeze of the hand.

Because leadership cannot occur except in relationship to others, a leadership act must include some kind of exchange. Every exchange between human beings has an element of communication in it; there is some message in every exchange. We "cannot *not* communicate" is the way that Watzlawick, Beavin and Jackson (1967, p.5) so neatly phrased it. Even refusing to respond to someone sends a message indicating "I will not answer," although it does not tell the other person why you will not respond.

Active Listening

Attending and responding are basic communication skills used in virtually every leadership situation. If you do not attend to what other people are saying, you will not understand them. If you do not respond to them, they will not feel understood or valued as a person. Gordon (1970, p.49) calls attending "active listening." Active listening is essential in the establishment of good working relationships. These are described in more detail in the chapter on communication.

Encouraging a Flow of Information

An adequate flow of information between people who are working together (the primary nurse and associate nurses, for example) is necessary for smooth operation in any setting. Without an adequate flow of information, many misunderstandings and omissions can occur. This is especially apparent in community settings where some members of the health care team may actually never see each other. For example:

> Operating without adequate communication, a community health nurse may be gathering resources for an older woman to return home from the hospital while the social worker is checking out suitable nursing homes for her. The patient and her family, of course, would be in a state of utter confusion until someone realized what was happening and improved communication between all of the people involved.

People are more likely to assume that the exchange of information is adequate when they see each other every day. This assumption needs to be thoroughly checked out before it is accepted. People may, literally, be only seeing each other and not actively listening at all.

A leader uses available *channels of communication* and creates new ones when they are needed. A leader also encourages others to do the same. In the previous example, for instance:

> The community health nurse could arrange to meet with the social worker, the older woman, and her family to discuss discharge plans. In fact, similar meetings should be held with all patients preparing for discharge. Some community health agencies have scheduled regular meetings with hospital discharge planning staff in order to create a new channel of much needed communication.

Just think about all of the people who can be involved in just one patient's care. You can see why adequate communication is so important when we are directing the care of many different patients or clients.

Directness and Assertiveness

An effective leader sends direct messages to others. Avoidance is ineffective (Barker, Tjosvold & Andrews, 1988), especially indirect, tentative messages or, even worse, the failure to send any message at all. The leader does not assume or hope that others will somehow understand what is expected of them. When the leader's messages are too tentative and indirect, the person who is expected to respond may not be at all sure what the message is. For example, imagine the following being said in a very soft, hesitant voice:

> Some people have told me that it is possible to do some harm, or at least no good, anyway, not to listen to a patient's complaint that something is wrong. Now, I do know that you really don't have much time, you're so busy and we've been so short-handed today, but if it's at all possible, if you could find some time somehow in your schedule. . .

Do you know what this team leader wants? Hasn't the leader wasted time hesitating and going around and around instead of making the simple but apparently necessary request to look into a patient's complaint? If you tend to be tentative instead of direct, practice simplifying your statements so that you get to the point directly.

Some type of insecurity is usually related to this tentative way of speaking. People joining a new group, for instance, are often uncertain about their roles in the group and so will try to avoid making statements that may antagonize other group members or make them seem out of place in the group. Another reason is that they believe that the other person is too fragile and may "fall apart" if they are not careful how they say something, particularly something negative (Satir, 1967, p.15). People in general are quite resilient and will probably appreciate a direct approach. In fact, avoiding negative responses can do far more harm than good in the long run because it denies that person an opportunity to change. Negative feedback can be expressed clearly and constructively, without harm to either person involved in the exchange.

Checking Perceptions

Checking out your perceptions with others is also important. Doing this increases your empathic skills and helps you avoid mistaken assumptions about the reasons for people's behavior. For example:

> If someone seems angry about an assignment, you should not change it until you find out why that person is angry. The anger could be unrelated to the assignment—the individual might have received a speeding ticket on the way to work. Or, perhaps the manner in which you gave the assignment, rather than the work involved, caused the anger.

Guessing is inaccurate and you will learn more by asking the right questions.

Feedback from the group can help you evaluate your effectiveness and serve as a guide for improving your leadership skills. It is hard to imagine a leadership situation in which feedback is not useful to the leader. Here is another example:

> Suppose that your team members are not showing up for team conferences. By yourself, you could probably come up with 100 possible reasons why this is happening, each reason suggesting a different solution. But how could you decide which of these is the right one? To avoid making assumptions, you can ask your team members how they see the situation. You can first state your problem and then say to them something like ''In order to avoid this happening again, I need to know why people are not coming to the team conferences.''

Providing Feedback

Group members need feedback for the same reasons that a leader needs feedback: to increase self awareness; to avoid operating on the basis of mistaken assumptions about other people's behavior; and as a guide for growth and change.

Negative feedback should be communicated without placing blame or attacking the person. The focus of the communication is on a specific *behavior*. For example:

> If you found an orderly feeding a patient the wrong diet, you would not say ''Hey, stupid! The patient can't eat that!'' which would insult the orderly. Instead, you could say, ''This patient is on a low-purine diet and cannot eat liver. Let's get the patient something else to eat.''

The second response is specific, it sticks to the problem, does not attack and allows for open dialogue that can lead to a solution of the problem (a very simple one in this case) instead of provoking a defensive response. It provides an opportunity for learning rather than for feeling bad.

You must respect the rights and dignity of your coworkers as much as you do the rights and dignity of your patients. Except in an urgent situation, look for a way to speak to the person privately. Yelling is not acceptable behavior and yelling in public creates bad feelings for everyone concerned. Many readers have probably witnessed such an incident at some time in school or at work. Such behavior embarrasses people, increases anger, builds defensiveness, and closes off communication.

Linking

Linking may be less familiar to you. Linking is first seeing and then expressing a connection between two separate ideas or statements. For example, when people in a group make separate, unconnected statements at a meeting, the group will probably go in several directions at once without accomplishing anything. The following is an example:

> One group member suggests providing a television for a bored, long term patient. The next person to speak follows this suggestion with an unrelated comment on the terrible weather. The leader then connects the two by commenting that if the weather were better, the bored patient could be taken outside every day but, in the meantime, what else could people suggest to alleviate the patient's boredom in addition to getting the patient a TV?

When someone assumes leadership and contributes the link between unconnected statements, the discussion begins to flow in one direction, building up energy as each statement is connected to the main flow of the discussion (Lifton, 1972).

You can also create links between people's ideas even when they are not actually together:

> A visiting nurse may complain about the number of clients she sees at home who have had their food stamp allocations reduced. You can answer, "A social worker in our agency has also expressed concern about the situation. Would you like to work with the social worker on the problem?"

Finding such links can be a creative endeavor. Linking can be a catalyst for action in many leadership situations.

Networking

The effective nurse deliberately networks with other people. Linking develops connections between ideas while networking develops connections between people. Once a relationship of trust and professional respect has been developed, the other person has a bias toward agreeing to your reasonable request rather than questioning it or avoiding a decision. This eases your way, making it possible to get things done without numerous bureaucratic barriers and delays. For example, if you have developed connections with the people in social service, it will probably be easier to speed a special request for placement of a client with an urgent need or to have something done late on a Friday afternoon when ordinarily they would say, "You will have to wait until Monday."

Networking facilitates the achievement of influence in a number of ways (Hosking, 1988). It not only smooths the way but also opens up channels to important information. Opportunities to share new ideas with colleagues is not only stimulating but provides information needed to get ahead at work and discover new job opportunities. Some of the most interesting and challenging positions are never advertised because they are filled with people from within the organization or with people known to those who are doing the hiring.

People like to talk about the "old-boy" networks of men in positions of power who share information and opportunities among themselves but prevent others from gaining access to these valuable resources (Christy, 1987).

Whether or not nurses should set up opposing exclusive networks is an interesting question. The point, however, is that a leader should be aware of the value of networking, develop her own networks, and gain access to existing networks. The sharing of information and opportunities with fellow professionals can have a synergistic effect: we can increase our energy supply of information and influence by sharing it. Many networking opportunities occur naturally but the leadership-oriented individual also *seeks out* ways to network.

ENERGY

If you have ever had an exhausting exchange with an agitated individual, then you have experienced the meaning of the phrase "feeling drained." The entity of which you felt drained is human energy. There are times when people feel "bursting with energy" as if they had an overflowing supply. Other times they are so low that they feel as if they are suffering an energy deficit. While we do know that a person can feel high or low in energy (Blattner, 1981), scientists cannot yet define exactly what this energy is or measure it accurately.

Neural and Emotional Energy

Human energy seems to be more than a purely physical phenomenon since our feeling states have a great effect on the amount of available energy we have. Consider, for example, how hard it is for a depressed person to just get out of bed in the morning. Compare this to a manic state in which a person can be active for hours and even days without pause. While this energy is usually described as being either physical or emotional, these are probably manifestations of the same energy field. It is believed that some kind of energy transformation can take place in people, changing the neural (electro-chemical) energy of the nervous system to emotional energy. Gruen (1979) has conducted some interesting research to test this idea:

> In a random sample of heart attack patients, the experimental group of patients who had psychotherapy during their hospital stay had shorter hospital stays, a feeling of increased vigor, and more activity with less anxiety four months after the heart attack than the control group of patients who did not have psychotherapy. The conclusion was that an increase in available energy resulted from the change in self-concept that occurred during therapy.

Gruen theorizes that somehow the person to person interaction of the therapy helped release this energy so that the patients could do more and felt more energetic—a release and transformation of energy.

Energy and Leadership Effectiveness

As you interact with other people, your energy level will have an influence on their response to you. For instance, one person's enthusiasm for a project can be infectious in the good sense of the word. If someone in a group gets really excited about an idea, the rest of the group often picks up the excitement and carries out the idea. For example:

A group of nurses and aides decided at a conference that one of their patients needed more social stimulation and would enjoy being with friends down the hall. The idea involved shifting several patients' units. Moving beds around usually evokes tired groans and much procrastination, but before the conference was over, one nurse went out and checked with the patients involved. The nurse came back saying "Yes, they want to do it." Before the chairs in the conference room were put back in place, there was a convoy of beds rolling down the hall. In fifteen minutes, everyone was settled in their new rooms and the glow of accomplishment was visible on the staff members' faces.

Something happens when an idea catches fire like this. The people involved seem to recharge from each other's enthusiasm and the energy level of the group rises dramatically. This is called "synergistic power," or the surge of energy that results when people exchange positive energy with each other (Craig & Craig, 1975; Claus & Bailey, 1977).

You can share your energy with people in many ways. Information can be thought of as an organized kind of energy which can be used and exchanged. It is the "fuel" that fires the imagination and provides the impetus to bring about changes in health care. A lack of energy and enthusiasm can work in the opposite direction. If no one believes an idea will work, then it will not work:

A favorite phrase on patient care plans is the direction to "spend time with the patient." If you are giving such an assignment and shrug or sigh when you say it (knowing it won't be done), if you skip reading that part of the care plan or do not check later to see what the results of doing it were, it will probably not be done. But if you emphasize spending time with the patient, citing why it is needed by this patient, explain what is meant by "spending more time," and if you are interested in the results of the interaction, you are far more likely to see it done.

Energy Flow and Reserves

A leader needs to have energy available for action. You can regulate your energy exchanges to some extent to ensure adequate reserves. Most people are at least subliminally aware when their energy reserves are low. They feel listless and weary and realize that they need to recharge. How people recharge seems to be an individual matter—the same experience can be restorative (positive) for one person and draining (negative) for someone else, as in the following example:

Some people love horror movies—the more terrifying the better—while others get scared and have bad dreams for days afterward. The enjoyment recharges one person in a positive manner while the other person has stored up a negative kind of energy that needs to be released in the bad dreams. Yet another person may be bored by horror movies and would not be recharged but loves to play tennis and feels exhilarated after a good match.

Some activities, like the tennis, seem to be both discharging and recharging activities. This whole concept of human energy and its positive and negative aspects needs to be further researched.

The availability of human energy may be related to states of health and illness. The results of Kirlian photography indicate that there may be measurable differences in energy levels between the sick and well person. There is a growing feeling, too, that people have resources of personal power and energy that have hardly been tapped. Even if we cannot actually use our psychic energy to move objects across the room (and who knows for sure that we cannot?), the sharing of the energy that is within each of us has a tremendous potential for impact on people.

Some people have difficulty using their energy their energy to its best advantage. They waste their energy doing things the hard way or in a disorganized fashion. An energy squanderer will do ten things to solve a single problem where one action would do just as well. On the other hand, using effective leadership techniques can reduce the number of draining experiences at work and help you keep your energy reserves up.

An Energy Inventory

You might try making an inventory of your energy reserves, discharges, and recharges to see where your energy is going. List all of your activities for one day. Include little things such as receiving a word of thanks from someone, and routine things such as meals. Mark them as sources of either positive (+) or negative (−) energy and rate the amount of energy involved on a scale of 1 to 5 with 1 being very low, 3 moderate and 5 very high amounts. A tremendously recharging experience would be +5 and a very draining experience would be −5. Your total would indicate a positive or negative balance for the day. Do you find yourself with a deficit at the end of the day? Are there negative sources that you could reduce or eliminate? Are there positive sources you could add or increase? Are you satisfied with the way in which you use your energy?

ACTION ───

The effective leader is decisive and action-oriented (Quillen, 1988). All of the components that came before this one—goals, knowledge and skill, self awareness, communication, and energy—are only of value if they are put to use.

Many of the actions mentioned will be discussed later in detail. Describing them here will give you a broad overview of what a leader does in order to influence others. Later in this chapter, you will find a checklist that summarizes the components of effective leadership and can be used to evaluate your own effectiveness as a leader.

By now, you have probably noticed some connections between the components. You will find more here and by the time you reach the end of this book, you probably will have found many new ones.

Initiating Action

A leader *initiates* action. Ideas, suggestions, and plans must be implemented in order to be effective. A good idea cannot have any influence if it remains only in your head. Even the best assessment and planning, whether a nursing care plan, community project, or some other plan, does very little good if it remains only a plan.

Many worthwhile proposals die of neglect because no one put any energy behind the proposals to bring them into action. For instance:

> You may hear a colleague say "Whatever happened to that idea we had about getting a mobile health unit?" In response, everyone shrugs and looks around at the others.

Someone had made a good suggestion, but no one had taken the initiative to pursue it any further.

A leader *confronts* himself and others. Confrontation is a powerful strategy used to present people with the way others perceive their actions. It should be a thoughtful reaction, not a thoughtless one that can degenerate into telling each other off. There are several ways in which you can confront an individual or group ranging from very gentle to very strong confrontations.

A leader does not sit back and watch a power struggle destroy working relationships or a client being put off by one agency after another. A leader takes action to solve these problems. Timing is also important. It is true that it is sometimes necessary to wait for the right opportunity to initiate action. But what happens much more often is that people delay too long before initiating action. Too much delay can mean losing an opportunity to act decisively.

Working with Others

A leader *guides* others, sharing knowledge and experience with them. The amount of guidance and direction varies according to the needs that arise in particular situations. A new nurse would need a lot of guidance in comparison to an experienced nurse, but even the most experienced benefit from some direction and from an exchange of ideas. A frequent exchange of ideas helps to prevent "going stupid". This is not a one-way exchange: the leader is also open to suggestion from others and eager to learn from others' knowledge and experience.

A leader *evaluates* the actions of herself and others. Nursing audits and peer review are formal evaluation procedures that are becoming established parts of nursing practice. Informal evaluation should take place constantly. Is your nursing care helping the patient recover or is it adding to the patient's distress? Has your leadership made it possible for your team members to work well together or has it resulted in disruptive behavior? An evaluation of what behavior has been productive and what has not been provides a guide for selecting strategies in the future. Evaluation done well can be a source of increased insight and can stimulate growth and development.

A leader *calls meetings* of all kinds. The meetings should have a specific purpose which could be to discuss plans or progress, organize work, work out solutions to problems, ventilate feelings, or share information. Getting people together as a group rather than dealing with them individually has several advantages. First, you can get the same message to everyone with less chance of the message being changed as it is transmitted. Second, you also may be able to get that tremendous joint action effect called synergic power with a group. Communication with everyone at once improves coordination, saves time, and often brings greater results.

A leader *mobilizes support systems*. You are not expected to do all of these things alone. In fact, there are many things you cannot accomplish singlehandedly. There are two kinds of support: actual assistance with a task and psychologic support. Your health care team provides the actual assistance with the work that needs to be done. Psychologic support can come from a number of sources including administrative backing of your activities, colleagues who say "I'm with you on this", and your patients who appreciate your skilled care. Support can also come from outside work and, last but not least, from yourself.

Critical Thinking and Problem Solving

A leader *critically analyzes* beliefs and practices. Critical thinking is related to evaluation but has a broader application. It is an open-minded but questioning approach toward beliefs, facts, and practices. Nursing practice is influenced by current beliefs and fashionable trends. Even "facts" can be inadequate or proven wrong by new evidence, as in the following examples.

Years ago, the germ theory revolutionized health care, but now we realize that it is inadequate by itself to explain the occurrence of illness in humans.

We once thought that premature infants should be given a high concentration of oxygen to assist respiration. However, it was discovered that too much oxygen for too long a time was responsible for the occurrence of retrolental fibroplasia in these infants.

What you learned in school or read in journals may also change as new discoveries are made. Even the facts can be wrong and the nurse leader must be ready and willing to challenge them.

A leader *problem solves* when confronted with a difficult situation. The problem solving process (collect data, define the problem, select strategies, take action, evaluate results) serves as a guide to dealing with a problem or difficult task. Problem solving is a systematic process that assists the leader in the analysis of a difficult situation and in the choice of actions. An effective leader usually thinks before acting.

A leader *plans and organizes* activities. Although planning and organization without action are not sufficient by themselves, they do contribute a great deal to the efficiency and effectiveness of an endeavor. Without them, people waste energy doing useless tasks, work at cross purposes or find themselves directionless, not knowing what to do next. Without good planning and organization, a job may be done twice or not at all. Poorly planned meetings are also time wasters. Good planning and organization are worth the time and effort involved. Formal planning is primarily a managerial responsibility and will be discussed in the next chapter.

Professional Activities

A leader *develops the structure of his or her own practice*. Leaders do not wait for someone else to tell them what to do. For example, a professional nurse does not wait for a physician's order before doing some health teaching, yet there are some nurses who still do this. Examples of ways in which nurses develop the structure of their roles are as follows:

A school nurse seeks opportunities for intervention; the nurse does not sit in the office hoping the teachers will remember that the nurse is there.

An infection control nurse visits the units, checks patients' charts, review reports, institutes surveys, and talks with personnel to keep on top of the situation. The nurse does not wait to be called in.

In order to do these things, a nurse must have both leadership ability and a clear idea of what nursing is. While there are many written definitions of nursing, it is suggested that the reader formulate a personal definition to live by, one you can use when someone asks you what nurses really do or why nurses should have more autonomy, authority, a salary increase, and so forth.

While nurses need to recognize the contributions of other members of the health team, they do not need to do this by diminishing their own contribution. Too often, nurses fail to realize they have expertise of their own:

> Nurses will call in a psychologist to a counsel a patient for a minor problem before they try to help the patient deal with the problem. They will also call in ''experts'' to teach their patients, diagnose a patient's response to a health problem, run a clinic, lead team conferences, and so forth.

Nurses can do all of these things and more. While it is appropriate to call on experts when they are needed, a unit leader needs a strong sense of professional identity and self confidence.

A leader *interprets the role* of the professional nurse to others: co-workers, clients, and the public. Developing structure emphasizes actual practice, while interpreting the role emphasizes telling people about it. If you listen closely, you'll find plenty of opportunities to inform people about what nurses can do. Here are just two examples:

> You might notice that teachers call on the school nurse to deal with head lice problems, but not with family problems that are keeping a child out of school.
>
> You may hear a community group bemoaning their difficulty getting someone to do camp physicals and have the opportunity to say, ''A nurse can do that.''

Does a leader *seek recognition*? There is some question about whether or not seeking recognition is a leadership function. A willingness to speak out in support of yourself, your group, and your profession is part of being a leader. But anyone who is obviously on an ego trip with only personal interests in mind is unlikely to be an effective leader. It seems that there are limits within which seeking recognition can be an effective leadership action.

Deciding to Act

A leader *takes risks.* A leader is not afraid of confrontation but is willing to make direct statements, question decisions, and, sometimes, break rules. Leaders choose their fights, they do not get trapped in them. Leaders decide for themselves when to take risks after weighing the consequences of doing so.

You probably take many small risks everyday without thinking about it. Sometimes the action is so necessary that you do not even pause to consider the risk to yourself until it is all over.

Every leadership action has some risk attached to it. It takes courage to stand up and speak out, to correct people when they are wrong, and to volunteer to take charge. Some readers will find this easy to do, having been accustomed to speaking up and taking charge and perhaps even taking over.

The need to risk holding back and trusting others to take responsibility and speak for themselves may be hard for these leaders. They may need to practice weighing consequences and choosing their battles in order to avoid scattering their energies and to reap the full benefit of their assertiveness.

Other readers may quake at the thought of confronting people and standing up for their rights. These readers may need extra practice in leadership techniques such as assertiveness and confrontation to build up confidence and get into the habit of speaking out. Ensuring adequate support systems and concentration on personal strengths before taking action may also increase assertiveness.

Whether you choose to act or not to act, you have made a decision. Deciding is often the hardest part. What will you gain? What will you lose? Which of these is most important to you? When you choose to lead, you are choosing to risk criticism and return confrontation. You are opening yourself up to challenges to your leadership. But choosing not to lead also has its risks; you risk a loss of autonomy, reduced opportunities to achieve self-actualization, and a loss of self-esteem. Confronting the risks of leadership is a choice to open up opportunities for more satisfying person-to-person interactions and for the possibility of greater rewards in your personal life and in your career.

THE LEADERSHIP EFFECTIVENESS CHECKLIST

Each reader will find areas of personal strength and weakness within the components of effective leadership. You may find, for example, that you are usually direct in your approach to people, but that you often fail to consider what they are trying to get out of a situation (their goals). Or, you may find that you are usually very sensitive to the needs and goals of others, but tend to be indirect. There are as many possible combinations as there are readers of this book.

As you were reading the chapter, you probably thought of times you had taken the actions described and times when you have forgotten or avoided these actions. Using the checklist in Figure 3–3 will help you in your self-analysis.

This is not one of those quick checklists where you add up your score and find out if you are "superior," "above average," or "fair." It is meant as a guide to serious analysis of your leadership ability. The idea is not to get a score of how effective or ineffective you are (this is better measured in terms of the results you've been getting) but to emphasize those strong points of yours that you can build on (especially those in the "Somewhat" column) and use to your best advantage and to show you where you can make some changes in your leadership in order to become more effective.

Now that you have read the chapter, think of a current or past leadership situation and analyze your actions in terms of the components of effective leadership, listed in Figure 3–3. You may want to return to this checklist after you have finished the book.

	VERY MUCH	SOME-WHAT	NOT AT ALL
A. GOALS			
1. Have you identified: Your personal goals? Group members' personal goals? Group goals? Environmental (such as organizational, community) goals?			
2. Are your goals congruent with the group's goals?			
3. Do you identify with the group, for example, use "we" instead of "I" and "you"?			
4. Do members of the group see you as identifying with the group?			
5. Have you clearly and specifically stated the group's goals including the: People involved? Target? Outcome?			
B. KNOWLEDGE AND SKILLS			
1. Do you have more knowledge and skill than the rest of the group?			
2. Do you feel confident of your knowledge and skill in this situation?			
3. Are you able to speak to the group on their level?			
4. Have you identified the needs and motives of the people in the group?			
5. Have you identified the sources of power and authority in the situation?			
6. Have you critically analyzed the situation including the leader, co-actor(s) and environment?			
7. Have you kept an open mind about the situation?			
C. SELF-AWARENESS			
1. Do you know what your own needs are? Have you found ways to meet these needs?			
2. Do you know what you expect to gain from this situation?			
3. Are you able to empathize with the people in the group?			
4. Do you see yourself as a leader?			
D. COMMUNICATION			
1. Do you know what channels of communication are usually used? Are you using them?			

Figure 3–3. Leadership effectiveness checklist.

	VERY MUCH	SOME-WHAT	NOT AT ALL
D. COMMUNICATION (continued)			
2. Is there an adequate flow of information?			
3. Have you created any new channels of communication?			
4. Are your communications open and direct?			
5. Do you attend and respond (listen actively) to what others are saying?			
6. Have you checked out your perceptions of the situation with the people involved?			
7. Do you see and point out connections (links) between the statements of different people?			
E. ENERGY			
1. Are you interested in the work of the group?			
2. Have you shared your interest and enthusiasm with the group?			
3. Do you really believe what you say to the group?			
4. Do you have enough energy for the task?			
F. ACTION			
1. Have you planned how to get the job done?			
2. Have you organized the work efficiently?			
3. Do you share your ideas with others?			
4. Do you call the group together often enough?			
5. Have you defined your nursing role and communicated with the group?			
6. Do you use the authority you have? Do you delegate it? Have you tried to increase it?			
7. Have you mobilized support systems?			
8. Are you willing to take risks? Have you taken any risks?			
9. Do you confront when it is needed?			
10. Do you initiate action when it is needed? Without delay?			
11. Do you seek feedback? Informally? Formally?			
12. Do you provide feedback? Informally Formally?			
13. Have you tried to improve your leadership ability?			

Figure 3–3. *Continued.*

SUMMARY

The components of effective leadership include clear, congruent and meaningful goals, adequate knowledge and skill, self awareness, effective communication, wise use of energy, and taking action.

An effective leader ensures that goals are clear, congruent and meaningful to the group so that it can proceed with its tasks.

The effective leader also has adequate knowledge and skill in leadership and in the leader's own profession. A thorough understanding of leadership makes it possible to analyze all aspects of a leadership situation and to choose the most effective strategy based on this analysis. A questioning, open-minded attitude enables the leader to critically evaluate information and to avoid the pitfall of "going stupid".

Through increased sensitivity to yourself and others, you can become more flexible and accepting of yourself and others. Self awareness can also improve your ability to develop close relationships with other people and to understand their behavior. As you learn more about your own unique characteristics, you can select the most appropriate leadership approaches to use and generally improve your effectiveness in interpersonal relations.

Adequate communication is at the core of effective leadership. Active listening, directness, checking out perceptions, giving feedback, and linking are all elements of good communication for effective leadership.

Energy can be shared with people as information, in the helping process, and in motivating people via synergic power. An adequate energy reserve is needed in order to be prepared to act.

Action is the sixth component of effective leadership. Leaders develop the structure of their practice and interpret their professional role to others. Leaders also initiate actions of many kinds including planning and organizing work, guiding and evaluating others, calling meetings, mobilizing support systems, taking risks, and confronting themselves and others. Leaders use the basic skills of problem solving, critical thinking and communication to carry out these actions most effectively.

REFERENCES*

Barker, J., Tjosvold, D. & Andrews, R. (1988). Conflict approaches of effective and ineffective project managers: A field study in a matrix organization. *Journal of Management Studies*, 25:2, 167–179.

Beal, G.M., Bohlen, J.M., & Raudebaugh, J.N. (1962). *Leadership and dynamic group action.* Ames, Iowa: Iowa State University Press.

Bennis, W. & Nanus, B. (1985). *Leaders: The strategies for taking charge.* New York: Harper and Row.

Blattner, B. (1981). *Holistic nursing.* Englewood Cliffs, N.J.: Prentice-Hall.

*Christy, K.A. (1987). Networks: Forming "old girl" connections among nurses. *Nursing Management,* 18, (4), 75–75.

Claus, K.E. & Bailey, J.T. (1977). *Power and influence in health care.* St. Louis: C.V. Mosby.

Craig, J.H. & Craig, M. (1975). Synergic power:

Beyond domination and permissiveness. Berkeley: Pro-Active Press.

Egan, G. (1976). *Interpersonal living.* Monterey, California: Brooks/Cole.

Gordon, T. (1970). *Parent effectiveness training.* New York: Plume Books.

Green, M. (1973). *Teacher as stranger.* Belmont, California: Wadsworth.

Gruen, W. (1979). Energy in group therapy: Implications for the therapist of energy transformation and generation as a negentropic system. *Small group behavior,* 10 (1) 23.

*Hollander, E.P. (1974). Leader effectiveness and the influence process. In Cathcart, R.S. & Samovar, L.A. *Small group communication: A reader.* ed. 2. Dubuque, Iowa: Wm. C. Brown.

Hollander, E.P. & Julian, J.W. (1978). *Studies in leader*

legitimacy, influence and innovation. In Berkowitz, L. Group processes. New York: Academic Press.

Holt, J. (1964). How children fail. New York: Pitman. In Greene, M. Teacher as stranger. (1973). Belmont, California: Wadsworth.

Hosking, D.M. (1988). Organizing, leadership and skilful process. Journal of Management Studies, 25, 147–167.

Kantor, E.P. & Lehr. W. (1975). Inside the family. New York: Harper & Row.

Krieger, D. (1974). The laying-on of hands as a therapeutic tool for nurses, speech presented at the American Cancer Society, New York City Division, Inc. In Symposium: A synthesis of community health resources for the rehabilitation of the cancer patient. New York: French and Polyclinic Medical School and Health Center.

Krieger, D. (1979). The therapeutic touch. Englewood Cliffs, N.J.: Prentice-Hall.

Laing, R.D (1969). Self and Others. ed. 2. New York: Penguin Books.

Lifton, W.M. (1972). Groups: Facilitating individual growth and societal change. New York: John Wiley & Sons.

*Mager, R.F. & Beach, K.M. (1975). Developing vocational instruction. ed. 2. Palo Alto, California: Fearon.

Ouchi, W.G. (1981) Theory Z: How American business can meet the Japanese challenge. Reading, Mass: Addison-Wesley.

Quillen, T. (1988). The ideal boss. Response, 1:7, 5.

Rogers, C.R. (1961). On becoming a person. Boston: Houghton-Mifflin.

Rogers, C.R. (1977). Carl Rogers on personal power. New York: Dell.

Satir, V. (1967). Conjoint family therapy. Palo Alto, California: Science and Behavior Books.

*Tannenbaum, R., Weschler, I.R. & Massarik, F. (1974). Leadership: A frame of reference. In Cathcart, R.S. & Samovar, L.A. Small group communication: A reader. ed. 2. Dubuque, Iowa: Wm. C. Brown.

Watzlawick, P., Beavin, J.H. & Jackson, DD. (1967). Pragmatics of human communication. New York: W.W. Norton.

Wick, R.J. (1977). Counseling strategies and intervention techniques for the human services. Philadelphia: J.B. Lippincott.

*References marked with an asterisk are suggested for further reading.

Chapter 4

OUTLINE

Effective Management
Defining Management
Practicing Management

Leadership
Planning
Time Management
Planning Current Work
Priorities
Timing and Sequence
Deadlines
Organizational Goals
Skill Mix of Staff
Characteristics of the Work
Planning Future Work

Direction
Work Assignment
Job Descriptions
Staffing and Scheduling
Technical Direction

Monitoring
Individual Staff Members
The Unit as a Whole
Monitoring Methods

Recognition and Rewards
Types of Rewards
Determining Rewards

Development
Two Schools of Thought
Encouraging Staff Development

Representation
Representing Staff Members
Representing Administration

Management Effectiveness Checklist
Summary

LEARNING OBJECTIVES

Upon completion of this chapter, the reader will be able to:

▷ Distinguish between leadership and management.

▷ Name and describe the components of effective management.

▷ Evaluate his or her own managerial effectiveness in terms of the components of effective management.

THE COMPONENTS OF EFFECTIVE MANAGEMENT

What makes a person an effective manager? First of all, leadership, which is the first component of effective management. The other components of effective management are: planning, direction, monitoring, recognition, development, and representation. Leadership is considered a fundamental prerequisite for effective management.

Each of these components of effective management is described and explained in this chapter. Together they summarize the most fundamental concepts of management. The details of management functions will then be discussed in later chapters.

EFFECTIVE MANAGEMENT

A manager works through others. For example, a nurse manager may not actually dispense medications, check fundi, make home visits, or give immunizations. The manager, however, is responsible for ensuring that this care is given and that it is done well. This is not a simple task. It takes a great deal of knowledge and skill to be an effective manager and we will look at some of the areas in which managers must be well prepared in order to be effective.

To be more specific, we will consider seven components of effective management practice. These components are leadership, planning, direction, development, monitoring, recognition and representation (Fig. 4–1). In other words, the effective manager:

1. Assumes *leadership* of the group.
2. Actively engages in *planning* the current and future work of the group.
3. Provides *direction* to staff members regarding the way the work is to be done.
4. Fosters the *development* of every staff member.
5. *Monitors* the work done by staff members to maintain quality and productivity.
6. *Recognizes* and rewards quality and productivity.
7. *Represents* both administration and staff members as needed in discussions and negotiations with others.

In this discussion of the components of effective management, it may be helpful to keep in mind the four major interacting elements in a management situation. These elements are an extension of the fundamental elements of a leadership situation, a situation which is more general than a

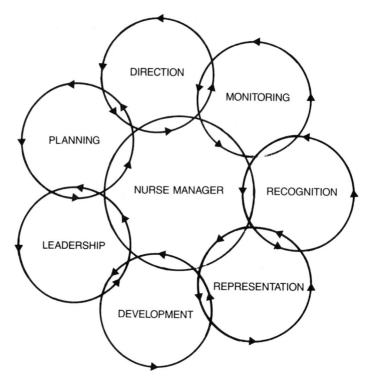

Figure 4–1. Components of effective management.

management situation. The fundamental elements of a management situation are the manager, staff members, the work, and environment (Fig. 4–2). Each of these elements has a powerful effect on the outcome. In this chapter we will concentrate primarily on the actions of the manager.

The contrast between an effective and an ineffective manager can be illustrated by a pair of comments often heard in a work situation. Managers are often heard to cry out in frustration "It would be easier to do the work myself!" while their subordinates are often heard complaining, "We do all the work. All our manager does is sit at a desk all day!" The ineffective manager frustrates himself or herself as well as staff members. The manager feels as if he or she is doing all of the work and getting little cooperation from staff members. The staff members, on the other hand, feel as if they are not only doing all of the work themselves but that their manager is making it harder for them to get it done. The effective manager, in contrast, makes it easier for staff to get their work done.

Defining Management

In 1916, Henri Fayol (Wren, 1972) wrote that the functions of a manager are to plan, organize, command, coordinate, and control (in French, *prevoir, organiser, commander, coordonner et controler*). Although often modified, (plan, organize, staff, direct, and control is one common modification), this

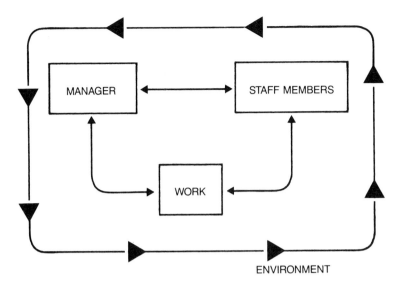

Figure 4–2. Elements of a management situation.

original list of functions appears regularly as the outline of management functions and is used as an organizer for many management textbooks. In fact, many managers have learned this list and will tell you that that is exactly what they do: plan, organize, direct, and control (Wren, 1972).

But Mintzberg (1975) says that while managers *say* that they plan, organize, direct, and control, what they actually *do* is quite different. Managers fill three different types of roles: interpersonal roles, informational roles and decisional roles. The interpersonal roles include ceremonial duties (such as attendance at an awards dinner), leadership, and the role of liaison. The informational role includes scanning the environment for any useful information and seeking ways to improve work methods. The decisional role includes deciding how to allocate resources (such as space or the amount of money available for giving raises), negotiating, and handling disturbances. Finally, the manager is also an entrepreneur, always alert to new ideas and new opportunities to expand and improve the effectiveness and profitability of the unit or the whole organization. As you read, you will see that the components of effective management are derived from both points of view represented by the ideas of Fayol and Mintzberg.

Practicing Management

From the outside, the manager's job looks easy. To staff members, it seems as if the nurse manager sits in the office writing reports, goes to many meetings, and occasionally makes rounds, asking questions about the work being done. The manager does not have to run from medications to monitors, respond to call lights, watch critical patients, get charting done, or new admissions stabilized. From all outward appearances, the nurse manager's job is easier than the staff nurse's job.

However, if you become a first-line manager (such as a head nurse, unit coordinator, or supervisor in community health), it will suddenly become apparent to you that you now have much more responsibility (Research Example 4–1). As a first-line manager, you are responsible for all of the care given by your staff. You will soon realize that it would be impossible for you to do all of this work yourself, even if you wanted to do it. If you had not thought about it before, you suddenly realize that, although you do have some authority over staff members, in another sense you are also dependent upon them to get the work done and that you will need a great deal of skill to do this well. Let us look now at each of the components of effective management in order to see what it is that makes a manager effective at working through others.

RESEARCH EXAMPLE 4–1. Tasks of First–Line Nurse Managers

What do first-line nurse managers do? Beaman developed a list of tasks done by nurse managers in acute care settings in Los Angeles. The questionnaire included tasks in each of the traditional functional areas of management: planning, staffing, controlling, directing, and organizing. Altogether, 109 questionnaires were mailed and 73 (67%) were returned.

When the responses were analyzed, Beaman found that 31 tasks had been selected by more than 50% of the people responding. The tasks included the following (some are combined):

▷ Assist inservice to prepare orientation schedule.
▷ Discuss the program of orientation with the new staff member.
▷ Decide when orientation is complete.
▷ Write counseling reports and discuss them with staff members.
▷ Discuss the need for termination.
▷ Terminate after approval has been obtained.
▷ Submit time schedule for three shifts.
▷ Assign patients, teams for day shift.
▷ Make recommendations about budget to nursing administration.
▷ Calculate nursing hours used and justify them.
▷ Call in extra help when needed.
▷ Prepare reports about budget variances.
▷ Make daily patient rounds.
▷ Attend and participate in first-line nursing management meetings.
▷ Conduct meetings with own staff for problem solving and learning.
▷ Set goals for individual unit.
▷ Participate in setting goals for the nursing department.
▷ Discuss unit problems with physicians regularly.
▷ Participate in all levels of quality assurance including designing the studies, collecting the data, and preparing reports.

The reader may want to compare these activities with the components of effective management discussed in this book.

LEADERSHIP

Because managers work through other people, their leadership skills are very important. In fact, some people actually believe that it is possible to be a generic manager, one who can effectively plan, direct, monitor, and evaluate any group of people, no matter what kind of work they do. Even if this is not true (it is particularly difficult to provide good direction or to evaluate outcomes if you do not know how to do the work yourself), this notion emphasizes the importance of the manager's leadership skills.

Without leadership skills, a manager may develop appropriate plans for the group, post a fair working schedule, and reward people fairly but still have difficulty getting people to work. This is because the manager has ignored the relationship aspects of the situation. Personality conflicts, communication problems, and immature groups are common problems that do not go away if they are ignored. In fact, they usually get worse. In short, it is possible to be a manager without being a leader but it is not possible to be a good manager without being a leader. Being an effective leader means developing self awareness, acquiring adequate knowledge and skill, using critical thinking, practicing good communication, recognizing and reconciling differences in goals, and using your energy wisely in taking action when it is needed. All of these are *prerequisites* for being an effective manager.

PLANNING

Planning is the component of effective management that is hardest to do and easiest to ignore. Because it deals primarily with the future, planning can be postponed unless deadlines are set or unless you make it part of your objectives for a particular period of time. In fact, if you do not specifically set aside time to do it or are required by your administration to do it, you probably will not do much planning despite its long term importance. Other more immediate demands can easily fill your day and leave no time for planning.

Planning is the essential link between good intentions and action (Kraegel, 1983). Without it, good ideas rarely become realities. Good planning requires a broad knowledge of the organization's operations and goals, detailed knowledge of your own department or unit, technical knowledge, and intuition, coupled with a keen awareness of changes and current trends affecting your area of health care.

The popular image of a manager who has time to sit quietly in the office thinking and planning has no basis in reality according to Mintzberg (1975) who found that a manager's work pace is unrelenting and that managers are bombarded with telephone calls, interruptions, problems, and crises all day long. People often call the manager's response to these immediate demands "putting out the brush fires." This firefighting can take up all of your time if you do not get control of it.

Most managers, then, spend most of their time responding to the immediate demands of their jobs. The planning that they do is often in their heads and involves tentative ideas of what they would like to see done next, either immediately or in the future.

Despite these obstacles, planning is an important component of effective management. There are several types of planning that need to be done. First, it is important to carefully plan your own time, called time management. Second, it is important to plan the work to be done by your group. Third, it is important to plan the future direction of your unit or department.

Time Management

"Work smarter, not harder," is the theme of time management. Time is finite and the effective manager must make the best use of the time available. Achieving an effective balance is probably the most difficult part (Dorney, 1988). Time management strategies help you organize and plan your time as much as is possible. There are some time demands that you simply will not be able to control such as a mandatory meeting, an outbreak of flu in the staff, or a patient's cardiac arrest, but you can manage these demands. You can, for example, determine whether or not the meeting is really mandatory and what you would gain or lose by not attending.

For a crisis, you need to have contingency plans. You need to have planned ahead of time how you can respond, what alternatives are available and which actions will be most effective. For example, should you request temporary personnel to replace your absent staff members or ask other staff members to work overtime? Should you fill in yourself? Each of these alternatives has its advantages and disadvantages and knowing these ahead of time will prepare you to respond quickly and efficiently during a crisis.

Time management includes eliminating unnecessary work, streamlining and organizing your work, and delegating work when possible. You may have to be quite creative in devising ways to make the best use of your time. Identifying and observing other people who manage their time well is another useful source of ideas about time management. The effective manager not only manages his or her own time as well as possible but also helps staff members do so. More details about time management can be found in Chapter 12.

Planning Current Work

Work done haphazardly is usually work done inefficiently. The work load is simply too great in most health care settings to allow this. In planning how current work is done, you need to consider several factors: priorities, timing and sequence, deadlines, organizational goals, skill mix of staff, and characteristics of the work.

PRIORITIES. Some work must be done before the day is over, no matter what else happens. Other work can be postponed. The work must be prioritized, i.e., done in order beginning with the most important and urgent tasks. But when necessary work is postponed, it is important that it not be forgotten. Physical care, for example, is often given priority over emotional care in acute care settings. Yet, the emotional needs of many patients may actually be the most acute need and the effects of its postponement will soon become apparent.

TIMING AND SEQUENCE. Some tasks must be done before others can be begun. For example, consents must be signed before preoperative medication takes effect and report given before patient care begins.

DEADLINES. Deadlines are imposed times by which a task must be done. The time may be specified within a physician order, by another department, or by upper-level management.

ORGANIZATIONAL GOALS. Priority goals of the organization, such as a renewed emphasis on risk management or on good patient-provider relations, should also be considered.

SKILL MIX OF STAFF. The ability and experience of staff members is also important. Some assignments simply cannot be given to auxiliary staff according to legal and professional standards of practice. Individual ability and experience must also be considered and you will want to make the best use of any specially skilled staff members.

CHARACTERISTICS OF THE WORK. Some nursing tasks require technical skill and precise timing, such as the administration of intravenous medications. Others require a high level of knowledge and judgment but have flexible timing, such as nutritional education. The timing of the first needs to be exact, the timing of the second needs to be flexible. The selection of the appropriate staff member to carry out these two different tasks should consider the abilities, preferences, and availability of the individuals involved.

This may seem like a large number of factors to keep in mind but they are all important. The effective manager considers each one in planning the daily and weekly work of the unit or team.

Planning Future Work

Planning future work is what most people think of when they hear the word planning. The effective manager plans for the future rather than waiting to see what the future will bring. Change is rapid in health care. Some nursing units or teams have been eliminated or reduced in some places. Some services may actually become altogether obsolete while others such as intensive care units have multiplied rapidly. The effective manager must be aware of these general trends as well as more specific, local ones that could affect the work, even the existence, of the unit. For example:

> The nurse-manager of the maternity unit watched the statistics for the unit carefully and realized that the number of births at the hospital was declining very slowly but steadily. Several neighborhood hospitals had been talking about closing their maternity units. It was clear that the population of the community was aging and could not support all of the existing services; some maternity units would soon close.
>
> The nurse-manager believed that the staff was highly skilled and provided excellent care but that the community did not recognize any differences between their services and those at other hospitals. The nurse-manager decided to embark upon a campaign to keep the unit open. The first step was to enlist the support of the staff nurses and then the obstetricians and pediatricians, who agreed to keep sending their patients to the unit. The head nurse met with the nursing staff to plan ways to make their unit particularly attractive to expectant parents so that they would request this particular hospital. With the staff, a plan was formulated to add birthing rooms, grandparent classes, and sibling visitation. Prenatal classes were videotaped so that women working outside the home could watch them at home or on their own time at the hospital and then meet for just one or two question and answer sessions. The new services were so well received that the local newspaper ran a story entitled "Local Hospital Caters to Needs of Expectant Moms."

Some plans may involve very complex organization-wide change while many others will be on a far smaller scale and involve such things as the introduction of an improved technique, new piece of equipment, new staffing patterns, a new flow sheet, and so forth. Whether on a small or grand scale, however, future planning is a very important part of the effective manager's functions.

DIRECTION

The effective manager provides direction to staff members. The amount of direction needed varies with the knowledge, experience, and initiative of individual staff members and the group as a whole. Everyone, however, needs some direction, no matter how small that amount may be. People need to know (1) what is expected of them, and (2) how to do it. The knowledgeable staff member will either know how to do the assigned task or how to obtain the needed information but will still need some direction about how the work has been divided among members of the team. The less experienced, less knowledgeable staff member will also need assistance with the how to do it part. This assistance does not necessarily have to come from the nurse-manager; it may be delegated to the more experienced staff members.

Work Assignment

Assigning work is one of the most fundamental managerial responsibilities. Only the most passive, laissez-faire manager might fail to make work assignments. Doing it effectively, however, requires consideration of a number of factors. In particular, ability of staff members and fairness of the assignment must be considered. Failure to do so is dangerous to patients and demoralizing to staff. Other factors to consider include efficiency, continuity, staff preferences, and learning opportunities for staff members.

Another important principle in making work assignments is to assign to strength, not away from weakness. The difference is subtle but important. Assigning to strength means that you select the person who can do a job well. Assigning from weakness means that you focus on avoiding staff weaknesses when delegating (Batten, 1988). For example:

> You know that Nurse X has had a great deal of difficulty being supportive to families of terminally ill patients and yet can handle a crisis situation with calm assurance and skill. If you assigned to weakness, you would avoid assigning Nurse X to any terminally ill patients whose families were frequently present and required much support. In doing this, you are very likely to give Nurse X a subtle message that Nurse X cannot be trusted with the care of grieving families, or even with the terminally ill. A more positive approach is to give Nurse X an assignment that requires dealing with patients in crises, an area where Nurse X excels.

The difference is very subtle but staff members are sensitive to these subtleties. Assigning to strength will contribute to positive esteem and higher morale among staff members while the opposite reduces esteem and morale.

Delegating work is rarely a simple task despite its being such a fundamental managerial responsibility. A number of conflicting demands may confront you when trying to make a fair assignment. These can include staff shortages, special requests from various staff members, and unpleasant or undesirable work that must be done. Some managers have difficulty delegating work at all. They try to do too much of the work themselves and wind up exhausted and frustrated, unable to fulfill their managerial responsibilities while trying to do other people's work. More detail on these and other dilemmas in making work assignments can be found in Chapter 18.

Job Descriptions

A job description is a formal, written listing of the work expected of an individual holding a particular position. A nurse aide's job description would be quite different from a nurse executive's job description, but they both should have job descriptions for several reasons.

A job description tells you what is expected of you in your position and what you can expect of other people in their positions. This information is particularly helpful when you are considering a new job and when there is some disagreement about what you are supposed to do in a particular position. You can also use a job description to clarify expectations when they are vague. A number of nurses who find themselves in newly created positions find it worthwhile to take the time to write their own job descriptions and obtain administrative approval for them. It is usually not necessary to do this in staff positions and you will find that some organizations have already developed very clear job descriptions.

Staffing and Scheduling

A great deal of time and effort has been put into devising workable staffing and scheduling patterns for nurses, particularly for nurses in acute care settings. The great number of different approaches (12 hour shifts, weekend staff, four day weeks, temporary pools, and job sharing are a few examples) gives us an idea just how complex and difficult it has been to find a cost-effective, quality-ensuring method of staffing units and scheduling work shifts.

Rapid turnover, retrenchment (the reduction in the total number of budgeted staff positions), nursing shortages, large proportions of auxiliary staff, use of temporary personnel, and the increased sophistication of nursing interventions all make staffing and scheduling a matter of achieving a delicate balance between patient, staff, and organizational needs. The needs and wishes of individual staff members, for example, have to be weighed against the needs of the unit as a whole. At times, you will wish that you had the wisdom of a King Solomon. Even when these decisions are centralized and computerized, requests for changes will have to be considered. The ability to distinguish between a true emergency and a desire to take it easy becomes very important and your fairness in approving and denying requests will have a great impact on the smooth operation of your unit.

One effective approach to reducing the number of conflicts arising from staffing and scheduling necessities is to use participative management. You will recall that participative management means including staff in decision making. The most democratic manager will allow staff members as a group to plan their own schedules; others will invite staff comments and suggestions and incorporate them in the scheduling or staffing routine. Whichever way you choose (your choice may be restricted by administrative policies), you will probably find that staff members have some creative ideas and that when their ideas are implemented, staff members will be far more committed to them and cooperative in keeping the unit adequately staffed than they would be under imposed routines. In other words, staff members can assume a great deal of responsibility for self-policing when given the opportunity.

Technical Direction

Giving technical direction is a somewhat tricky business. Some nurse managers give far too much with the result that they interfere with the functioning of their units by constantly "suggesting" better ways to do things. In the extreme case, this can immobilize the unit. Staff members feel as if they should not take a single step without the manager's approval. Also, there is usually more than one correct way to do something and the manager who steps in too often may be correcting individual style more than substantial mistakes.

The opposite, of course, is the nurse manager who gives no technical direction at all, often in the belief that people should take the initiative to learn on their own. While this is true, it can be carried to extremes and staff members can be deprived of the information needed to perform well.

The quantity of nursing literature and changes in nursing care have been increasing geometrically. It is difficult for staff members to find time to sift through all the information that pertains to their work (Broadwell & House, 1986). The nurse manager is in a good position to do some preliminary sifting, sorting and condensing of information, channeling information to the group and eliminating the obviously irrelevant and repetitious material. A great deal of information also circulates within any organization and you can help your staff deal with it all by summarizing the main points and clarifying how changes will affect the unit.

The means by which information and direction are shared is also important. The effective manager avoids taking over for other people. A typical way in which this is done is "Let me show you how to do it" (Lashbrook, 1986). This approach is usually well meaning but often irritating to the professional staff member because of its implied message, "I can do this better than you can." The goal in giving direction and technical assistance is to inform without criticism, implied or direct.

The climate within which people work influences the way in which they seek information. In some work settings, admitting a need for information is equal to admitting personal inadequacy. The result is that learning needs are concealed and that people seek information indirectly and surreptitiously. In contrast, an open, trusting climate encourages people to freely and spontaneously seek and share information without any concern for being put down. In fact, information seeking and learning are rewarded in this environment.

MONITORING _____

Once you have given directions to staff members, can you then sit back and wait for results? Of course not. The effective manager monitors the

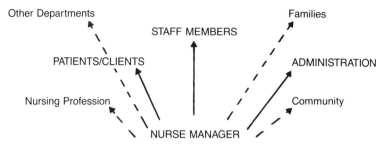

Figure 4–3. Constituencies of the nurse manager.

staff's progress at regular intervals. But that is not all that a manager needs to monitor. The first-line nurse manager has responsibility to several constituencies. The three major constituencies are: the staff, the patients or clients, and the administration (Fig. 4–3). In addition, the first-line nurse manager must also consider other groups such as other departments or units, the patients' families and significant others, the nursing profession, and so forth. We will focus, however, on the three major constituencies whose interests are the major concern of the nurse manager in deciding what should be monitored.

The patients' or clients' major concern would be with the quality of the care given by the staff. The organization's major concern would be with the effectiveness of the staff and the resulting satisfaction of the clients. The staff's major concern would be in serving the clients well and in being treated well by the organization. Some of these interests are primarily served by the monitoring function of the nurse manager; others are primarily served by the representation function which is the final component of effective management.

The nurse manager is concerned with the adequacy of functioning of individual staff members. The nurse manager is also concerned with the adequacy of the functioning of the unit as a whole. To ensure this adequacy, a number of different aspects of the individual staff member's and the unit's functioning should be monitored. Some of these are listed below to give you an idea of what might need regular scanning by the nurse manager.

Individual Staff Members

The following is a list of some items to consider in monitoring the work of individual staff members:

▷ Absenteeism
▷ Late Arrivals, Early Departures
▷ Adherence to Professional Standards
▷ Adherence to Standards of Ethical Behavior
▷ Conformity to Legal Standards of Practice
▷ Excellence in Provision of Patient Care
▷ Excellence in Recording Patient Care and its Outcomes
▷ Ability to Work with Other Staff Members
▷ Pursuit of Professional Growth
▷ Leadership

The type of unit, type of care given, ability and experience of the staff, and similar factors will help determine how often each of the items needs to be monitored. Some, such as absenteeism, require daily scanning. Others, such as adherence to professional standards, require weekly or monthly scanning unless a problem has arisen that alerts you to the need for more frequent monitoring.

The Unit as a Whole

The following is a list of some items to consider in monitoring the unit as a whole:

▷ Patient Census
▷ Number of Clinic Visits, Home Visits
▷ Incidence of Infection
▷ Incidence of Falls, Decubiti, and so forth
▷ Injuries to Staff
▷ Relationships with Other Departments
▷ Comparison with Other Units
▷ Cost Overruns
▷ Staff Requirements
▷ Compliance with Regulatory Requirements
▷ Compliance with Professional Standards (such as National League for Nursing or the Joint Commission on Accreditation of Hospitals)

Monitoring Methods

There are a number of ways to collect the information needed to monitor the activities and outcomes on your unit. Direct observation is one of the most important. As you make your rounds, you can make on-the-spot suggestions and corrections as needed (discussed in detail in Chapter 21 on providing informal feedback). You can also ask individual staff members to tell you how they are progressing. This is particularly useful when a staff member has experienced some difficulty that you are trying to resolve together, when a new or particularly complex task is being done, or when evaluating progress toward objectives that were set during the initial phase of the formal evaluation procedure.

There are also more formal methods of monitoring. Peer review procedures and chart audits are often used to monitor adherence to standards of care. Formal employee performance appraisals are held at regular intervals to inform employees about the degree to which they are performing at expected levels. These formal evaluations should also serve as the means by which decisions about pay raises and promotions are made. Finally, numerous reports can be obtained or generated regarding the incidence of accidents or infections, budget overruns, or other occurrences of which you need to keep track. Comparisons with the statistics for other units and with previous years for your unit usually give you an idea of areas where improvement is occurring or, conversely, where there is a problem developing. If the purpose of monitoring can be summarized in one sentence, it is to identify such trends and problems early while they are still small and to prevent them from becoming big problems.

RECOGNITION AND REWARDS

The purpose of giving recognition and rewards is to retain good employees, and to motivate them to continue to be as productive as possible. In other words, the effective manager uses rewards to encourage desired behaviors. It would seem that people who do the best work should receive the most rewards and that employers would reward the behavior that is most desired. But this is not always the case. Often there is a great deal of subjectivity in rewards systems and some paradoxical reasoning (more accurately, lack of reasoning) in the ways rewards are given. Before considering these, however, let us look first at what kinds of rewards are available to the first-line nurse manager.

Types of Rewards

The effective manager uses as broad a range of rewards as possible. The positive ones include raises and promotions but there are many others that, while they are less dramatic, also serve to reward desired behavior. In fact, one author has said this even more strongly. "The weight of managers' feedback," says Huntsman, "has credibility beyond a manager's wildest dreams" (1987, p. 52). Simple positive feedback is often overlooked or underestimated as a means to reward desired behavior. Recognition by one's peers is another which the nurse manager can foster by announcing achievements at staff meetings and using the organizational newsletter to recognize achievements. It is also possible to reward staff members by giving them challenging assignments and seeking interesting opportunities either within the unit or somewhere else within the organization.

Negative rewards are also available to the nurse manager. Termination of employment is the most extreme example of negative rewards. Other examples include negative feedback, a very necessary component of the manager's repertoire, and the omission of challenging assignments or other special recognition for those who have not earned it.

Determining Rewards

To the non-management person, a manager's ability to give or deny rewards can make the manager seem quite powerful. In reality, however, you will find that a manager faces a number of restrictions in giving these rewards. Both the policies and preferences of upper-level management (the first-line manager's bosses) are some of the most common and sometimes severe restrictions. In some organizations, first-line managers only evaluate staff members. The recommendations for raises and promotions come from higher up the management chain and may or may not agree with the first-line manager's evaluation. Almost every organization restricts the number of promotions and the amount of salary increases that can be given.

Upper management is not the only source of restrictions on the first-line manager's decisions about giving rewards. Managers must also carefully consider the effect of the way in which they are given. If staff members see them as having been given in a fair and objective manner, rewards can be a very effective motivator. But if they seem to be subjective, staff can become destructively competitive, apathetic, or confused in regard to what is really expected of them.

There is a common saying that "the squeaky wheel gets the grease." If this is true on your unit, that is, if it is true that the staff member who demands attention or who would complain loudly if dissatisfied gets more than the quieter staff members, it will be obvious to staff members and will be the source of much resentment and lower motivation. Somewhat paradoxically, the complainer is being rewarded for complaining while the non-complaining, more cooperative staff members receive no reward. This is an example of what one writer calls the "folly of rewarding A while hoping for B" (Kerr, 1986, p. 417). The manner in which rewards are given is probably as important as the size and frequency of the reward.

DEVELOPMENT

Two Schools of Thought

Staff development is not found in the traditional lists of manager functions such as Fayol's plan, organize, command, coordinate, and control or the many variations of that list.

There seems to be two schools of thought about staff development. The first is that staff members are a valuable resource of the organization. As a valuable resource, they should be developed to their fullest extent. Staff development is considered a wise investment in the future growth and development of the organization. The second, opposite, point of view is that little should be spent on staff development. If a particular expertise is needed, go out and look for someone who already has that expertise. Staff members are kept as long as they are useful; when they are no longer useful, they are discarded.

The first school of thought about staff development clearly resembles Theory Z (Ouchi, 1981). Employees are expected and encouraged to remain with the organization a long time. When the employee's skills become obsolete, employees are retrained, not discarded. The result is a far more loyal staff with a higher degree of security and a much higher level of commitment to the organization. Employees feel valued and they function accordingly. This approach also encourages employees to work cooperatively while the second approach encourages competition and fosters a climate of insecurity. Under that second "use and discard," approach, staff members often feel threatened and are far more concerned about their own future than about the future of the organization.

Encouraging Staff Development

The effective manager takes responsibility not only for his or her own development but also for development of individual staff members and for the group as a whole. Staff development is a long-term building strategy as distinguished from training which is designed to meet a more specific, immediate learning need (Bernhard & Ingals, 1988). The ways in which staff development can be supported are numerous and will vary somewhat according to what your organization is willing to support financially.

Capable staff members should be encouraged to continue their education, particularly if the organization assists them in paying their tuition. All staff members should be encouraged to attend continuing education programs, even if they are not required for license renewal in your state. The educational gain, not license renewal, should be the major motivator for attendance at continuing education programs. If it is at all possible, staff members should be given time off for continuing education rather than asking them to use vacation time to pursue continued learning. They can also be encouraged to attend programs given within the organization.

Some nurse managers have, unfortunately, developed the habit of attending all of these programs themselves, forgetting to encourage other staff members to attend as well. Sending staff members to these programs is usually perceived as a reward or a sign of positive regard from the manager.

Much learning can also take place within the unit or team itself. People who do engage in continued learning activities should be encouraged to share their new knowledge with the rest of the staff in both formal and informal ways. This can be done through informal discussion or it can be formally planned for conference time or staff meetings. Problem solving conferences should also be designed to be learning experiences. Different staff members, for example, may be assigned to prepare for the conferences on a rotating basis to share the work and to share the leadership experience that this provides. Some groups of nurses have also formed lunchtime or after work discussion groups to network and share information.

One final comment about staff development. A frequent complaint about staff development programs is that what is taught is often not put into practice after the person has returned to work. This complaint is often heard about leadership and management workshops but it applies to all types of continuing education. Typically, the staff member or manager returns from the workshop full of enthusiasm for the new approach or ideas developed at the workshop only to find it so difficult to implement them that the enthusiasm quickly dies and is soon forgotten. Sharing workshop experiences with other staff members can help prevent this loss but the nurse manager should also actively assist the staff member in applying the new ideas to the work setting.

REPRESENTATION

Like staff development, representation is another component of effective management not found in the traditional organize, plan, control, and direct list. And yet, as Mintzberg (1975) points out, a manager can spend a great deal of time representing his or her group of staff members. How your manager represents you is a matter of vital interest to most employees. It can also be a source of conflict for the nurse manager who finds herself or himself in the middle — between staff and the upper management people to whom the nurse manager must report, two of the three constituencies mentioned earlier. We will first consider the many different ways in which the manager represents staff members and administration and then look briefly at the way in which conflict can arise in fulfilling this representation function.

Representing Staff Members

The first-line manager typically represents the staff in discussions with other departments and with upper management, speaking on behalf of the staff's needs, requests, and rights. The following are examples of how this occurs in some ordinary situations:

> For security reasons, the administrator of a large city hospital was considering the enforcement of limited visiting hours. Keeping visiting hours confined to five hours in the late afternoon and early evening would make it possible to control the flow of people in and out of the hospital. When this was announced, the nurse manager of the pediatric unit said that the nursing staff would find this restriction on parents nontherapeutic and therefore strongly inadvisable. The head nurse of the oncology unit agreed and the idea was reconsidered and then dropped.

> The physical therapy department decided to open at seven a.m. so that their staff could finish and go home early. The rehabilitation unit coordinator, however, pointed out that this would mean the night shift staff on the nursing units would have to begin morning care and there was not enough personnel on this shift to do so. The physical therapy department had to give up their plan to begin at seven.

> A small county public health unit had expanded its services to include primary care. This change meant an extension of the working day to include some evenings and Saturday work for the existing staff. The public health nursing supervisor successfully negotiated overtime payments for the public health nurses who would be working more than their regular forty hours per week and made the overtime voluntary instead of mandatory.

In the three examples given above, the nurse managers were acting primarily as *advocates* for their staff members.

Another important role in representing one's department is to act as a *coordinator*, ensuring adequate communication and smooth operations between different departments within the organization and with outside agencies (such as the need to be consistent in care given at home and in the inpatient unit of a hospice program). A third important role is to act as the *promoter* for the unit, convincing others of the value and quality of the work done by the unit and seeking opportunities to expand or to improve the function of the unit. This last role is a new but important one for most nurses. It is also in keeping with the competitive spirit of the times. Patient education is an area that provides a good example of this promoter role:

> The Coordinator of Patient Education was shocked to see that the proposed budget for the patient education department had been cut in half for the next year. Two diabetes educators and one childbirth educator would lose their jobs if this budget was implemented. The Coordinator demanded an explanation and was told that the hospital would no longer support departments that did not contribute to the organization's profits. At the very least, the patient education department would have to support itself, i.e., bring in enough money to cover the cost of operating the department.
>
> This new requirement demanded a radical change in thinking for the patient educators. They had thought of themselves as professionals who provided a needed service but had not considered the cost of the individual patient teaching that was their primary activity. After a series of brainstorming and planning sessions, the group as a whole decided that they would do more group teaching, design more self-learning materials, and use the closed circuit television system more effectively. They also planned to do a series of programs for the community for which a reasonable fee would be charged. The Coordinator began planning and publicizing these programs, and also planned to market their services to corporations who would pay for their health promotion programs. In addition,

the Coordinator made an increased effort to provide needed services to as many units and departments in the hospital as possible in order to gain their support for the continued operation of the patient education department.

Representing Administration

Everyone who works has at least one boss and many people have more than one boss. The first-line manager, for example, usually reports to second-line managers, such as supervisors, assistant directors, or directors of nursing. As a first-line manager, you would be expected to contribute to the achievement of the organization's goals and to carry out whatever functions and tasks have been delegated to you by upper management. The manager is expected to support the organization's policies and procedures. When these are incorrect or ineffective, however, the effective manager takes the responsibility of challenging them and working to change them.

A very common situation in which the manager is expected to represent administration is when a new policy is put into practice. This policy could be anything from a change in signing-in procedures to a change in the way that families are informed when a patient dies. Whatever the change is, the nurse manager is expected to inform staff members of the change, explain the policy and then to ensure that it is implemented.

First-line managers are also expected to represent administration in communicating such personnel decisions as granting raises, promoting people, and firing people. When the decisions have been made in a participative manner in which the manager's recommendations are given serious consideration, this responsibility causes little conflict between representing administration and representing the staff. However, when the manager does not agree with the decision, this responsibility can cause a tremendous amount of conflict in which you are caught between your responsibility to administration and to the staff. Choosing sides and supporting one against the other is not the best approach because it may lead to long term alienation from the other side. An authoritarian administration may force you into such a position. A better way to handle the situation is through the negotiation of your differences with either or both sides in the issue.

MANAGEMENT EFFECTIVENESS CHECKLIST _____

Like the Leadership Effectiveness Checklist, this list is meant to provide you with a way to review your management effectiveness in a deliberate and thoughtful way (Fig. 4–4). It is not a short little quiz that will give you a score but a review of the major points in the description of the effective manager. If you are not in a managerial position at the present time, you may want to read it now for a review of this chapter but save it as self evaluation tool for the time when you do occupy a managerial position.

SUMMARY _____

Management is often defined as planning, directing, coordinating, and controlling but it includes more than this. The components of effective management include leadership, planning, giving direction, developing

	VERY MUCH	SOME-WHAT	NOT AT ALL
A. LEADERSHIP			
1. Have you reviewed the leadership checklist?			
Are you . . .			
Developing self awareness?			
Acquiring adequate knowledge and skill?			
Using critical thinking?			
Practicing good communication?			
Recognizing and reconciling differences in goals?			
Using your energy wisely?			
2. Do you give your attention to both the human (relationship) and business (task) aspects of your responsibilities?			
B. PLANNING			
1. Do you set aside time for planning?			
2. Do you manage your time by . . .			
Preparing for emergencies and crises?			
Making the best use of your time?			
Helping staff members manage their time well?			
3. Do you plan current work and consider . . .			
Priorities?			
Timing and Sequence?			
Deadlines?			
Organizational Goals?			
Skill Mix of the Staff?			
Characteristics of the Work?			
4. Do you plan for the future of your department?			
C. DIRECTION			
1. Do you communicate clearly to staff . . .			
What is expected of them?			
How to do the work?			
Do you do this in a non-threatening manner?			
2. Do you ensure that everyone has a job description?			
3. Do you prepare schedules that are . . .			
Fair and adequate to meet the needs of the unit?			
Developed in consideration of staff suggestions?			

Figure 4–4. Management effectiveness checklist.

	VERY MUCH	SOME-WHAT	NOT AT ALL
D. MONITORING			
1. Do you monitor . . .			
The care given by your staff?			
Individual staff members' performance			
The budget?			
Operation of the unit as a whole?			
2. Do you monitor in a systematic manner?			
3. Do you use a variety of formal and informal monitoring methods?			
E. REWARDS			
1. Do you utilize a variety of both positive and negative rewards?			
2. Do you use rewards to reinforce only the behaviors that are desired and not other, less desirable behavior?			
F. DEVELOPMENT			
1. Do you encourage staff development by . . .			
Rewarding it?			
Making opportunities available?			
Supporting implementation of what is learned?			
2. Have you furthered your own professional growth and development?			
G. REPRESENTATION			
1. In representing staff members and the unit as a whole, do you function as . . .			
An advocate?			
A coordinator?			
A promoter?			
2. Do you support administration actions and represent them fairly to your staff?			
3. Do you enforce administration policy?			
4. When an administration action or policy is ineffective in some way, do you work to change it?			
5. When differences between your staff and the administration occur, do you work to negotiate an acceptable settlement?			

Figure 4–4. *Continued.*

staff, monitoring operations, giving rewards fairly, and representing both staff members and administration as needed.

The effective first-line manager sets aside time for planning. The time of both manager and staff should be put to the best use possible and this can only be done with planning and organization. Planning of current work requires consideration of a number of factors including priorities, timing and sequencing of work, deadlines, organizational goals, the skills of the staff, and characteristics of the work. The future of the unit should be well thought out in terms of currents trends, both general and specific.

Staff members need to know what is expected of them and how to carry out their assigned work. The effective manager sees to it that staff are well informed about the operation of the unit, and that staffing and scheduling plans are both fair and adequate.

The work of individual staff members, the quality of the care given by the unit as a whole, and a number of other factors are monitored on a regular basis by the effective manager. Both formal and informal methods can be used including direct observation, peer review, formal performance appraisals, a variety of specific reports, the budget, and so forth.

Recognition can be either positive or negative. The first-line manager actually experiences a number of restrictions in carrying out this managerial responsibility, particularly from upper management. The effective manager also carefully considers staff response to reward distribution, attempting as much as possible to reward desired, not undesirable, behavior.

Both the manager and staff members should continue to grow and develop as professionals. The effective manager not only provides a number of opportunities for this growth and development but also ensures that the environment of the unit is conducive to implementation of new ideas and provides challenges to capable staff members.

Finally, the effective manager actively represents his or her staff, acting as an advocate, coordinator and promoter in dealings with other departments, upper management, and other agencies. When conflicts arise between the needs, requests, and rights of staff members and the wishes of administration, the effective manager attempts to negotiate a fair and equitable agreement between these two important constituencies.

REFERENCES*

Batten, J.D. (1988). Leading by expectation. *Management World, 17,* 35–36.

*Beaman, A.L. (1986). What do first-line nursing managers do? *Journal of Nursing Administration, 16,* 6–9.

*Bernhard, H.B. & Ingals, C.A. (1988). Six lessons for the corporate classroom. *Harvard Business Review,* 88:5, 40–48.

Broadwell, M.M. & House, R.S. (1986). *Supervising technical and professional people.* New York: John Wiley.

*Dorney, R.C. (1988). Making time to manage. *Harvard Business Review,* 88:1, 38–40.

Huntsman, A.J. (1987). A model for employee development. *Nursing Management, 18,* (2), 51–54.

*Kerr, S. (1986). On the folly of rewarding A while hoping for B. In Williamson, J.N. (ed.) *The Leader-Manager.* New York: John Wiley.

*Kraegel, J.M. (1983). *Planning strategies for nurse managers.* Rockville, Md: Aspen Systems.

*Lashbrook, S.B. (1986). Management as a performance system. In Williamson, J.N. (ed.) *The Leader-Manager.* New York: John Wiley.

*Mintzberg, H. (1975). The manager's job: Folklore and fact. *Harvard Business Review.* 53, 49–61.

Ouchi, W.G. (1981). *Theory Z: How American business can meet the Japanese challenge.* Reading, Mass: Addison-Wesley.

Wren, D.A. (1972). *The evolution of management thought.* New York: Ronald Press.

*References marked with an asterisk are recommended for further reading.

Chapter 5

THE CONTEXT: A CHANGING ENVIRONMENT

Chapter 5

OUTLINE

Evolution of the Health Care System
The Early Period
Scientific, Technologic, and Social
    Expansion
Growth and Prosperity
Skepticism and Disillusionment

Health Care Finances Today
Retrospective Payment
Impact of Prospective Payment

Marketing
Definition
Marketing Techniques
Importance to Nursing

The Image of Nursing
Image Problems
Image Improvement

Summary

LEARNING OBJECTIVES

Upon completion of this chapter, the reader will be able to:

▷ Trace the evolution of the current U.S. health care system.

▷ Assess the impact of prospective payment and a business orientation on health care and nursing leadership and management.

▷ Apply some basic techniques to the marketing of a particular type of nursing service.

▷ Discuss the impact of today's image of nursing on the nursing profession and on nursing leadership.

THE CONTEXT: A CHANGING ENVIRONMENT*

Change has become a cardinal feature of the way we live. Social, political, economic, and technological changes have been especially rapid in the past twenty-five years, affecting the health care delivery system, governmental roles in the lives of individuals and communities, our expectations of health care, and the role of women in society. All of these have had a great impact on the nursing profession and all have implications for the leadership roles and actions we must take to ensure professional survival and growth in an increasingly complex world.

In this chapter, we will look first at those broad changes in society which particularly impact on the health care system and on the nursing profession. It is a fairly long story but one that helps us understand the current situation in health care. Several of the important issues facing us today, including marketing and the image of nursing, will be discussed. It is these trends and issues that shape the environment in which we work, the context in which we provide leadership and management.

EVOLUTION OF THE HEALTH CARE SYSTEM _____

The Early Period

Social welfare programs as we know them today did not exist in colonial America. Any help or assistance that was available came from family, friends, neighbors, or church members. Health care was given primarily by lay practitioners using a variety of remedies and treatments selected by trial and error, and by folk recommendations rather than by research. Health care was not yet organized and the hospitals and community agencies that are so familiar to us today did not exist.

The modern health care system really began in the mid-nineteenth century. In the United States, the casualties of the Civil War focused attention on the need for hospitals, surgeons, and nurses. Most health care still remained outside the walls of any organized institution and in the hands of the individual practitioner.

The establishment of the nation's first large hospitals, Bellevue in New York and Massachusetts General in Boston, marked the beginning of the institutionalization of health care. By the early 1900's sanitation had been

---

*Co-authored by Patricia Lund, R.N., Ed.D. and Ruth M. Tappen, R.N., Ed.D.

substantially improved. Various voluntary organizations were established, such as the Mental Health Society in 1909 and the American Cancer Society in 1913. Some organized charities, such as the Red Cross, began to be recognized for their contributions to the health and welfare of the population (Spradley, 1985). Most nurses then worked independently as a private duty nurse would do today. Hospitals primarily used student nurses rather than employing graduate nurses to staff their wards. In many cities, visiting nurses were bringing badly needed care to the homes of the poor and ill. By 1910, the larger visiting nurse associations were adding prevention to their services but these preventive measures were soon taken over by the nurses in the developing local public health agencies (Buhler-Wilkerson, 1985).

Scientific, Technologic, and Social Expansion

Science and technology made rapid advances in the period from 1900 to 1940. Vitamins were discovered in 1912, insulin in 1922, and the 1940s saw the introduction of antibiotics. With the availability of effective antibiotic therapy, the nature of the nation's health problems changed dramatically. Improved sanitation, widespread immunization, and antibiotic therapy lessened the threat of infectious disease and chronic diseases (heart disease, cancer, stroke) assumed greater importance.

As more effective technology was developed, the hospital became the favored workplace and began to attract more paying patients. Up until this time, there was no reason for a private patient to go to a hospital because it could not offer any more than the care and services that could be given in a person's own home. Physicians as well as nurses made house calls and private nurses were readily available to work in the home.

The financial troubles of the Depression gave birth to many economic changes including the beginnings of commercial health insurance. A group of Dallas schoolteachers arranged a prepaid plan to provide them with up to 21 days of hospitalization a year for 50 cents a month. This idea was supported by the American Hospital Association which feared a loss of income because people were having trouble paying their bills. The idea quickly gained popularity.

Before World War II, 20 percent of Americans were covered by health insurance; by the 1960s, 70 percent were covered (Torrens, 1978). Today it is an expected part of the employer benefit package. However, most people do not realize how expensive it is. To give an example, Iacocca (1984) claims that approximately $600 of the cost of each automobile and truck manufactured goes towards paying workers' health care benefits. Today, health care insurance pays for approximately 27 percent of all health care costs while out of pocket payments (those made by the individual or family) account for 33 percent. The government, through various programs, pays 40 percent, the largest proportion (Sheridan, 1983).

At about the same time (1935), Congress passed the well known Social Security Act. This Act provides aid to people who are totally disabled, blind, the aged poor, and families with dependent children, now known collectively as the Supplemental Security Income (SSI) program. Social Security also provides pensions to the retired on the basis of contributions made during their working years. This marked the beginning of federal government involvement in social welfare programs.

After the war, many new families were formed. Nineteen forty-six has been identified as the year that the first Baby Boomer was born, a demographic phenomenon of high birth rates which continued through 1964. This population has been attracting attention by its sheer size and progress through the life span. Concern has been expressed about meeting and financing their increasing health care needs in the future as they become the older generation.

The Hill-Burton Program began in 1946 with the purpose of increasing the number of hospital beds in rural areas and redistributing physicians to equalize the availability of medical care. This program extended into the 1960s with the Hill-Harris amendment, providing for the modernization or replacement of public and nonprofit facilities in both urban and rural areas. These bills have been criticized for having concentrated too much on construction and not enough on health care delivery and distribution (Rydman and Rydman, 1983). They were not at all effective in achieving physician redistribution. With Social Security and the Hill-Burton act, the federal government became "firmly and irreversibly part of the American health care system" (Hyman, 1975).

Growth and Prosperity

The New Frontier began in 1961 with the inauguration of President Kennedy who encouraged the development of a sense of altruism. A positive attitude toward helping the people of the world was exemplified by the Peace Corps. The theme of his successor, President Johnson, was the Great Society. People believed that we could conquer health and social problems the same way that we "conquered" space. The application of our vast knowledge and resources would lead us to the envisioned Great Society.

One successful offshoot of space exploration was a tremendous expansion in research and technological development, much of which was applicable and adaptable to health care. Sophisticated monitoring devices became available, making intensive care units possible. New materials and compounds had been developed and found their way into replacement joints and other devices.

In this era of growth and prosperity, the concept of comprehensive medical insurance for older adults finally gained popular support. Compromises were made and in 1965 two separate programs were created, Medicare and Medicaid. Medicare is a federally supported program for the elderly or disabled social security recipient, financed by Social Security payroll deductions. Medicaid is a program for the financially indigent, administered by the states with a combination of federal, state and local funding (Wing, 1976).

Skepticism and Disillusionment

The controversial war in Vietnam and the resignation of President Nixon and several of his top aides following the hearings and trials of the Watergate case increased public skepticism of governmental actions and policies. President Ford signed the National Health Planning and Resources Development Act designed to replace all previous planning programs, including the Hill-Burton program. This Act set forth specific guidelines for health planning and construction of new facilities in which cooperative arrangements among facilities, the elimination of duplication of resources, the identification of priority goals, and the encouragement of the development of Health Maintenance Organizations (HMOs) were the goals. The intent was to influence the supply and demand of services on a statewide level, with input from regional groups known as Health Systems Agencies. Despite substantial budgetary cuts almost yearly, some were still in operation in the late 1980s.

Disillusionment with the unfulfilled promises of the Great Society and its hastily enacted programs (Schlesinger, 1988), perceived loss of the war in Vietnam and the recognition of our dependence on the world's economy affected the way people looked at themselves. Suddenly we were vulnerable and imperfect, facing complex social and economic problems for which there were no simple solutions. It had proven easier to send a person into space than to solve the problems of poverty and ill health here on earth.

Meanwhile, taxes, especially social security taxes, continued to rise and health care costs continued to climb, reaching $248.1 million in 1980 or 9.1 percent of the gross national product. This had increased from $41.9 million and 5.9 percent of the gross national product in 1965, the year in which the Medicare and Medicaid legislation had been approved (Pear, 1986). People began to talk about the limitations of the nation's resources and our ability to continue to finance these programs. In 1980, Reagan was elected president on a platform of fiscal restraint and a return of initiative to the states known as the New Federalism. This concept implies a reduced federal government obligation to serve and protect those who are not capable of helping themselves, providing a "safety net" to assist during crises but not providing full assistance for everyone who is in need. Self-reliance had again become a theme. Much of the responsibility for meeting health and welfare needs was supposed to be returned to state and local government and private, religious, and corporate philanthropy (Jones, 1985).

To reduce taxes and balance the federal budget, spending cuts were deemed necessary. With rapid technological advances, increased government support, and a growing cohort of aged people putting pressure on the Social Security system, health costs continued to increase and became a prime target for reduction measures. An increase in emphasis on prevention, health maintenance, and care outside the hospital is predicted for the future, (Christman, 1987) but how it will be paid for and how effective it will be in reducing our overall expenditures for health care remains to be seen.

In the 1980s, people generally began to accept the concept of self-responsibility for health, particularly in regard to changing health behaviors. Healthier diets and the benefits of exercise were accepted as good ideas. Once an accepted, even glamorous behavior, smoking was banned in many public places because of its deleterious effect on people's health.

But the limits of self-reliance began to become clearer as the 1980s came to an end. The staggering burden of providing care for a family member with Alzheimers' and related diseases has been well publicized and people find the prospect of cognitive loss and the resulting dependency a frightening prospect. Current services are fragmented and unresponsive (Weiler, 1987), and the number of people with severe dementia is expected to increase by 60 percent by the year 2000. Many questions have been raised about our health care system's ability to respond to these needs.

Any complacency left over from the previous decade has been shattered by the growing realization that any member of society could be exposed to AIDS, a disease virtually unknown before 1980. Infectious diseases had *not* been conquered completely, and our health care system is again being challenged to meet the needs of people with another health problem. Infusions of both private and government funds have been needed to support the demand for both research and new health care services for people with AIDS. An estimated $1.1 billion was spent on AIDS care in 1986 and predictions run from $8 billion to $16 billion by 1991 (Buchanan, 1988). A gradual realization that some health problems are so big, so widespread, and so demanding of resources that only an all-out effort of both government and private sectors could meet the challenge, has come to health care professionals and the public alike. In fact, the AIDS problem has reminded us that such health problems do not respect national borders and are really an international concern.

HEALTH CARE FINANCES TODAY

Retrospective Payment

Up until this time, private insurance and some government programs simply reimbursed the providers of health care services, especially hospitals, on the basis of what it had cost to provide these services. This meant that there was no incentive for either the consumer or health care provider to be cautious about expenditures or to seek lower cost or alternative methods of care and treatment. Health care was given as ordered with little questioning of physicians' decisions either by the hospital, insuror, or consumer.

Private insurors and others who pay the bills, including the employers and unions who pay the premiums for health care benefits, began to question the cost of health care. They began to encourage outpatient procedures, second opinions before surgery and more (but still limited) preventive measures such as screening tests. Employers also began to encourage employees to attend health education and fitness programs. In the past, most health insurance plans had really been "sick insurance" with few benefits related to primary prevention.

Medicare has had to regularly increase both the monthly premiums paid by its recipients and the deductible charge for each hospitalization. Also, many services such as dental care, routine eye care, medications, or nursing visits with physicians' orders are not covered by Medicare, an unpleasant surprise to the consumer. Many elderly, therefore, carry an additional insurance policy to cover costs not included in Medicare. Of particular concern is the extremely limited coverage of long term care costs by Medicare or private insurors. By its nature, long term care can continue for months or years and drain a family's finances completely. The experiences of many AIDS patients and the frail elderly are examples of the burdens of long term care.

Impact of Prospective Payment

As was mentioned earlier, payment was made to providers on a cost basis, paying whatever costs had been generated. This created an incentive for overutilization of some health services (Shaffer, 1985). With inflation and a growing number of aged who, as a group, are high users of health care, it could be expected that costs would continue to soar unless some changes were made.

Finally, in an attempt to control costs, Public Law 98-21, the Social Security Amendments of 1983, was passed. This bill, which some believe has the potential to completely revolutionize the health care system, provides for *prospective* rather than retrospective reimbursement for hospitals. The payment system was gradually phased into hospitals beginning in 1983 and focuses on setting payment levels ahead of time. Under this system, 467 different diagnosis-related groups (DRGs) were identified. Medicare data from prior years (beginning with 1982) were utilized by the federal Health Care Financing Administration to determine a fixed payment for each DRG. A hospital is paid a flat rate for the treatment of a patient with a given diagnosis. This provides an incentive for efficiency: if the hospital can deliver the care for less than the DRG price, it can keep the difference. If the cost of the care exceeds the DRG rate, the hospital must absorb the loss. Rates are set in advance of the year in which they are in effect and are considered fixed, based on past cost data. Capital costs and costs of educational programs such as schools of nursing are no longer reimbursible costs.

What are the implications of this change in health care financing? First, it firmly moves the delivery of health care into the context of the business world where the ability to compete is essential to survival. Actually, health care is the largest business in the United States from the perspective of the gross national product and expenditures. In the course of having to become more business-like and competitive in their operations, some hospitals have failed and it is anticipated that a more will eventually close.

The prospective payment system greatly increases the incentive to discharge patients more rapidly. But moving patients out faster, sometimes before they are ready to leave, can cause a decrease in the hospital's daily occupancy rate and a resulting decrease in revenues while fixed costs (utilities, mortgages or salaries) continue to accumulate (Shaffer 1985). This new system's impact is not limited to hospitals. It has brought more acutely ill patients to nursing homes and into home health care and it is being extended to other sectors of the health care system.

More hospitals are becoming part of larger multi-hospital systems. In 1984, one out of three hospitals belonged to a multi-hospital system (Ermann & Gabel, 1984). That number has since doubled and some people believe that we may no longer have community hospitals in the future because they will be replaced by either vertically integrated or horizontally integrated health care systems (Johnson, 1983). The *vertical systems* would evolve from the joining or expanding of the community hospital with other types of health care organizations into multifaceted organizations serving a broader range of the community's health care needs. The *horizontal systems* would emerge from the regional or nationally owned chains of hospitals. As these large corporations become dominant in health care, we will have to learn how to influence corporate decision making in order to ensure nursing its rightful place within the corporate power structure (West, 1987). An example of the vertically oriented system is the Montefiore Medical Center in New York which is spread over eight different sites and offers a variety of services including a hospice and the unique Loeb Center, the first institution staffed entirely by registered nurses. Another form is the VAP (value-adding partnership) in which the separate organizations remain independent but work closely together to manage the flow of services to each other's advantage (Johnson & Lawrence, 1988).

What impact will these changes have? As hospitals and other health care organizations are forced to become more business-like and competitive, their boards of trustees may become more actively involved in the actual operation of the institution and the chief executive officer, other administrators, and managers will be held more accountable than ever. Physician behaviors will be monitored more closely because they account for 70 percent of the decisions regarding how each health care dollar is spent (Maraldo, 1983).

These changes are causing major shifts of power within individual health care institutions and within the entire health care system. Change and power shifts usually cause discomfort and there has been tremendous discomfort and strain in the health care system as new challenges arise and new strategies for coping, surviving, and thriving are sought and implemented.

Hospitals are seeking ways to diversify their services, venturing into new fields such as adult day care, wellness programs, surgicenters, sleep disorder clinics, pain clinics, cardiac rehabilitation, nutrition and the like (Spitzer, 1987). Some have even ventured into the catering and office cleaning services to better utilize their staffs during offpeak hours.

Home care is becoming increasingly important. As patients under the DRG system are discharged "quicker and sicker" and home care is seen as a less costly alternative to hospitalization, there is a huge market for personal assistance, professional nursing, and physical and occupational therapy services to be tapped. However, reimbursement for these services is also a problem. Few insurance policies or government programs cover out of hospital services as generously as they covered hospital services in the past.

Health care administrators are being forced to monitor costs more carefully than ever. They are also monitoring patterns of patient care. Because of its labor-intensive nature, nursing especially must document what it does, how it does it, and what difference it makes to the patient and to the patient's length of stay. Nursing departments will have to clearly identify what they do in a particular organization if they have not done so before. While it may initially seem to be a cost saving to cut professional nursing hours, the rising acuity level of the patient populations requires a high level of skilled care and giving less professional level care may increase the length of stay and drive up costs even further (Williams, 1987).

The resulting emphasis on efficiency and productivity forces nurses to sharpen their approaches to planning nursing care. With shorter lengths of stay and tighter reimbursement policies, it becomes even more important to ensure that nursing assessments, diagnoses, goals and plans are realistic, measurable, and achievable in the time allotted for care and that discharge planning be initiated at the time of admission so that there may be continuity of care into the home and community. Stevens (1985) goes so far as to suggest that nursing can no longer afford a philosophy of ideal care. She has proposed a resource-driven model of care, a model in which you begin with the amount of resources available and then proceed to set the goals. In other words, it would be necessary to first consider the amount of funds available for the patient's care, then the goals most appropriate for that patient and affordable for the institution, and then work toward the product, a patient discharged at a higher level of wellness. This resource-driven model is far more business-oriented than service- or patient-oriented.

The nursing profession can take advantage of the current climate in health care. Nursing can be the link between quality and cost. It will be necessary to identify revenue producing areas and those areas that can be subsidized by the revenue producers. It will also be necessary to identify areas where lesser skills may be safely and effectively substituted, using the skills of the professional in the most efficient and effective manner in terms of patient outcomes, as well as in budgetary terms. Major budgetary and staffing analyses need to be done within nursing departments so that there is data available to provide the basis for the "system-smart" allocation of scarce resources (Shaffer 1985). In order to thrive under a prospective payment system, one must have sufficient knowledge of the system to be able to make correct decisions as well as the courage to act upon these decisions.

It is a time of challenge and opportunity. New roles for nurses may be invented (Clark & Quinn, 1988; Spitzer & Dauvivier, 1987). Quality must not be lost in the quest for efficiency and the interests of marketing cannot be allowed to overrule the interests of the patient. Nursing comprises 50 percent of most hospital budgets. This means that the nurse leader-manager is in a crucial, pivotal position in the institution. To perform well, you will need a knowledge base in planning, financial management, computers, organizational dynamics and leadership. The nurse leader-manager will be participating in strategic planning, marketing, budgeting and negotiating more than ever before and needs to be prepared to do these things well.

MARKETING

In the past, any marketing that was done was done to attract nurses, physicians, and other professionals to the staff. The physicians, in turn, brought the patients to the institution. Today's consumer is more sophisticated, however, and may request a specific agency or institution. Marketing techniques have been ignored by nurses in the past and only recently began to be used by physicians, dentists, and lawyers, after the Supreme Court ruled that the learned professions are subject to antitrust law and lifted the bans against advertising in the 1970s (Sheridan, 1983).

Definition

Marketing is the successful selling of a product or service (Stevens 1985a). It is a strategy used to gain the competitive edge. It can be further defined as the effective management of exchange relations with various markets and publics (Kotler, 1982). Ideally, it should be more than a promotional or selling effort. When marketing its services, the organization should try to identify and respond to the needs, preferences and perceptions of its consumers (Alward, 1983a; Stuehler, 1980). It should also have done some planning and have a clear idea of what its goals are before embarking upon a marketing campaign.

Institutions compete with each other for consumers in many ways. Advertisements for hospitals, HMOs, home health agencies, and other health care organizations are not at all unusual any more. Many now have marketing specialists on their staffs and some have entire public relations departments. In fact, the public relations staff often has a great deal of influence on the planning and decision making within these organizations. They may strongly influence decisions as diverse as the next community education program, the addition or deletion of a particular department or the color scheme of the new stationery and logo for the institution. The future of the nursing department within an organization is naturally linked to the fate of the organization as a whole and so nursing leaders and managers need to recognize the usefulness of marketing the services offered.

Marketing Techniques

Seven components of an effective marketing campaign have been identified by Kotler and Levy (1978):

1. *Product definition.* The definition of the service, policy, or product which emphasizes what basic consumer needs will be met or served by that product.
2. *Definition of the target group.* The population which will be the primary or sole recipient of the marketing communication. No one service can be all things to all people so the target group must be carefully defined.
3. *Differential marketing.* The design of different marketing campaigns to reach the diverse groups within a target population (often called segmentation).
4. *Customer behavior analysis.* What are the motives underlying the behavior of the target population?
5. *Integrated market planning.* The coordination and total responsibility for a specific item being marketed.
6. *Multiple marketing tools.* How will the message be communicated? Will several approaches be tried?
7. *Continuous feedback and periodic audit.* The ongoing process of assessing whether the marketing strategies designed to meet the stated goal are effective.

These components of an effective marketing campaign actually resemble many of the aspects of a good community assessment and contain a number of points about good planning and good leadership in general. The major difference is that they focus on effectively *selling* the product or service of your organization.

How have health care organizations become involved in marketing? Some have done this through newspaper and magazine advertising to the lay public, featuring primary nursing, a new emergency room, executive fitness programs, ambulatory surgery, special programs for senior citizens and the like. Maternity facilities have been advertised effectively on videotape on local television channels showing family-centered scenes where the older child meets his new sibling. Radio spots have also been utilized, featuring new educational programs, public services, and attention-getters, such as the x-raying of children's candy on Halloween.

A recently introduced managerial and marketing technique in health care has been the *product-line management system* where the knowledge and energies of several disciplines are united to develop and manage a comprehensive program. Maternity services may typify this:

> Pre-pregnancy classes are offered along with prenatal care, expectant parent and La-maze classes, and tours of the facility. Services often emphasized for the intrapartal period are family-centered care, rooming-in, and the availability of birthing rooms with the backup of a full surgical suite. If a special care nursery is available in a facility, it may be advertised in the maternity product line by emphasizing the full scope of services and preparation for care of the newborn with minimal disruption of the family unit. Post discharge services including home visits by the postpartum unit nurses, follow-up postpartal care and contraception clinics, postpartum exercise classes, and infant stimulation classes may also be advertised, depending upon the needs and wants of the target population. A pleasant maternity experience may leave the new mother with positive feelings about the institution and its staff. This, in turn, may bring repeat business from that family—to the emergency room, the pediatric unit, or, perhaps, to the maternity unit again.

Women, by the way, are the major consumers of health care services and they are the ones who make most of the decisions about where family members will obtain their health care (Hospitals, 1985).

Trauma centers are also well advertised, from dramatic pictures of helicopters arriving on the hospital's helipad to operating room scenes. A comprehensive center may advertise its specialized vascular services and follow-up care such as physical therapy. Less frequently advertised are the occupational and speech therapies, burn units, and those that are thought to be less attractive or possibly upsetting to the public. One unfortunate example of this type of selective advertising is the hospital that serves primarily older adults yet deliberately seeks young patients for the photographs for its brochures. Comprehensive cancer centers are another example: here the emphasis in advertising is on the screening and sophisticated diagnostic equipment available.

The unique feature of product-line management is the integrated approach to its many constituent disciplines. The "top" person may or may not be the vice president of nursing; it may be the vice president of public relations or of personnel. Nurse managers involved in such systems comment on how different it is to be the "top nurse," the person responsible for articulating what nursing is and can accomplish to peers from other disciplines. These nurse managers are actually marketing nursing to other colleagues as well. The product-line approach may become more popular as its effectiveness is demonstrated.

From a marketing point of view, health care is a product. This product has three components to consider in marketing it effectively: the physical characteristics of the institution, the services offered, and the personnel who provide those services. It is generally thought that the personnel are the most important component to the patient market and their families, at least after they have entered the system (Sapienza and Kahn, 1980). The image projected by the nursing staff and the public relations skills of its members will clearly have an impact on these markets.

It is also important to identify submarkets or target populations with similar needs, preferences, perceptions, attitudes and behaviors because each subgroup requires different marketing strategies and skills. This concept of identifying subgroups is known as segmentation of the population (Alward, 1983).

Importance to Nursing

Why should nurses be cognizant of marketing principles? The answer is to secure professional survival and growth in a competitive age. Nursing has both internal and external markets or "publics" (Camunas, 1987). The internal market is the nursing division of the parent organization and its patient population. Other internal markets within an institution may be its medical staff, the laboratory, the trustees and other departments. External nursing markets include the families, visitors, communities, donors and supporters, suppliers, regulators and other agencies, particularly those who refer patients to your organization. These nursing markets or publics are the constituencies that we discussed in the previous chapter.

Participation in marketing could be thought of as an extension of the assessment process. Nurses are in closer patient contact than other members of the health care team, and in an excellent position to assess patient needs and evaluate how well existing services can meet them. A broader assessment is like case finding for your employer or perhaps for yourself as a nurse entrepreneur. Defining new markets is the first step, occurring hand-in-hand with product identification. Nurses are also well situated to work on the identification of the target groups. Marketing campaigns cannot succeed if unmet needs or desires are not identified. This is an area where nurses practicing at the bedside or visiting people in their homes can contribute particularly significant information to the marketing plan of their organizations.

The nurse manager cannot market nursing skills and expertise internally or externally without the support and commitment of the nursing staff. To be committed to these marketing goals, the entire staff must understand the purpose and rationale behind them and how they can be carried out. In other words, the nurse manager would have to take the leadership in guiding the staff in understanding and carrying out the marketing plan.

THE IMAGE OF NURSING

What image has nursing projected to the public and to other colleagues over the years? You may not have thought of it this way before, but if nursing care is the product that we deliver, then it is important that this product be well accepted. To be well accepted, nurses must, among other things, project an image of wellness, self-confidence, and professionalism.

Image Problems

Most individuals enter the nursing profession with a personal commitment, having made a definite choice to pursue this career. Often, however, long practicing nurses are heard complaining about their work, their hours, and their salaries without committing themselves to the kind of action that could alter their personal or collective status. Some also become angry, apathetic, or burned out and give visible signs of this by exhibiting low energy, little enthusiasm, and even professional sabotage. How often do we hear nurses recognizing and praising the accomplishments of their colleagues?

Signs of chronic disillusionment, such as complaining and back-biting and image inconsistencies such as smoking, obesity, and sedentary life styles are personal and organizational "image wreckers" (Smith 1984). These behaviors do not help nurses project themselves well. Think about it. Would you want to be cared for or take health instruction from a complaining, dissatisfied nurse or one who displays signs of poor health habits? What would your impression be?

An interesting study by the National Association of Nurse Recruiters (1980) found that low professional image, lack of professional image, lack of professional recognition, and lack of career mobility for nurses has contributed to nursing shortages. Having a reputation as being one of the three main career options (secretary, teacher or nurse) that were open to women before the women's liberation movement may also be hindering efforts to recruit the best people into the field. Furthermore, these fields are still erroneously seen by the public as offering low salaries and little career advancement. In the past they were thought of as being appropriate training grounds for a future wife and mother, a job to hold "until" marriage and children came along. Married women who worked were seen as providing a second income for the purchase of "extras" rather than as people who were supporting themselves and family members with their salaries.

Image Improvement

Nurses need to move toward a positive, assertive orientation of personal control and empowerment and away from a defensive survival mentality. Old behaviors of unprofessional dress, subservience, and negative attitudes cannot be continued in a competitive age. Professional business women are examples of the personal and collective success of people who had to market themselves vigorously with a limited number of earlier role models. They, like some nurses, have been risk takers and role breakers (Grissum and Spengler, 1975) in the most positive sense. They did not have traditions to fall back on but had to create their own roles and images, thinking positively and marketing themselves in the world of business (Smith 1984).

When a positive self image is combined with appropriate marketing techniques, a favorable public image can be projected. This positive image can include such things as a professional manner, good public relations at the bedside, in the home, and in the community, and providing services in a manner in which you would want to be served.

A positive nursing image can contribute to your organization's image development and marketing. Just as other service industries, such as the airlines, market their services using positive staff images, so can the health care industry market its services. The nursing staff can indirectly become the agency's largest sales force (Smith, 1984).

The media are known to have a profound influence upon the public's opinions. Nursing's media image does not yet portray the nurse lobbyist, clinician, practitioner, educator, researcher, and manager. Nursing should not passively accept such inaccurate portrayals in the media. The scope and depth of nursing roles should be shown accurately. While individuals and professional associations have tried to make these changes, nurses can also work to reach out to young people who are making career decisions and to their guidance counselors to provide accurate information about the myriad of opportunities in nursing.

It is also important to present a united front to the public, especially when we are working in the political arena. Rather than expending our energies fighting each other, we need to stand back occasionally and see how we appear to others. It is time to look ahead to the future of the profession, to pay attention to society's projected needs, and to plan future services in conjunction with these projected needs.

SUMMARY

In the discussion of the evolution of the health care system, mention was made of the development and growth of hospitals which became the favored workplace for health care; the influence of scientific and technological advances; the effect of the introduction of antibiotics; and the introduction of health insurance, Medicare and Medicaid. Government involvement in health care has gradually increased but the costs have also increased to the point where concern is being expressed about the limitations of our resources in continuing to provide for everyone's health care needs. In response to this concern, a system of prospective payment has been introduced that has had a significant impact on many facets of the health care system, particularly on attitudes toward competition, productivity, and marketing.

Marketing was defined as successful selling of a product, in this case, health care. The components of effective marketing technique include definition of the product and of the target populations, and an analysis of the population's behavior, needs, and desires. A number of different marketing strategies were described.

Nursing's image problems include negative attitudes on the part of some members of the profession, and a perception that nursing offers few opportunities for advancement, that it is solely a woman's job and that nurses fill primarily subservient roles. Presenting a positive, assertive, united front to the public was suggested to improve nursing's image. Encouragement of positive images in the media that portray the breadth and depth of nursing roles is also important in improving the image of nursing.

REFERENCES*

*Alward, R.R. (1983). A marketing approach to nursing administration: Part I. *Journal of Nursing Administration, 13,* (3).

Ashley, J. (1976). *Hospitals, paternalism and the role of the nurse.* New York: Teachers College Press.

Bartkowski, J.J. & Swandby, J.M. (1985). Charting nursing's course through megatrends. *Nursing and Health Care, 6* (7).

Brink, S.D. (1986). Health care in the 1990's: A buyer's market. *Hospital and Health Services Administration, 31,* (5), 16–28.

Buchanan, R.J. (1988). State Medicaid coverage of

AZT and AIDS-related policies. *American Journal of Public Health,* 78:4, 432–436.

Buhler-Wilkerson, K. (1985). Public health nursing: In sickness or in health? *American Journal of Public Health, 75.*

*Camunas, C. (1987). Using public relations to market nursing service. *Journal of Nursing Administration, 16,* (10), 26–30.

*Cipriano, P.F. (1986). Certification: Self-regulation for specialty practice. In *Patterns of specialization: Challenge to the curriculum.* New York: National League for Nursing.

Christman, L. (1987). The future of the nursing profession. *Nursing Administration Quarterly, 11,* (2), 26–30.

Clark, L & Quinn, J (1988). The New Entrepreneurs. *Nursing and Health Care,* 9, 7–15.

Curran, C. (1985). The corporate connections: Multihospital systems rekindle commitment. In *Patterns of education: The unfolding of nursing.* New York: National League for Nursing.

Ermann, D. & Gabel, J. (1984). Multihospital systems, issues, and empirical findings. *Health Affairs,* 3 (1), 51.

Grissum, M. & Spengler, C. (1976). *Womanpower and health care.* Boston: Little, Brown and Company.

Heaney, R.P. & Barger-Lux, M.J. (1984). Today's crisis in university-provided education in the health professions. *Educational Record,* 65 (4).

Iacocca, L. (1984). *Iacocca—An autobiography.* New York: Bantam Books.

Johnson, R.L. (1983). Era of responsibility: Competition, challenges. *Hospitals, 57,* 75–82.

Johnson, R. & Lawrence, P.R. (1988). Beyond vertical integration: The rise of the value-adding partnership. *Harvard Business Review,* 88:4, 94–101.

*Jones, P.A. (1985). Reaganomics: Health policy and politics. In R.R. Wieczorek, *Power, politics and policy in nursing.* New York: Springer.

*Kotler, P. & Levy, S.J. (1978). Broadening the concept of marketing. In P.J. Montans (Ed.) *Marketing in nonprofit organizations.* New York: AMACOM.

McBride, A.B. (1985). *Orchestrating a career in nursing.* Pleasantville, New York: Sigma Theta Tau Regional Assembly, Pace University.

———. (1980). NANR analyzes nursing shortage. *American Journal of Nursing, 80,* (4).

Maraldo, P. (1983). *Reimbursement for nurses in the primary care arena: A cost saving for health care.* New York: National League for Nursing.

Pear, R. (1986). Spending for health care in 1985 rose at lowest rate in two decades. *New York Times,* July 30.

Peplau, H. (1985). Is nursing's self-regulatory power being eroded. *American Journal of Nursing, 85,* 141.

*Piemonte, R.V. (1985). Credentialing: The thread between licensure, accreditation, and certification. In *Patterns in education: The unfolding of nursing.* New York: National League for Nursing.

Rydman, L.D. & Rydman, R.J. (1983). The United States health care delivery system. In W. Burgess & E. Ragland *Community Health Nursing: Philosophy, process and practice.* Norwalk, Conn.: Appleton-Century-Crofts.

Sapienza, A.M. & Kahn, R.A. (1980). Impacting the product: staff involvement in a health care marketing strategy. *Hospital Topics, 58,* 24–27.

———. (1985). Schools alarmed by downturn in applications: "Pool is down in quality," some say. *American Journal of Nursing, 85,* (11)

Schlesinger, M. (1988). The perfectibility of public programs: Real lessons from large-scale demonstrations. *American Journal of Public Health,* 78:8, 899–902.

Shaffer, F.A. (1985). Prospective payment: A strategic plan for nursing power. In R.R. Wieczorek (ed.) *Power, politics and policy in nursing.* New York: Springer.

*Sheridan, D.R. (1983). The health care industry in the marketplace: Implications for nursing. *Journal of Nursing Administration,* 13, (9).

Smith, B.A. (1984). Toward a more profitable nursing image. *Nursing Success Today, 1,* 18–23.

*Spitzer, R.B. & Dauvivier, M. (1987). Nursing in the 1990's: Expanding opportunities. *Nursing Administration Quarterly, 11,* (2), 55–61.

Spradley, B.W. (1985). *Community health nursing: Concepts and practice.* Boston: Little, Brown and Co.

Stevens, B.J. (1985a). *The nurse as executive.* Rockville, Md.: Aspen Publications.

Stevens, B.J. (1985b). Tackling a changing society head on. *Nursing and Health Care,* 6, (1).

Stuehler, G. (1980). How hospital planning and marketing relate. *Hospitals, 54,* (9).

———. (1979). *The study of credentialing in nursing: A new approach.* Vol. I. Kansas City, Mo.: American Nurses Association.

Torrens, P. (1978). *The American health care system: Issues and problems.* Saint Louis: C.V. Mosby Co.

Walker, L.A. (1987). What comforts AIDS families. *The New York Times Magazine,* June 21, 1987.

*Wasserman, C.G. (1985). Marketing: A strategy for power in arenas of competition. In R.R. Wieczorek, *Power, politics and policy in nursing.* New York: Springer.

Weiler, P. (1987). The public health impact of Alzheimer's Disease. *American Journal of Public Health,* 77:9, 1157–1158.

West, M.E. (1987). Nursing and the corporate world. *Journal of Nursing Administration,* 17, (3), 22–33.

Williams, P. (1987). Economic responsibility and viability of the nursing department in the prospective payment environment. *Nursing Administration Quarterly,* 11, (2) 30–34.

Wing, K.R. (1976). *The law and the public's health.* St. Louis: C.V. Mosby.

———. (1985). Women: Target of new marketing efforts. *Hospitals, 59,* (8).

---

*References marked with an asterisk are recommended for further reading.**

UNIT I LEARNING ACTIVITIES _____

▷ Interview a nurse or other health care worker from a culture different from your own. Make up a list of open-ended questions after re-reading the section on cultural differences in Chapter 1. You might want to ask about the person's reasons for working, types of satisfaction gained from working, aspirations, status of nurses in other countries, and so forth. Compare the answers with your own cultural perspective and with information about your respective cultures found in the literature.

▷ Role play a staff meeting in which you are the first-line manager who must resolve a productivity problem. Paperwork is not being done on time by your staff and your supervisor is pressuring you to make sure that all charting is 100 percent complete and accurate. Try using Ouchi's Theory Z approach in the first role play and then use Miller's Behavioral Management approach in a second role play. Evaluate the effect of the selected approach on the outcome.

▷ Read the original account (available in most libraries) by Lewin, Lippit and White of the research that provided the basis for the authoritarian, democratic, and laissez-faire styles of leadership. Critique their account of the research. (You can do this with the Research Example instead, but the original account is preferable.)

▷ At the end of a day spent in a clinical setting, evaluate your leadership effectiveness using the checklist at the end of Chapter 3. Identify three areas of particular strength and three in which you need to improve. Develop a personal plan for improvement in the areas of weakness and for ways to capitalize on your strengths.

▷ Using the Management Effectiveness checklist, observe a head nurse, supervisor or other management-level individual in a clinical setting. Evaluate this person's effectiveness as a manager, considering ways in which the environment, type of work and characteristics of the staff impact on this person's effectiveness.

▷ Plan a debate on either (1) The value of marketing nursing services or (2) The use of a business orientation vs a caring orientation in nursing management. Research the subject thoroughly and draw up a list of *pro* and *con* arguments. If possible, debate the issue with a colleague in front of an interested audience.

Unit II

PLANNING AND
DECISION MAKING

Chapter 6.   Critical Thinking
Chapter 7.   Problem Solving and Goal Setting
Chapter 8.   Project Planning
Chapter 9.   Financial Management
Unit II Learning Activities

Chapter 6 ▬▬▬▬▬▬▬

OUTLINE ▬▬▬▬▬▬▬▬▬▬▬▬▬▬▬▬▬▬▬▬

The Purpose of Critical Thinking
Complex Judgments and Decisions
Selective Attention
Making Connections
Taking a Stranger's Viewpoint

Critical Analysis
Uses of Critical Analysis

Questions for Critical Analysis
  I. What Is the Central Issue?
 II. What Are the Underlying
     Assumptions?
III. Is the Evidence Given Valid?
 IV. Are the Conclusions Acceptable?

Summary

LEARNING OBJECTIVES ▬▬▬▬▬▬▬▬▬▬▬▬▬▬▬▬

Upon completion of this chapter, the reader will be able to:

▷ Use an inquiring approach in analyzing questions of importance in nursing practice and leadership.

▷ Identify the central issue in a problem or argument.

▷ Apply a set of criteria to determine the validity of evidence presented in support of an argument.

▷ Evaluate the accuracy, applicability, and value stance of a given conclusion.

CRITICAL THINKING

Critical thinking is both an attitude and an approach. It is a willingness to give fair consideration to every idea, but to accept an idea only after you have thought about it. It is an inquiring way of looking at the world.

The purpose of this chapter is to assist you in the development of this spirit of alertness and open-mindedness and in encouraging others to develop this spirit. Health care professionals cannot be dogmatic. A person with a closed mind misses many opportunities for positive growth by rejecting all new ideas. The opposite is the person who accepts the useless along with the useful idea and has trouble distinguishing between the two. You could compare this person to an old-fashioned grain sifter that keeps the chaff and lets the valuable part, wheat, pass through.

Leaders and managers need to have what could be called semipermeable minds when confronting new ideas: open to possibility but questioning certainty. It is in this spirit that they ask "Why?" when no one else does and "Why not?" when everyone else fails to see a possibility.

THE PURPOSE OF CRITICAL THINKING

We will consider first some of the ways in which critical thinking can be of use to a health care professional, particularly to the nurse leader-manager.

Complex Judgments and Decisions

Like other professionals, nurses make many judgments for which there are no simple answers, both in giving care and in managing others. Nurses deal with complex human beings and work in some very complex systems. Neither are completely predictable. The uniqueness of each person and of each situation demands a newly formulated assessment, not an automatic, preprogrammed one.

Decisions confront us constantly in nursing practice. The use of triage in an emergency room is realistically based on the assumption that someone has to decide whom to treat first. The staff nurse has to decide which call light to answer first. The community nurse often must decide what to tell a patient and his or her family about the illness and prognosis.

Nurse leaders and managers also find themselves constantly faced with the necessity of making decisions. Does this new policy make sense? Which staff member's suggestion is the best one? Who is right in this disagreement? Questions like these require critical analysis to help the leader-manager see all sides of the issue and make the best decision.

Critical thinking makes the assumptions behind a decision more evident. It is often necessary for a leader-manager to confront colleagues about their avoidance of an issue. What is the assumption behind the confrontation? Usually, it is the belief that it is worthwhile for a person to suffer some temporary discomfort to ensure future improvements. Philosopher Maxine Greene raises an interesting question about even this assumption. She asks, "Who has a right to make other human beings 'likeable and happy and productive'?" (1973, p. 56). This is a decision you and your colleagues have to make.

Selective Attention

A second reason why critical thinking is important is the vast number of messages directed at people through television, radio, newspapers, books, and journals, as well as in person. We are bombarded with political promises, bureaucratic doubletalk, persuasive advertisements, bandwagon appeals, and meaningless verbiage mixed in with useful facts and thoughtful discussions. It can be difficult to decide what to accept and what to reject as erroneous messages can often sound very convincing. Try reading the following paragraph quickly and see if you can make any sense out of it:

> In particular, initiation of critical subsystems development presents extremely interesting challenges to the subsystem compatibility rating. In this regard, an overview of the entire installation performance is further compounded when taking into account the philosophy or commonality and standardization. On the other hand, any associated supporting element presents extremely interesting challenges to the philosophy of commonality and standardization (Scientific Report Writer, n.d.).

If the complexity of this paragraph puzzled you or made you feel as if you were a poor reader, then you were not thinking critically. This paragraph is a sample of computer-generated sentences put together in a completely random fashion. It is all chaff and no wheat, completely nonsensical. You need to be able to separate the wheat from the chaff in any information you receive, and critical thinking can help you do this (Gay & Edgil, 1982).

Making Connections

Critical thinking has a creative side to it. Creative thinkers look for alternative solutions and new ideas even when the currently accepted ones are satisfactory (Lipman, 1985). Have you ever found new relationships between different pieces of information or between different experiences? Greene calls this *making connections* (1973, p. 159). Doing this brings more meaning to what you observe and learn. It can also lead you to the discovery of new meanings, as in the following example:

> Physiology, sociology, and psychology may seem like separate worlds, but they are all attempts to explain the same phenomenon—man. This becomes more apparent when you look for connections. Listen to a person's heartbeat and at the same time watch that person's expression and body language. If you listen too long, the expression may become worried, the body position less relaxed, and the heartbeat more rapid. A connection between concepts in physiology, sociology, and psychology can explain what has happened but each one separately will not provide a complete answer.

Making connections helps to eliminate the feeling that you have learned many little bits of unrelated information. When these bits become related to each other and to your experience, they then become more meaningful and easier to remember.

This process can lead to completely new connections. Many important scientific discoveries, such as the revelations about the role of interferon in fighting disease, or the transmission of AIDS, or even the relationship between some antihypertensive medications and the prevention of baldness, were made this way. Not every new connection is quite as important as these, but each adds creativity and the excitement of discovery to your practice.

Taking a Stranger's Viewpoint

Thinking critically and creatively is what Greene describes as taking a stranger's viewpoint. She compares it to the way you look at familiar surroundings after being away from them for a long time. When you first come back, you see more details and more features and are much more aware of routine activities. Greene describes this way of seeing things in the following way:

> To take a stranger's vantage point on everyday reality is to look inquiringly and wonderingly on the world in which one lives (p. 267).

When you compare the idea of taking a stranger's viewpoint to an automatic acceptance or rejection of every idea that comes your way, you can see how much of a difference this can make. You can use the information in the next section on critical analysis as one way to adopt that stranger's viewpoint and see your world from a different perspective.

CRITICAL ANALYSIS _____

The term *critical thinking* refers to the questioning approach discussed so far. *Critical analysis* is a related term used to describe a set of questions you can apply to a particular situation or idea. It is a process that will assist you in separating the wheat from the chaff.

The set of questions involved is actually a set of criteria for judging an idea, not sequential steps. You may not always need to use each question or criterion, but you do need to be aware of all of them in order to select the most relevant.

Uses of Critical Analysis

Critical analysis is useful in a variety of different situations. You can critically analyze any of the following:

Leadership and management practices may actually lead to the very behavior they are trying to prevent when not subjected to critical analysis before use.

Organizational policies and practices may be illogical and inconsistent unless critically analyzed.

Nursing practices, whether infant stimulation, palliative care, neonatal intensive care, contracting with a client, or virtually any other practice, should be critically analyzed.

Nursing issues, such as the definition of nursing, two levels of licensure, external degrees, cost effectiveness, and so forth warrant critical analysis.

Research reports, should be critically analyzed to decide if the results are applicable to your practice.

Rumors, gossip, and advice, although not ordinarily listed together, all need critical analysis before you accept or reject them.

Journal articles and other written materials warrant critical analysis.

Leader actions, from planning to evaluation, can be made more objective and creative if you use critical thinking.

Questions for Critical Analysis

A number of scholars have developed schemes to help people think critically. From these schemes, a set of questions and criteria, shown in Table 6-1, have been developed to help you progress along the road to being a critical thinker and a sharper, more aware, and effective leader and manager (Ennis, 1962; Dressel & Mayhew, n.d.; Nickerson, 1986).

These questions will seem abstract and perhaps unrelated to everyday experience unless you engage yourself in the process of critical analysis. It is suggested that you choose a practice or belief that disturbs you in some way and test it with each question as you read this section. You could, for example, critically analyze demand versus scheduled feeding of infants, or arguments in favor of a strictly authoritarian approach to child rearing, or the popular belief that many old people become "senile". In this way, you can see how critical analysis can work for you.

QUESTION I. WHAT IS THE CENTRAL ISSUE?

To get at the meaning of the central issue, restate it as a pro and con in your own words. To use popular beliefs about aging as an example, you could restate the question as: Does mental ability decline with age? If restating is too difficult, it may be easier to identify a main theme. You can also try reorganizing the ideas into a new pattern. A creative reorganization often results in new insights and new perspectives on an issue.

TABLE 6-1. Critical Analysis Questions

   I. What is the central issue?
  II. What are the underlying assumptions?
 III. Is the evidence given valid?
    1. Are stereotypes or clichés used?
    2. Are emotional or biased arguments used?
    3. Are the data adequate and verifiable?
    4. Are important terms clearly defined?
    5. Are the given data relevant?
    6. Is the problem or issue correctly identified?
  IV. Are the conclusions acceptable?
    1. Is the conclusion accurate?
    2. Is the conclusion applicable?
    3. Is there any value conflict?

The issue of prison reform provides a good example of the need to search for the central issue:

> Actually, there seem to be several underlying issues operating in debates about prison reform. One of these issues is the question of whether the inmates are "bad" or "sick." If you think that they are bad, then they should be punished and prisons should be miserable places to be (and most certainly are). But, if you think of the inmates as sick or troubled, then they should be given treatment, which requires a therapeutic environment.

A major theme or issue in prison reform, then, would be punishment versus treatment as the approach to handling prisoners.

QUESTION II. WHAT ARE THE UNDERLYING ASSUMPTIONS?

Some underlying assumptions are personal, others are culture bound. In either case, assumptions are unstated beliefs that influence conclusions. People make assumptions all the time and often act on them without realizing it.

Greene (1973) says that you cannot really be self-aware until you examine your preconceptions (assumptions). Do you, for example, assume that old age is a time of loss and deterioration or do you see it as a time of joy? Greene especially emphasizes the need to be aware of the models or paradigms we use in constructing our world. This textbook can be used as an example of the way in which models are used to construct our perceptions of the world:

> This book is based on the open systems view of the world and on a concept of people as holistic beings who strive toward growth and self–actualization. This is an optimistic view of human beings, and you could find many people who disagree with this way of looking at people.

QUESTION III. IS THE EVIDENCE GIVEN VALID?

Most of the time, some kind of evidence (whether fact or fiction) is given to support a point of view. In either case, it can be accurate or inaccurate. Stereotypes, clichés, biases, appeals to emotion, and obvious contradictions are warning signals that you should look closely at the evidence given. For example, the public's vague belief that aging brings with it an increase in wisdom but that many old people have declining mental abilities is an obvious contradiction that requires further analysis. Relevant, verifiable, and consistent evidence given to support a clearly stated conclusion is a sign that an argument is well supported. These concerns are summarized in the following six points.

1. *Look for the use of stereotypes or clichés.* Every time phrases that overgeneralize about people (e.g., "typical parent," "the aged," "middle-aged man," or "cancer patient") are used, there is the danger of stereotyping. When this is done, you lose sight of the uniqueness of the individual who happens to be a parent, an employee of a certain age, or a patient stricken with cancer. Nurses are, fortunately, working on becoming more aware of cultural, racial, and other stereotypes, but many are still in use.

Clichés are overused expressions. People tend to use them without thinking about what they mean or imply. "You're old enough to know better," and "Why don't you take it like a man," are clichés that could easily have a counterproductive effect if directed at a distressed staff member.

2. *Look for the use of emotional or biased arguments.* An emotional

appeal can be very persuasive and is often used for this reason. The term *senility*, for example, has far more emotional overtones than the term *cognitive impairment*. Arguments are also biased when they present only supporting evidence and no opposing viewpoint.

Even professional issues have emotional components. A long-standing issue in nursing shows this:

> The reaction of some nurses to proposals that the bachelor's degree (B.S.N.) be required for licensure in the future was one of anger and anxiety. They were afraid that they would find themselves treated as second-class nurses if such a requirement were approved, even though the promised grandfather clauses would protect their licenses. Given the existence of these grandfather clauses, the argument that the proposal is unfair to currently practicing nurses who do not have B.S.N. degrees has a strong emotional component.

The use of bias or emotion may be quite subtle and hard to recognize. Although such an appeal is often effective, a critical thinker should be alert to its presence in order to avoid being persuaded for the wrong reasons.

3. ***Look for the use of adequate and verifiable data.*** Critical thinkers do not depend on intuition, emotion, or hunches alone (Lipman, 1985). Instead, they seek some objective data to support an argument. First, decide whether the data given consist of fact, opinion, or a combination of the two. Often the information and research available on a subject are inadequate, so it is necessary to rely on judgment. Even so, you can distinguish between a heavily biased opinion and a well-thought-out judgment based on a combination of experience and whatever knowledge is available. Although you can have more confidence in the second case, it is still important to keep an open mind because future information may contradict even the expert's best judgment. For example, hypertension used to be called the executives' disease, but statistical analyses have shown that it is also a poor man's problem related to factors other than occupation.

Even research is not necessarily conclusive. The continuing debate about what really motivates an employee, despite considerable research on the subject, is one example. The artificial sweetener debate is another good example of inconclusiveness. Although the evaluation of research is too complicated a subject to go into here, it is safe to say that most research findings are tentative (often raising more questions than answers) and subject to error even though statistics are used to estimate the amount of error (Thomas, 1982). Probably the best questions to ask in considering the acceptability of research findings are the following:

▷ Could you repeat the investigation and get the same results?
▷ Does the design allow for collection of the type of data that are really needed to answer your question?
▷ Are the results applicable to your situation?

4. ***Determine if important terms are clearly defined.*** We often use terms in a careless, offhand fashion. Vagueness should be avoided (Flew, 1977). Have you ever had an argument with someone only to find that the main disagreement was in the way you each defined a term? The following example shows how important definitions can be:

> A Clinical Nurse Specialist proposed to begin a cardiac rehabilitation program on two cardiology units. Colleagues in several departments assisted in the development of the plan

and agreed to participate. The Director of Nursing and Medical Chief of Cardiology approved the plan.

The Clinical Nurse Specialist finished preparing the educational materials and protocols for gradual increases in activity just before implementing the program. At this point, the Hospital Administrator approached the Clinical Nurse Specialist and stated that the rehabilitation program could not begin without the approval of the Board of Trustees.

Upon hearing the term cardiac rehabilitation, the Administrator had pictured a large outpatient clinic with elaborate exercise equipment and its own new staff. In contrast, the Clinical Nurse Specialist had actually planned an inpatient program, designed to assist patients with cardiac problems to improve their level of functioning and prepare them for discharge, using existing staff and equipment from several departments under the Clinical Nurse Specialist's supervision. Neither the Clinical Nurse Specialist nor the Administrator had clearly defined for the other person what they meant by the term cardiac rehabilitation.

Many nursing terms are vaguely defined. A classic example of this is the term *nursing need*. Is it something that nurses need or is it an identifiable need for nursing care (Block, 1974)? Another example is *assessment*, which is used to refer to the collection of data, the diagnosis of the problem, or both. When terms are clearly defined, it becomes much easier to determine the relevancy of the data, which is the next point in judging validity.

Health care givers also use a lot of jargon, often without being aware that they are using it. Not only do they abbreviate everything from SIDS to TPN, they also use words that are currently in fashion and words that have fallen out of fashion (Ingle, 1976). For example, the term *client* is preferred by many because it implies health and less dependence than the term *patient*.

5. *Make sure the data are relevant.* An argument may be so persuasive that you do not notice that the evidence given is not directly related to the question. While you might think that this is rare, actually it is not unusual. In fact, side issues or irrelevancies may be brought up purposely to draw your attention away from the main point, especially if they are persuasive. This often happens in disputes, and the leader-manager should avoid being sidetracked or drawn into irrelevant arguments when negotiating a settlement.

The same irrelevancy of the data collected shows up in many different situations. Another example is the following:

The major objective of a class for people with hypertension would be to help them control their high blood pressure by means of diet, medication, exercise, stress reduction, and so forth. Yet, at the end of the course, participants are asked if they enjoyed the course and to define such terms as systolic and diastolic. Neither of these factors is relevant to the question of blood pressure control. What is relevant is whether or not they carry out their treatment program correctly and whether this results in a lowering of their blood pressure.

6. *Determine if the problem or issue is correctly identified.* This last point is related to the previous two. All three of these points are important when working through the problem-solving process. The following is an example of a problem that may need to be redefined:

Both professional caregivers and parents have been trying to find ways to slow down hyperactive children. Rogers (1970) believes, however, that the hyperactive child is an evolutionary emergent, that is, the next step in our evolution as humans, and actually more in tune with the rapid pace of change than the rest of us are. If Rogers is correct, we have been working on the wrong problem.

Problems and issues may also be oversimplified. When people reduce a complex issue to a simple yes or no question, there is a danger that important aspects of an issue will be ignored. The following is an example:

> The shortage or surplus of nurses is a perennial issue that needs continual redefinition. "Do we need more nurses?" is too simple a question to encompass such a complex situation. There is, for example, a difference between counting the number of actively employed nurses and counting every nurse in the country, including those who will never return to nursing practice. There is also a difference between a new nurse with a two-year degree and an experienced nurse with a high level of competence in a particular specialty area.
>
> Is there a shortage in one part of the country and a surplus in another? Is "need" measured by the number of job openings or by the number of nurses who could be utilized to improve the current standard of health care?
>
> These and other questions need to be answered before deciding whether or not we have a real shortage or surplus of nurses.

QUESTION IV. ARE THE CONCLUSIONS ACCEPTABLE?

This question of acceptability has three parts: accuracy, applicability, and value stance. Each of these represents a different perspective on the question of acceptability.

1. *Accuracy of the conclusion.* The first concern is with the correctness or accuracy of the conclusion. Is that conclusion based on the facts given? Sometimes they ignore the facts, as in the following example.

> A researcher asked families if they would take care of an elderly family member who became ill. Almost exactly half of the families said that they would, and the other half said that they would not. The researcher, who believed that *every* family should be willing to help, concluded that *most families will not* take care of their elderly family members if they become ill. The researcher's conclusion was not based on the facts alone but on a perception of the facts.

You also need to ask if the facts or supporting arguments are sufficiently valid. The points in question III will help you make this decision.

2. *Applicability of the conclusion.* Is the conclusion applicable to your situation? Some ideas or solutions will fit only one situation; others can be adapted to a variety of circumstances. For example:

> An experimental drug treatment project may be successful primarily because the clients were handpicked or had volunteered for the program and because the staff was so enthusiastic about the new treatment. If this is true, how well will this treatment work in your agency when it becomes an ordinary routine used for a wide variety of drug abuse problems?

3. *Existence of any value conflict.* The third aspect of the question is the extent to which the conclusion or solution conflicts with your personal and professional values. To take an extreme example, a lobotomy may effectively calm certain highly agitated individuals, but can you accept it as a treatment of mental illness if you believe in the right to self-determination and free will?

Restraints, total life support systems, abortions, the rights of AIDS patients, withholding diagnosis of a terminal illness, and fostering independence are just a few of the issues that can arise in your professional practice that may challenge your values and beliefs. The accuracy, applicability, and value stance of a conclusion are all important aspects to consider in deciding its acceptability. A critical thinker considers each one of these before accepting a conclusion.

SUMMARY

Critical thinking is defined here as an inquiring way to look at the world. This approach includes such actions as seeking new connections between ideas and using a set of criteria to judge the acceptability of an idea. The four criteria include identifying the central issue, identifying the underlying assumptions, analyzing the validity of the evidence given, and deciding whether or not the conclusion is acceptable, applicable, and congruent with your value system.

REFERENCES*

*Block, D. (1974). Some crucial terms in nursing: What do they really mean? *Nursing Outlook, 22,* 689.

Dressel, P. & Mayhew, L.B: (n.d.) *Critical thinking in social science.* Mimeo, n.d.

Ennis, B.H. (1962). A concept of critical thinking. *Harvard Educational Review, 32,* 81.

*Flew, A. (1977). *Thinking straight.* Buffalo, N.Y.: Prometheus Books.

Gay, J.T. & Edgil, A.E. (1982). Critical reading. *Nursing and Health Care, 3,* (5), 266.

Greene, M. (1973). *Teacher as stranger.* Belmont, Calif.: Wadsworth.

*Ingle, D.J. (1976). *Is it really so?* Philadelphia: Westminster.

Lipman, M. (1985). Thinking skills fostered by philosophy for children. In Segal, J.W., Chipman, S.F. & Glaser, R. (eds): *Thinking and learning skills.* London: Lawrence Erlbaum

*Nickerson, R.S. (1986). Reasoning. In Dillon, R.F. & Sternberg, R.J. (eds): *Cognition and instruction.* New York: Academic Press.

Rogers, M. (1970). *An introduction to the theoretical basis of nursing.* Philadelphia: F.A. Davis.

————. (n.d.). *Scientific report writer: a computerized nonsensical report writer.* Origin unknown.

Thomas. L. (1982). The art of teaching science. *New York Times,* March 14. 78.

---

*References marked with an asterisk are suggested for further reading.

Chapter 7

OUTLINE

Problem Solving
Purpose
Steps in the Process
    Step 1. Assessment: Collect Data
    Step 2. Diagnosis: Define the Problem
    Step 3. Plan: Select Strategies
    Step 4. Implementation: Take Action
    Step 5. Evaluation: Evaluate Results
Individual Approaches to Problem Solving

Setting Goals and Objectives
Essentials of Management by Objectives
    Writing Objectives
    Implementing Objectives
    Evaluating Outcomes
Advantages and Disadvantages of the
    Goal-Setting Approach

Summary

LEARNING OBJECTIVES

Upon completion of this chapter, the reader will be able to:

▷ Compare and contrast problem solving and the nursing process.

▷ Use the problem-solving process in a leader-manager situation that requires a solution to a problem.

▷ Write objectives for both individuals and working groups that are appropriate and include observable outcomes.

▷ Define Management by Objectives and list its advantages and disadvantages.

PROBLEM SOLVING AND GOAL SETTING

Decisions . . . choices . . . problems . . . we face these every day. Often we are obligated to respond to them whether or not we have a real answer. How do people logically and systematically make decisions? In this chapter we will consider the most basic of the decision-making processes, problem solving and goal setting. The next chapter will continue with the more complex processes of planning and decision-making needed in the very complex, multifaceted situations faced by nurse managers and leaders in health care organizations.

PROBLEM SOLVING

Problem solving is simply a series of steps designed to help you organize information available in order to come up with the best possible solution to a problem (Table 7–1). It is a deliberate, thoughtful way to deal with an immediate situation that is creating some kind of difficulty for which there is no ready-made solution. Instead of reacting to a problem without thinking it through, problem solvers try to first sort out the complexities of the situation and then to bring some thought and organization to their actions to resolve the problem (Golightly, 1981; Kaufman, 1979).

Purpose

Problem solving itself does not supply the answer. It is only the *process* through which you arrive at an answer. Its major usefulness is in providing guidelines or structure for you when you are faced with a problem. It is also the basis of the nursing process, which is probably quite familiar to you. Looking at Table 7–1, you can see that problem solving is simply the more general application of the same familiar steps. *Nursing process* refers to the use of these steps in relation to a patient, client, or group, while problem solving refers to any kind of problem, whether it is related to your patients, to your coworkers, or to repairing your car. You might say, in other words, that problem solving is the *generic* process that can be applied to any number of different kinds of problems.

The steps in problem solving are also used in crisis intervention. The deliberateness of the process can help the person or group undergoing a crisis bring some order to what seems like an uncontrollable situation. After listing everything wrong, trying to formulate a statement summarizing the problem, and then listing every possible alternative solution, the crisis

TABLE 7–1. Comparison of the Problem Solving and Nursing Processes

	I	II	III	IV	V
Problem solving	Collect data	Define problem	Select strategies	Take action	Evaluate
Nursing process	Assessment	Diagnosis	Plan	Implementation	Evaluation

begins to seem more manageable and less overwhelming. By the time you reach the listing of solutions, you will feel at least partially in control of the situation again and able to respond more constructively and calmly.

Problem solving can have a calming effect. "Let's problem solve," is very often a useful response from the leader when a person or group is angry, upset, or confused about how to handle a problem. You can help a client problem solve, you can lead a group through the process, and you can problem solve for yourself.

Steps in the Process

A common source of stress in a work situation will be used to illustrate how to use each of the steps in problem solving:

Imagine that you find yourself in the following situation. Several incidents in the past two weeks have given you the impression that your supervisor is unhappy with your work. You are a new employee and have heard fellow nurses describe past incidents with new employees, saying, "You haven't been here long enough to see how fast the heads roll." At this point, you are afraid that you may be the next to be fired.

In such a situation, the most difficult thing to do may be to remember to problem solve. It may seem that problem solving would be too slow when action is required to save your job, but action without thought may have worse consequences than no action. Action that is both quick and deliberate is needed. This is one reason why a leader or facilitator is so valuable in getting people to begin problem solving in a high-anxiety situation.

STEP 1. ASSESSMENT: COLLECT DATA. List as much information concerning the problem as you are able to do at this time. You may not have all the data you need to complete the process; you can and should seek more on an as-needed basis as you proceed through the process. If your data are unreliable or too incomplete to define the problem, you will have to get more before proceeding. Sometimes you can include getting more data as one of your selected strategies for resolving the problem. Remember, however, that you are gathering data for a specific purpose and that when you have sufficient information to confirm or delete your hypotheses about the situation, you should proceed to the next step and not continue to gather unnecessary information.

The data list for this work problem could include the following information:

1. The supervisor frowns at my charts.
2. The supervisor does not make eye contact with me.
3. Other nurses are given special assignments; I have not been given any.

4. A coworker overheard that I was "being observed," and told me this.
5. I have not been evaluated since I began this job.
6. No one has told me that I am doing a good job. (You should also note here that no one told you the opposite, either.)
7. I believe that I am functioning adequately but feel anxious about the extent to which my performance is seen as satisfactory by the supervisor.

It is important to state the data as *objectively* as possible, saving interpretation for the next step. You can do this by describing observed behavior instead of your interpretation of that behavior. The following statements illustrate the difference between interpretative and objective data statements:

INTERPRETATIVE The supervisor does not like the way I chart.

OBJECTIVE The supervisor frowned when reading my charts but said nothing.

STEP 2. DIAGNOSIS: DEFINE THE PROBLEM. Once you have collected a reasonably adequate amount of data, you can begin to analyze it. Look especially for patterns in the data as well as for clues to the underlying dynamics of the situation, remembering that there are often multiple rather than single factors at work when a problem arises. Then prepare a summarizing statement of the situation in which you define the problem as specifically and objectively as possible. This summary should not include the solution to the problem. The difference is illustrated below:

SOLUTION STATEMENT (Premature)   I should demand an evaluation.

PROBLEM STATEMENT (Appropriate) I do not know how I am being evaluated.

Jumping to the solution is tempting, especially when urgently needed, but it keeps you from exploring new avenues and selecting the best of the available alternatives. It also prevents you from ensuring that your diagnosis is correct before applying a solution.

Let us return to the work situation. Your data so far, although stated objectively, are still somewhat vague. But there is evidence of several patterns running through the data. The first pattern is a general sense of being concerned about your position. There are also clues that point to some kind of dissatisfaction from your supervisor. The second pattern is a vagueness in the data. Almost all the information is indirect or inferred and open to different interpretations. From this analysis, the problems may be defined as follows:

1. Possible supervisor dissatisfaction with my work. Insufficient data to confirm or deny this possibility.
2. Feeling of concern related to my impression that the supervisor may be dissatisfied and to lack of evaluative feedback.

Sometimes it is not possible to immediately define the problem, but only to come up with several alternative hypotheses. If this occurs, it is necessary to gather more information on each hypothesis before selecting one to follow through in the planning step (Elstein, Shulman & Sprafka, 1978).

STEP 3. PLAN: SELECT STRATEGIES.   Write down every appropriate action that you can think of. Do not discard any of these strategies irrevocably until you have considered *all* the possibilities. This is a form of individual *brainstorming* (a term used to describe making every possible suggestion whether wild, weird, or brilliant, without judging how good they are until the brainstorming session is over).

After listing all of the possible actions, select the strategies that, in your judgment, will be the most appropriate and effective strategies for the situation, that is, select the strategies most likely to work. Your leadership skills and experience will help you make the decision. Two examples from other leadership situations:

1. A strike could solve a disagreement with administration over where nurses can park their cars, but it is too strong a measure. A memo, on the other hand, although more appropriate, may be too weak if this has been a long-standing disagreement.
2. It would be inappropriate to tear down a colleague's defense mechanisms in the middle of a crisis. There is a better time to confront someone with his or her use of defense mechanisms.

In real life, many of these distinctions are more subtle than the examples given here.

To return to the work situation, here is a list of possible strategies to resolve the problem:

1. Resign before I am fired.
2. Demand an evaluation as my right.
3. Ignore the problem; it might go away.
4. Transfer to another unit.
5. Try to improve my performance.
6. Compliment my supervisor so my supervisor will like me.
7. Ask my coworker what was meant by saying I was "being observed."
8. Seek feedback from coworkers on my performance.
9. Request an evaluation from my supervisor.

After completing the list, analyze the potential effectiveness and appropriateness of each strategy:

1. Resigning is too drastic a move at this time.
2. Demanding an evaluation is also too strong, because no one has yet refused to do one.
3. Ignoring the problem is ineffective, because it will neither reduce your anxiety nor tell you where or what the problem is.
4. A transfer is a milder form of withdrawal from the problem, but you will still not learn as much about yourself or others if you do not explore the problem before requesting a transfer. Because you do not know yet why this problem has occurred, you would not have learned how to prevent it from occurring in the future or how to handle it if it happened again.
5. Trying to improve your performance would probably not solve the problem at this point, because you do not know exactly how it needs to be improved. This strategy could be effective later if you determine from further data collecting that your performance was not yet satisfactory. A

self-evaluation might provide some reassurance and would also prepare you for a formal evaluation.

6. Complimenting the supervisor might help, but if it is too obvious it may alienate your supervisor or your coworkers and it will not resolve your anxiety. Flattery is an inappropriate strategy.

7. 8, & 9. Since part of the defined problem was insufficient data, talking to your coworker, seeking feedback, and requesting an evaluation from your supervisor can all help fill this need. An evaluation can take some time to prepare so talking with coworkers and requesting informal feedback from your supervisor can provide you with more immediate information and perhaps reduce your anxiety level enough so that you can function well in the meantime.

In this example, a combination of strategies looks like it will be most effective.

STEP 4. IMPLEMENTATION: TAKE ACTION.   Now you are ready to act. You have selected the strategies that in your judgment are most likely to be effective and appropriate for resolving the problem. As you put your plan into action, the responses you get will tell you whether to proceed or to go back and think through the process again. The results can be surprising.

Gathering more data is a common strategy and one that is needed in the imaginary work situation. In the example, you planned to get more information and evaluative feedback from your coworkers, to do a self-evaluation, and then to ask your supervisor for an evaluation:

> Although you cannot be certain that the supervisor will see it the same way, you conclude from your self-evaluation that you have done well in the last three months. A list of your strengths will also be a good selling point during the formal evaluation process.
>
> The next day, you talk to some coworkers and find out that they think you have been "making waves." They point out that you have been adding nursing diagnoses to the patient problem lists in the charts, and only physicians and social workers have been listing problems in this institution. You have also been consulting with other departments about your patients' problems, which has traditionally been the head nurse's role. Your coworkers suggest that you keep the head nurse better informed about your activities, but indicate that they approve of your patient advocacy.
>
> Your request for more feedback from the supervisor results in some clarification of what you thought was happening. The supervisor frowns at your charting because your handwriting is so small the supervisor cannot read it. You have not been given a special assignment because you are still a new employee, but so far you are performing well. A formal evaluation is usually done in consultation with the head nurse after six months, but the supervisor agrees to prepare an interim report and share it with you and the head nurse the following week. You feel relieved, promise to write more legibly, and decide to communicate more with your head nurse, saying that you are ready to take on special assignments along with the rest of your colleagues.
>
> The formal evaluation confirmed that you are doing above-average work. Your list of strengths not only gave you confidence, but was also added to the evaluation done by the supervisor and head nurse.

STEP 5. EVALUATION: EVALUATE RESULTS.   At each step you need to critically analyze the data you are collecting, evaluate the responses that you are getting, or both. Thinking about what you are doing and what results you are getting should be a continuous process so that you can revise your plan where needed as you go along. The evaluation can be subjective as well as objective, including not only the measurable results but also any feeling of accomplishment or satisfaction from having resolved the problem successfully. Your evaluation should also provide clues for future action. For example, would you proceed the same way next time? Did you find a better way?

To return to the work situation one more time:

> Your original diagnosis was an accurate guide to action because you tried to avoid interpreting the data and kept an open mind despite some anxiety. The selection of strategies was correct. If you had resigned or transferred to another unit, you would probably have heard how satisfied the supervisor was with your work when you left the unit. If you had ignored the problem, your anxiety might well have increased and eventually interfered with your performance. It turns out that, while there is still plenty you can learn about your work and your leadership skills, you are doing well and can feel satisfied with both your performance and your evaluation.
>
> In the future, you will ask people right away to explain what they mean when they use a vague term like ''being observed,'' instead of worrying about it. You will also confront a problem and ask for feedback sooner but feel that you used these strategies quite well this time.

Individual Approaches to Problem Solving

Long ago, Benjamin Franklin described his personal method for making decisions: list all factors for and against a particular decision, assign weights to each factor, sum these weights for each list, and then see whether the pro or con comes out best.

Franklin's method bears a great deal of similarity to our modern day problem solving. In fact, some research has indicated that people generally use one fundamental, perhaps even innate, approach that does not change easily, even when they are taught a different method. One extensive study found that people generate hypotheses early in the problem-solving process and do not wait until all the facts are in before coming up with some solutions. These researchers also found that different people are best at solving different types of problems. (Elstein, Shulman, Sprafka, et al, 1978). You may, for example, be particularly adept at solving problems with recalcitrant equipment, while your colleague is particularly good at working out creative staffing patterns when a temporary staff shortage occurs. One's profession also seems to affect the content of that person's problem solving (Holzemer, 1986). For instance, a nurse may focus on different aspects of a situation than a physician.

People also have a tendency to oversimplify or choose a solution that worked in the past (Prescott, Dennis, & Jacox, 1987). The number of factors that affect a situation can become quite complex in their interrelationships. Often there is no single, obvious reason why a problem occurred nor one simple action that can solve the problem (Elstein, Shulman & Sprafka, 1978). This desire for simplicity is strong enough that people will try to make new facts fit old hunches in order to avoid having to redefine the problem. You should be alert for this when problem solving with others.

SETTING GOALS AND OBJECTIVES _____

Essentials of Management by Objectives

The purpose of using goals or objectives is to set out clearly what direction your work should take and what specific accomplishments (outcomes) are expected within a given period of time. In other words, the objectives serve first as a guide to the planning of your work and later as a guide to evaluating your work. Problem solving is done to deal with a specific problem or situation; setting goals is done to plan future work.

The essentials of this approach are quite simple: set meaningful goals written in the form of objectives, carry out the objectives, and evaluate how well the objectives have been met. This procedure assumes that a thorough collection of data and definition of the needs of the work situation have already been done.

WRITING OBJECTIVES. Assuming that you have adequate data, the first step is to write a set of objectives for a given period of time. The objectives should begin with an action verb and describe an activity that can be measured or at least observed. When possible, they should be specific, be time-bound, and state a measurable or observable end result in order to increase the objectivity of the evaluation done at the end point.

The objectives should also be *meaningful* and either *congruent* with the goals of the system in which you are working or deliberately aimed at changing its goals. Meaningful goals are those which describe some kind of change or progress in the work being done or an entirely new direction. Meaningless objectives tend to describe routine activities or no action at all, such as "Have a positive attitude toward work."

Most of your objectives will be congruent with the goals of the system in which you are working. But when changes are needed, your objectives may be deliberately in conflict with some of your team's or organization's goals. If you find that all or most of your objects are in conflict with those of the team or organization, you need to consider this carefully and question whether or not you should move to another team or organization.

The time set for completing the objectives depends on the nature of the work being planned, the proportion of the work day set aside to work on the objectives, and other factors that will affect the speed with which the work can be done. Common time frames used in most health care organizations are one month, three months, six months and one year.

Objectives may be used as the basis upon which a formal evaluation is made in the management system known as *management by objectives* (*MBO*). When objectives are used as a part of a formal system of management, they are written not only for individual employees but also for larger work groups, including committees, departments, and the organization as a whole (Trexler, 1987). (See Table 7–2 for some examples.) Congruence between these different levels of objectives is sometimes difficult to achieve.

Individual Objectives. If your organization uses MBO, you may be given a set of objectives, asked to write your own objectives, or asked to write them with your immediate supervisor. Of course, there is a great difference between being encouraged to set your own objectives and being handed a

TABLE 7–2. Examples of Individual and Group Level Objectives

Level	Objective
Individual staff nurse	Complete a course in infection control in the home.
Nursing team	Review all cases for the past six months in which occurrence of infection is documented.
Nursing supervisors	Update all policies and procedures related to infection control.
Home health agency (organizational level)	Reduce incidence of infection in current agency caseload.

predetermined set of objectives. The first method increases motivation and encourages self-management; the second is nonparticipative, discourages self-management, reduces motivation, and may primarily be a means for control (Levinson & LaMonica, 1980).

Whether or not you have an employer who uses MBO, you can develop your own objectives to guide career planning and professional growth. The following is an example:

> Imagine that you have begun working in a new position in a critical care unit. For the first few weeks, your primary objectives would be to learn the new job and become acquainted with the people with whom you are working and the organization in which you are now working.
>
> At the end of three months, you feel more comfortable with the work that you are doing and have also become familiar with the informal ways of working within this particular organization. At this point, you can either go along with the routines of the job and accept whatever changes in assignment are made for you or you can decide on the direction you would like to see your career take and set objectives for yourself that will take you in that direction.

If you decide to set your own course, there are several questions to ask yourself:

1. How can I improve my practice?
2. What do I want to gain from this position?
3. What do I want to be doing a year from now?
4. What do I want to be doing five years from now?

The specific objectives that you write will depend on your answers to these questions, your overall goals, and your current position. Both short-term and long-term objectives are helpful. For example, you may want to learn how to assemble, use, and adjust the new respirator that is going to be used on your unit within the next month. This would be a short-term objective. You may also want to write a protocol for the use of the new respirator by the end of the month, implement full use of the respirator in three months, and complete an evaluation of its effectiveness in six months or a year.

Long-term goals may need to be broken down into steps. For example, a year from now you may want to have completed a course to become a clinical specialist in critical care. You can develop a time line to follow in working toward this long-term objective as follows:

1 month: Obtain information about courses and programs available.

3 months: Complete application to selected program.

6 months: Begin course in critical care nursing.

1 year: Complete first course.

You can see that it would take longer than one year to fulfill your long-term objective or goal to complete an entire clinical specialist program. The short-term objectives serve as check points on your way to your long-term objective.

Work Group Objectives.   As the leader or manager of a variety of working groups, you will also find objectives useful as guides for planning and evaluating the work of these groups. The criteria for writing objectives are the same, but their scope and content will differ. The following objectives would be appropriate for a task force or committee:

1 month: Invite a speaker on home care services to the next meeting.

3 months: Select a method for surveying the availability of home care services in the community.

6 months: Survey the availability of home care services in the community.

1 year: Prepare a report on the availability of home care services in the community.

It is less common and yet probably more important for health care teams to develop a set of objectives, because they can very easily become immersed in their daily routines and lose sight of future goals or direction for improvement and change. The following list is one example:

1. Increase the number of complete discharge plans.
2. Invite people from other agencies to client-oriented conferences.
3. Plan, organize, and initiate a support group for families of developmentally disabled children.
4. Design a new crash cart system to decrease current response time.
5. Revise outpatient chemotherapy procedures to decrease waiting time and increase patient comfort.

IMPLEMENTING OBJECTIVES.   Once the objectives and time frames have been determined, the next step is to carry out the work indicated. The objective itself defines the general action and the expected outcome, but does not tell you exactly how to go about carrying out the action. For example, the health care team objective of including people from other agencies in client-oriented conferences tells you that people should be invited but it does not tell you exactly which people, how many people, or how to extend the invitation. The objective serves as a guide, telling you what to do but not how to do it.

Some of the examples given have included an indication of the time in which the objective is expected to be completed. Time lines are particularly helpful in working out the specific objectives leading to a long-term goal. When the objective is a complex one, it may also be necessary to break it down even further into separate steps or components in order to have an adequate guide for your work and for evaluating your progress as you go along.

The objectives and time estimates are meant to be a flexible guide, not unbendable demands. Circumstances change and external factors can interfere with fulfilling an objective within a projected amount of time. For example, if you need one more course to complete a clinical specialist program but the course is cancelled at the last minute, you cannot be expected to fulfill the objectives in the previously estimated amount of time. You might, however, be expected to investigate the possibility of an alternative way to complete the program requirements on time.

EVALUATING OUTCOMES. Evaluation of accomplishments is based on the degree to which this outcome was met. This outcome may or may not have been very specifically described in the objective:

> For example, one of the health care team objectives was to increase the number of completed discharge plans. If 25% of the discharge plans were completed before setting this goal, then an outcome of 50% now completed would indicate that the objective had been met. However, if the objective had stated that all (100%) of the discharge plans would be complete, then a 50% completion rate would not have fulfilled the objective.

The degree to which the individual or work group has control over all of the factors that affect the fulfillment of the objective is a source of concern in the evaluation phase of MBO, especially when the objectives are used as the basis for formal evaluation of employees and affect decisions about raises, promotions, and so forth. For example:

> Your team's goal of reducing waiting time in the immunization clinic to a half hour or less seemed reasonable until an unforeseen outbreak of measles occurred in the high schools. The resulting flood of high school students going to the health department for immunization would make it virtually impossible to meet your team's goal, at least until the outbreak was brought under control.

The concern about external factors that can influence the progress of work toward a stated objective has led to the development of a somewhat more complex MBO system. In this system, any major obstacles that stood in the way of completing the objectives within the given time are listed separately to recognize the possibility of their occurrence. The types of support and resources that are needed from others in order to fulfill objectives are also listed separately at the time that the objectives are set in order to increase the fairness of using the objectives as evaluation criteria.

Advantages and Disadvantages of the Goal-Setting Approach

Management by objectives, or MBO, is a well-known approach to planning and evaluating the work done in organizations (Drucker, 1977). Although it is usually described as a tool for managers, it can also be used by leaders who do not hold the title of manager. In fact, MBO can be used by any individual or group at any level in the organization, or by the organization as a whole. It can be used as a total system of management throughout the organization, including financial management (Deegan & O'Donovan,

1984), but this requires a real commitment to the purposes and philosophy of MBO that does not always occur.

Depending on the way in which it is used, MBO can be either a useful management system or just another imposition on the staff's time and energy. One of its major advantages is that it can direct attention and energy where they are most needed and, in this way, help people to set priorities and be more productive. If it is used as a total management system at all levels within the organization, the objectives should actually be set before individual departments are even organized (Deegan, 1977). The objectives, which are set at various levels throughout the organization, then determine how work should be organized and what work has the highest priority. They serve as a planning guide and encourage goal-directed behavior rather than random activity. They can also help people avoid getting so caught up in the daily routine that they lose sight of their long-term goals.

MBO can be used with either an authoritarian or participative management style. When individuals and work groups set their own objectives, the result is usually a greater degree of acceptance of the objectives and a high level of motivation to meet the goals. The participative style also encourages self-direction and professional growth. The mutually agreed-upon objectives become a means for communicating expected standards of work and help each staff member sort out what needs to be done. Well-written objectives can clearly communicate what everyone is expected to accomplish.

Another advantage to MBO is that it provides an opportunity for everyone involved in a particular job to know what is expected. Using these same objectives to evaluate performance helps to eliminate the subjectivity that is so often a problem in evaluation.

On the other hand, MBO can be a meaningless exercise if the objectives are not used after they are written. The quality of the objectives usually deteriorates under such circumstances, leading to further disillusionment and eventual abandonment of the system (Deegan, 1977). In order for goal setting to be an effective approach, the objectives must be meaningful in the first place, referred to frequently for feedback on the amount of progress being made, and, finally, used as the standard by which performance is evaluated. It is very important, however, that all of the factors influencing whether or not objectives are met be thoroughly analyzed, as was mentioned above, or the objectives will become an overly demanding and rigid standard, appearing to staff as a punishment rather than a guide.

When MBO is used in an authoritarian manner, it becomes an additional set of controls over employees and is quickly perceived as such. The objectives may become a source of unrealistic demands, especially if goals are set higher and higher each year. They may also become a threat when used as an evaluative tool without initial discussion and acceptance by the employee. You can see that these uses undermine the advantages of clearer guidelines, higher motivation, and improved productivity for which MBO is used in the first place. MBO can be rigid and confining and can result in unfair evaluations. The program can also become an empty, time-consuming routine if the objectives are not meaningful or if people do not take them seriously and use them. The use of objective writing and goal setting as a management system is a potentially effective approach, but it is only as good as the objectives that are written and the manner in which they are used.

SUMMARY ———————————————————————————————————

The nursing process and the problem-solving process are based upon the same progression of events: collect whatever data are needed, define the problem, select appropriate strategies for dealing with the problem, take action, and evaluate results. Problem solving is particularly helpful in bringing a sense of order and manageability to a problem, clarifying the situation, and calming people during a crisis. Many people have a tendency to try to define the problem immediately rather than waiting until the facts are known, and to oversimplify the problem in an attempt to make it more manageable. There are also differences in approach based on the amount of knowledge and experience an individual has with a particular type of problem.

Goal setting and objective writing may be used as the basis of a total management system, called Management by Objectives (MBO). The objectives serve as a guide to planning the work, setting priorities, and evaluating effectiveness. Objectives should begin with an action verb and include observable outcomes. The objectives may be long-term or short-term; be individual, group, or organizational; and used in an authoritative or participative manner. When using objectives to evaluate outcomes, it is important to recognize the effects that organizational and external factors may have had on an individual's or a group's success in meeting the objectives. Some systems also include the resources and support needed to achieve the objectives in order to make the evaluation fairer.

REFERENCES* ———————————————————————————————

*Deegan, A.X. & O'Donovan, T.R. (1982). *Management by Objectives for hospitals.* Rockville, Maryland: Aspen Systems.

Deegan, A.X. & O'Donovan, T.R. (1984). Budgeting and management by objectives. *Health Care Management Review,* 9, (1).

Drucker, P. (1977). *People and performance: The best of Peter Drucker on Management.* New York: Harper and Row.

Elstein, A.S., Shulman, L.S., & Sprafka, S.A. et al. (1978). *Medical problem solving: An analysis of clinical reasoning.* Cambridge, Massachusetts: Harvard University Press.

Golightly, C.K. (1981). *Creative problem solving for health professionals.* Rockville, Maryland: Aspen Systems.

Holzemer, W.L. (1986). The structure of problem solving in simulations. *Nursing Research,* 35, 231–235.

*Kaufman, R. (1979). *Identifying and solving problems: A systems approach.* La Jolla, California: University Associates.

*Levinson, H. & LaMonica, E.L. (1980). Management by whose objectives? *Journal of Nursing Administration,* 10, (2), 22.

Prescott, P.A., Dennis, K.A., & Jacos, A.K. (1987). Clinical decision making of staff nurses. *Image,* 19, (2), 56–62.

Trexler, B.J. (1987). Nursing department purpose, philosophy, and objectives: Their use and effectiveness. *Journal of Nursing Administration,* 17, (3), 8–12.

———————————————————

*References marked with an asterisk are suggested for further reading.

Chapter 8

PROJECT PLANNING

Chapter 8

OUTLINE

Planning
Types of Planning

Phase I: Developing the Plan
Establish the Purpose
Analyze the Situation
Problem Analysis
Situational Variables
Anticipated Response to Change
Formulate Objectives
Generate Alternative Solutions
Brainstorming
Nominal Group Technique
Synectics
Analyze the Options and Select a
Course of Action
Simulation
Scenarios
Pilot Projects

Phase II: Presenting the Plan
Obtaining Approval
Making a Presentation
Content
Delivery

**Phase III: Implementing and
Monitoring the Plan**
Planning the Implementation
Schedules
Gantt Charts
PERT Charts
Critical Path Method
Directing Implementation
Monitoring Implementation
Evaluating Outcomes
Revising and Updating the Plan

Summary

LEARNING OBJECTIVES

Upon completion of this chapter, the reader will be able to:

▷ List and explain the three phases of planning.

▷ Outline a plan for a health-related project.

▷ Identify the situational variables that would affect a project plan.

▷ Suggest ways to generate creative alternative solutions.

▷ Use a simple rating system to evaluate alternative solutions.

▷ Present a project plan in a persuasive manner.

▷ Use a Gantt or similar chart to monitor implementation of a project.

PROJECT PLANNING

Project planning is the focus of this chapter. The process is divided into three major phases: developing the plan, presenting the plan, and implementing and monitoring the plan (Fig. 8–1).

The specific steps in developing the plan include establishing the purpose or mission of the project, analyzing the situational variables that will affect the project, formulating objectives, generating alternative courses of action, analyzing these alternatives, and selecting a course of action. That first phase alone is a lot of work and requires patience when there is a strong desire to get something done.

In the second phase, the plan must be presented to whomever has the final authority to approve the plan and provide the money to carry it out. This person is often called the *sponsor*. In the third phase, the approved plan is implemented, the implementation is monitored, and the outcomes are evaluated so that the plan can be revised and updated as needed (Byson and Delbecq, 1979; Nutt, 1984).

Although project planning is a far more elaborate and complex undertaking, its basic sequence of events has its foundations in the problem-solving process. You will probably recognize this kinship to problem solving as you progress through this chapter. As you read this chapter, you may want to refer back to Figure 8–1 from time to time to keep the three major phases of project planning and the specific steps within them clear in your mind. What is presented here should be helpful to you in all of your planning activities as a leader-manager.

PLANNING

Whether it is done on small scale to get a project underway or on a broad, organization-wide basis, planning is one of the distinguishing characteristics of the effective manager.

Planning is a dynamic, future-oriented process. It is quite complex and involves a whole set of interrelated actions and decisions (Sloma, 1984). The phases and specifics of the process can be compared with the logic of the basic problem-solving process, but they involve a great number of complex managerial activities that are usually not necessary for problem solving.

Types of Planning

Strategic planning is marketing-oriented planning for the future of an entire organization. *Project planning* is the process applied to a particular project within an organization or in cooperation with other agencies (Dychtwald & Zitter, 1988; Lukacs, 1984).

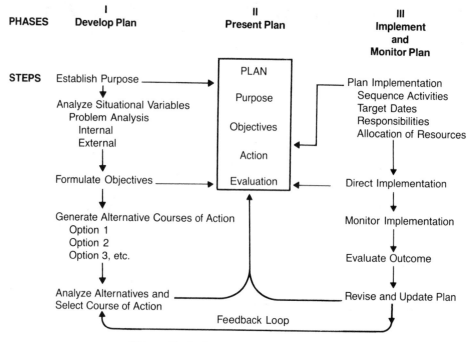

Figure 8–1. Project planning model.

In actual practice, many projects are implemented with very little planning. Many of the steps that we will discuss in this chapter are skipped or done in great haste.

A common shortcut is adopting a plan that has worked well somewhere else. This ignores the uniqueness of each organization, the community within which it operates, and the population it serves. Other common shortcuts are to jump right to generating options or asking just a few key people for their opinions and then moving immediately into implementation. Some people admire this "bold" approach, mistaking precipitate action for decisiveness. This often leads to expensive or even fatal mistakes in projects.

PHASE I: DEVELOPING THE PLAN

Establish the Purpose

The first step in planning is to clearly establish the purpose or mission of the entire process. Failure to do so will lead to much confusion, frustration, and wasted effort. It is *not* necessary, however, to be very specific about the objectives of planning at this point. In fact, it would be premature to specify the objectives so early in the process.

Most planning is initiated when a *performance gap* of some type is recognized. This gap may be an existing one or one that is likely to occur in the near future. The performance gap becomes the *raison d'être* of the planning process; it is the spark that sets fire to the latent interest in planning.

Planning may be reactive or proactive. *Reactive* planning is done in response to an existing problem. The problem may be an increase in errors or incident reports, competition from another agency, a drop in the number of patients, an increase in the cost of staff or equipment, or failure to achieve approval by a regulating agency. Any of these would provide sufficient impetus to initiate planning.

Proactive planning, on the other hand, is planning done in anticipation of such problems occurring in the future, before the problems occur. It may be done in anticipation of changing needs or to promote growth and excellence within the organization. A major advantage of proactive planning is that it can be done in an atmosphere of calm instead of chaos. However, more attention must be given to keeping interest and support sufficiently high to move ahead without the pressure of an immediate need or an impending crisis. The main disadvantage of reactive planning, on the other hand, is that urgency can lead to carelessness and haste (the "Do something, anything fast!" mentality) (Cerne, 1988; Nutt, 1984).

Planning, then, is initiated when either a current or anticipated need or performance gap is recognized. Meeting this need or closing the gap becomes the purpose or mission of the planning process. A statement of the purpose should be general until a thorough assessment of the situation has been done. Keeping the statement general allows the planner more flexibility. This is especially necessary if the perceived problem differs from the actual problem that is found when an assessment is done.

The statement of purpose may be for a relatively simple performance gap such as "To reduce the waiting time between collection of lab specimens and reporting of the results." Or, it may be for a relatively complex problem such as the following community health example:

> As federal and state money for health care services became increasingly difficult to obtain, the City Council became concerned about its responsibility to provide health care for the indigent population. They were particularly concerned about the huge and rapidly increasing cost of the city hospital's emergency service. It was generally assumed that many of the visits were actually nonemergency in nature and that a cheaper alternative could be found.
>
> The City Council appointed a committee with representatives from the Council itself, the city hospital, and the health department. The stated purpose of the committee was "to develop a more efficient plan for meeting the primary and emergency health care needs of the city's indigent population."

Note that the stated purpose is very broad and did not even mention the emergency room problem that was the original impetus for this planning project. We will return to these two examples of the lab specimens and the emergency department several times later in this chapter.

Analyze the Situation

This is the major assessment phase of the planning process. Although it is often necessary to collect additional data at later stages, it is here that the focus is on data collection. The assessment has several purposes and can become quite complicated.

What kind of information is needed? As the planner, you will need three major kinds of information: information to confirm (or question) the identified problem; information to identify the factors that affect the problem; and an estimate of the anticipated responses to change.

PROBLEM ANALYSIS. Information is needed to verify the purpose that has been identified in the previous stage and to assist in setting the goals in the next stage. It is not unusual for the problem to have been misidentified. It is especially common for a symptom to have been mistaken for the core problem. It is important to find the source of the problem and to distinguish it from the signs that signal its existence.

SITUATIONAL VARIABLES. Information about the situation (environment) in which this need or performance gap has arisen is necessary for developing the alternatives later on. In order to do this thoroughly, a holistic approach that encompasses as many important variables as possible is clearly preferable.

It is difficult to develop a list of all the possible factors that would be applicable to any situation and yet be specific enough to help the planner. There are several systems frameworks that attempt to do this. One example, adapted from Nadler (Nutt, 1984), includes function, inputs, outputs, sequence, context, physical catalysts, and human catalysts in the assessment (Table 8–1). The laboratory example will be used to illustrate its application to a project planning situation:

1. *Function.* Purpose or use. The general function of the lab is to accurately and efficiently process specimens whereas the function of the nursing unit in regard to lab tests is to ensure that appropriate specimens are sent and that the results are interpreted and communicated as necessary.
2. *Outputs.* The product produced by each system involved. The lab pro-

TABLE 8–1. System Framework for Analyzing Environmental Variables

Function:
  What is our purpose?
Outputs:
  What is our product?
Inputs:
  What is needed to produce the product?
Sequence:
  In what order are the inputs needed?
Context:
  What is the effect of the environment on our functioning?
Physical Catalysts:
  What additional things would make the work easier, faster, and of higher quality?
Human Catalysts:
  What additional people would make the work easier, faster, and of higher quality?
Interrelationships:
  How should the various parts fit together to provide an integrated, functional system of operaton?

duces printed test results. The nursing unit produces health care for its patients.

3. *Inputs.* Whatever is needed to produce the output. The lab needs appropriate specimens, adequate staff and equipment, and a certain amount of time in which to process the specimens. The nursing unit needs to know how to collect and send the specimens and needs to receive the results in a clear, interpretable, and timely fashion.

4. *Sequence.* The order in which things must be done. The lab cannot process specimens until they are received and logged. The nursing unit cannot act on the results until they have been received.

5. *Environment.* The context in which the function takes place. The nursing unit receives information from multiple sources, only one of which is the lab. Although it appears much quieter than the nursing unit, the laboratory experiences periods of high activity and multiple demands for immediate results, which distract technicians from processing the nonemergency specimens.

6. *Physical Catalysts.* The objects that would make the work easier, faster or of higher quality. The equipment for processing the specimens is adequate but there is no computer equipment on the nursing stations to receive laboratory results directly.

7. *Human Catalysts.* Any people who could make the work easier, faster, or of higher quality. Clerks enter patient records on the nursing unit. Telephone calls and verbal requests take precedence, however, so recording is often not done until late afternoon. Until the records are entered, the nurses on the unit must sort through the printouts from the lab to find the results for a particular patient. No one in the lab seems to be particularly interested in what happens to the results once they leave the lab.

8. *Interrelationships.* The connections between the various parts of the system or systems. The lab computer cannot communicate with the nursing unit computer. The recording must be done manually, and nursing personnel often find themselves caught in the middle between lab personnel irritated with them over frequent calls for results and physicians impatient with results that are slow in coming. Also, nurses must delay nursing decisions until the results arrive. This leaves patients waiting for care.

A second approach to assessment comes from Kola and Kosberg (1981). Their approach includes assessment of a service in terms of demand, resources, and priorities. This approach is especially helpful when more than one organization is involved in the planning process and when your organization has a strong community health orientation. The City Council example will be used to illustrate its use:

1. *Demand.* Who is seeking this type of service? How often do they require the service? How are they paying for it? In the emergency care example, it is important to know how many people reside in the city, how many of these residents are unable to pay for care, what services are needed, how many people use emergency services, and how many of the visits to the emergency department are actually for nonemergency purposes.

2. *Current Resources.* To what extent is this service currently available?

What funding is available? Can other agencies offer the primary care services currently being sought from the emergency department?

3. *Adequacy of Resources.* Do current services meet the demand? Is there sufficient staff, expertise, and money available to offer the service? For example, are sufficient nonemergency services available? Are they adequately funded and staffed? Do they meet accepted standards of care? Is the staff adequately trained? Are the services accessible and well-received by clients? Is there continuity of care?

4. *Priorities.* How important is this service? What need is most urgent? What is the major concern of the population unable to pay for health care?

Continuing the City Council example:

There are three sources of primary care for the indigent in the city: a health department pediatric clinic, a federally funded center that serves all ages in one specifically defined catchment area, and a private, nonprofit agency that serves the elderly but is dependent on outside funding and is in danger of closing.

Clients find it easier to go to the emergency room because it is open twenty-four hours a day and serves all ages. Cost to the city for care at any of the clinics is under $100 per visit, but an emergency room visit averages $200 per visit. The clinics are underutilized, whereas a visit to the emergency room can involve a wait of up to three hours.

ANTICIPATED RESPONSE TO CHANGE. Information is also needed about the probable response of the environment in which the change (i.e., the plan) will take place. This information will be especially useful in the implementation stages. It also affects the choice from among the alternatives generated, because some may be appropriate in terms of solving the problem but would be impossible to actually implement given the current situation.

The elements to be considered may be divided into the factors or forces that would support change and those that would inhibit change (as is done in Lewin's model, explained further in Chapter 19). Among the factors to be considered are the nature of the change itself; the environment in which the change will take place (such as type of decision-making generally done, openness to change); availability of resources needed to bring about change including time, money, and information; and the people and organizations who will support, oppose, or ignore the attempt to change. These people may include staff members, clients, administrators, the people in the regulatory agencies who govern funding for some services, and many more.

Much of the data about anticipated responses to change will have to be fairly general at this stage. At this point it is especially helpful to identify the *stakeholders* in the situation. The stakeholders are those who have an interest, or a stake, in the outcome of the planning process (Nutt, 1984). Because it is a more complicated situation, the City Council example will be used to illustrate the identification of stakeholders:

The City Council appointed a Planning Committee to deal with the problem of overuse of the emergency room and the burgeoning costs that had resulted. The following people have a clear interest in the outcomes of the Planning Committee's work:

The Planning Committee itself would not want the public embarrassment of failing in its assigned task nor does it want to anger or upset anyone important in the community or on the City Council.

The clients, at this point, seem to prefer the hospital emergency room, although they do not like the long waiting hours.

The City Hospital wants to continue to receive the substantial revenue generated by the emergency room use, but the staff is overburdened by the number of patients.

The primary care clinics all need to increase their utilization, but each also wants to maintain its identity, territory, and clients.

Taxpayers in the city will have to monetarily support whatever outcome occurs.

Funding Agencies want to see their contributions well-used but are also affected by political considerations.

The City Council wants the problem solved, but without too great an expenditure since members will have to answer to voters in the next election.

Formulate Objectives

Now that the need or performance gap has been fully assessed, it is possible to develop specific objectives for the project. The objectives should be written as measurable outcomes so that they can later serve as guidelines for evaluation in the final stages of this process.

There are two important points to keep in mind while writing objectives within the planning process. The first, and often the most difficult, is to avoid writing solutions into the objectives. People often are not aware that they are doing this unless it is pointed out to them by someone else. An example of this might be helpful:

An appropriate, although not necessarily a realistic, objective for the indigent care project would be ''To continue to provide nonemergency primary care on a twenty-four hour basis.'' The same objective, written in such a way that the means by which it will be carried out are mistakenly included would be, ''To keep the three existing primary care clinics open on a twenty-four hour basis.'' By specifying the solution, this second objective eliminates other alternatives, such as twenty-four hour telephone consultation with emergency room backup.

The second point about writing objectives is the level of specificity on which they are written. Some are so specific that it would be necessary to write hundreds for a complex project, while others are so broad that they offer little guidance to the rest of the planning process. The following is an example of this difference:

Too Broad: To improve the health of the city's medically indigent population.

Too Specific: To publicize the existing pediatric clinic.

About Right: To reduce the nonemergency use of city hospital's emergency department by 50% in the next year.

You may have noticed that the overly specific objective actually states a solution, which is somewhat premature at this point.

Generate Alternative Solutions

Now it is finally time to focus on solutions to the problem. Creativity, open-mindedness, expertise, and an adequate assessment are all vital to this step.

Too often the alternatives are only variations of the current situation rather than completely different solutions. The planner's leadership skills become particularly important in creating a climate of discovery and positive thinking. When monetary resources are scarce or the performance gap is long-standing and no amount of tinkering with it has had any effect, the sponsor, planning committee (or its equivalent), and other stakeholders may be pessimistic about a positive outcome.

Brainstorming, the nominal group technique, and synectics are often recommended for use at this stage. Other activities include consultation with inside and outside experts, a search of the literature, and a survey of clients and other stakeholders if there was insufficient data collected in the assessment stage. It is also important to avoid the tempting alternative of imitating someone else's solution. This is somewhat analogous to borrowing someone else's shoes: they rarely fit well.

Brainstorming. Brainstorming is designed to encourage creativity. The purpose of the brainstorming session is to encourage people to break out of old, rigid patterns of thinking.

The rules are simple. Every idea put forth by a group member is acknowledged by recording it on a chalkboard or flipchart. The group doing the brainstorming is told that all ideas relevant to the subject are to be received without criticism or challenge of any type. Limitations and restrictions are to be ignored for the moment, but other members of the group may expand on an offered idea. Wild, crazy, unrealistic ideas are encouraged, because they may contain the nucleus of a realistic solution or a stimulus to another idea that can actually be implemented.

The session may be ended after a given amount of time or when the group has clearly exhausted its ideas. The leader, however, should encourage the group to generate as many ideas as possible and ensure that all have participated. Some people may have difficulty "letting loose" in a work situation, so this should be taken into consideration.

The composition of the brainstorming group is another point to consider. Each member must have sufficient background information and expertise to participate intelligently. On the other hand, a fresh perspective is quite valuable and may come from people with little prior contact with the problem. Too large a group will limit individual participation and may inhibit creativity. A group larger than fifteen people is probably too large, but the dynamics of the group are more important than the actual number. It is important that the group see this as a serious undertaking, not a silly exercise, and that you do it only if there is a possibility that a creative new approach could be accepted.

After the brainstorming, the ideas are evaluated in terms of what would work most effectively. This is done without reference to the originator of the idea (not easy to do in some groups). Any critique should be constructive and without implied criticism of the idea's originator. The final product should be a small list of the best approaches for achieving the outcomes specified by the objectives (Beal, Bohlen & Raudabaugh, 1962).

NOMINAL GROUP TECHNIQUE. This is a more formal way to encourage creative thinking. It is particularly useful in an organization that is very formal or in a group where status and power differences are likely to lead to the dominance of a few and the consequent loss of potential contributions from other group members (Delbecq and Van de Ven, 1971).

Unlike brainstorming, this is a quiet procedure. The leader introduces the subject and explains the ground rules. Group members are asked to think carefully about the problem and then make a list of possible solutions without discussing them with anyone else. When participants are finished writing, the leader then asks that each group member, in turn, read one item from his or her list and records it on a chalkboard or flipchart. Alternatively, the leader may collect and read the suggestions in order to keep their sources anonymous. This continues until all of the ideas have been recorded. The ideas are then discussed in terms of how they might provide a solution to the problem and how they may or may not work. Finally, the group is asked to create a list of preferred options as was done after brainstorming.

SYNECTICS. Synectics is a third approach to generating creative ideas within a group (Prince, 1970). One of the fundamental ideas of synectics is that new ideas need to be nurtured, protected, and given a chance to develop before they are subjected to evaluation. Ironically, the opposite usually happens in a group. People often are automatically critical of embryonic ideas, responding to them as if they should be born fully developed instead of ready to be developed.

For example, if someone suggested that the laboratory (from the earlier example) hire a team of couriers to deliver test results to the units, the typical immediate response would be that hiring a team of new employees is too expensive. Avoiding this usual response, a more encouraging reply would be to ask for more information about the couriers. How many would be needed? Would they be part of the existing courier system? Could we use electronic "couriers" instead? Could the new computer system act as the courier? These responses encourage further thought rather than inhibiting it.

Each of us is, to differing degrees, sensitive to criticism, especially in front of a group of our colleagues and supervisors. This sensitivity inhibits some people to the point where they will offer no suggestions in groups. Others will shoot down their own ideas before other people have the chance to do it. Still others become aggressive and attack tender new ideas to avoid being attacked themselves. These attacks can be quite subtle. They can, for example, be disguised as "helpful suggestions" or "concerned questions," but their effect is to kill the new idea. Obviously, none of these defensive or offensive responses enhances creativity.

In contrast, the synectic response encourages creativity by nurturing the new idea and protecting its source. The group is asked to build upon each other's ideas rather than tearing them down. Instead of challenging a new idea, group members try to contribute to its development. Questions and comments that would nurture rather than discourage an idea include the following:

1. May I add to your suggestion? I think we could also do. . . .
2. Let's see how this could work.

3. Can you elaborate on your idea? Tell us how you see. . . .
4. Your suggestion has possibilities. Let's talk about how this could be done.

Such an approach not only gives the new idea a chance but encourages other people to present their ideas. Without this approach, many potentially worthy ideas die in their formative stage. Brainstorming and synectics have similar goals. Brainstorming focuses on bringing out the greatest variety of ideas possible, while synectics focuses on protecting and developing ideas that are brought up within the group.

Analyze the Options and Select a Course of Action

Now it is time to be analytical. In this step, each option is evaluated as thoroughly as possible *before* it is implemented. You are trying to predict how well each one will work without actually doing it. This means that you will be relying upon a great deal of informed judgment in making these decisions. This is a crucial step, but one that is usually done too quickly.

As we saw in the last section, a typical response is premature criticism. Refraining from this until each idea has been given full consideration is quite difficult. In fact, the sponsor, in particular, may become quite impatient at this point and wish to get on with the implementation of his or her favorite option.

There are several methods available for making these judgments as accurately and objectively as possible. The fundamental notion is to simulate in some way the actual implementation of each option. Ways to simulate the options include paper-and-pencil or computer simulation; scenarios; and pilot projects (De Geus, 1988; Nutt, 1984). Each has its advantages and disadvantages.

Simulation. Paper-and-pencil simulation is the most common way to analyze the pros and cons of each option. Each option is analyzed in terms of its requirements and anticipated outcomes. The requirements (resources needed) differ somewhat depending upon the project, but most projects will require some space, staff, equipment, supplies, specialized expertise, legal or regulatory approvals, and time in which to accomplish the implementation. All of these requirements and outcomes are calculated or predicted as accurately as possible for each option, and then the options are rated according to the least difficulty in implementation for the greatest gain after implementation.

A simplified example of this kind of rating can be illustrated using the laboratory example:

> Four options were generated by the group formed to solve the problem of slow reporting of results: a new courier system; adding this task to those of the existing courier system; adding a new computer system; and using the hospital-wide computer system after it has been installed. Each option was rated in terms of the requirements for new equipment, staff, and expertise and an estimate of the resulting improvement in communication between the laboratory and the nursing units. Each criterion was rated on a scale of 1, most effective (low requirement, high improvement), to 3, least effective (high requirement, low improvement).
>
> As you can see in Table 8–2, the new or existing courier systems would require far less equipment than the computer system but far more staff in terms of numbers of people added to carry out this project. Actual cost figures can be calculated for both of these

TABLE 8–2. Example of a Simplified Rating System

	New Courier System	Existing Couriers	Computer System	Computer System after Hospital System is Installed
Requirements:				
Equipment	1	1	3	1
Staff	3	2	1	1
Expertise/ Training	2	1	2	2
Outcomes:				
Time in reporting results	1	2	1	1
Total Rating	7	6	7	5

Rating System: 1   most effective (low requirement, high improvement)
               to
            3   least effective (high requirement, low improvement)

categories, noting that most of the computer expenditure occurs only once but that staff is a continuous expense. (Both require some types of "maintenance" in the form of repairs for the computer and benefits for employees.)

Expertise requirements are higher for the options that are completely new. Use of the existing courier system seems to be least costly to implement but less effective in the long run since the delivery of laboratory results will have to compete with other important tasks.

The final decision was to use the existing courier system until a new hospital computer system was fully installed, at which time this option could be implemented with the lowest requirement demand and a better outcome than use of the existing courier system.

This type of rating system is somewhat oversimplified, but it does help to reduce the subjectivity of the decision-making process.

Computer simulation programs are available for some common decision-making processes but will not be available for many others. However, the calculation of projected costs of most projects can be done by entering the data onto an electronic spreadsheet and then changing the numbers (such as the cost of staff) to reflect the needs of each option. The spreadsheet then shows you how much each option would cost in terms of expenses such as staff. One way to visualize this is to think of the spreadsheet as answering financial "What if . . . " questions, such as "What if I add five more employees—how much will that increase the budget?" "What if I purchase new equipment? Which will cost more?"

SCENARIOS. Scenarios are especially useful when the human and organizational factors in project implementation are likely to be more important considerations than cost. It is a valuable analytical tool when one of the major concerns about implementation of various options deals with people's response to change (Will people accept this new routine? Are they willing to try it? Can they figure it out? How much resistance will there be?)

What is a scenario? A scenario is similar to role playing except that it can be done without actually limiting specific roles to specific individuals. The implementation of each option may be acted out or just walked through mentally by the people who are analyzing the options. Again, imagination and creativity should be encouraged because the purpose of creating the scenario is to find the unanticipated advantages and disadvantages of each option. The scenario is a means by which we can ask, "What would happen if we actually implemented this option?" before the choice is made.

The City Council problem of providing primary care for the medically indigent would lend itself well to the development of a scenario:

Suppose the planning committee had generated five options: (1) develop a new free-standing primary care clinic, (2) open a clinic within the hospital emergency department, (3) develop a primary care clinic within the emergency department of another hospital, (4) ask the health department to add primary care services to their well-baby clinics or (5) expand the nonprofit agency now serving the elderly.

A scenario would then address important questions about each of the options, such as the following:

1. How would clients be referred to the new clinic? By whom? What will persuade them to go there? How will they respond?
2. Where would the new clinic be located? How would clients get to the new site? Can they find it? Is there public transportation available?
3. Who (i.e., what agency) will operate the clinic? Does this agency have the necessary expertise? How will the staff at the clinic serving the elderly, for example, respond to the addition of pediatric clients? Where will the funding come from? How much will the clients be asked to pay? Will federal funds be diverted from the existing clinic? Will the city's voters support this new expenditure?
4. What kind of care will be given at the new clinic? How is it different from current services? Will an entire family see the same health care team? Can they fill prescriptions at the center?

Members of the planning committee would take the roles of the city council, voters, clients, staff, administrators of the clinic, and so forth to work through each of these stakeholders' responses to each option. For example, a committee member would assume the role of a pregnant woman with two preschool children, one ill and one needing immunizations, and then "walk through" the services of each option beginning with the telephone call to make an appointment and ending with follow-up care.

Working through a scenario may seem complicated but it raises a lot of questions that would otherwise be neglected in planning. It is usually a stimulating experience once participants become involved in the process.

PILOT PROJECTS.   Pilot projects are actual small-scale representations of the suggested options. They have the advantage of most closely reflecting the reality of implementing an option, but they can be very expensive in both time and money. A pilot project may also not be as realistic as is often assumed. Since a great deal of interest and enthusiasm is often put into the pilot project, it may be more successful than the full-scale option would be over a longer period of time. It is expensive to pilot more than one or two options, so a premature decision as to which option is most favorable may occur. Despite these drawbacks, the pilot project is a powerful means of analyzing an option.

Using the previous examples, it is easy to see the advantages and disadvantages:

A few weeks' trial of a new courier system for the laboratory would be very informative. It would provide actual time figures on how much faster results can be relayed to the nursing unit.

A trial run of the new clinic would be far more expensive and probably require a year or more of operation to assess its impact on the use of the emergency department, but it would provide very useful information. Imagine, however, the cost of year-long trials for each of the five options!

The reader may have noticed that the existence of criteria for analyzing the value of each option has been implied in the examples given. Selection of criteria upon which to evaluate each option should go back to the purpose and objectives of the planning process. The criteria may include cost reduction without a loss of quality, more efficient use of staff time, and an improvement in the quality of care given. Whatever criteria are chosen, it is important that they be clearly spelled out and agreed upon before the analysis of the options is done.

Once the alternatives have been evaluated and the best option selected, we can move to the second phase of planning, presenting the plan. (You may want to refer back to Figure 8–1.)

PHASE II: PRESENTING THE PLAN

Obtaining Approval

Although occasionally you may proceed directly from developing the plan to implementing the plan, most often you will have to present the plan for approval from administrators, planning councils, or participating agencies before you can proceed. Some of those to whom you present the plan may have acted as sponsor of the planning, having initiated and supported your work up to this point. Even with this support, however, the sponsor usually retains his or her right to approve, modify, or reject the completed plan.

In order to achieve this approval, you will have to be persuasive. Sometimes it is necessary to be very persuasive. At other times, this is just *pro forma*, that is, a matter of following established procedures and lines of authority with approval virtually assured ahead of time. When approval is not assured, however, you will want to make the proposal as attractive and acceptable to the sponsor as possible. It may be helpful to think of this part of the process as "selling" your proposal. It is your job now to somehow get the sponsor to "buy" your plan. The quality of the work you have done up to now will, of course, have a great influence on the decision, but the way in which you sell your plan may be the deciding factor.

Making a Presentation

Making a presentation is really an exercise of your leadership. We will look at two aspects of a presentation: the substance or content of the proposal and the technique or delivery of the proposal.

CONTENT. In order to be credible, your proposal must be well supported, not only by your carefully thought-out arguments, but by facts.

Accurate statistics, however simple, are very persuasive. You could, for example, survey post-coronary patients, asking them four or five simple questions about the causes of myocardial infarction and prevention of further damage. It is safe to predict that many will not have these answers and that your survey would strongly support the need for patient education. Your own survey should then be further supported by other statistics from the literature on patient education.

The examples used throughout this chapter so far offer other possibilities for the use of figures to support a need. In the laboratory example, for instance, even a one-day survey of the time gaps between sending specimens and receiving the results would strongly support the need for a new system. Statistics would be even more important in the City Council example, where the number of nonemergency visits and the total cost of these visits would be essential information in your proposal.

When presenting information, Boettinger (1979) suggests that you *never underestimate the intelligence of your audience nor overestimate their knowledge of the subject.* In other words, do not talk down to them or assume that you can fool them. On the other hand, do not assume that they already know as much as you have learned in the process of developing the plan.

Boettinger also suggests a framework that you may find helpful for organizing your presentation. This framework follows the way your audience needs to think about the proposal. First, describe the problem as it currently exists, then describe the situation in more detail, and, finally, present your plan for the resolution of the problem (or prevention of the problem in proactive planning). The outline of the framework is as follows:

1. Statement of the Problem
2. Development of the Situation
3. Resolution of the Problem

The second part, Development of the Situation, is the stage at which you provide the more detailed description of the problem. One way is the historical approach, in which you trace the problem back to its origins (avoiding placing blame on any particular people) and then trace its development up to the current situation. This provides the background people need to understand the situation. Sometimes your audience will know this background very well, in which case you can be brief. Do not omit this section, however, because it establishes a common understanding of the situation. Other approaches include beginning with a description of the crisis, or potential crisis, or presenting the situation as an opportunity, a challenge to the organization. The "crossroads approach" is another one useful in presenting a proactive plan. In the crossroads approach you depict the organization as having come to a crucial juncture at which it can either forge ahead of or fail behind its competitors. Whichever way you choose, your presentation should achieve a gradual unfolding as you reveal layer after layer of the situation and the factors that are affecting it (Boettinger, 1979).

The third and last part of your presentation is your description of how to resolve the problem, that is, your carefully prepared plan. Most people in the audience have not carefully worked through all the steps of the process, generating and then weighing each option carefully. Since they have not, one effective way to present your plan is to share this process with them, mentioning each option and demonstrating why each was rejected and why the selected one is the best choice. If you do not do this, the audience's natural reaction will be to attempt to discover a new solution or to argue with your selection. Sharing the decision-making process avoids this second guessing, provided that you considered the needs of each stakeholder in preparing the plan.

DELIVERY.   The people to whom you are presenting the plan may be as few as two or as many as several hundred in a community project. Usually the plan is prepared in written form, which includes the purpose, objectives, proposed action, and means for evaluation (as shown in the middle section of Figure 8–1). You will then probably be asked to present and explain it. The manner in which you present the plan can have a substantial effect on the fate of your proposal. The following are some characteristics of a well-presented proposal.

1. *It is persuasive.* Emphasize the ways in which the plan meets the needs, concerns, and goals of the sponsor and other stakeholders. These could be to save money, improve the organization's image, provide better care, meet a pressing need, eliminate a performance gap, and so forth.
2. *It is concise.* People become impatient with unnecessary detail and overly long explanations. Busy administrators appreciate it when you get to the point directly. A descriptive slogan, symbol, or title for your project, especially for a large-scale project, can catch and hold attention. For example, a clean-up campaign can be called Project Pride or a proposal for a day-care center in your hospital can be called KinderCare.
3. *It is professional.* Sloppy work may be rejected before the quality of your ideas has been given a chance. Your proposal should be clear, well-organized, and appropriately formal but not humorless, unenthusiastic, or pedantic. It should be presented with confidence that is supported by your having done your "homework" before presenting the plan. You can admit to the inevitable gaps in information without being apologetic or defensive. You can also list the shortcomings of previous attempts to solve the problem without putting other people on the defensive.
4. *It is personalized.* Personalizing the proposal is important because it is a way to engage your audience. You can talk about how the plan will affect the stakeholders, especially the sponsor. For example, you can say that when a new computer system is installed, Ms. X will be the project director, Mr. Y and Ms. Z will spend one-half of their time working on the installation for the next six months, and the nurses on Units 1, 2, and 3 will then be able to do x, y, and z in half the time. Specific examples also help. For example, you can say "Let's follow Patient X through the new Primary Care Clinic. When he first telephones the clinic for an appointment. . . . " It is much easier for your audience to identify with Patient X or Mr. Y than with two hundred clients or a whole project staff.

   Another way to personalize your presentation is to give credit where it is due to the people who have contributed to the plan. People want to be recognized for their contributions and are more inclined to support a project to which they have had some recognized input (a basic tenet of participative leadership).
5. *It is imaginative.* A descriptive analogy, attractive audiovisuals, charts,

graphs, a memorable title, and personalized examples are just a few of the ways in which you can exercise some imagination and creativity. This lends uniqueness to your presentation and firmly captures your audience's interest and attention.

PHASE III: IMPLEMENTING AND MONITORING THE PLAN

This last phase is not always carried through directly by the planner or sponsor. For the sake of some simplicity here, however, it will be assumed that the planner continues to be the leader of the project now that it is about to become a reality.

Technically, the first step of this phase is still a planning step. The implementation must be planned in terms of the sequence of activities, target dates for completion of various tasks, and assignment of responsibility for continuing these activities. Once this is done, the leader of the project will direct the actual implementation, monitor implementation, evaluate outcomes, and revise the plan as needed. These last steps involve a broad range of general leadership and managerial knowledge and skills dealt with in other sections of this book, so they will only be introduced here.

Planning the Implementation

This step can be very detailed if the project is a complicated one involving many people and many different activities over a long time. A number of useful techniques have been developed to organize and keep track of all these details. Among these are Gantt charts, PERT, and Critical Path Method (Longenecker & Pringle, 1981; Special Projects Office, 1958; Spiegel & Hyman, 1978). Each of these methods provides a way to organize and later monitor the implementation activities of a unit, team, project group, or even the whole agency. They can also be used to organize and monitor routine work, especially project-oriented work.

The project leader's major concerns at this point are:

1. The activities and the sequence in which they must be done.
2. The target dates for completing each activity.
3. Assignment of responsibilities to particular individuals.
4. The allocation of resources.

Allocation of resources focuses primarily on selecting staff, securing space and equipment, and working within a given budget. Although the budget is considered in a separate chapter, it must be kept in mind during implementation of the plan because it can be a strict constraint on the resources available to you.

SCHEDULES. Schedules are probably the simplest and most familiar of the methods described here. A schedule organizes work on the basis of time and assigned staff members, leaving out details of the tasks to be done. Their simplicity makes them easy to construct and use, and they form the basis for the more complex methods. A routine schedule would list staff assignments to a pediatric unit for the next month, including days off and vacation time. A project schedule differs somewhat in that it usually lists the tasks instead of the staff, with dates for starting and completing them.

GANTT CHARTS. Gantt charts are really highly developed schedules in which the tasks are more detailed and there is some indication of their relationship in time (Table 8–3). These charts usually do not indicate which tasks depend on the completion of earlier ones. They derive their name from their developer, Henry L. Gantt, an early management theorist (Longenecker & Pringle, 1981).

Table 8–3 illustrates a simple Gantt chart that could be used for implementation of a new courier system in the laboratory example. Note that two activities, developing the new reporting slip for results and hiring couriers, will be done at the same time, but that hiring is scheduled to be completed sooner. Note also that a column has been added to indicate the people responsible for completing each task. Although not always included, this is vital information for the entire project staff. A chart such as the one illustrated can be useful in reminding you of the multiple tasks that need to be done and in monitoring whether or not project activities are progressing on time.

PERT CHARTS. PERT charts provide more detail on the relationships between the various activities of a particular project. A PERT chart graphically illustrates the sequence of events and their interrelationships, using *circles for events* and *arrows for the activities* leading up to those events (Nutt, 1984; Special Reports Office, 1958; Speigel & Hyman, 1978). This is confusing when you first try to create a PERT chart. Figure 8–2 illustrates a simplified PERT chart for the same courier system shown in Table 8–3. Under each arrow is the time that it is expected to take to complete that activity.

The PERT chart is more systems–oriented than the Gantt chart. From the PERT chart, you can see how the work must flow from one event to the next and how one activity depends on another. It helps the project leader and staff see the project as a whole with interrelated parts, each contributing to the final outcome. On the other hand, the Gantt chart is easier to construct and simpler to follow. These charts can become far more complex than the ones illustrated, and some require the use of the computer.

TABLE 8–3. Gantt Chart. Example Illustrating Implementation of a New Courier System

Task	Assigned Responsibility	Jan	Feb	Mar	Apr	May	June
A. Develop new report forms	PQ KL	-------------------->					
B. Hire couriers	AM	------>					
C. Train couriers	CB		------>				
D. Pilot new system on two units	PB KL			------>			
E. Implement on all units	PB KL				------------------->		
F. Evaluate	AM						---->

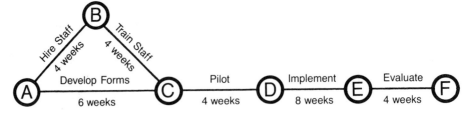

A. Decision to begin project

B. Staff selected

C. Staff trained; forms developed

D. Pilot completed

E. Implementation for two months

F. Evaluation completed

Figure 8–2. PERT chart. Example illustrating implementation of the same courier system shown in Table 8–3.

CRITICAL PATH METHOD. This method is very similar to PERT except that it also identifies the critical path, that is, the path that takes the longest time to complete. Returning to Figure 8–2 for a moment, you can see that path A-B-C is estimated to require eight weeks, whereas path A-C requires only six weeks to complete. Path ABC is the *critical path*, because it is the one most likely to delay completion of the project.

Another helpful device in planning for implementation is to calculate not only the most likely but also the *most optimistic* and *least optimistic* estimates (usually 20% more or less than the most likely amount of time) of time needed to complete the project. These outside estimates can make the charts a more realistic projection of what may occur and prevent unrealistic expectations about completion of the project. Many activities depend on one another for completion, with a great number of variables, many outside the control of the project leader, affecting the outcome. For example, a low unemployment rate would make it difficult to find couriers, or there might be a delay in printing the forms due to a printers' strike.

Whichever method you use, by the end of this step you should have a clear plan of action that informs you and the project staff as to what needs to be done and by when. Along with this plan should be a congruent budget. The budget and your plan of action become the guidelines for directing and monitoring implementation.

Directing Implementation

Once the previous steps have been completed, the actual implementation of the project can begin. The project still needs the support of the sponsor and the direction of the planner (or designated leader) because it is new and represents a change, however welcome or unwelcome. At this point, the skills needed are primarily those of the leader involved in bringing about change. The plan now becomes a reality.

Monitoring Implementation

No matter how well the planning was done, some unforeseen problems are likely to occur and must be rapidly identified and resolved by the leader. Supervision of staff is always necessary, as is working within the budget. These must be considered continuing responsibilities. The major focus of monitoring that is unique to a new project, however, is referral back to the original design to ensure that it is being followed, (except where conscious revisions were made) and to evaluate whether or not the project is being implemented according to the schedule devised. The Gantt, PERT, and Critical Path Method charts are helpful in this regard.

Evaluating Outcomes

There are several different kinds of evaluation. *Formative* evaluation is ongoing and done as the project is being implemented. This formative evaluation is usually the responsibility of the project leader. At the end of the implementation phase, however, a *summative* evaluation is also needed to determine how well the project has succeeded in meeting the objectives set back in the first phase of planning. This evaluation is usually more formal and more exhaustive than the ongoing evaluation, and it may well determine whether or not the activities initiated will be continued. Evaluation is dealt with in more detail in Chapters 21 and 23.

Revising and Updating the Plan

This final step demonstrates the circularity of the planning process and of the development and implementation of any new project. Continuous revision, improvement, enhancement, and updating of any project are signs of a healthy, growth-oriented organization. The process may lead back to revision of the objectives, the action plan, even the purpose of the original plan.

Although we have moved through an orderly sequence of steps through the three phases of the project planning process, you can see that a return to any one of them is possible at any point within the process.

SUMMARY ————————————————————

Planning is a dynamic, future-oriented process consisting of three major phases: (1) *developing the plan*, (2) *presenting the plan*, and (3) *implementing and monitoring the plan*. During the development of the plan, the purpose or mission of the project is established and a thorough assessment of the context in which the project will be implemented is done. Then the specific objectives for the project are formulated, and alternative approaches to reaching those objectives are generated. Each option or alternative is thoroughly analyzed before one is selected. At this point, the plan is presented for approval. Once accepted, the details of how it will be implemented are worked out, and then the actual implementation can take place. Monitoring should occur throughout the implementation phase. Evaluation of the outcomes is done in terms of the degree to which the original objectives were met and the plan is revised and updated accordingly.

REFERENCES*

Beal, G.M., Bohlen, J.M. & Raudabaugh, J.N. (1962). *Leadership and Dynamic Group Action.* Ames, Iowa: Iowa State University Press.

*Boettinger, H.M. (1979). *Moving mountains: The art of letting others see things your way.* New York: Collier Books.

Byson, J.M, & Delbecq, A.L. (1979). A contingent approach to strategy and tactics in project planning. *Journal of the American Planning Association, 45,* 167–179. (Reprinted in Kraegel, 1983.)

Cerne, F. (1988). Plan today for tomorrow's work force. *Hospitals,* July 5, 68.

Delbecq, A. & Van de Ven, A. (1971). A group process model for problem identification and program planning. *Journal of Applied Behavioral Science, 7,* 466–492.

De Geus, A.P. (1988). Planning as learning. *Harvard Business Review, 88,* 70–74.

Dychtwald, K. & Zitter, M. (1988). Developing a strategic marketing plan for hospitals. *Healthcare Financial Management, 42,* 42–50.

Kola, L.A. & Kosberg, J.I. (1981). Model to assess community services for the elderly alcoholic. *Public Health Reports, 96,* 458–463.

*Kraegel, J.M. (ed). (1983). *Planning strategies for nurse managers.* Rockville, Maryland: Aspen Systems.

Longenecker, J.G. & Pringle, C.D. (1981) *Management* (5th ed). Columbus, Ohio: Charles E. Merrill.

Lukacs, J.L. (1984) Strategic planning in hospitals: Application for nurse executives. *Journal of Nursing Administration. 14* (9), 11–17.

Nutt, P.C. (1984). *Planning methods for health and related organizations.* New York: John Wiley.

*Prince, G.M. (1970). *The practice of creativity: A manual for group problem solving.* New York: Collier Books.

*Sloma, R.S. (1984). *No-Nonsense Planning.* New York: The Free Press.

Special Projects Office (1958). *PERT: Program evaluation research task: Summary report.* Washington, D.C.: Bureau of Naval Weapons, Department of the Navy. (Cited in Nutt, 1984).

Spiegel, A.D. & Hyman, H.H. (1978). *Basic health planning methods.* Rockville, Maryland: Aspen Systems.

*References marked with an asterisk are recommended for further reading about various aspects of project planning.

Chapter 9

FINANCIAL MANAGEMENT

Chapter 9

OUTLINE

Importance of Financial Management
Effect on Your Work
Blaming the Budget
Planning
Power and Authority

Responsibility for Financial Management
Chief Executive Officer
Governing Board
Chief Fiscal Officer
Managers
Budget Committee

Types of Budgets
Incremental Budgeting
Zero-Base Budgeting

The Budget Process
Phase I: Planning
Phase II: Preparation
Phase III: Modification and Approval
Phase IV: Monitoring

Summary

LEARNING OBJECTIVES

Upon completion of this chapter, the reader will be able to:

▷ Explain why financial management is important to the nurse leader-manager.

▷ Identify the individuals within an organization who usually have responsibility for budget preparation, approval, and monitoring.

▷ Distinguish zero-base budgeting from incremental budgeting.

▷ Read and explain a simple budget summary for a nursing unit.

FINANCIAL MANAGEMENT

The nurse today who believes that it is not necessary to be aware of the financial side of health care is very much like the proverbial ostrich that sticks its head in the sand and hopes that what it cannot see will not hurt it. The budget of a health care organization determines how many nurses will be hired, how much they will be paid, and even, to some extent, what they will be asked to do. In health care organizations with decentralized budgeting you may soon become involved in preparing and monitoring a budget. This has come as a surprise to many new nurse managers who are left to learn by trial and error how to prepare a good working budget.

In this chapter, we will consider why financial management is an important subject, and we will consider the budget itself: who is responsible for it, and the sequence of events in budgeting.

IMPORTANCE OF FINANCIAL MANAGEMENT _____

Why are financial management and, more specifically, the budget of a health care organization, of importance to the professional person?

Effect on Your Work

The financial management of the organization affects many aspects of work in the organization. It affects the salaries offered, the number of people available to do the work, and the quality and quantity of equipment and supplies available (see Table 9–1). The following are some examples of important organizational decisions based primarily on budgetary factors:

A hospital with limited revenues has decided to close its obstetrical unit because it is rarely filled and is operating at a loss to the hospital. The hospital has offered to find positions in its medical or pediatric units for the nurses with a specialty in obstetrics.

A home health agency has chosen to serve only private pay and Medicare clients, because Medicaid does not pay as much per visit as it actually costs to make the visit. The agency also limits the time allowed per visit in order to increase efficiency and profits.

A nursing home keeps staffing levels to the minimum required by law in order to reduce costs and increase profits.

Decisions like these affect both the people working in the organization and those who are served by the organization. You can also see that such budgetary decisions reflect the goals and values of the organization.

Blaming the Budget

The budget itself is just a document. It is a piece of paper listing numerous figures distributed according to a series of decisions made by designated

TABLE 9–1. Components of the Operating Budget

Costs (Expenses)
  Payroll: salary, vacation, holidays, social security, education, unemployment, other fringe benefits.
  Supplies: office supplies, treatment supplies, and so forth.
  Overhead: building maintenance, water, electric.
  Other: mortgage interest, loans, insurance.
Revenue (Income)
  Patient Sources: private pay, Medicaid, Medicare, other insurance.
  Contributions: philanthropic, grants-in-aid, research and program grants.
  Other: interest, rent, sale of equipment.

people within the organization. But once it is complete, the budget frequently has a great deal of power ascribed to it (Dillon, 1979). In this game of *blaming the budget*, power and authority are ascribed to the budget itself rather than to the people in the organization who have created the budget and subsequently enforce adherence to it.

The budget is frequently used as an excuse for unpopular decisions. For example, you might be told that "The budget won't allow us to hire more nurses" or that "The budget says we cannot modernize the nursery this year." Although it is true that some figures in the budget are not within the administration's control, much of the allocation of funds to one department or the other within the organization certainly is. You would not think so, though, when you hear administrators blaming the budget.

Planning

Financial management requires planning in the form of predictions about how much money the organization will bring in during the next year and how much it will need to spend in order to continue operating. Health care organizations depend upon an adequate money supply for their continued survival and growth. Those that use their money efficiently and effectively thrive, while those that do not may cease to operate entirely (Sweeny & Wisner, 1975).

The people who prepare the organization's budget must look ahead and consider such trends as economic inflation, recession, community needs, public demands, availability of qualified staff, changes in health care methodology, and competition from other organizations. Failure to consider any of these factors can result in an inadequate budget and eventual depletion of resources.

Whether the goals of the organization are stated directly or implied by the allocation of funds for certain projects and the lack of funds for other projects, the budget is a *statement in monetary terms of what the organization and its various departments expect to be doing in the next year*. Any new service or activity that has money specifically allocated for it in the budget is far more likely to be carried out than one for which you have to make a special request for funds during the year. This can be true even for a relatively small amount of money. Simply knowing when budgets are being prepared, and by whom, and getting your pet project included in the budget can be a very important step in accomplishing your goal.

Power and Authority

Money is an important source of power, particularly when it is in limited supply. Those people within the organization who have some authority to say how this resource will be allocated have a great deal of power over the operation of the organization. Their decisions greatly affect the growth or stagnation of various departments and the direction of the organization as a whole.

Another important point is that departments that can show that they bring money into the organization generally receive more favorable attention from administration and a larger share of the next year's budget. In other words, the profitable areas are encouraged to grow while the nonprofitable ones languish. This poses a particular problem for nursing departments in many hospitals owing to some peculiarities in budgeting procedures.

Despite its dominance in terms of sheer numbers, far surpassing any other health care discipline, nursing often has wielded less power than would generally be expected owing in part to the way in which its finances are handled. Nursing is often treated as an *expense-only* unit within the hospital budget. Put simply, this means that separate records are kept of all the expenses (money spent) for nursing for such things as salaries and supplies, but the revenue generated by nursing (money paid to the hospital for nursing care) is a part of the daily room charge considered general revenue and not credited to nursing.

Nursing care is actually the major service offered by the hospital, but the nursing department is often not credited with bringing income into the hospital. So it *appears* to be a source of great expense, frequently targeted for cutbacks when money is in short supply. The end result is that nursing's power and influence in the organization are limited (Bruttomesso, 1985; Higgerson & Van Slyck, 1982).

A comparison with other departments, such as respiratory therapy or physical therapy, illustrates this difference. Every treatment given to a patient by these other services can be recorded and billed separately. The result is that these and other departments can show that they generate an income, even a profit, that offsets the cost of running these departments. It has been difficult for nursing to do this.

With the general trend toward corporate health care, larger and larger multihospital, multiagency corporations are being formed. In these multi-agency systems, your particular facility may be only one of many owned by a corporation seeking to make its operations as efficient as possible. Many activities formerly done in each agency are done at the centralized corporate level to increase efficiency and reduce cost. For example, a very large corporation can bargain for lower prices on supplies bought in large quantities. Other activities that affect nursing, such as the development of policies and procedures or the planning of in-service programs, may also be done at the corporate level rather than in your individual facility.

There are a number of other ways to reduce cost by centralizing activities, and the reader should not assume that other services are immune to their impact. For example, several national laboratories are contracting with hospitals to do all of their lab work and virtually eliminate the in-hospital laboratory as we know it. These laboratories are able to do this at a lower per-unit rate because of the efficiency of doing a very high volume of work on the very expensive machines and the reduction of the number of people in higher paid managerial positions. The attractive projected budget savings persuaded hospitals to contract with these corporations. The same approach will be tried with other departments if this proves to be a successful approach.

RESPONSIBILITY FOR FINANCIAL MANAGEMENT

Budgeting is a management responsibility. In authoritarian-style organizations, the process is highly centralized, so that only a small number of people at the higher levels of administration are involved in preparation of the budget. In others, it may be widely decentralized, involving all the managers within the organization, who in turn seek input from their staffs. Whichever way is used, the final authority for the organization-wide budget rests with the governing board and chief executive officer (CEO), who may actually prepare the final master budget in very small agencies. We will focus here on the division of responsibility typically used in the participative approach (Bean & Laliberty, 1980).

Chief Executive Officer

Whether called the President, Executive Director, or another name, the CEO has general responsibility for the overall budget. The CEO sets the process in motion, determines the extent of involvement of others in the organization, assigns responsibilities, and sets deadlines.

The long-range goals of the organization must be determined before decisions can be made about allocation of resources. For example:

A hospital may have a long-range goal of expanding into the area of home care services to broaden its financial base, or it may have decided to concentrate on the specialized intensive care services offered only by that facility.

A health department may have a long-range goal of expanding beyond its current function to offer comprehensive primary care or to add mental health care to its array of services.

Forecasting future needs and demands in the health care market is an important part of the process of determining these long-range goals. Internal factors also affect the budget goals: proposed changes in departmental activities, expansion or renovation of existing facilities, and addition of new services and equipment affect the way the organization's money will be spent. All of these must be taken into consideration when giving direction to preparation of the budget.

Governing Board

Although the members of the governing board or board of trustees are not usually involved in the actual preparation of the budget, they are responsible for working with the CEO in setting the long-range goals of the organization, in recommending changes in the budget, and in giving final approval to the organizational budget.

Chief Fiscal Officer

This individual, often called the Comptroller, provides the information on past budgets and expenses needed to begin the process of preparing a new budget (Kiser, 1988; Needles, Anderson & Caldwell, 1984). A set of budget guidelines is also prepared to assist managers in completing their portion of the budget. These guidelines include explanations of the budget forms and reporting procedures used; formulas for calculating the cost of fringe benefits; cost and income figures for the past year; predictions of the rate of inflation and other costs increases (for anything from new equipment to the cost of electricity); and, of course, the deadlines for submitting budget requests.

The fiscal officer and his or her department are also responsible for providing an analysis of the financial health of the organization and predicting its future financial status. They are responsible for the continuous management of the financial aspects of the organization, from paying employees and suppliers to collecting payments from patients or third-party payers.

Managers

In the decentralized, participative approach to budgeting, every department head and manager is responsible for preparing his or her section of the budget in detail. This "mini" budget should reflect the needs of the department and be congruent with the organization's goals. All of the "departmental" budgets prepared at this level are finally combined into the master budget. To keep the subject relatively simple, we will concentrate primarily on the components of a budget that would be prepared by a nurse manager.

Budget Committee

When a participative approach is used, the CEO often appoints a budget committee with representatives from various departments. This committee becomes a forum in which negotiation, coordination, and consolidation of the budget take place (these also take place "behind the scenes" in most organizations). The differences in power and influence among the various departments become clear as these negotiations take place. The composition of the budget committee varies from representation from each department to a small group of high-level executives. A nursing budget committee may also be formed for the same purposes within the nursing department itself.

The individual budget from each manager must be evaluated in terms of its congruence with the long-range goals of the organization and the ability of the organization to provide the funds requested by each of the departments. An organization cannot spend money it does not have! It is easy to imagine that each department will request what it considers its fair share of the budget, but that in times of restricted resources the organization will not necessarily have sufficient money to give each department what it wants.

TYPES OF BUDGETS

We will consider two different approaches to preparing the budget: the incremental approach and zero-base budgeting.

Incremental Budgeting

Incremental or historical budgeting is the traditional process in which budgets, divided into the components shown in the operating budget outline in Table 9–1, are prepared every year on the basis of what was spent the year before (Berman & Weeks, 1979). The two most basic components of the budget are *income* by its source (contributions, private payment, Medicare, Medicaid, and other third-party payers) and *expenses* (salaries, benefits, equipment, supplies, overhead, staff education, and so forth).

The budget process begins with an analysis of the income and expenses of the previous year. Special attention is given to departments and categories that were substantially over budget or under budget and the reasons for these deviations (variances) from the previous budget. These are taken into consideration in projecting the next year's income and expenses.

These deviations often cause problems for departments. For example, a department that was unable to find enough qualified staff in a particular budget year may find the unfilled staff lines taken out of the budget for the next year "because you managed all right this year without them" or will find that its efficiency ironically means that extra funds go to a department that was not so efficient and ran over its budget. On the other hand, running too far over budget also leads to serious questions about the efficiency and quality of management of the department unless the manager can clearly demonstrate that the deviance was due to circumstances that could not have been predicted or to changes made by the administration. In other words, the manager must show that the cost overruns (unbudgeted expenses) were justified.

Budgeting projections are also based upon plans to expand or limit services, add new staff, and so forth. Any of these actions requires a change in the budget, usually an increase, which is the reason why this budget is called an incremental budget. In incremental budgeting, the projected changes in costs and income are simply *added* to the previous year's budget.

After this analysis of the organization's past budget and future plans, dollar figures are assigned to all departments and to all categories on both the income and expenditure sides of the budget. In some organizations, individual departments are given some flexibility in allocating funds to various categories. In other organizations, departments are restricted to using funds only as designated in the budget unless a modification is requested and approved. For the organization as a whole, the income or credit side of the budget is supposed to equal or surpass the expense or debit side of the budget. This balancing of the budget is not generally required of each department within the organization, but it is highly desired, and we may see more demands for it in the future.

Zero-Base Budgeting

Zero-base budgeting is designed to require even more justification from each department regarding any funds budgeted to it for the next year. This approach is based on the idea that no expense should be assumed to be absolutely necessary. The result is that every expenditure must be justified as essential to the function of the organization. In theory, at least, the zero-base budget begins with a blank slate every year: No expense from last year can be repeated for the next year without giving reasons why it is still necessary.

The use of the *decision package* is the core of the zero-base budgeting process and the feature that particularly distinguishes it from the traditional incremental process (Pyhrr, 1973). Decision packages consist of several basic elements: a listing of all current and proposed objectives or activities of a given team, nursing unit, or department; alternative ways of carrying out these activities; the different costs for each alternative; the advantages of continuing the activity; and the consequences of discontinuing the activity. The following is a sample from a decision package (without cost figures) for an inservice department:

Objective:	Provide CPR (cardiopulmonary resuscitation) instruction for all employees.
Advantages:	Every employee will be prepared to respond immediately to an emergency situation. Will save lives and reduce insurance premiums. Additional benefit to employees.
Disadvantages:	Time away from work for CPR class. Cost of part-time CPR instructor.
Alternative 1:	Require each employee to acquire CPR instruction from a community organization.
Major Advantage:	No cost to organization.
Major Disadvantage:	Employee resistance and resentment of control of off-duty hours.
Alternative 2:	Do not require CPR.
Major Advantage:	No cost; no employee resentment.
Major Disadvantage:	Potential loss of client life, increased insurance rates, and lawsuits.

All the listed activities, such as providing CPR instruction in the example above, are ranked or prioritized, from the most essential ones required to maintain minimal operation of the nursing unit to those that are nonessential but desirable if sufficient money is available to support them. The packages are then compiled for the entire organization and further prioritizing is done on the basis of organization-wide goals and resources.

In comparison with incremental budgeting, zero-base budgeting requires more thought and planning. More attention is given to activities and expenses that are usually assumed to be essential but may actually be avoidable. Zero-based budgeting encourages the participative approach, because information from people at all levels is needed to adequately analyze and prioritize the activities of each unit or department. The process can help to eliminate padding the budget and encourage more discussion of future plans and priorities, but it also requires more time to complete than the incremental budget. Zero-based budgeting's major advantages are that it encourages planning, may help to reduce costs, rationalizes expenditures, and increases employee understanding and support of the budget.

THE BUDGET PROCESS

Phase I: Planning

As was mentioned earlier, the planning phase is an important part of the overall financial management of a health care organization (see Table 9–2). No facility operates in a vacuum: The current economic picture, growth of competition, regulatory changes, and other factors have an impact on the

TABLE 9–2. The Budgeting Process

Phase 1 Planning	Phase 2 Preparation	Phase 3 Modification and Approval	Phase 4 Monitoring
1. Set short- and long-term goals.	1. Translate objectives into projected costs and revenues.	1. Prepare preliminary master budget from all department requests.	1. Prepare monthly summaries of departmental expenses and revenues.
2. Form budget committee.	2. Write justifications for all requested expenses.	2. Compare projected costs with estimated revenues.	2. Compare actual expenses with budgeted expenses.
3. Prioritize objectives.	3. Eliminate lowest priority objectives as necessary.	3. Eliminate lowest priority items until budget is balanced.	3. Investigate any variance above 5%.
4. Analyze past performance.	4. Present proposed budget.	4. Approve final master budget.	4. Readjust budget and/or improve performance as necessary.
5. Predict future costs and revenues.		5. Communicate final budget to all departments.	5. Continue to monitor on monthly basis.
6. Develop budget guidelines.			

future costs and income of every organization. It is important that the nurse manager be aware of these trends and their effect on nursing within the organization. It is also important to know what the priorities of the organization are. Are future growth and expansion an important goal? Or are short-term profits considered more important (Anderson, 1986)? Are employees considered a valuable resource to be nurtured and developed, or are they considered a short-term resource to be pushed to their limits for as long as they can endure it? Priorities must be established, specific guidelines developed, past performance analyzed, responsibilities assigned, a budget committee selected, and deadlines for completing the budget established. Once this is done, a draft of the budget can be done.

Phase II: Preparation

Each manager develops objectives for his or her department as illustrated in the discussion of zero-base budgeting. These objectives must then be translated into probable cost and revenue figures according to the guidelines prepared by the accounting department. Most of the calculations required to do this involve predictions about the staff and supplies needed to do the work and the amount of patient service or patient days and associated income that will be generated. A few examples of the types of calculations required are given below.

1. *Full-time equivalents.* A full-time employee is generally one who works 40 hours a week, every week. One full-time equivalent, or FTE, is whatever combination of part-time employees it takes to equal the work of one full-time staff member. For example, one half-time employee and two quarter-time employees equal one FTE for the purpose of calculating staffing requirements, although one could ask whether they are actually equivalent in the way in which they fulfill the job responsibilities.

2. *Actual hours worked.* When preparing the budget, it is important to recognize that most permanent employees are actually paid for more days than they really work. Typically, an employee is allowed a certain number of sick days, vacation days, and holidays within a year. These days are *paid but not worked*, and so any calculations of staffing requirements must take them into consideration. For example, a full-time hourly staff member working 40 hours a week is paid for 2,080 hours a year (annual paid hours = 40 hours per week × 52 weeks per year = 2,080). When sick days, holidays, vacations, and so forth are subtracted, however, we see that the staff member actually works only 1,800 hours a year (Hoffman, 1984; Roehm & Labarthe, 1987).

3. *Minimum staffing requirements.* Let us say that your rehabilitation unit has a capacity of 30 patients but that the average number of occupied rooms (average daily census) is 25. An analysis of the patients' care requirements has resulted in the estimation that each patient needs an average of 4 nursing hours in a 24–hour day. The resulting calculation is that the patients on your unit as a whole usually need 100 nursing care hours per day:

    4 hours per day needed by each patient × average patient census of 25 = 100 hours required per day

In a 365–day year, then, 36,500 nursing care hours would be needed on this unit:

365 days per year $\times$ 100 hours needed per day = 36,500 nursing care hours

If we return to the estimation that each staff member actually worked 1,800 hours a year, your unit would require an estimated *minimum* staffing of 20.3 full-time equivalent staff members giving direct care:

36,500 care hours/1,800 hours worked per staff member per year = 20.3 staff members needed

These figures can also be found in summary form in the formula at the bottom of Table 9–3.

4. *Staffing budget.* We will continue the example of staffing a rehabilitation unit to develop a simplified annual staffing budget for this unit. It was estimated that 20.3 full-time staff members or the equivalent would be needed to give direct care. In addition, a head nurse, assistant head nurse, and unit clerk will be needed to provide the management and support services for the unit (see Table 9–3). Fringe benefits, including social security taxes, state and federal unemployment taxes, continuing education costs, membership in professional organizations, health insurance, shift differentials, and retirement benefits are calculated by the facility at a rate of 20% of the annual salary (this procedure will vary from one institution to another). The grand total for the rehabilitation unit, $654,050, is the amount budgeted only for the personnel who work on the rehabilitation unit. A separate summary sheet would be used for other expenses such as office supplies, medical supplies, equipment, and overhead (repairs, maintenance, electricity, and so forth).

If your organization uses zero-base budgeting, you would also have to calculate the cost of optimum staffing at a higher level of nursing hours per patient and compare it with the cost of minimum staffing, using a mix of registered nurses and auxiliary personnel. Then one of the staffing patterns is selected on the basis of which one provides the most effective use of the organization's dollars and which pattern the organization can afford given other demands for available funds.

TABLE 9–3. Annual Staffing Budget Summary

Staff	A. FTE*	B. Salary	C. Fringe @20%†	D. Total A(B + C)
Rehabilitation Unit				
Head Nurse and Assistant Head Nurse	2	31,335	6,267	75,204
Unit Clerk	1	10,600	2,120	12,720
RNs	20.3‡	23,240	4,648	566,126
				654,050

*Full-time equivalent.
†Benefits, including shift differentials.
‡Average daily census 25 $\times$ estimated care requirements 4 = 100 hours per patient day $\times$ 365 = 36,500 annual hours/1800 actual hours worked = 20.3 FTE.

Although often considered a nuisance by nurse managers, many organizations require written explanations or justification of budget requests. Using the rehabilitation unit as an example, you would be expected to justify (explain) why an all-RN staff would be superior to a mix of personnel and why the optimum all-RN staffing level would be better than the minimum all-RN staffing level. These justifications are not just busy work. They provide the administrators with a brief written explanation of the rationale behind your budget requests and are an opportunity to communicate the needs of your unit before budget decisions are made.

The budget, whether zero-based or not, may also include a breakdown of monthly costs and revenues as well as the totals for the year. The completed budget, along with the written justifications, is then submitted to the agency budget committee. The budget committee reviews the proposed departmental budgets and makes its recommendations to the administrators who make the final decisions.

Phase III: Modification and Approval

The budget requests for your unit must compete with the requests from other nursing units and other departments in the institution. The total amount requested from all departments is compared with the amount of revenue reasonably expected to be earned in the next year. Budget requests often have to be reduced somewhat to balance expected costs and revenues. Generally, the lowest priority items are cut first, although when resources are very limited, even high-priority items must be eliminated. Skillful politicking can result in low-priority items being retained at the expense of higher-priority items. Once this difficult task is completed, the final budget is prepared, approved by the administrator and governing board, and sent to each department to serve as the financial guide for the coming year.

Phase IV: Monitoring

Financial management is far more than the annual rite of preparing the budget. The budget is a working document, a guide to the financial component of unit and department management, and a yardstick by which the effectiveness of this management is evaluated.

Monthly summaries of expenses and income are usually distributed to every manager and should be carefully reviewed, for two reasons. The first is to catch possible errors made by the accounting department. For example, expenditures made by other departments may erroneously (sometimes carelessly, occasionally deliberately) be charged to your unit. It is important to spot these errors and to be sure that they are corrected.

Second, the monthly summaries usually report both the budgeted amount and the amount actually spent for each category. Any differences between these two figures should be checked, especially those that are 5% or more over the budgeted amount (generally 10% under the budgeted amount in the case of revenues). Sometimes the variance appears because a large expenditure was made in one month (for example, the purchase of a new monitor) and will not appear again for the rest of the year. When averaged over the year, this expense should equal the budgeted amount. In other cases, however, you might note that expenses are over budget for items such as supplies or temporary personnel and that these need to be brought under control or the budget needs to be adjusted, depending on the situation. This regular surveillance should be continued every month.

There is another important aspect of monitoring that goes beyond the surveillance of the monthly summaries. This is an in-depth analysis of various financial aspects of your unit's operation. There are any number of different factors worthy of analysis. You could, for example, analyze the cost of using disposable versus reusable supplies or the difference between leasing and buying a very expensive piece of equipment (computerized monitors, the unit ice machine, a copier, and so forth). The effectiveness of an all-RN staff in comparison with a mixture of aides, practical nurses, and registered nurses is a perennial issue that has a financial aspect. The cost saving use of nurse practitioners compared with physicians is another question that frequently comes up in community health, as does the cost of making home visits versus clinic visits. Attention to issues of accountability and efficiency can also help to improve care despite limitations in resources (Cerne, 1988). In larger organizations, you can usually request the assistance of the budget or accounting office in doing these analyses.

The results of these financial analyses frequently can be used to support your arguments in favor of needed improvements, better treatment of nursing staff, and increased recognition of the contribution of nursing to the overall success of the organization. One example is the cost of staff turnover in the organization. Although there are many reasons for a staff member to leave an employer, a major one is dissatisfaction with working conditions (salary, opportunities for advancement, and so forth). The cost of replacing just one nurse can be quite substantial. This cost includes advertising and recruiting activities, interviewing, processing the application, moving expenses, orientation (salaries of instructional staff, supplies, staff time, and so forth), and a temporary replacement until the position is filled. All together, this could cost your organization $1,500 or more per new nurse hired (Hoffman, 1985). In a large organization that hires 100 nurses in a year, turnover alone would cost the organization $150,000 a year. Suggestions for action to improve conditions and reduce this expense should fall on receptive ears and lead to improvements in work conditions for the current staff. These financial analyses are time-consuming but often provide persuasive data to support your requests for changes in the budget or management of the unit.

Financial management as a whole is a complex but important subject. Every professional nurse who assumes responsibility for exerting leadership at work needs a basic understanding of the subject. This understanding will help you to do such things as respond intelligently when told that the budget will not allow a change to be implemented or to prepare a budget to accompany a plan for a new service, for a new project, or for your unit as a whole.

SUMMARY

The financial management of a health care organization affects the work of every professional in that organization. Finances need to be considered when doing any kind of planning. Those who control the budget control an important source of power within the organization.

Responsibility for financial management begins with the governing board and administration of the organization. When participative management is used, it extends to every manager and his or her staff.

The incremental type of budget is built upon past budgets, whereas zero-base budgeting is based upon objectives for the coming year and demands that every expenditure, no matter how basic, be justified. The budgeting process begins with these objectives, which are then translated into projected costs and revenues, modified as needed, approved, and then monitored throughout the year for any variance from planned costs and revenues.

REFERENCES*

Anderson, B. (1986). Budget principles for nurse managers. *The Director of Nurses as Manager: Concepts and Practice for a Changing Role.* Florida Association of Homes for the Aging Fourteenth Annual Meeting, Miami, Florida.

*Bean, J.J. & Laliberty, R. (1980). *Decentralizing hospital management: A manual for supervisors.* Reading, Massachusetts: Addison-Wesley.

Berman, H.J. & Weeks, L.E. (1979) *The financial management of hospitals.* Ann Arbor, Michigan: Health Administration Press.

Bruttomesso, K.A. (1985). Variable hospital accounting practices: Are they fair for the nursing department? *Journal of Nursing Administration, 15,* (10), 8–13.

Cerne, F. (1988). Hospitals not immune to high cost of stress. *Hospitals* (October 5) 69–70.

Dillon, R.D. (1979). *Zero base budgeting for health care institutions.* Rockville, Maryland: Aspen Systems.

Higgerson, N.J. & Van Slyck, A. (1982). Variable billing for services: New fiscal direction for nursing. *Journal of Nursing Administration, 12,* (6), 20.

*Hoffman, F.M. (1984). *Financial management for nurse managers.* Norwalk, Connecticut: Appleton-Century-Crofts.

Hoffman, F.M. (1985). Cost per RN hired. *Journal of Nursing Administration, 15,* (2), 27–29.

Kiser, J.J. (1988). The role of the financial manager: How much has it changed? *Healthcare Financial Management, 42,* 72–76.

Needles, B.E., Anderson, H.R., & Caldwell, J.C. (1984). *Principles of accounting.* Boston: Houghton Mifflin.

Pyhrr, P.A. (1973). *Zero base budgeting: A practical management tool for evaluating expenses.* New York: John Wiley.

Roehm, H.A. & Labarthe, S. (1987). Six steps to managing unit costs. *Nursing Management, 18,* (2), 58–62.

Sweeney, A. & Wisner, J.N. (1975). *Budgeting fundamentals for nonfinancial executives.* New York: AMACOM.

---

*References marked with an asterisk are suggested for further reading on the subject of financial management.

UNIT II LEARNING ACTIVITIES _____

▷ Problem solving and reasoning are processes of great interest to cognitive psychologists. At the library, find information about typical patterns found such as satisficing, rigidity or the bias to seek confirmation. Once you are confident that you understand one of these concepts, listen and observe people attempting to solve clinical problems until you have collected two or three examples of these patterns. Describe the patterns and analyze the effect they had on the problem solving.

▷ Select a recently completed project with which you are well acquainted. Evaluate the planning that occurred or did not occur and what effect planning had on the outcome of the project. Who were the sponsors, stakeholders, and planners? How many of the phases and individual steps of planning were actually carried out? Can you identify which approach was used for each step? What could have been done to facilitate planning and enhance the outcome?

▷ With a small group of colleagues or classmates, try using brainstorming and/or the nominal group technique to identify a health care delivery problem and devise three to five alternative strategies to improve health care delivery on the given situation. Subject each of the alternatives to the scenario and simulation approaches to evaluation. Critique the value of each approach in helping the group select one of the alternatives.

▷ Ask permission to photocopy an annual operating budget for a nursing care unit or small community health agency. (The budget should not include individual salary figures to protect confidentiality). Compare the budgeted distribution of available funds to the organization's goals. Then try to work out a different distribution assuming 20% *more* available funds and 20% *less* available. Analyze the effect each would have on the quality of the nursing care given.

Unit III

ORGANIZING

Chapter 10. Health Care Organizations
Chapter 11. Organizing Care
Chapter 12. Time Management
Chapter 13. Computer Applications
Chapter 14. Collective Bargaining
Unit III Learning Activities

Chapter 10

OUTLINE

Types of Health Care Organizations

Organizations as Complex, Open
  Systems
  Wholeness and Individuality
  Hierarchy
  Complexity
  Openness
  Pattern

Organizational Structure and Function
  Structural Configurations
    Bureaucracy
    Matrix Organizations

Function
  Formal and Informal Goals
  Formal and Informal Levels of Operation

Patterns of Relationships in
  Organizations
  Power and Authority in Relationships
  Relationship Games
    Paternalism
    Karpman Triangle
    "I Told You So"
    Bear Trap

Summary

LEARNING OBJECTIVES

Upon completion of this chapter, the reader will be able to:

▷ Differentiate the various types of health care organizations.

▷ Describe the characteristics of a health care organization as a complex, open system.

▷ Distinguish formal and informal organizational goals.

▷ Work at both the formal and informal levels of an organization.

▷ Compare the structure and function of a typical bureaucratic organization with a matrix organization.

▷ Recognize the relationship games played within an organization.

HEALTH CARE ORGANIZATIONS

U p to this point, the organization as a whole has often been mentioned but the organization itself has not been the focus of our attention. We turn now to consideration of large numbers of people in complex systems in which health care professionals work.

These larger systems are much more complex than the small groups and teams that usually demand our attention. They are actually suprasystems made up of many smaller, interrelated systems and subsystems. They are important because the way in which they are structured, their overall climate, and their patterns of interaction have a great deal of influence on the way people function within them. In fact, you could say that organizational well-being is directly related to employee well-being (Stennett-Brewer, 1987).

A very broad perspective is needed when studying organizations. It is not possible to observe directly everything that happens in these systems. It is possible, however, to identify and evaluate their structures, functions, and patterns of relationships once you know what to look for, and to learn how to function more effectively within these larger systems.

This chapter describes the different types of organizations in which health care professionals work. It then considers the characteristics of the organization as an open system, the different ways in which organizations can be structured, how they actually operate compared with their formal design, and some typical patterns of relationships that are found within them.

TYPES OF HEALTH CARE ORGANIZATIONS

Nurses practice in many different types of organizations. Most of these are health care organizations such as hospitals, clinics, health maintenance organizations, home health care agencies, public health agencies, nursing homes, community mental health centers, and neighborhood health centers. Others are organizations in which health care is just one of many functions, a service offered to the clients or to the people employed by the organization. Schools, camps, day care centers, prisons, and businesses of all kinds are some examples of this second category.

Health care organizations vary widely in the type of services they offer, the people they serve, and the way in which they are financed. Some are highly specialized, offering only preventive services, counseling, or treatment of a specific disease such as diabetes or AIDS. Others, such as general hospitals, offer a wide range of services from prenatal classes to ambulatory surgery and intensive care. Despite this wide range of services, however, the organization that offers truly holistic health care is rare.

Many health care services are designed for a very specific, limited population. They may be available only to employees of a particular company or to children in a particular school district. Some are designed only for the aged, for women, or for people with a particular problem such as alcoholism or drug abuse. Some are available only to the poor, while others are available only to those who can afford them or who are enrolled in a particular kind of health plan. These limitations frequently result in people being excluded and being unable to obtain a needed service.

Health care organizations can also be classified as for-profit or not-for-profit according to the way in which they were formed and are financed. Those that are operated for profit are also called *proprietary* organizations. The money needed to form and operate these organizations comes from the same sources as any other business: the sale of bonds or shares (stock) in the company and operating income. Payment for the services that they provide comes from private insurance, government reimbursement, or out of the pocket of the person receiving the care. Because they are operated for a profit, proprietary organizations usually cannot survive for long if they are losing money. They also provide little or no service for those who cannot pay unless these services are reimbursed by the government.

The not-for-profit, or nonprofit, category includes *voluntary* organizations and *public* agencies and institutions. Interestingly, most of the early hospitals in the United States were voluntary community hospitals rather than religious or public hospitals as in England and most of Europe (Williams & Torrens, 1984). After the Industrial Revolution, donations to charitable organizations grew, and more paid staff were added to the volunteers whose work had supported these early institutions. The interests of the donors had an influence on what services would be made available just as governmental goals and policies do today.

In the 1950s, nonprofit service agencies funded by the government began to replace many of the charitable organizations. Services were given primarily to those who were entitled to them by income, age, or defined need as specified in laws and in the regulations developed from these laws. Recently we have seen the emergence of not-for-profit health care that is based on competition rather than charity or public service. Nonprofit health care organizations are now competing with one another and with for-profit organizations to get and hold their share of the health care market (McLaughlin, 1986).

The term *not-for-profit* does not mean that these organizations do not have to be concerned with their financial well-being (Young, 1982). Although they have no stockholders hoping for profits, they still must be concerned with having adequate money to expand, to be prepared for inflation or for hard times, and to be able to pay back money borrowed for new buildings, equipment, and so forth. Some prefer to use the terms *fund balances* or *excess of receipts over expenditures* rather than the term *profits* to avoid confusion with the proprietary health care organization's profit-making orientation (McLaughlin, 1986). The differences between the two types of organizations are often blurred, particularly in day-to-day operations, because both provide needed services and both must maintain some degree of financial health.

The second category of not-for-profit health care organizations is the *public* or government-operated agency or institution. These organizations are directly supported and operated by funds from the local, state, or federal government. Their services are often free or offered at a reduced rate to those who cannot pay the full cost (the medically indigent). Although these organizations are not operated for a profit, their administrators are directly answerable to the sponsoring government agency and boards. Indirectly they are answerable to elected officials and the taxpayers who provide the money for their support. The amount of support they receive is strongly influenced by public opinion and the prevailing political climate. Shifts in the political climate have a direct impact on these organizations and their staffs.

Official public health agencies had their beginning in the local (and often temporary) health boards that were formed to handle sanitation and quarantine procedures on a community-wide basis. Much later in United States history, public health agencies became involved in personal health services to individuals and families. City and county hospitals also appeared fairly late (in the early 1900s) and were established to provide care for those who could not obtain or pay for care elsewhere.

At about the same time, the large state mental institutions were being established by state governments. Federal health care organizations include the military health care system, the Veterans Administration hospitals and clinics, and the Indian health services. Generally speaking, services established by local governments for those who cannot pay for their own care have always been severely underfinanced and understaffed. This causes a great deal of frustration for the health care professionals in these organizations who can see the need for their services but are limited by the resources available (Williams & Torrens, 1984). Unlike either the proprietary or voluntary segments of the health care system, the publicly financed organizations cannot select their target populations, and often find themselves charged with responsibility for some of the most difficult and complex health problems. In planning health promotion and prevention campaigns, for example, the health department can find itself attempting to reach the segments of the population that are most negatively disposed to health promotion messages because those with motivation have already been reached by the other segments of the system (Frederiksen, Solomon & Brehony, 1984).

ORGANIZATIONS AS COMPLEX, OPEN SYSTEMS ———————

Wholeness and Individuality

An organization is more difficult to comprehend in its entirety than is a group or individual. As large and complex as they are, however, organizations also have characteristics as a whole that are different from and greater than the sum of their parts. This means, for example, that even when many people join or leave, the organization as a whole can continue to function and retain its identity. It also means that a change in one part of the organization has an effect on the whole. For example, a change in the operating hours of the hospital laboratory could affect the work of inpatient units, the operating room, ambulatory surgery, and the clinics.

Organizations also exhibit individuality. They are not all alike by any means (Mintzberg, 1981). Like groups, they can be characterized by a certain climate or emotional atmosphere (Appelbaum, 1986). It is both interesting and informative to ask people who work in an organization to describe its atmosphere or personality. People may describe their organization as "open and informal," "schizophrenic," "suffering from growing pains," "old and traditional," or "hungry" (looking for more clients or money). You may find some differences if you ask several people, but a definite pattern usually emerges from the answers to this question.

You can also identify some of these characteristics by observing people's behavior and your own responses to the organization. Some organizations have a climate that is warm and friendly, open to new people and new ideas. Others present themselves as cold, hostile to new ideas, and suspicious of new people.

Imagine what your first impression of these two mental health centers would be:

First Organization: When you approach the door, a guard blocks your way until you explain that you are a community health nurse here to consult with the psychologist treating one of your clients. When the guard finally says, "Go ahead," you enter a bare lobby and head for the glass window at the far end. The switchboard operator slides back the glass and says "Yes?" You repeat your explanation and the operator slides the glass closed without another word. A minute later, the glass is opened and the operator says, "Room 203, on your left," and slides the window shut again.

Second Organization: As you approach the door, the guard steps forward and says, "Good morning, may I help you?" Upon hearing your explanation, the guard opens the door for you and directs you to the receptionist seated at a desk in the center of a lobby that contains some old chairs and small pots of flowers. The receptionist smiles at you, pages the psychologist and tells you to make yourself comfortable, the psychologist will be out in just a moment.

Can you imagine how differently clients would feel about walking into these two places?

The work climate of health care organizations can differ in other ways as well. For example, research studies have shown that the level of anxiety among staff members varies from department to department and from one organization to another. The degree of alienation in the staff has been found to differ substantially from one organization to another. Effective leadership interventions can influence the prevailing climate. Respect for the dignity and worth of the individual employee, open communications, administrative support, and taking action on problems as needed have been found to affect the climate of the organization in a positive way (McClure, 1972; Revans, 1972).

This difference in climate has important implications not only for leadership and management action but also for selecting an organization in which you want to work.

The powerful and pervasive effect of the organizational climate on the perceptions and behavior of people within that organization is described in Research Example 10–1, "Being Sane in Insane Places."

RESEARCH EXAMPLE 10–1. Being Sane in Insane Places

In this provocative and frequently quoted study, Rosenhan (1973) asked whether the characteristics that lead to a diagnosis of mental illness are really found in the patients themselves or in the organizational context, that is, in the environment. Eight "sane" people (three psychologists, a graduate student, a pediatrician, a psychiatrist, a painter, and a housewife), five men and three women, presented themselves at the admissions offices of hospitals in five different states. Each person complained of hearing strange voices that were often unclear or sounded "empty" or "hollow." All eight were admitted immediately and placed in a psychiatric ward. Seven were diagnosed as schizophrenics.

Once on the psychiatric wards, these pseudopatients, as the researcher calls them, no longer claimed to hear voices and behaved as they usually did. Except for giving false symptoms and false names, they related their own ordinary life events when asked for their life history. But once they had been labeled as sick, the label stuck—all were discharged with the diagnosis of schizophrenia in remission after an average stay of 19 days (the range was 7 to 52 days).

Many of the real patients detected the pseudopatients and accused them of being journalists or evaluators checking up on the hospital. But there was no evidence that any staff member—including the psychiatrist, nurses, and attendants—ever questioned the assumption that they were genuinely ill, despite patient records describing them as friendly, cooperative, and exhibiting no abnormal behavior.

The researcher found that the staff's perceptions of the pseudopatient's behavior, no matter how normal it was, was so strongly shaped by the diagnosis that it was considered disturbed. An example of this effect is the staff's response or, more accurately, nonresponse to the fact that the pseudopatients took notes. The staff never questioned this behavior, although the real patients did. One physician told a pseudopatient that he did not have to write down the name of his medicine but could ask if he forgot it. Another pseudopatient had the comment, "Patient engages in writing behavior" written in his chart. Apparently, the writing was presumed to be part of the disturbance.

The researcher also found that the source of any disturbance was always assumed to be the patient and not the staff's behavior or the effect of the environment. For example, when a pseudopatient was found walking the halls, a nurse asked him if he was nervous. Actually, he was bored. The researcher concludes that the staff's perceptions of behavior were controlled by the situation. The organizations themselves had a climate in which the behavior of their inmates was easily misperceived.

Hierarchy

Complex organizations are made up of many levels of systems and subsystems given names such as divisions, areas, units, departments, groups, and teams. These different levels form a hierarchy within the organization.

In most organizations, people are ranked according to their function and the amount of authority that they have. This hierarchy can be thought of as a pyramid having the smallest number of people with the greatest amount of authority at the top and the largest number of people with little or no authority at the bottom, as shown in Figure 10–1. People are also ranked according to the amount of status and salary paid.

Some organizations have a structure and climate that encourage the free movement of information up and down the hierarchy. Others have limited communication networks in which very few people know what is happening or feel as if they had anything to say about what is happening.

While it illustrates the existence of the hierarchy, the pyramid actually oversimplifies the structure and the patterns of interaction that occur within an organization. Although it would not be as clear, a hierarchy of intersecting circles would be a more accurate model of most organizations. Some of these variations will be discussed later in this chapter.

Complexity

The number of interacting levels of groups just described is one indication of an organization's complexity. As the number of people in a system increases, the number of different relationships possible between people increases geometrically. For example, there are 4 different relationship combinations possible in a group of 3 people; 9 in a group of 4 people; and 9801 in a group of 100 people.

Most organizations have multiple rather than single goals that may be in conflict with one another (Huse & Bowditch, 1973). For example, cost cutting done to increase the profits of a proprietary organization may conflict with the goal of delivering high-quality care.

Openness

Every open system, including an organization, affects its environment and is affected by its environment. For example, hospitals located in high-crime areas may experience higher demands for their emergency services, especially for treatment of traumatic injuries, and this demand affects the emergency department's need for staff. The organization may welcome its clients, heal them, and send them away feeling better; or it may reject or harm them, sending them away feeling worse.

An organization exchanges information and energy with its environment. It can provide the specialized skills and information needed to promote or restore health. These skills are exchanged for money and recognition.

This exchange is influenced by many factors in the environment such as the number of other organizations offering the same services, the actual and perceived need for the service, and government regulation. Some organizations cannot find sufficient skilled staff to offer needed services. Others find that their service is not valued and that people are not willing to pay for it. In still other cases, insufficient knowledge is available about a problem to be able to offer satisfactory care. All of these factors and many more interact to produce a very complex health care system.

Pattern

Like other systems, organizations have identifiable rhythms and cycles. For example, health care organizations operate 24 hours a day, every day of

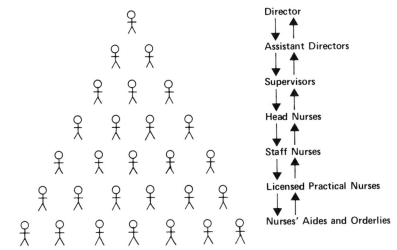

Director
Assistant Directors
Supervisors
Head Nurses
Staff Nurses
Licensed Practical Nurses
Nurses' Aides and Orderlies

A TRADITIONAL NURSING HIERARCHY IN HOSPITALS AND LARGER NURSING HOMES

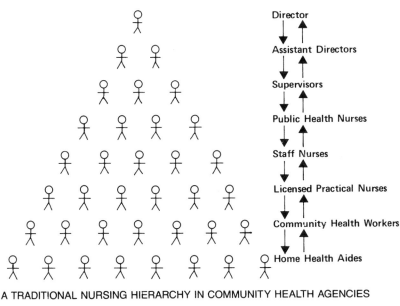

Director
Assistant Directors
Supervisors
Public Health Nurses
Staff Nurses
Licensed Practical Nurses
Community Health Workers
Home Health Aides

A TRADITIONAL NURSING HIERARCHY IN COMMUNITY HEALTH AGENCIES

▼ indicates direction in which orders flow and authority is delegated

▲ indicates direction in which requests flow

↓↑ information, power, and influence may flow in either direction

Figure 10–1. Traditional nursing hierarchies in organizations.

the year. Within those 24 hours, the day shift is usually the busiest and the night shift usually has the least number of people working.

The most typical growth pattern for organizations is early, rapid growth followed by a slower rate of growth, or even no growth, in the late stages of its life cycle. Some organizations experience spurts of new growth later in the life cycle, but eventually all of them experience a decline and cease to exist. Organizations can develop and increase their effectiveness, but all do not succeed in doing this (Levitt, 1988; Meyer, 1977). Some typical patterns are also discussed in the last section of this chapter.

Ideally, organizations function according to agreed-upon procedures and carry out their stated goals. However, they do not actually operate in this simple and straightforward manner. Instead, there are many informal ways in which the work actually gets done. Being able to recognize the difference between these two levels and how they affect the functioning of the organization is part of learning how to work effectively within an organization. These two levels of operation are discussed later in this chapter.

ORGANIZATIONAL STRUCTURE AND FUNCTION

Structural Configurations

A new or small organization usually has a very simple structure consisting of a small number of people including a chief executive officer (CEO) at the top of the hierarchy, very few or no people in the middle ranks, and the most employees at the bottom forming the *operating core*, to use Mintzberg's term (1983) as shown in Figure 10–2. Supervision and coordination are done directly from the top by the CEO, who acts as the dominant leader and manager of the whole organization. Orders usually come from the top, and much of the communication within the organization can be and usually is quite informal.

As the organization grows larger, this simple structure no longer works well. The operating core of employees becomes too large for direct supervision by one or two people at the top. The work is divided up into smaller components, and many leadership and management functions are delegated

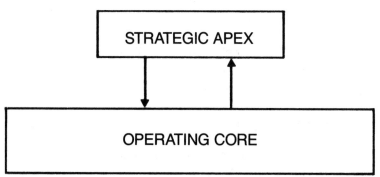

Figure 10–2. Structure of a small new organization. (Adapted from Mintzberg [1983].)

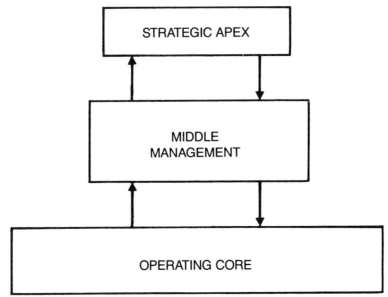

Figure 10–3. Structure of growing organization. (Adapted from Mintzberg [1983].)

to people lower in the hierarchy, forming a level of middle-management people (Fig. 10–3).

The organization may become even more complex as two other components are added: support staff and technical staff. *Support staff* provide services to the employees of the organization. In a large hospital, this includes the people who run the cafeteria, the print shop, audiovisuals, and the housekeeping department. They provide services to the staff rather than to the patients or clients themselves. The second component is the *technical staff*. These people are expert in particular areas and act as internal consultants to the operating core. Examples of technical staff in a hospital would include hospital planners and the inservice education department. This complex organization now has all five components of Mintzberg's model (Fig. 10–4).

There are a number of ways in which the working relationships between people within and between the five components can be formally structured. We will look at two of the more extreme varieties, the strict linear structure of the bureaucracy and the more fluid and circular structure of the matrix organization.

BUREAUCRACY.   Some degree of bureaucracy is characteristic of the formal operation of virtually every organization. Even deliberately informal work groups often take on some of these characteristics. This happens because these arrangements known as *bureaucracy* are designed to promote smooth operations within a large and complex group of people.

Max Weber (1969) said that a bureaucracy has the four following characteristics:

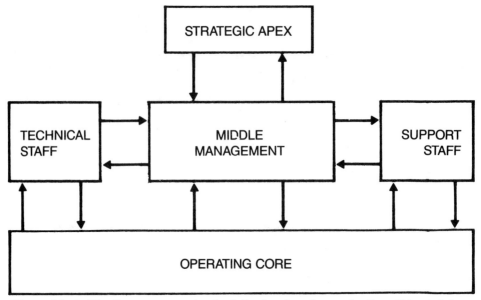

Figure 10–4. The five components of a fully developed organization. (Adapted from Mintzberg [1983].)

1. *Division of Labor*: specific parts of the job to be done are assigned to different individuals or groups. For example, nurses, aides, physicians, dietitians, and social workers all provide parts of the health care needed by one patient.
2. *Hierarchy*: all employees are organized and ranked according to their degree of authority within the organization. For example, administrators and directors are at the top of most hospital hierarchies while aides and maintenance workers are at the bottom.
3. *Rules and Regulations*: acceptable and unacceptable behavior and the proper way to carry out predictable tasks are specifically stated, often in writing. For example, procedure books, policy manuals, by-laws, statements, and memos prescribe many types of behavior from acceptable aseptic techniques to vacation policies in health care organizations.
4. *Emphasis on Technical Competence*: People with certain skills and knowledge are hired to carry out specific parts of the total work of the organization. For example, a community mental health center will have psychiatrists, psychologists, social workers, and nurses to do different kinds of therapies, and clerical staff to do the typing and filing.

In the traditional bureaucracy, the emphasis is on the vertical relationships or *chain of command*. In the chain of command, the CEO at the top delegates authority to people in middle management and so on down the line. People in the technical and support staff components have relatively limited power and authority compared with those in the center who have *line authority*, which extends all the way down to the first-line manager.

There are varying degrees to which an organization can be bureaucratized. A highly controlled and bureaucratized approach is based on the belief that employees must be told what to do, that they must be closely supervised to ensure that they will do it, and that some employees are more skilled and responsible than others and should, therefore, have authority over the others. An organization that is managed according to these beliefs (which hearken back to the management theories of Fayol and Taylor discussed in Chapter 2) would have many detailed rules and regulations, close supervision of employees, and little autonomy allowed individual employees, even professionals capable of functioning independently.

People generally respond negatively to the word bureaucracy. One reason for this is that in most bureaucratic organizations, with their long lines of delegated authority and decision making, you often cannot identify exactly who is responsible for having made a certain decision or created a certain unpopular rule. Arendt (1977) calls this "rule by nobody" because the source of these decisions and rules is faceless. No one person takes full responsibility for outcomes, and nobody seems to know where these rules and decisions originated. In extremely bureaucratic organizations, employees believe that they are being controlled by impersonal rules and regulations. Having no influence on decisions within the organization leads to a feeling of powerlessness and alienation.

One of the greatest frustrations people experience in trying to relate to a bureaucratic organization either as employees or as clients is the diffusion of responsibility and subsequent refusal to make a decision. For example, to get something done in some organizations, you need the approval of six different people on six different forms, and each of the six people refuses to give you approval until the other five have given theirs. This is not true of every bureaucratic organization, but it is one very common outcome, known as "bureaucratic red tape."

An extreme division of labor extends the rule-by-nobody even to responsibility for the end product of the organization. For example, when 6, 8, or even 20 people in one health care organization have given care to a patient, how can you say who is responsible for the outcome? Another problem arises from an extreme division of labor: how can people derive any satisfaction or pride in their work when it is difficult to identify their contribution? The following is one example of this fragmentation:

> In a child health clinic, a nurse observed that one youngster was flushed and restless and had some abdominal pain. The child was immediately referred to a physician who diagnosed the problem as appendicitis.
>
> The child was admitted to the hospital and prepared for surgery. The operating room nurse and recovery room nurse both offered support and reassurance when the child seemed frightened by this new experience and strange environment.
>
> Several nurses cared for the child on the pediatric unit until the child was sent home. The child recovered quickly at home and returned to school in 2 weeks.
>
> However, the clinic nurse's original assessment was not confirmed to the nurse until the child returned to the clinic a year later. The operating room and recovery room nurses never found out whether or not their intervention had left the child less fearful, and the nurses on the pediatric unit never found out whether or not the child did well at home and in returning to school.

Each of these care givers had an important but limited part in the child's care. The lack of involvement in the whole process and of feedback about the child's progress to recovery meant that not one of them received timely confirmation of the ultimate effectiveness of their intervention. This resulted in a failure to meet their needs for recognition and self-actualization, both important sources of motivation.

MATRIX ORGANIZATIONS. There is no single, widely accepted alternative model for organizations that eliminates the problems of bureaucracy and yet promotes the smooth and efficient operation of a large organization. Some approaches have been suggested to alleviate these problems and increase the effectiveness of the organization, including the concept of the matrix organization (Lawrence, 1979; McKelvey & Kilmann, 1975; Drucker, 1977).

It has been increasingly recognized that organizations need to be not only efficient but also adaptable and innovative. Organizations must be prepared for uncertainty, for rapid changes in their environment, and for rapid, creative responses to these challenges. In addition, they need to provide an internal climate that not only allows but also motivates employees to work to the best of their ability.

The matrix organization emphasizes increased flexibility of the organizational structure, increased participation in decision making, and more autonomy for working groups or teams. For example, rigid department or unit structures are reorganized into semi-autonomous teams composed of professionals from different departments and disciplines. Each team is given a specific task or function to carry out (examples would be a hospital infection-control team or a child protection team in a community agency). These teams are given much more authority than is ordinarily the case in a bureaucratic organization. The teams themselves are responsible for much of their own self-correction and self-control, although they usually have a designated leader. Together, team members make decisions about work assignments and how to deal with any problems that arise. In other words, the teams supervise or manage themselves to a much greater extent than in a bureaucracy.

On the other hand, many of these teams find themselves with two or more managers to whom they must report. Two or more managers may also complete their evaluation forms and make salary and promotion recommendations. The chain of command can be very confusing, and direction and expectations can be quite ambiguous. If not managed well, this leads to conflicts over territory, power struggles, and duplication of effort. If managed well, though, the matrix organization provides many more opportunities for pooling needed talents and skills and can provide a climate that fosters innovation and creativity.

Many of the teams and project groups that are formed within a matrix organization are ad hoc groups that continue only for the life of a particular project. People can be assigned to more than one of these groups at the same time if the projects do not require their full-time attention. Some of these teams are temporary task forces put together to accomplish a specific task within a given amount of time. People with the various skills needed to complete the task may be drawn from many different parts of the organization to form the team. An advantage of ad hoc groups is the greatly increased flexibility to respond to changing needs of the organization; a disadvantage is the potential disruption of the departments or areas from which people are taken to form the team. The creation of temporary task forces may also threaten some people's feelings of security if these needs are not met in another manner.

As you can imagine, working on such a team would require much more agreement among team members than is required in more traditional departments. The increased participation in decision making by each employee reduces the feelings of powerlessness and alienation that can arise in bureaucracies.

Supervisors and administrators can also be given different functions in a matrix organization. Instead of spending their time watching and controlling other people's work, they can become planners and resource persons. Providing the conditions required for the optimum functioning of the teams becomes their most important responsibility. They are expected to ensure that the support, information, materials, and budgeted funds needed to do the job well are available to the team. They also need to provide more coordination between the teams so that the teams are working toward congruent goals, cooperating rather than blocking each other and not duplicating effort.

Very large organizations can also be divided into functional areas that operate as if they were smaller organizations. This reduces the complexity of each division. It allows each division to be better integrated when integration of the organization as a whole has become virtually impossible because of its great size, complexity, and diversity. However, communication between divisions may become more difficult. The matrix organization provides an alternative to the bureaucratic organization but has some of its own disadvantages as you can see.

Function

The classic approach to organizations was to study only the formal organization. But it eventually became apparent through research such as the Hawthorne studies discussed in Chapter 2, for example, that too many important factors were being ignored. You need to know about and use both the formal and informal functions of the organization in order to be effective. Knowing about just one of these levels would give you only part of the picture. In fact, it has recently been emphasized that the formal and informal levels are really intertwined with one another and that the actual function of the organization includes both (Mintzberg, 1983).

FORMAL AND INFORMAL GOALS. There are two kinds of goals in an organization, the *official stated goals* and the *unstated operative goals* (Perrow, 1969).

The formal, official goals of an organization are the goals that appear in public statements about the organization. They are the ones you would be told about if you asked a representative of the organization what its purpose was or the goals you would find in an official statement of the purpose of the organization.

Official goals tend to be general, public spirited, and idealistic. They are designed to sound benevolent and impressive. The following are some examples:

▷ Promote the health and well-being of the clients we serve.

▷ Protect the people of this city.

▷ Foster a spirit of cooperative concern for those in need of our services.

It is usually easy to determine the official goals of an organization. Most organizations want the public to hear about their official goals, making an effort to publicize them because they promote the desired image of a public-spirited organization. However, the official goals do not fully explain the behavior of an organization, much of which is directed toward achieving another set of goals, the operative goals.

The informal, operative goals of an organization are those the organization is actually pursuing in its day-to-day operation. They are usually not verbalized and tend to be less rational and public spirited than the official goals.

Operative goals are not only different from the official goals but often are in conflict with them. They focus primarily on the survival and growth of the organization rather than public benefit.

Health care organizations depend on their environments for a continuous supply of clients, money, and personnel. Without these, they cannot continue to exist. These needs are reflected in their operative goals, which are commonly aimed at efficiency rather than effectiveness, quantity rather than quality, maintenance of a positive public image, achieving financial gain, avoiding public criticism, and avoiding legal problems, especially expensive and embarrassing lawsuits. The personal needs and ambitions of people who have power and authority in the organization also affect the operative goals.

Operative goals are more difficult to determine than official goals because they implicit. In fact, stating them directly can provoke denial and insistence on the official goals.

Careful observation of behavior in the organization is needed to identify the operative goals. In particular, you need to look at the decisions that are made; what kind of behavior is rewarded; and the actual, unstated priorities that are implied by these actions. Some typical operative goals that exist in health care organizations include financial gain, efficiency, quantity over quality, public image, avoiding criticism, avoiding lawsuits, and meeting individual needs.

Financial Gain.   The basic system drive to continue existence often leads to the priority of financial gain over more idealistic goals. Even not-for-profit health care organizations pursue financial gain, sometimes at the public's expense. For example:

> Some hospitals have told people who obviously can afford the extra cost that there are no semiprivate rooms available so that their higher-priced single rooms are not left empty and unproductive (Citizens Board, 1972). Other hospitals refuse care to people who cannot pay, insist on payment in advance for surgery, or refuse to release patients who cannot pay their bills, keeping them extra days while the bill becomes even higher.

The pursuit of profits can subvert care giving goals. The recurring nursing home scandals, for example, demonstrate that the goals of increasing profits for the organization's owners can result in neglect of clients' needs.

There are many sources of profit in the health care industry. These include the profits of the companies who manufacture and sell the drugs, equipment, and supplies. Others profit indirectly from health care and may exert influence on the organization's operative goals. One example is the lawyers, bankers, architects, planners, real estate salesmen, and various consultants who benefit when an existing hospital expands (Nichols, 1976).

Efficiency.   Efficient operation means greater output per dollar spent. This goal is not always congruent with quality care. The individual client is divided into separate parts, each to be treated skillfully and efficiently by a specialist in taking care of that part. Unfortunately, this approach fails to consider the interrelationships of these parts and the person as a whole.

Staffing patterns often reflect the operative goal of improving efficiency. The functional mode of organizing nursing care (in which one person gives all of the medications, another does all of the treatment, and so forth) is one example. Another example is the hiring of the person with the least amount of skill, such as a nursing assistant, rather than the person who can do the job best but commands a higher salary.

Staff nurses frequently find themselves praised and rewarded for completing assignments and charting on time rather than for their perceptive observations or professional judgments, another example of the priority of efficiency over providing effective care.

Quantity Over Quality.   The priority of quantity over quality leads to the "numbers game" in organizations. Departments are asked to report the number of things done rather than how well they are done, and are rewarded for producing quantity rather than quality.

This tendency translates into reporting how many people a nurse practitioner can see in one day rather than the effectiveness of the care. Inservice educators are rewarded for holding many classes attended by large numbers of individuals rather than for the amount of learning that took place. Public health nurses find their agencies reporting the number of home visits made and looking for ways to increase the number that can be made in one day rather than evaluating the effectiveness of these visits and the number of family members that were served on one visit.

Other departments have the same experience. Getting food trays to patients quickly often seems to be more important than the ability to make a restrictive diet palatable. Seeing many patients in physical therapy is more likely to be rewarded than the ability to motivate patients to continue their exercises after discharge.

Public Image.   A positive public image is important because it affects the number of clients and contributors that the organization can attract. This can conflict with the official goals. For example, what happens to an individual patient is much less apparent to a hospital's potential clients and benefactors than an attractive, modern building, so money needed for additional staff may be spent on renovation and landscaping instead.

On the other hand, you can also take advantage of this operative goal. For example, to gain support for a birthing room, you can point out that it would be the first birthing room in the community, that many people have asked for one, and that it would receive favorable publicity when the organization announces its introduction.

Avoiding Criticism.   Many health care organizations will go to great lengths to avoid criticism that would tarnish their public image or otherwise threaten their existence. For example:

A county health department hired a pediatric nurse clinician to conduct child health clinics. The clinics were well attended, and the parents were very satisfied with the family-centered care they received. In fact, they were so satisfied that many reduced their pediatrician visits, which provoked a strong protest from area pediatricians. In response to the protest, the pediatric nurse clinician's clinics were limited to families who could not pay for a private physician.

As with the previous example, you can often use the goal of avoiding criticism to help you bring about a needed change in the organization's operations.

Avoiding Lawsuits. Concern about legal repercussions is sometimes used as a convenient excuse to constrain health care professionals. For example:

Ambulatory patients who have every functional capacity needed to take their own medications are usually not permitted to do so because of concern about legal responsibilities.

Efforts to expand nursing roles in health care organizations have been blocked by concern with encroaching upon medical practice.

Community health nurses may not be permitted to make a second home visit when the client does not have a physician.

This operative goal can also be turned to your advantage. For example, if discharge planning is inadequate, you can point out that the organization could be held legally responsible if patients are given insufficient information about self-care before discharge and injure themselves as a result.

Meeting Individual Needs. The personal needs, desires, and ambitions of people with power and authority in organizations often influence decisions. For example:

Some caregivers meet their own needs by encouraging clients to be dependent on them long after they could be independent.

Surgeons may perform unnecessary operations to keep their skills sharp or their practices busy.

An administrator may propose purchasing expensive equipment because the administrator wants to be part of technologically advanced organization.

These individual needs can set in motion operative goals that are in conflict with not only the official goals but also with some of the other operative goals of the organization.

FORMAL AND INFORMAL LEVELS OF OPERATION. Like the formal goals of the organization, the formal level of operation is the official, stated structure and function of the organization. If you asked an administrator to describe the organization to you, the administrator would probably describe this formal level of operation. The description would include the way in which employees are divided into groups, the kind of work each group does, and who supervises the work of each group. Here is an example from an ambulatory care center:

This is the main clinic in which we have our administrative offices as well as our comprehensive ambulatory care clinic. Clients can see the physicians, nurses, social worker, dietitian, or community worker as needed here. We have three satellite clinics staffed by nurse practitioners and a social worker. We also have an outreach team that is based here at the main clinic but travels to different locations each day of the week and responds to emergency calls. Clients who need to see a physician or dietitian must come to the main clinic. Also, the bookkeeping and billing are done from the main office, but people can call the satellite clinics to make appointments.

The description would go on to say who is in charge of each clinic, who manages the entire organization, the specific services offered, the fees charged, the hours each clinic is open, and so on.

If you expressed interest in further information, the administrator might give you a *table of organization.* This is a diagram showing the formal relationships between employees of the organization, the way in which they are grouped together, and who reports to whom (Fig. 10–5).

On the formal level, communication flows along the established lines shown in the diagram; for example, from the administrator to the assistant administrator to the director of the main clinic to the supervisors to the rest of the staff and back again. This is often referred to as the *proper channels of communication.*

It is often said of these organizational hierarchies that the orders come

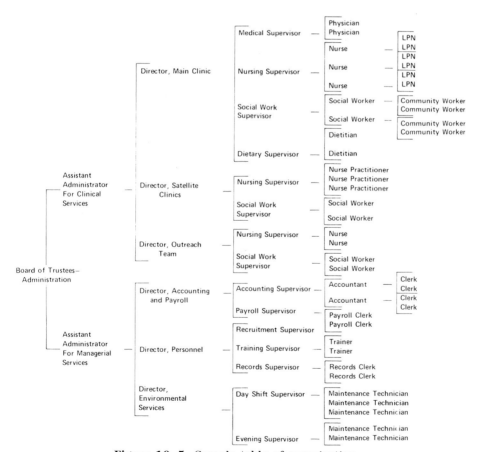

Figure 10–5. Sample table of organization.

down and the requests go up. The board of trustees delegates authority to the administrator who in turn delegates some authority to the assistant administrators and so on down the line. Staff members at the bottom of the pyramid have authority over no one except perhaps the clients served by the organization (who do not even appear on most tables of organization). Work assignments and directions are also passed down the line in the same way.

The informal level of operation includes all those unwritten, unofficial relationships that develop in an organization but are not reflected in the official structure of the organization. It includes norms and traditions about the way people work together, and it has a strong influence on what actually happens in an organization, existing alongside, and intertwined with, the formal level of operation. They are not necessarily in harmony with each other, however.

The informal level of operations exists even in the most highly controlled organization. For example, you may find that some rules and regulations are circumvented, that the hierarchy is ignored, that someone high up in the hierarchy has very little power or influence, or that lines between specific jobs are blurred in actual operation. Alternative paths are created by which requests are made and filled without multiple approvals; tasks are completed quickly, and messages are communicated across and around the so-called proper channels of communication. The following is an example of informal communications in a highly controlled organization:

> A prison is a highly controlled organization in which its clients (the prisoners) are not even allowed to leave without permission. There are many restrictions placed on both the guards and the prisoners about who can visit, what possessions the prisoners are allowed, and so forth. At the same time, some prisoners are able to buy and sell drugs, liquor, and sex, all absolutely forbidden by the formal organization. They are able to do these things through the informal level of operation that exists even in prisons.

Because they exist within the same system and affect the same people, the formal and informal levels of operation are interrelated aspects of the organization as a whole. These two levels can be complementary and facilitative or in conflict and obstructive of each other. When they are complementary, the informal level can provide a way of dealing with barriers such as the regulation in the following example:

> If you visited a small town and were told that a local law required horses to wear bonnets on Sunday, you would probably laugh about the archiac law and leave your horse bareheaded, if you had one. You would not expect anyone to say anything to you about your horse, not even the police, whose formal duty is to enforce the law. Informally, you would know that you are not expected to obey that particular law.
> At the same time, you would also know that there are other laws that you are expected to obey and that you would definitely hear about it if you did not obey them.

In this example, the informal level complements the formal level by providing a socially acceptable way of dealing with an absurd regulation: ignore it. It facilitates operations by ignoring or revising formal relationships, rules, and regulations. When complementary, the informal level can humanize the impersonality and inflexibility of a large, bureaucratic organization.

The informal level of operations also provides a lively and efficient informal communication network commonly known as the grapevine. Although best known for spreading rumors, it is not always a negative force in an organization. The grapevine provides employees with needed information that the formal system is slow or neglectful about sharing with them. It is also useful as a way to test a new idea or change without having to go through the frequently cumbersome formal level of operations.

Informal role expectations can be blended with formal ones so that people are not overly restricted by formal job descriptions. This blurring provides flexibility but can also cause some confusion, especially for the new employee who does not yet understand the informal system. Blurring of roles can also lead to increased territorial conflicts between individuals or groups within the organization.

The informal level can provide support for people in an organization that fails to provide support on the formal level. However, when this is extended to protecting inept employees, it can reduce the organization's effectiveness. Another way in which the informal level can reduce effectiveness is when employees informally agree to limit the amount of work they do and put pressure on their coworkers to do the same.

A conflict with the formal level in a crucial area can lead to serious problems. The following is an example:

> Officially, nurse aides are not allowed to give medications to patients, but occasionally a busy nurse will informally ask an aide to take an oral medication to a waiting patient or to stay with the patient who takes a long time to swallow several tablets.
>
> One day, an aide gave a medication to the wrong patient, who experienced some serious side effects from the drug. As required, the incident was reported and both the nurse and the aide were fired for failing to obey the official rules.

Incongruency between the informal and formal levels can also lead to some difficulties for those who do not understand the two levels. The following is an example:

> A community health agency officially prohibited payment for overtime, but staff members often had to stay late to finish their work. Informally, their supervisors allowed them to leave early when things were quiet or when they had an appointment in order to compensate for the extra time they had worked.
>
> The director of the agency was aware of this informal procedure and tacitly allowed it to continue because it resulted in staff members feeling that they were being treated fairly. However, when a naive staff member demanded to be given earned compensation time in the middle of a very busy week, the staff member was told that there was no such thing as compensation time and that staff members were not allowed to work overtime and so could not possibly have earned any compensation time.

This staff member made the mistake of trying to deal with an informal procedure as if it were a formal regulation. As a result, no staff member was granted any compensation time until the formal and informal levels had been clearly differentiated again.

Many efforts to bring about improvements or changes have failed because the person planning them thought it could be done by just setting up a formal procedure. The following example illustrates the difference between using only the formal level and using both:

> Two different nurses working in a large city hospital had what they thought were good ideas for improving patient care in that hospital. The first nurse had some ideas for improving the patient assessment form and asked the head nurse how a suggestion was supposed to be sent to the Director of Nursing. The head nurse told the nurse to put the

idea in writing, including reasons why the nurse thought it would improve nursing care, and to give two copies to the supervisor who would keep one and send the other to the director.

The nurse typed a three-page report explaining the idea and how it would increase efficiency and promote better patient care. The nurse gave the report to the supervisor as directed.

Three months later the nurse received a note from the director expressing appreciation for the suggestion and saying that it would be shared with the head nurses and supervisors to find out if they thought it would work. By the time the nurse received this note, the idea was almost forgotten. It was apparently received without enthusiasm because it was never implemented.

The second nurse followed the procedure that other people had used successfully in that hospital. The second nurse talked with the head nurse and one of the supervisors at lunch one day about an idea for improving admission procedures and why the nurse thought it would work. Both seemed interested so the nurse asked them, "How can we try this out?" They suggested that the nurse ask to be included on the agenda for their next meeting and come to explain the idea to the group.

The nurse asked the head nurse and supervisor to help plan the presentation. They worked out the details of the plan with the assistance of one of the hospital's inservice educators. At the meeting, the idea received sufficient support to try it out on several units to see if it would work.

The first nurse used only the formal channels of communication and the idea moved along them without gathering any support or having any impact. The nurse failed to observe how the informal level operated in the implementation of an idea and neglected to find out who was interested in the idea or to attempt to interest people in the idea in order to gain some support.

In contrast, the second nurse had observed that many ideas came from the head nurses and supervisors and that the people the nurse talked to were often interested in new ideas. This is only the first phase in bringing about a change but it is an important one. Without the use of the informal

---

▷ How much money is spent on decor, landscaping, public relations, and other amenities?

▷ Are employees expected to become involved in community activities? Is this involvement rewarded?

▷ How do people dress? Is formality expected or is informality preferred?

▷ Is socializing with coworkers encouraged or discouraged?

▷ Are ethnic or sexist jokes encouraged, tolerated, or frowned upon?

▷ What types of status symbols are evident? Do badges, uniforms, office furniture, titles, or special privileges indicate people's status in the organization?

▷ Who is most likely to receive a promotion or raise in pay? Is it people who have seniority, advance preparation, excellent evaluations, or "connections" with people in powerful positions?

▷ Where do the most important discussions and decisions take place? Do they take place in formal meetings, informal situations, or in private meetings with administrators?

▷ Are there any "touchy" or taboo subjects such as unions, the work of a particular physician, or certain inadequacies in the operation of the organization?

Figure 10–6. Assessment of the informal function of an organization. (Adapted from Del Bueno [1987].)

level of operation it is very likely that the second nurse's idea would also have been ignored.

A sampling of the kinds of information you would seek in trying to understand the informal goals and level of operations in an organization can be found in Figure 10–6 (Del Bueno, 1987). Observation and analysis of the informal level of an organization should be an important aspect of your assessment of any organization. As was illustrated in the examples, knowledge of the informal level of function can contribute considerably to your effectiveness within that organization.

PATTERNS OF RELATIONSHIPS IN ORGANIZATIONS

Power and Authority in Relationships

Authority is a specific type of power that originates in the official position a person holds within the organization. It exists only because other people are willing to accept and obey the decisions made by the person in authority (Merton, 1969). It is an important but by no means the only source of power and influence in organizations.

Every individual in an organization has some resources for power and influence, but the amount of authority a person has is related to that person's position in the hierarchy. There is a purpose for this unequal distribution: the relatively small number of people with authority are expected to exert some control over the way the rest of the organization functions.

Health care organizations typically have a board of some kind — known as the board of directors, trustees, or governors — at the top of the hierarchy. Board members are often influential businesspeople, professionals, or community leaders. They are legally and ethically responsible for the operation of the organization but usually delegate most of this responsibility to the administrator. This does not always happen: Sometimes board members get involved in everyday operations. This may occur in a crisis, such as a big lawsuit or when some members have difficulty delegating their authority. An amusing example of this difficulty in delegating authority was a board whose members questioned the brand of grape juice being served and complained about the color of the paint being used (Perrow, 1969).

Generally speaking, however, the function of board members is to set general policies, not to get involved in the day-to-day operation of the organization. Health care is a highly complex and technologically advanced field, and the professional administrator usually has the time and training needed to thoroughly assess the situation and make these decisions.

Another element of the authority structure of hospitals is the medical staff, often called the "shadow organization" because it has its own admission requirements, hierarchy, rewards, and sanctions. The staff are a dominant force and yet are neither employed nor controlled by the health care organization. Often they are not even loyal to the organization (Trent, 1986). Can you imagine such an unusual arrangement in any ordinary business? Many abuses of power by physicians have been documented, including power plays to control the functions of the organization, exploitation and domination of nurses, and discrimination within medical staffs (Citizens Board, 1972; Nichols, 1976).

The board, administrator, and medical staff usually form a triad of power and authority at the top of the organizational hierarchy. Several trends are challenging and changing this triad. More physicians are being employed directly by organizations. Governmental regulation has become an increasingly powerful influence on health care organizations as it has moved toward more evaluation, restrictions, and control of the health care delivery system. Consumer representation on planning and advisory boards also has had the potential for increasing organizational responsiveness to people's needs but so far has not really fulfilled its potential (Merton, 1969; Longest, 1984).

Nurses have also challenged the traditional organizational triad. Nursing service administrators are leaders of the largest group of health care professionals in most health care organizations (approximately 50 percent of the staff of most hospitals). At the present time, most are still immediately below the triad at the top of the hierarchy, but many have moved up into these influential positions and are no longer satisfied with the limited amount of power and authority that they had in the past.

Nursing service administrators today often find themselves in the middle, between conflicting expectations. They are expected to support the interests of the nursing staff in their relationships with other departments of the organization. From the nursing point of view, the director of nursing (or vice-president in charge of patient services) should be an advocate rather than a "policeman" of the nursing staff. At the same time, they are expected to represent the board and administrator (often the medical staff as well) in their dealings with the nursing staff. The expectation of the organizational triad is that they will direct and control the nursing staff, but the director of nursing needs the cooperation of the nursing staff to do this effectively. Remembering that it is the board and administrator who hire, evaluate, and give salary increases to the director of nursing, you can see that the director walks a "rather delicate tight-rope" in trying to work effectively with both groups (McClure, 1972, p. 146).

After considering the conflict faced by nurse administrators, it may not surprise you that they are often described by nurses lower in the hierarchy as the source of most of their problems. Staff nurses rate lack of support from nursing service administration, inadequate staffing, and restrictions on giving the best patient care as some of their major problems. All of these problems can be influenced, but not necessarily controlled, by the director of nursing (Funkhouser, 1977).

There has been some interest in changing nursing's position in the typical hierarchy. One proposed model is to create a nursing staff similar to the medical staff so that a hospital would have a board of trustees at the top and, immediately below the board, a board of medical examiners, a board of nursing governors, boards of other professions, and the hospital administration (Johnson, Hoppel, Edelman, & Brown, 1983). The board of nursing would handle such matters as credentials, standards, and cooperation between staff and private practitioners. This model seems to promote a proliferation of administrative-level personnel. If not carefully designed, it may lead to problems similar to those caused by the separate medical staff.

Another model suggests contracting for nursing services in which the nursing staff takes responsibility for scheduling and self-management, including peer review (Dear, Weisman, & O'Keefe, 1985). This model supports primary care and the expansion of the nurse's role, including increased discharge planning and follow-up after discharge.

Before concluding this section, it is important to point out that nurses are neither powerless nor at the bottom of the hierarchy. Depending on the particular organization, nurses have positional authority over other nurses, practical nurses, aides, orderlies, and people from other professions and departments. It is also worth noting at this point that many other health care professionals (such as physical therapists, dietitians, social workers, and so forth) are located in similar positions in the organizational hierarchy. They face much the same kinds of conflicts as nurses do in dealing with the expectations of people above and below them in the hierarchy and, at the same time, promoting the practice of their professions.

No single person's power or authority in an organization is absolute. Each person, no matter how high up in hierarchy, is susceptible to the power of others either within or outside of the organization. Nor is anyone, no matter how low on the hierarchy, completely without power. While people at lower levels of the hierarchy have little or no authority, they have other sources of power that can counterbalance the authority of people above them in the hierarchy. For example, people in high-level positions depend on their staffs to carry out their decisions. A head nurse could not carry out all of the work that must be done if the staff left.

Research on organizations has shown that people at all levels in organizations tend to attribute more power to others than to themselves (Lindquist & Blackburn, 1974). In a survey of one university, for example, the faculty felt that the students and administration had most of the power, the administrators felt that the faculty and students had most of the power, and the students felt that the faculty and administrators had all of the power. It may help you to remember this when you are dealing with persons above or below you in the hierarchy of your organization: these people probably feel much less powerful than they seem to you.

Relationship Games

Games are a repetitive and unproductive pattern of relating to others. Like individual people, organizations also play these games. There are several that they are especially likely to play.

PATERNALISM.   Many organizations treat their employees as though they were children instead of mature adults. One of the problems with this approach is that it is likely to provoke childish behavior such as rebelliousness or dependency in return. It also has a tendency to inhibit the growth and development of employees and subsequently affects their ability to contribute to the best of their ability. An authoritarian or directive type of management in which employees are allowed little or no voice in decision making because their supervisors think that they know what is best for them and do not expect them to be able to make wise decisions is just one of the many ways in which paternalism occurs in organizations.

Paternalism can appear to be benevolent. For example, many organizations show interest and concern for what happens to their employees outside of working hours. However, when this commendable concern is extended paternalistically into telling or even requiring employees to conduct their lives in a certain way, it is no longer benevolent.

Paternalistic organizations are also likely to give their employees turkeys on Thanksgiving or to hold expensive celebrations on such occasions as the anniversary of the organization. The paternalistic aspect of this becomes more apparent when you realize that many employees would prefer to make their own decisions about how to spend the money used to hold these celebrations rather than being given a piece of birthday cake and balloons to take home from work.

The examples given so far are of the milder form of paternalism. Organizational paternalism can become much more restrictive and suffocating. Ashley's 1976 history of hospitals' paternalistic treatment of nurses provides a good background for this more serious kind of paternalism:

> Until the 1950s, many hospitals employed only a limited number of graduate nurses and used student nurses for most of the hospital nursing staff positions. Nurses were poorly paid and poorly educated women who accepted society's definition of them as servants and physicians' helpers. For example, it was considered more important for nurses to get meals served while the gravy was still hot than for nurses to know anything about their patients' needs. Physicians continually exerted control over nurses and nursing education, denying their value at the same time that they depended on nurses to care for their patients 24 hours a day. Many of the nurses who held positions of authority in hospitals supported this definition instead of fighting it, which reinforced the pattern of poor self-image and passivity that others have capitalized on since the 1900s.

Although much has changed since then, there is still some passivity and low self-esteem evident in the behavior of nurses, and the approach of many health care organizations (and some physicians) toward nurses is still paternalistic.

Calling the other's game by refusing to respond in a childish manner is one way to confront paternalism (for an example, see Chapter 15, on communication). However, a planned change strategy may be necessary to change the way an organization treats its employees.

KARPMAN TRIANGLE.   This is another counterproductive game that service organizations play with both clients and employees. There are three different roles to choose from in the Karpman Triangle: victim, persecutor, or rescuer (see Fig. 15–1). Participants switch from one role to another around the triangle to play this game.

This counterproductive game (which is explained in more detail in Chapter 15) consists of moving from one role to another around the triangle. It can be played by the organization as well as by individuals. The following example shows how an organization can play the different roles in relation to clients:

> A health department decided to offer free immunizations to people who were going to travel in foreign countries, most of whom could afford to pay for this service (rescuer). When they were overwhelmed by the crowd of people appearing at their door for the first travelers' clinic, the health department announced that further clinics would be cancelled, claiming that people who could really afford to pay for the service were taking advantage of the health department (persecutor).

Organizations also play these games with their employees, as is shown in the following examples:

> An agency had very harsh personnel policies, including the immediate dismissal of any employee caught taking home even a pencil (persecutor). When questioned about these extreme policies, a spokesperson for the agency said it was necessary because so many of its employees were not interested in the welfare of the organization (victim).
>
> Because of inadequate planning for summer vacations, a hospital suffered a serious shortage of maintenance workers and asked its maintenance workers to work two double shifts a week all summer to cover the shortage (victim). These employees had a union contract, so they were paid time and a half for the extra shifts. When this group was due for a salary increase in the fall, the hospital said it would not grant an increase because the maintenance workers had taken so much overtime all summer (persecutor).

As with paternalism, refusing to play any of these roles is one way to counteract this game. It is often necessary, however, to use planned change strategies to change an organization's pattern of relationships with its employees.

"I TOLD YOU SO."   This is another potentially destructive game that some organizations have developed (consciously or unconsciously) in response to pressures to promote more women and people from minority groups into positions with some authority within the hierarchy. Instead of selecting the individual from these groups who has the best qualifications for the job, an individual who lacks the ability, education, or experience needed is chosen and placed into a position that he or she is not prepared to fill. The almost inevitable result is that many fail to carry out the responsibilities of their new positions effectively. Their failure provides the organization with an excuse for continuing its inequitable promotion practices, and gives the people who oppose the equitable promotion of women and minorities a chance to say, "I told you so."

It can be very difficult for individuals who are offered a promotion to a position beyond their present capabilities to reject that attractive, even flattering, offer unless they are aware that they are being set up for failure. Once such a person is in the position, it is often possible for co-workers to offer sufficient help and support for that person to succeed despite the trap that has been set.

BEAR TRAP.   This is another trap into which the unsuspecting prospective employee may fall. The bear trap is set by organizations that enter into agreements with people seeking employment and later do not honor those agreements. Although it is natural for representatives of an organization to make known only its more positive aspects to someone they wish to hire, some go beyond this to what can only be called misrepresentation of the conditions of employment. An organization's success in doing this is greatly enhanced by the naiveté and eagerness of the job applicant.

Typically included in this trap are promises of an exciting and challenging job, fast promotions, job security, and impressive flexibility regarding working conditions and transfers between departments. The following are examples of some common traps set by organizations.

> Miss K., a new graduate nurse, chose a particular agency because they promised her 2 weeks of vacation in December for her wedding. She began working at the agency in July

and was generally satisfied with the position until she was told that no one is ever allowed to take time off in December or January and that her request for time off was denied.

Another prospective employee, Mr. S., who requested a staff position in the emergency department, was promised a transfer there after completing the required 3 months on a general medical or surgical unit of the hospital. After completing the three months, he was told that there were no openings in the emergency department. He finally left the hospital after 2 years during which no opening in the emergency department ever came up at a time when he could be transferred, although he knew of at least two new nurses who had been added to the emergency department staff while he worked for that hospital.

An experienced nurse administrator, Mrs. R., was hired by a large agency after a 6-month search for someone with her expertise. She accepted the position primarily because she was promised a great deal of freedom and autonomy to hire her own staff and to develop the services to be offered on the basis of an assessment of client needs. After beginning work, she found that the agency actually already had a rough plan for the project, which she was expected to implement immediately without conducting a needs assessment. She was also given a list of 12 current employees from which to choose her 9 staff members because the agency could not afford to hire additional staff. This was hardly the freedom and autonomy that she had been promised.

Astute questioning and observation of both managers and staff members during employment interviews can substantially reduce the possibility of falling into such traps after accepting a position (perhaps rejecting what might have been a better offer) and committing your time and energy to that position. Any agreements made should be obtained in writing. Once in the trap, you have to decide whether you are going to fight for change and for fulfillment of the promises made, accept the organization's failure to fulfill its agreements with you, or resign.

SUMMARY

Health care organizations vary in the type and comprehensiveness of services offered and in the type of populations served. They may also be categorized as either not-for-profit (voluntary, publicly financed) or for-profit (proprietary).

Organizations are complex suprasystems made up of large numbers of people grouped hierarchically into smaller systems and subsystems. Because of their size and complexity, they frequently have multiple purposes, goals, and functions. They also have identifiable characteristics, including their climate and structure, and exhibit patterns of behavior such as growth, activity cycles, and patterns of interactions.

The official goals of an organization are the stated goals. The operative goals are the unstated ones that the organization is actually pursuing in its day-to-day operation. The operative goals are usually harder to identify and are generally less idealistic. Financial gain, efficiency, quantity over quality, maintenance of a positive public image, avoidance of criticism, and avoidance of lawsuits are common operative goals in health care organizations.

The formal level of operation is the official, stated structure (represented by the table of organization) and function of the organization. The formal level often has the bureaucratic characteristics of a hierarchy, division of labor, rules and regulations, and emphasis on technical competence.

There are alternate models such as the matrix organization, which emphasizes flexibility, innovation, project orientation, temporary groups, and multiple managers.

The informal level of operation in an organization includes the unwritten, unofficial relationships, norms, and traditions that develop within an organization. These may complement and support the formal level, or they may be in conflict with it. It is important to know and use both levels of goals and operations in order to work effectively within an organization.

Authority, which is derived from holding certain positions within the organizational structure, is generally greatest at the top of the hierarchy and lowest at the bottom. However, other sources of power are available to people in low-authority positions. Paternalism, the Karpman Triangle, "I Told You So," and the Bear Trap are unproductive relationship patterns often found in health care organizations. In paternalism, the organization acts as parent to the employee "children"; in the Karpman Triangle, the organization plays the roles of victim, rescuer, or persecutor; in "I Told You So," the organization promotes unqualified people expecting them to fail; and in the Bear Trap, the organization enters agreements that are not honored. Confrontation and change strategies can be used to repattern these organizational behaviors.

REFERENCES*

Appelbaum, S.H. (1986). The organizational climate audit . . . or how healthy is your hospital? *Hospital and Health Services Administration*, 29, 51–70.

*Ashley, J. (1976). *Hospitals, Paternalism and the Role of the Nurse*. New York: Teachers College Press.

*Citizens Board of Inquiry into Health Services to Americans: (1972). *Heal yourself*. Washington, D.C.: American Public Health Association.

*Del Bueno, D.J. (1987). An organizational checklist. *Journal of Nursing Administration*, 17 (5), 30–33.

*Dear, M.R., Weisman, C.S. & O'Keefe, S. (1985). Evaluation of a contract model for professional nursing practice. *Health Care Management Review*, 10, 65–77.

Dalton, M. (1929). Formal and informal organizations. In Etzioni A. (ed) *Readings on Modern Organizations*. Englewood Cliffs, New Jersey: Prentice-Hall.

Drucker, P.L. (1977). *People and Performance: The Best of Peter Drucker*. New York: Harper and Row.

Frederiksen, L.W., Solomon, L.J. & Brehony, K.A. (1984). *Marketing Health Behavior: Principles, Techniques and Applications*. New York: Plenum Press.

Funkhouser, G.R. (1977). Quality of care: Part II. *Nursing '77*, 7 (1), 27.

Greene, M. (1977). Self-consciousness in a technological world. In Fitzpatrick, M.L. (ed) *Present Realities/Future Imperatives in Nursing Education*. New York: Teachers College Press.

Huse, E.F. & Bowditch, J.L. (1977). *Behavior in Organizations: A Systems Approach to Managing*. Reading, Massachusetts: Addison-Wesley.

Johnson, L.M., Happel, J.R., Edelman, J. & Brown, S.J. (1983). Nursing Administration Quarterly Forum. *Nursing Administration Quarterly*, 8, 30–46.

*Jongeward, D. (1973). *Everybody Wins: Transactional Analysis Applied to Organizations*. Reading, Massachusetts: Addison-Wesley.

Jongeward, D. & Seyer, P.D. (1978). *Choosing Success: Transactional Analysis on the Job*. New York: John Wiley.

Lawrence, W.G. (1979). *Exploring Individual and Organizational Boundaries*. New York: John Wiley.

Levitt, T. (1988). The innovating organization. *Harvard Business Review*, 88 (1), 7.

Lindquist, J.D. & Blackburn, R.T. (1974). Middlegrove: The locus of campus power. *American Association of University Professors Bulletin*, 60, 367.

*Longest, B.B. (1984). *Management Practices for the Health Professional*. Norwalk, Connecticut: Appleton & Lange.

McClure, M. (1972). *The reasons for hospital staff nurse resignations*. Unpublished doctoral dissertation. New York: Teachers College, Columbia University.

McKelvey, B. & Kilmann, R.H. (1975). Organization design: A participative multivariate approach. *Administrative Science Quarterly*, 20 (1), 24.

*McLaughlin, C.P. (1986). *The Management of Nonprofit Organizations*. New York: John Wiley.

Merton, R. (1969). The social nature of leadership. *American Journal of Nursing*, 69, 12.

Meyer, M.W. (1977). *Theory of Organization Structure*. Indianapolis, Indiana: Bobbs-Merrill.

Mintzberg, H. (1981). Organization design: Fashion or fit? *Harvard Business Review, 59,* 103.

Mintzberg, H. (1983). *Structure in Fives: Designing Effective Organizations.* Englewood Cliffs, New Jersey: Prentice-Hall.

Nichols, B. (1976). Oklahoma crude: Everything's gushing up hospitals. In Kotelchuck, D. (ed) *Prognosis Negative.* New York: Vintage Books.

*Perrow, C. (1969). The analysis of goals in complex organizations. In Etzioni, A. (ed) *Readings on modern organizations.* Englewood Cliffs, New Jersey: Prentice-Hall.

Revans, R.W. (1972). Psychological factors in hospitals and nurse staffing. In Levine, E. (ed) *Research on nurse staffing in hospitals.* Washington, D.C.: U.S. Department of Health, Education, and Welfare.

Rosenhan, D.L. (1973). On being sane in insane places. *Science, 179,* 250.

Stennett-Brewer, L. (1987). Organizational stress diagnosis and hospital employee assistance programs. *Hospital Topics,* 65 (2), 25–31.

Tausky, C. (1978). *Work Organizations: Major Theoretical Perspectives.* Itasca, Illinois: Peacock Press.

*Trent, W.C. (1986). Some unique aspects of health care management. *Hospitals and Health Services Administration, 31,* 122–132.

Weber, M. (1969). Bureaucratic organization. In Etzioni A, (ed) *Readings on Modern Organizations.* Englewood Cliffs, New Jersey: Prentice-Hall.

Wolf, G.A., Lesic, L.K. & Leak, A.G. (1986). Primary nursing: The impact on nursing costs within DRGs. *Journal of Nursing Administration,* 16 (3), 9–11.

Zander, K. (1985). Second generation primary nursing: A new agenda. *Journal of Nursing Administration,* 15 (3), 18–24.

*References marked with an asterisk are recommended for further reading.

Chapter 11

ORGANIZING CARE

Chapter 11

OUTLINE

Organizing the Delivery of Nursing Care
  Case Method
    Advantages
    Disadvantages
  Functional Method
    Advantages
    Disadvantages
  Team Nursing
    Advantages
    Disadvantages
  Primary Nursing
    Advantages
    Disadvantages

Staffing and Scheduling
  Determining Staffing Needs
    Patient Census
    Acuity and Complexity of Care
    Patient Classification Systems
    Staff Mix
    Productive Versus Nonproductive Time
  Issues in Staffing and Scheduling
    Flextime
    Specialization
    Temporary Personnel
    Budget
  Developing a System

Summary

LEARNING OBJECTIVES

Upon completion of this chapter, the reader will be able to:

▷ Compare and contrast the four most common methods of organizing nursing care (case, functional, team, and primary).

▷ Debate the advantages and disadvantages of these four ways of organizing nursing care.

▷ Describe the descriptive, checklist, and time-based systems of patient classification.

▷ Discuss the various factors that affect staffing and scheduling decisions.

ORGANIZING CARE*

In this chapter, we will focus on the various approaches devised to deliver nursing care effectively and efficiently to patient populations. We will consider first the four most common ways to deliver nursing care: case method, functional method, team nursing, and primary nursing. Each has certain advantages and disadvantages in terms of effect on staff members and the quality of care. Most health care organizations make adaptations in whichever approach they use, some quite creatively. These adaptations need to be critically analyzed because some are successful but others may defeat their original purpose.

The second major nursing management concern addressed in this chapter is staffing and scheduling. The variability in patient needs, difficulty in predicting crises, and need to staff inpatient units and even home health services on a 7-day-a-week, 24-hour-a-day basis has made this a subject of much discussion in the nursing literature and among nursing staff as well. Effective staffing and scheduling can facilitate the delivery of a high level of care; poor staffing and scheduling can create management headaches, exhausted staff, and threats to patient safety.

ORGANIZING THE DELIVERY OF NURSING CARE ⸻

There are four common ways to organize the delivery of nursing care: case, functional, team, and primary nursing (Brown, 1980; Rowland & Rowland, 1980). Each can be modified to meet the goals of a particular organization, its staff and its patients.

Case Method

The case method is the assignment of one nurse to the total care of one or more patients or clients. The assigned nurse is responsible for providing all the nursing care that is needed.

The work of the private-duty nurse is one example. Community health agencies use this method to assign cases to individual nurses, and intensive care units often use a modified version of this method for delivering nursing care. It is also used extensively for student assignments.

ADVANTAGES. Although it is the oldest of the four modes, many still consider the case method the ideal way to deliver nursing care. It is simple and direct in comparison with the others, does not require the complex assignment planning that some others do, and has clear lines of responsibility.

*Co-authored by Ruth M. Tappen, R.N., Ed.D. and Phyllis George, R.N., M.A.

Its primary advantage, though, is that the care given is comprehensive, continuous, and usually holistic. The likelihood of the care being fragmented, discontinuous, or full of serious gaps is greatly reduced.

DISADVANTAGES.   With so many advantages, why is the case method not used universally? The major difficulties are related to the number and complexity of health care problems and the settings in which care is given. The case method is less efficient than other methods because it uses highly skilled, higher-paid professionals to do work that can be done by less-skilled, lower-paid people. It cannot be used to assign patients or clients to ancillary staff members. In addition, with the number of specialties that have developed in the health care field, it is very difficult for an individual professional to be knowledgeable in all areas and to provide the most expert care for patients or clients with a wide variety of needs.

There are also some disadvantages that relate specifically to inpatient and intensive home care. Around-the-clock care cannot be done by one person. Inpatient units are organized in such a way that interaction with many different departments is necessary for obtaining such services and supplies as drugs, linens, meals, laboratory tests, and various therapies. Having a large number of different nurses independently interacting with each of these departments leads to confusion. In such complexly organized settings, more coordination seems to be needed.

Functional Method

The functional method is based on a division of labor similar to an assembly line. Individual care givers are assigned to do specific tasks rather than assigned to certain patients or clients.

Assignments are based on efficiency: tasks are given to the lowest-skilled, lowest-paid worker who is available and able to do the work. The usual result on inpatient units is that one nurse is assigned to be in charge of the unit; another nurse administers all medications; a practical nurse takes blood pressures; and an aide takes temperatures, passes out meal trays, and so forth.

In a home health care agency, use of the functional method would mean that a nurse would visit a client to counsel, teach, or carry out complex care techniques, and a home health aide would also visit to assist with bathing and personal care. Nursing care in the home is rarely divided into as many discrete pieces because of the inefficiency of multiple visits.

ADVANTAGES.   The major advantage of the functional method is its efficiency. This method makes it possible to use more unskilled or lesser-skilled people to get the work done. When care givers are given the same assignments on a regular basis, each person becomes quite adept at them and can finish the tasks quickly.

This makes it easy to give clearly defined assignments and to check later to ensure that they were completed. Once the tasks are defined and the assignments are made, there is usually very little overlap or confusion about who is expected to do a particular job. In this way time required for coordination of staff members is minimized. It is interesting to note that even when team or primary nursing is the usual mode for delivering care, organizations frequently fall back on the functional method if a serious shortage of staff occurs.

DISADVANTAGES. The functional method may not be as efficient as it is generally thought to be. From the point of view of getting the work done (efficiency), the need for coordination may be kept to a minimum; but the need for it is increased from the point of view of the recipient of this care (effectiveness). Consider, for example, how inefficient it is to have three different staff members enter a room, one to give a medication, the second to take a blood pressure reading, and a third to check a dressing.

An even more serious drawback of this method of care is the extreme fragmentation of care that results. The functional approach is mechanistic and impersonal, and emphasizes the more technical aspects of nursing care. Both staff and patients are likely to be dissatisfied with the way care is given.

For the staff, the work becomes repetitive and boring. Doing the same disconnected tasks prevents them from experiencing the satisfaction of seeing anything done from beginning to end. For example, if a patient has a quick and uneventful recovery from surgery, no one staff member can take pride in having assured the patient's comfort and prevented postoperative complications. The patient, too, is confused and sometimes irritated by the large number of people going in and out of the patient's room or home, each one doing only one or two things and refusing to do others because it is someone else's job. Potentially more serious is the fact that communication between staff members may be minimal so that no one is aware of everything that is happening to an individual patient. Although the nurse in charge is theoretically responsible for all care given, responsibility is so diffused among various care givers that a serious gap in care can occur without anyone realizing it. Holistic nursing is virtually impossible under the functional mode.

Team Nursing

Team nursing is the delivery of nursing care by a designated team of staff members including both professional nurses and nonprofessional (ancillary) staff. Several elements are considered necessary:

1. The leader of the team should be a registered professional nurse not a practical nurse. The team leader is delegated authority to make assignments for team members.
2. The leader is expected to use a democratic style in interactions with team members.
3. The team is responsible for the total care given to an assigned group of patients or clients.
4. Communication among team members is built in and essential to the success of team nursing. This includes written patient care assignments, nursing care plans, reports to and from the team leader, team conferences, and frequent informal feedback among team members (Kramer, 1971; Kron, 1981; Lambertsen, 1953).

Team nursing was designed at the end of World War II to make the best use of the limited nursing staff available and alleviate the problems created by the functional method. As more workers with minimal on-the-job training were hired in the health care field, it became necessary to reorganize the delivery of care. It was also hoped that the use of team nursing would increase both staff and patient satisfaction and improve the quality of care.

The team leader has a pivotal role and is expected to supervise ancillary staff closely and to provide informal training for them as needed. The leader is also expected to be thoroughly acquainted with the needs of every patient or client assigned to the team, even if not directly involved in their care. In hospitals or nursing homes, the head nurse or nurse manager selects the team leaders and designates the scope of the team's responsibility. The nurse manager is also responsible for overall management of the nursing unit, meeting the more formal education needs of staff, and formal evaluation. In community settings, the supervisor usually fulfills these roles.

ADVANTAGES. Although team nursing was not designed to make up for inadequate staffing, it does make it possible to deliver quality care using a relatively large proportion of ancillary personnel. In comparison with the functional method, it is far more satisfying to both patients and staff when it is done well. The abilities of each staff member are more likely to be recognized and fully used. The increased amount of cooperation and communication among team members can raise morale, improve the functioning of the staff as a whole, and give team members a greater sense of having contributed to the outcomes of the care given. Especially in hospital settings, most nurses working on teams find that they know both their patients and fellow staff members better than when using the functional method.

Although patient care is still divided among several people, it is far less fragmented than in the functional method because of the increased communication and extensive coordination efforts of the team leader. The team nursing approach allows comprehensive, holistic nursing care when the team functions at a high level of maturity.

DISADVANTAGES. One of the greatest disadvantages of team nursing is that it is so often done poorly. It is far more than simply dividing staff into equal groups and then assigning an equal number of patients to each group. Yet this method is often called team nursing even though it usually is much more like the functional method in everything but name.

Team nursing requires a great deal of cooperation and communication from staff. It demands even more of the team leader, who spends much time coordinating and supervising team members and who must be highly skilled both as a leader and as a practitioner. Not every nurse practicing today is prepared for these roles.

Some efficiency is lost because of the demands for increased interaction among staff members. The number of people attending the same patient under the functional method is not substantially reduced in team nursing.

Although the team leader is a professional nurse, a large proportion of the staff is not, and much of the care is given by persons other than nurses. In contrast, both the case method and primary nursing emphasize care given by professional nurses.

Primary Nursing

Primary nursing incorporates the case method's concept of assigning total care and responsibility for one patient into a modality designed for inpatient care but adaptable to ambulatory care. Every patient has a designated primary nurse who is responsible for planning the care and ensuring that the plan is implemented around the clock, seven days a week. When the primary nurse is not at work, the implementation is delegated directly to an associate nurse, but the primary nurse is still accountable and in some institutions may be called on if a serious problem arises (Marram & Barrett, 1979). Primary nurses are accountable for the *outcomes* of the nursing care given, not just for the fact that care is given (Zander, 1985).

When primary nursing is implemented, the inpatient unit is usually divided into districts or modules with a primary nurse assigned to each district. The nurse manager of a patient care unit assigns the direct care of the patients to the primary care nursing staff. The primary nurse does all initial assessments and develops care plans for all assigned patients. The primary nurse may have other staff members to call on for assistance. She or he will organize the work and assign parts of it to other staff members. Aides know that their primary job is providing personal care for patients, assisting the staff nurse with patients with complex care needs, keeping water pitchers filled, answering call lights, and conveying messages to the primary nurse about patients' needs.

Primary nurses may help one another with development and implementation of care plans. She or he also does complex treatments, coordinates the nursing care plan with other disciplines (including the physicians' medical care plan), administers medications, counsels patients and their families, plans for discharge, provides needed education, and evaluates the efficacy of the interventions.

ADVANTAGES.   Primary nursing has many of the advantages of the case method. Nurses have more autonomy than in the functional or team approaches and are challenged to work to their full capacity. They spend less time in coordinating and supervising and more in direct-care activities. The primary nurse is also more accountable because responsibility is focused rather than diffused.

After becoming accustomed to this mode, primary nurses generally believe that they are more effective working under this system. In fact, many studies have shown that both cost and turnover are reduced, although evidence of its impact on the quality of care is still inconclusive (Fairbanks, 1981). Nurses also gain more satisfaction from being involved in the entire care of a patient and being able to give more holistic care.

Patients also seem to appreciate the more personalized and holistic care that can be given in primary nursing. They are especially pleased to be able to say, "This is my nurse." People from other disciplines also appreciate the fact that they can consult with one particular, identifiable nurse who knows all about the patient.

DISADVANTAGES.   As with team nursing, most of the disadvantages of primary nursing come from problems with implementation. Although proponents argue that it is no more costly than other ways to deliver care, its detractors point out that it requires a much higher proportion of professional nurses to ancillary personnel. It has also been noted that, even with primary nursing, the hospitalized person is cared for by at least six nurses (three nurses to cover the three 8-hour shifts in a day and another three associates to substitute for them on their days off).

Primary nursing demands increased independence, accountability, and the ability to make thorough assessments and plan care accordingly. Unfortunately, not every nurse is prepared for this, especially those accustomed to the functional method's routine. Some are threatened by these additional demands; others find that they need additional education before assuming the primary nurse role. This may include experienced nurses (Mutchner, 1986). Ancillary workers often feel a sense of loss when their direct-care activities are reduced or eliminated under primary nursing.

One of the major differences between primary nursing and team nursing is the conceptualization of the way care is given, especially by whom. Team nursing was developed to include ancillary personnel in care-giving roles appropriately and emphasizes the supervising, teaching, and coordinating functions of the nurse. Primary nursing focuses on the nurse as the caregiver and does not clearly define the roles of ancillary personnel. In fact, there is much disagreement over the issue of licensed practical nurses assuming the primary nurse role, and many variations of primary nursing have arisen from attempts to make appropriate use of ancillary personnel in primary nursing.

STAFFING AND SCHEDULING

Determining Staffing Needs

The major factors in determining the staffing and scheduling decisions include patient census, complexity of care, patient classification, staff mix, and accounting for productive versus nonproductive time. The issues that influence these decisions include flextime, specialization, use of temporary personnel, and the influence of the budget.

PATIENT CENSUS. Obviously the number of patients on a unit is a major factor affecting decisions about how to staff. All other factors being equal, a unit of 20 patients requires more staffing than a unit of 12.

The census of any unit can vary from one day to the next and can mean the difference between adequate staff one day and inadequate staff the next. What was adequate staff at the start of the shift can become a severe shortage as the shift progresses:

> Evening shift staff in a hospital are often dismayed when they learn that the census is low at the start of the shift: They know that they could receive multiple emergency admissions that will fill the empty beds and require a great deal of time and attention.

Census numbers alone are not sufficient to determine staffing needs (Vail, Morton, & Rider, 1987). Staffing only by census can leave a unit woefully short of staff. The Joint Commission on Accreditation of Hospitals requires a defined system rather than dependence on patient census for determining staffing needs. Twelve critically ill patients may have more nursing needs than 20 less acutely ill patients. For this reason, attempts have been made to assess the acuity and complexity of patient care needs and to classify patients according to the number of hours of nursing care needed.

ACUITY AND COMPLEXITY OF CARE. One of the questions that must be answered before staff can be appropriately assigned to care for a particular group of patients is, "Exactly what kind of care do they need?" In other words, how many patients have IV lines running? How many need to have medication? How many need assistance with basic tasks like bathing, toileting, feeding themselves, getting in and out of bed? How many have special skin care needs, are confused and disoriented, need to be taught how to care for themselves because of a condition they have not had before (for example, diabetes, hypertension, or a colostomy)? How many will require fresh postoperative care? How many are complex conditions? Answering these questions in an organized way produces an *acuity index*, which enables the nursing unit manager to determine quickly how many staff members are needed, and then how many should be registered nurses, licensed practical nurses, or aides.

In contrast, the DRG prospective payment system, which tells the nurse the number of days for which the hospital will be reimbursed for a particular patient, is based on the medical diagnosis of the patient. It does not take into account what the patient's actual self-care deficits or nursing needs are. It does not consider, for example, what kinds of disabilities the patient has, what will interfere with his learning to care for himself, or what other problems he has that may not be indicated by his DRG allocation but which may affect the number and kinds of nursing needs he will present.

Many hospitals and agencies have experimented with patient classification systems in which the acuity index is assessed for every patient on every shift. Each patient is rated on the basis of a number of factors that affect the amount of nursing care he or she needs, such as:

▷ Feeds self with little or no assistance versus requires total assistance.
▷ Ambulatory versus bedbound.
▷ Receiving oral medication versus intravenous medication.
▷ Requires special wound care or isolation.
▷ Needs teaching of a specific self-care function.
▷ Is confused and disoriented.
▷ Needs vital signs measured every 15 minutes versus every 2 hours or every 4 hours.

The patient can then be assigned to an acuity or complexity category that will indicate how many actual hours of nursing care he will need during a particular shift. When that information is collected for every patient on the unit, the total number of hours of care required will give an indication of the number and type of nursing staff needed on the unit for that shift. However, if the scoring system used becomes too detailed or must be done too often, it can demand too much of the nurse manager's time and divert attention away from other responsibilities (Research Example 11–1).

PATIENT CLASSIFICATION SYSTEMS. There are three major types of patient classification systems: the descriptive, the checklist, and the time-based systems (Lewis & Carini, 1984).

Descriptive Systems. The descriptive type is simply a set of narrative descriptions of the various degrees of acuity or complexity of care required by a particular patient. These degrees range from minimal care, or Category I, to extensive care needs, or Category V. A minimal care or Category I patient could be described as one who is ambulatory, can perform all activities of daily living independently, is receiving only routine medications and

RESEARCH EXAMPLE 11–1. How Often Should Patient Classification Ratings Be Done?

Is it necessary to do patient classification ratings every shift? Kinley and Crone-wett (1987). conducted a study of the ratings of 621 nonrandomly selected patients on the medical-surgical and pediatric units of a 411-bed hospital in New England.

A time-based patient classification system called AIM was used at this hospital. AIM uses a rating scale that results in scores using PCUs worth 6 minutes each. The researchers compared the patient ratings done by each of the three shifts during a 24-hour period with the mean (average) rating for that day. The Pearson r correlations were very high, ranging from 0.95 to 0.99 for the whole sample and 0.91 to 0.99 for individual units. They also found that the evening shift's rating came closest to the mean.

What do the results tell us? The researchers say that it is possible that nurses copied the ratings given by previous shifts but add that some precautions were taken to avoid this possibility on one of the units and that this unit had the same high correlations. They conclude that there is no reason to rate patients' level of care more than once a day, pointing out rather persuasively that it costs a hospital with an average patient census of 350 approximately 9500 hours of nurse time per year to do the ratings three times a day versus only 3200 hours to do it once a day. This results in a gain of 6300 hours that can be used for other purposes. (This figure is based on an estimated 90 seconds per rating plus 10 seconds of unit secretary time to calculate the mean.)

treatments, requires only minimal emotional support, and needs only brief explanations or instructions that are readily understood. At the opposite end is the Category V patient, who requires highly complex and intensive levels of care. This type of patient needs almost constant monitoring, frequent complex medications and treatments (such as Swan-Ganz catheters, ventilators, hyperalimentation, and central venous pressure monitoring), assistance with all activities of daily living, and intensive psychotherapeutic intervention and/or education (Lewis & Carini, 1984).

Although these descriptions can be made quite specific, they force patients into only five categories, demanding a lot of judgment on the part of the nurse doing the rating. Variability between raters can be a problem, with some raters being very optimistic about a patient's level of need and another "padding" the ratings to make the unit's workload look impressively high. On the other hand, the descriptive system has the advantage of being quite simple. It is probably still the most commonly used system in the United States (Halloran & Vermeersch, 1987).

Checklist System. The checklist system produces a score for each patient based on a separate rating of the patient's acuity or complexity of care level in a number of different categories. Common categories reflect many of the same factors that are clustered together in the descriptive system: teaching, monitoring, emotional support, personal care, medications, treatments, and so forth. Typically, within each of these categories the patient is rated on a scale of 1 to 5. The total score from each of these ratings comprises the patient's level of care.

This system reduces some of the subjectivity of the descriptive approach and provides a greater range of ratings for a patient population. The ratings are still somewhat arbitrary because they are not based on any empirical evidence of how much more demand is placed on the nursing staff by, say, a Category IV patient than a Category II patient.

Time-based Systems.   Time-based systems of patient classification have a more solid empirical base but are more complex. Acuity or complexity levels of various patients are determined by the amount of time required to complete a wide range of specific nursing interventions. A time-based unit of measure such as the relative value unit (RVU) or patient care unit (PCU) is then assigned to each nursing intervention or to each patient need (Kinley & Cronenwett, 1987; Thomas & Vaughan, 1986).

> Typically, the RVU has an arbitrarily set value of 6 or 10 minutes. This means that a patient who needs 60 RVUs would need 360 minutes (6 hours) or 600 minutes (10 hours) of care in a day, depending on the given value of the RVU.

Specific interventions also can be classified according to the lowest level of nursing personnel who can perform the task. Dispensing medications, for example, cannot be done by a nursing assistant, but most personal care can. Analysis of the total RVUs in each category of personnel can then be used to determine the staffing mix (i.e., how many nurses, licensed practical nurses, and nursing assistants are needed) for a unit.

The time-based methods of patient classification and staffing need determination may remind the reader of Frederick Taylor's management approach. The system has some of the same advantages and disadvantages of Taylor's (Chapter 2) approach. It is a relatively objective and quantitatively specific method that can be made quite reliable (consistent among different raters), but it is very mechanistic. It divides the patient into very small, discrete categories of need that may reflect neither the whole of the patient's needs nor the degree of coordination and integration that must be done by the nurse with primary responsibility for the patient's care. Most of these classification systems also neglect to take into account the degree to which the effectiveness of support services such as pharmacy, dietary, and social services impinges on the efficiency and effectiveness of nursing services. Further development of these systems and judicious interpretation of their scores may help to overcome these limitations.

A major advantage of the time-based system of patient classification is that it provides a valuable data base for nursing administration. The data allows analysis of the relative staffing needs of various units and a degree of flexibility in responding to changing staffing needs that has been difficult to achieve without this information. A further advantage, one that may be used more and more in the future, is that patients can be billed according to the amount of nursing care that they required during their stay. This allows nursing to be separated from the room and board ("hotel") charges that have obscured the value of nursing care in inpatient settings for so long (Thomas & Vaughan, 1986).

STAFF MIX.   Once the level of needs of the unit's patients is known, another factor is the mix of staff members assigned to care for patients: How many RNs, LPNs, and aides have been assigned to work on that unit? Who is best prepared to take care of the particular needs each patient has?

In some institutions, nonprofessional staff have been eliminated and replaced with a lesser number of professionally prepared staff. The idea behind this is that RNs can provide more complex kinds of care than either an LPN or an aide and so can be assigned to a broader range of functions. In other institutions, the prevailing wisdom has it that professional staff are very expensive and their skills can be used more efficiently if the nonprofessional tasks are done by nonprofessionals. In that case, fewer RNs are available to care for patients and there will be relatively more LPNs and aides. Both approaches have disadvantages. In the case of the all-professional staff, nurses may be spending considerable time doing relatively routine tasks that could be done by nonprofessional staff and therefore have less time for the tasks that require the skills of a nurse. In the opposite situation, there may not be enough professional staff available for the tasks that require a nurse's skill. Either way, the nursing needs of the patient may or may not be adequately addressed.

The use of the acuity index can help in determining the proper staff mix. The unit with a high acuity or complexity index may be able to make the most efficient use of a high proportion of RN staff because those patients have a high number of complex care needs. There should also be some ancillary staff to assist with routine tasks. If, on the other hand, the acuity index indicates that patients have a high proportion of chronic care needs requiring routine kinds of maintenance care, the unit may operate more efficiently with relatively more paraprofessional staff, with RNs needed primarily to plan and manage care, carry out the higher level assessments and complex interventions, and develop appropriate discharge plans.

Finding the right staff mix can influence the lengths of stay for patients on the unit and keep the length of stay within DRG guidelines. It also affects the quality of care patients receive and how quickly they get better.

PRODUCTIVE VERSUS NONPRODUCTIVE TIME. In planning for staffing, consideration must also be given to demands on staff time that are not directly related to patient care. Inservice programs and performance appraisals, for example, are necessary for ensuring quality of care, but they take time away from the direct care of patients. Time is also spent on a number of other tasks and functions that are not direct patient care, including charting, counting narcotics, giving reports, waiting for elevators, getting supplies, and traveling for home visits. Nonproductive nurse time can also be affected by an institution's organization of support services (such as who serves meal trays), even the placement of laundry chutes and nursing stations. Some hospitals make up for this time by paying staff for eight hours of work and then requiring each shift's charge nurse to come in a half hour early to inventory narcotics and receive report. This solution eases the hospital's budget, but it means that the nurses are involuntarily donating their time to cover an inadequate staffing budget. Someone else has to be assigned to a nurse's patients whenever the nurse has a day off, calls in sick, or attends an inservice program. Some types of nonproductive time can be predicted and planned for, while others cannot. For example, if a 20-bed unit can be adequately staffed by eight people (four nurses, two licensed practical nurses, and two nursing assistants), more than eight staff are actually needed to cover for days off, sick days, and so forth.

Issues in Staffing and Scheduling

FLEXTIME. Some health care organizations have experimented with assigning staff on the basis of fluctuating time schedules. This may take the form of 4-day weeks of 10-hour shifts or 3-day weeks of 12-hour shifts. These longer shifts make it possible to have more staff on duty during especially heavy need hours of the day, such as early in the morning or at suppertime. It also allows staff to work shorter weeks and have more consecutive days off, which some people have found helpful in keeping them fresh for the job.

In some home care agencies, the nurse may adjust the hours worked to suit the needs of the patients, making it possible to provide a broader range of services. For example, flexible working hours may make it easier for the nurse to provide early morning or evening teaching to a new diabetic who is learning to give himself insulin, but who also needs to go to work.

The option of flextime may pose organizational and management challenges. If flextime is instituted to expand the service hours of an agency, it will be necessary to provide longer hours of supervision and clerical support. Providing adequate staff to cover all needs that may arise could be more costly and pose difficult logistical problems.

SPECIALIZATION. One way to increase the efficiency of staff assignments is to group patients with the same diagnoses or nursing needs. The nurses assigned to the unit develop experience in caring for patients with a particular problem or having undergone a particular type of procedure. Spinal cord injury units and open-heart surgery teams are examples of this type of specialization. Because the staff is taking care of patients with similar needs so consistently, they are efficient at identifying the common needs those patients are likely to have and at providing for specific interventions in the care plan. This may be seen as a good way to provide cost-efficient quality care. Many aspects of care become routine and can be accomplished in less time than it would take the nurse who is not so accustomed to caring for these particular patients. It may even be possible to discharge the patient in less time if teaching is begun and completed sooner and the patient becomes independent in caring for himself or herself sooner.

Some hospitals are developing a large number of specialty care units (such as alcohol-abuse treatment units and diabetic treatment centers) rather than trying to offer care for every type of patient who might be admitted to the general hospital. In this way, they establish a reputation for providing better care than the general hospital can provide for patients with those special needs.

While the medical profession has been specialized for some time, nursing has begun to develop its own specialities such as critical care, gerontological nursing, trauma care, or maternal and child health. These nurses become experts in providing nursing care for patients with a particular set of needs. There is some debate, however, over the benefits of specialization. The following is an example of a debate in a public health agency:

> The current method of assignment in this agency is generalist, that is, each nurse is responsible for all the nursing care given in the assigned geographical area. The nurse receives all the referrals and makes all initial visits for patients who require nursing care in

conjunction with a medical regimen. In addition, the nurse is responsible for all the health guidance and public health care that is required by individuals or groups in the assigned geographical area, including immunization and well-baby clinics, contact investigations for TB, and consultation on the best location for long-term care for elderly clients.

Recently this agency has been piloting a new method of assignment in two of its field offices. In each office, a team of two nurses has been assigned to provide all public health and health guidance care for the entire geographical area served by the field office. The remaining staff has been given larger geographical areas than previously in which they are responsible for only the care of patients with a diagnosis requiring supportive home care or rehabilitation and teaching.

In some respects, community health nurses have retained a generalist focus long after their hospital or institutional counterparts have specialized in the care of patients with particular needs. They have been expected to be expert in many technical procedures formerly the province of institutional settings only but now frequently occurring in the home, as well as the principles and practice of preventive health care and public health procedures. The specialist assignment is seen as an opportunity for community health nurses to become more expert in one area of nursing in the community, with the expectation that the care given will be of higher quality, the satisfactions greater, and the frustrations less. But many find great reward in the generalist role and worry that they will become bored and stale confining their practice to one arena.

TEMPORARY PERSONNEL. In some situations, such as staff vacancies or periods of unexpectedly high demand for services, additional staff may be hired or assigned temporarily to supplement existing staff. If this does not meet the demand, temporary staff may be hired directly drawn from the organization's own temporary pool, or contracted from a registry or temporary agency. The ability to fill staffing needs on a demand basis will depend on the availability of budgeted funds and of temporary staff in the community. Some nurses are willing to forfeit benefits and advancement opportunities in return for the higher wages and greater time flexibility of temporary staff work. However, many question the quality of care provided by temporary nurses who do not know the patients well, often are not specialists in the particular area to which they are assigned, and have little commitment to the unit or to the organization.

BUDGET. The institution's or agency's budget may determine to a considerable extent, how staffing will be done. Allocations in the budget for overtime, temporary staff, negotiated changes in salary scales, unexpected increases in census, or patient referrals allow greater flexibility to adjust staffing as needed. Failure to allow for such contingencies in the budget may make it impossible to respond adequately to the fluctuations in patient need, leaving patients inadequately cared for and the staff frustrated and worn out.

Developing a System

Every health care organization needs to develop a responsive system for staffing its units, preferably one that is based on a well-developed patient classification system. Although the number of beds on a unit may not change, the acuity and complexity levels will undoubtedly fluctuate from day to day and week to week.

Any hospital staffing system must take into account the 24-hours-a-day,

7 days-a-week nature of the need for staff. Some institutions establish a policy of every third weekend off and mandatory rotation to ensure adequate staffing for the less popular working hours. These policies ignore the needs and preferences of the staff members. Others hire sufficient staff and develop their own pool of temporary staff to maintain the needed flexibility and, at the same time, to keep their staff satisfied.

The organization's mission and goals also affect staffing. A home care agency that does not provide emergency services and uses alternate support systems for their clients on evenings and weekends will not need to plan for as much staff flexibility but still must be prepared to handle a large influx of new referrals. An on-call system may be adequate to meet infrequent needs for extra staff, but it is easily abused and creates personal difficulties for staff members. Maintaining staff on call and paying overtime can also be a very expensive alternative and may push staff to physical and mental extremes of exertion and fatigue. The same can be said for making a habit of asking staff to work double shifts, an inexcusable action in anything but a real emergency. A reordering of staff priorities can also be used to handle minor increases in demand on staff but cannot be continued on a indefinite basis.

Both the organization's management philosophy and budget have a great deal of influence on its staffing policies. Staffing is a complex function that does not yield to easy or consistent formulas, especially those that are borrowed from other organizations. An understanding of the principles discussed in this chapter will help you to take an active part in designing an effective staffing systems for your unit and for your employing organization.

Summary

Case, functional, team, and primary nursing are common ways to organize nursing care. The case method involves total care for one or more patients by one nurse. It does not allow for 24-hour coverage or roles for ancillary personnel. The functional method is an assembly-line division of tasks often selected for its apparent efficiency but resulting in fragmented care. Team nursing focuses on the coordination and supervision of care given by the team, including ancillary staff. Primary nursing returns to the focus on the nurse as care giver with associate nurses covering the other hours of the day. Both team and primary nursing are more difficult to implement than the functional or case methods.

Many factors must be considered in planning the staffing of a nursing unit or health care organization, including the acuity or complexity of patient care, the mix of ancillary and professional staff, the issue of specialization versus generalized practice, and the different ways in which people's schedules can be made more flexible to meet the needs of both the staff and the institution. Other factors include the number of patients on a unit (census), limitations imposed by the budget, allowing for the effect of nonproductive time, and the use of temporary personnel.

Patient classification systems include the descriptive type, which simply categorizes patients according to level of care needed; checklists; and time-based systems that calculate the amount of time needed to carry out specific procedures and express these amounts in standard units. This data base is then used to create a staffing system to suit the individual organization. Staff nurses, clinical specialists, and nurse managers should be involved in the development of the classification schemes and staffing systems.

REFERENCES*

Adams, R. & Johnson, B. (1986). Acuity and staffing under prospective payment. *Journal of Nursing Administration*, *16* (10), 21–25.

Brown, B.J. (1980). *Nurse Staffing: A Practical Guide.* Germantown, Maryland: Aspen Systems.

Eliopoulos, C. (1983). Nursing staffing in long-term care facilities: The case against a high ratio of RNs. *Journal of Nursing Administration*, *13* (10), 29–31.

Fairbanks, J.E. (1981). Primary nursing: More data. *Nursing Administration Quarterly*, *5* (3), 51.

Grohar, M.E. (1986). A comparison of patient acuity and nursing resource use. *Journal of Nursing Administration*, *16* (6), 19–23.

Halloran, E.J. & Vermeersch, P.E. (1987). Variability in nurse staffing research. *Journal of Nursing Administration*, *17* (2), 26–34.

Kinley, J. & Cronenwett, L.R. (1987). Multiple-shift patient classification: Is it necessary? *Journal of Nursing Administration*, *17* (2). 22–25.

*Kramer, M: (1971). Team nursing—A means or an end? *Nursing Outlook*, *19* (10), 648–652.

Kron, T. (1981). *The Management of Patient Care.* Philadelphia: W.B. Saunders.

Lambertsen, E.C. (1953). *Nursing Team: Organization and Functioning.* New York: Teachers College Press.

*Lewis, E.N. & Carini, P.V. (1984). *Nurse Staffing and Patient Classification.* Rockville, Maryland: Aspen Systems.

Marram, G.D., Barrett, M.W. & Bevis, E.O. (1979). *Primary Nursing: A Model for Individual Care.* St. Louis: C.V. Mosby.

*Mutchner, L. (1986). How well are we practicing primary nursing? *Journal of Nursing Administration*, *16* (9), 8–13.

Rowland, H.S. & Rowland, B.L. (1980). *Nursing Administration Handbook.* Germantown, Maryland: Aspen Systems.

*Thomas, S. & Vaughan, R.G. (1986). Costing nursing services using RVUs. *Journal of Nursing Administration*, *16* (12). 10–16.

Vail, J.D. Morton, D.A. & Rieder, K.A. (1987). Workload management system highlights staffing needs. *Nursing and Health Care*, *8*, 289–293.

Vaughan, R.G. (1985). Comparing acuity among hospitals: Who has the sickest patients? *Journal of Nursing Administration*, *15* (5), 25–28.

van Servellen, G.M. & Mac Leod, V. (1985). DRGs and primary nursing: Are they compatible? *Journal of Nursing Administration*, *15* (4), 32–36.

Wolf, G.A., Lesic, L.K. & Leak, A.G. (1986). Primary nursing: The impact on nursing costs within DRGs. *Journal of Nursing Administration*, *16* (3), 9–11.

Zander, K. (1985). Second generation primary nursing: A new agenda. *Journal of Nursing Administration*, *15* (3), 18–24.

*References marked with an asterisk are suggested for further reading.

Chapter 12

TIME MANAGEMENT

Chapter 12

OUTLINE

The Tyranny of Time

Setting Your Own Goals

Organizing Your Work
Lists
Tickler Files
Schedules and Blocks of Time
Time Lines
Filing Systems

Setting Limits
Saying ''No''
Eliminating Unnecessary Work
Keeping Goals Reasonable
Delegating

Streamlining Your Work
Keeping a Time Log
Reducing Interruptions
Recurrent Crises
Categorizing Activities
Finding the Fastest Way
Automating Repetitive Tasks

Enhancing Productivity Through
Leadership

Summary

LEARNING OBJECTIVES

Upon completion of this chapter, the reader will be able to:

▷ Set short and long term personal and career goals.

▷ Analyze activities at work using a time log.

▷ Organize and streamline work to make more effective use of available time.

▷ Set limits on the demands made on one's time.

TIME MANAGEMENT

Busyness seems to be a characteristic of our society today. Even if you have not yet worked in a health care setting as an employee, you may have observed the hectic pace in many of these organizations or experienced overscheduling for yourself in your personal life. Such a sense of being "swamped," controlled, or pressured by time or the lack of time can lead to an increase in errors, omission of important tasks, and generalized feelings of stress and ineffectiveness. For this reason, we will look at ways to manage time in the workplace. The chapter begins with consideration of our cultural time perspectives followed by a discussion of ways to organize, limit, streamline, and enhance productivity to most effectively use your time at work.

THE TYRANNY OF TIME

In our society, calendars, clocks, watches, newspapers, television, and radio all remind us of our position in time, how much of it we have used and how much we have left. How often do you look at your watch in a day? Do you divide your day into blocks of time? Do you have separate activities planned for each hour or even for every few minutes or do you see the minutes, hours, and days as part of the whole of your life? Our perception of time is important because it affects our use of it and our response to it.

Webber (1972, 1980) has collected a number of interesting tests of people's perception of time. You may want to take a few minutes to try some of these:

1. Do you think of time more as a galloping horseman or as a vast, motionless ocean?
2. Which of these words best describes time to you: sharp, active, empty, soothing, tense, cold, deep, clear, young, or sad?
3. Is your watch fast or slow? (You can check it with the radio.)
4. Ask a friend to help you for this test. Go into a quiet room without any work, reading material, radio, food, or other distractions. Have your friend call you in somewhere between 10 and 20 minutes. Try to guess how long you were in that room.

(Interpretation of your answers can be found on page 234.)

Most Western societies have conceptualized time as linear, moving forward like an arrow. Other cultures perceive time as circular, measured in seasons and important events instead of hours, minutes, and seconds. Time is seen as continuous and repetitive: if you have missed an opportunity, it will come around to you again someday. In the Western mode of thinking, however, it is emphasized that once a particular time has passed, it will

233

never be repeated again. If you were sick, for example, and missed a New Year's Eve celebration, there is no way that you can recapture that opportunity. You can celebrate another new year but it will be a new one, a different New Year's Eve.

In some Western countries, people like to brag that their trains are so punctual that a person can set his or her watch by them. Computers can complete operations in a fraction of a second, and we can measure speeds to the nanosecond. Time clocks that record the minute we enter and leave work are commonplace, and few excuses for being late are really considered acceptable. Time sheets and schedules are a part of most health care givers' lives. We are expected to follow precisely set schedules and meet deadlines for virtually everything we do, from distributing medications to getting reports done on time. In community health, nurses are asked to account for their time from entering the office to leaving in the evening, specifying travel time, clinic time, home visits, meetings, recordkeeping, and so on. Many of these agencies then produce vast quantities of computer-generated data that can be analyzed in terms of the proportions of time spent on various activities. It's no wonder, then, that some of us seem obsessed with time.

Individual personality, culture, and environment all interact in influencing our perceptions of time (Matejka & Dunsing, 1988). If you are a highly achievement-oriented person, for example, you are more likely to have already set some career goals for yourself and to have a mental schedule of deadlines for reaching these goals ("become assistant administrator in 8 years"). Each of us also has a different endogenous tempo (Chapple, 1970). Some of us have fast tempos, others have slow ones. We can change our tempos to some extent in response to a variety of contexts (Davis, 1982). A fast-paced environment, for example, will influence most of us to work at a faster pace despite the difficulty or discomfort experienced if our endogenous tempo is much slower.

Now we can turn to interpreting your answers to the questions from Webber. A person who has a circular concept of time would compare it to a vast, still ocean rather than a galloping horseman, characteristic of the linear perception emphasizing speed and motion forward. A fast-tempo, achievement-oriented person would describe time as clear, young, sharp, active, or tense rather than empty, soothing, sad, cold, or deep. These same fast-tempo people are likely to have fast watches and to overestimate the amount of time that they sat in a quiet room (Webber, 1980).

Many health care professionals are linear, fast-tempo, achievement-oriented people. Simply working at a fast pace, however, is not equivalent to accomplishing a great deal. Much energy can be dissipated in hurrying about, stirring things up, but actually accomplishing very little. The rest of this chapter considers ways in which you can use your time and energy to the best effect. We will begin with goal setting, a preliminary step in time management.

SETTING YOUR OWN GOALS _____

How can you get somewhere if you do not know where you want to go? Many time management books and seminars begin with an exploration of short- and long-term personal and career goals. The assumption behind this preliminary step is that most people concerned with the management of their time must make some choices as to which activities to continue and which to postpone or drop altogether. A thoughtful analysis of your personal and career goals provides the *guidelines by which to decide how to spend your time*. It is assumed that the proportion of time that should be spent on any particular activity, whether work or play, is an individual decision, one that is best made on the basis of your own goals.

What do you see yourself doing five years from now? What would be your ideal? Would it be becoming a supervisor? Or would it be recognition as a highly skilled practitioner in your specialty area? Would you prefer to have increased your family time or developed a special talent? Each of these choices would require a very different plan for spending your time over the next five years. Shorter-term goals have the same potential variety: they may be anything from developing a healthier personal lifestyle to getting along better with your boss or asking for a raise.

The correct way to state goals or objectives was discussed in Chapter 7. In this case, the content of the goals is far more important than the style in which they are written. They should genuinely reflect what you want to do and what kind of a person you wish to be rather than what you think you *should* want. Being self-aware and honest with yourself is a prerequisite to setting your own goals.

Lakein (1973) suggests that you draw up a list of your goals. Divide these into three lists: your lifetime goals, what you wish to accomplish in five years, and what you want to accomplish in the next six months (Fig. 12–1). You may want to divide them again into personal and career goals to ensure

My personal and career goals for the next 6 months are:

My personal and career goals for the next 5 years are:

My lifetime goals are:

Figure 12–1. Goal setting. Write as many goals as you can under each heading. Then select the three most important ones under each heading and cross out the others.

Six-Month Goals:

1. _____ 2. _____ 3. _____
Actions _____ _____ _____
_____ _____ _____
_____ _____ _____
_____ _____ _____
_____ _____ _____

Five-Year Goals:

1. _____ 2. _____ 3. _____
Actions _____ _____ _____
_____ _____ _____
_____ _____ _____
_____ _____ _____
_____ _____ _____

Lifetime Goals:

1. _____ 2. _____ 3. _____
Actions _____ _____ _____
_____ _____ _____
_____ _____ _____
_____ _____ _____
_____ _____ _____

Figure 12–2. Actions needed to accomplish your goals. Fill in the top three goals from each category in Figure 12–1. List the separate steps you need to take to meet each of your selected goals, and set tentative, realistic target dates for completion of each action.

some emphasis on both or you may prefer to be more holistic and write just one list as shown. Then, select the three most important goals from each list. Include only those on which you are really willing to spend some time and energy, crossing out all of the others listed.

Next, list the actions needed to achieve each of the nine goals (Fig. 12–2). Finally, try to set some target dates for their completion. Make these target dates realistic estimates to avoid their becoming additional time pressures.

The goals that you have listed now become your guidelines for determining what is a priority when you are allotting your time to various activities. The following sections will offer some suggestions to assist you in finding time to pursue these goals.

ORGANIZING YOUR WORK

Now let's turn to some specific ways to use time more effectively to move toward achievement of those personal and career goals. It seems that some people are naturally more organized than others, but a conscious effort can help anyone avoid time-wasting disorganization. Whether it is just eliminating extra steps or avoiding serious delays in finishing your work, organizing your work can reduce the amount of time spent doing things that are neither productive nor satisfying.

Lists

One of the most useful organizers is the "Things to Do" list. You can prepare this list either at the end of every day or first thing in the morning before you do anything else. Do not include the routine tasks that you do every day because they make the list too long and you will do them without a reminder. If you are a first-line manager, for example, it is not necessary to list the routine tasks of making assignments, giving report, doing rounds, and so forth. Instead, put the unique tasks of the day on the list: preparation for a care-planning conference, telephone calls to families, discussion of a new project with the director of nursing, a stop at the library to research an unfamiliar diagnosis, or preparation of an employee evaluation. These are the postponable tasks that may never be done or will be done poorly in a last-minute rush if you do not plan the time to do them. You may want to prioritize them, starring those that must be done that day. If you find yourself postponing an item for several days, decide whether it should be given priority the next day or dropped from the list as unnecessary.

The list itself should be in a form most convenient for you: on your desk calendar if you spend your day in an office, in your pocket, or on a clipboard if you spend most of your day on a nursing care unit, in a clinic, or in clients' homes. Checking the list several times a day for reminders will quickly become a good habit. Your daily list may become your most important time manager.

Tickler Files

Tickler files are long-term lists in a manner of speaking. The basic principle of a tickler file is that you create a reminder system of approaching deadlines and due dates for yourself. For example, at the beginning of a school semester, you generally find out when exams will be given and the dates assignments are due. Many students find it helpful to enter all of these dates on a semester-long calendar so that they can see in a glance what is due each week and can look ahead to see what is coming in the next few weeks. Putting all these items on one calendar can also show you where tests and assignments cluster around the same time. This situation would require preparation further in advance or a change in the due dates to meet these multiple deadlines. Unlike the daily list, the tickler file may contain some regular assignments (such as an important committee meeting or the monthly summaries written for long-term care patients) that could be forgotten otherwise.

Using a tickler file, you can anticipate coming deadlines and remind yourself when to begin preparation for a particular task. You might, for example, have an important report, the annual unit budget, due on the first of July. Since you know that it takes about six weeks to finish the budget, you can write a note to yourself on your tickler file to begin work in the middle of May, allowing yourself enough time to get it done.

Schedules and Blocks of Time

Without a schedule you are much more likely to drift through a day or jump from one activity to another in a disorganized fashion. Assignment sheets, worksheets, flow sheets, and care plans are all designed to help you plan and schedule your time effectively. The care plan is the general design for care of each individual patient or family. Assignment sheets indicate the patients or clients for whom each staff member is responsible. Worksheets are then created to organize the daily care that must be given to the assigned patients or clients. Flow sheets are lists of items that must be recorded for each patient.

Effective worksheets and flow sheets schedule and organize your work day. They provide reminders about various tasks and when they have to be done. The danger in them, however, is that the more they divide the day into discrete segments, the more they also fragment your work and discourage a holistic approach. If the worksheet becomes the focus of your attention, your attention can be directed away from the whole picture.

Some activities must be done at a certain time. These will structure your day or week to a great extent, and their timing may well be out of your control. However, in every job there also are tasks that can be done whenever you want to do them, so long as they are done on time. There will also be some unstructured time that you can schedule to suit you.

There are several points to consider in scheduling this discretionary time at work. First of all, certain tasks have earlier deadlines than others and these deadlines must be considered in your scheduling. Second, priorities in patient care, your own personal priorities, and your employer's priorities must be considered in deciding what to do first and how much time to spend on a particular task. Third, some activities are best done all at once. For these activities, you need to set aside *blocks* of time during which you can concentrate on the task. It is difficult, for example, to write an evaluation by doing it five or ten minutes at a time. By the time you reorient yourself to the task, the five or ten minutes is over and nothing is accomplished. Doing such tasks all at one time or in several substantial blocks of time is a much more efficient use of your time. Finally, consider your own energy levels when scheduling your activities. A task that requires intense concentration should not be done at 4 PM if that is a time when your energy flags. As much as it is possible, you should work *with* your energy levels, not against them.

Some people go to work early just to have a block of uninterrupted time in which to do a complicated task. Others take work home with them for the same reason. The drawback in doing this, however, is that you are extending your working hours at the expense of rest and leisure time. You may also be wasting time during your scheduled work hours, time in which you could have gotten the task done if you rescheduled other activities, reduced interruptions and avoided putting off difficult or unpleasant work.

Time Lines

Although they are primarily a technique used in the planning process, time lines are also useful in time management. Time lines are usually project-oriented, illustrating graphically the activities and deadlines that must be met to complete a project as planned. If your work is primarily project-oriented, a set of these time lines (one for each project) would be a helpful time organizer (see Table 8–3 and Fig. 8–2 in Chapter 8 for an example). If your work is not project-oriented, however, it probably would be more useful to develop a single time line for the 6-month, 5-year, and lifetime goals that you have set for yourself, including the major activities needed to achieve those goals.

Filing Systems

Filing systems are particularly important to people with a great deal of paperwork, especially those at the coordinator or manager levels. However, every professional maintains some types of papers such as licenses, certificates, continuing education activities, and current information for their specialty area. Keeping these papers organized in easily retrievable files rather than in disorganized stacks saves a great deal of time whenever you have to find a particular piece of paper or information. Do not let unsorted papers accumulate. Instead, put them into files (manila folders, for example) immediately so that you can find them when you need them again.

SETTING LIMITS

Saying "No"

To set limits, it is necessary to know what your priorities are and to stick with them, saying "no" to nonpriority demands on your time. For many people, it is very difficult to say "no" and to stand firm. This assertiveness and determination is an important component of time management.

Is it possible to say "no" to your boss? It may not seem so at first, but actually many requests from your manager or supervisor are negotiable. You may, for example, be asked to represent your nursing care division on a hospital safety committee. The invitation is flattering in that it is an indication that your supervisor has recognized your ability. If you have ambitions toward entering management in this organization, then this opportunity will probably help you move toward your goal. If, on the other hand, your ambitions are focused on becoming a clinical specialist, membership on the committee would not further your goals and you can, politely and somewhat regretfully, thank your supervisor and decline the invitation.

Can you refuse a burdensome patient assignment? Not in such a direct manner, but you can confront your supervisor effectively regarding the problem. This is particularly true if you have been given more work than others on your team. You can also confront the issue of understaffing or poor scheduling.

There are psychological needs that can interfere with effective limit setting. For some people, ambition keeps them from saying "no" to any opportunity, no matter how overloaded they are. We call these people "workaholics" but may fail to see the symptoms in ourselves. Other people fear displeasing others, especially their supervisors. They are afraid to question an assignment or to negotiate for a more reasonable workload such as accepting a new task only when relieved of an old one. Still others have such a great need to be rescuers that they continually give of themselves, not only to clients but to their coworkers and supervisors without replenishing themselves, until they are exhausted.

People who accept too much work not only hurt themselves but can be a problem to others. Out of sheer sensory overload or fatigue, their work will be inefficient and is much more likely to be careless and sloppy, an unacceptable situation in a health care setting. It is the responsibility of the team leader or nurse manager to avoid overloading these staff members despite the temptation to do so.

Eliminating Unnecessary Work

Some work has become so deeply embedded that it appears to be required, although it really is unnecessary. Some nursing routines fall into this category. Vital signs, baths, linen changes, dressing changes, irrigations, and similar basic tasks are more often done according to a schedule rather than need, which may be much more or much less than the routine.

Many meetings fall into this category (Bech, 1988). If you are the leader of the group, then it is fairly easy to cancel unnecessary meetings, but if you are a member of the group, it may require a combination of diplomacy and persuasiveness to eliminate such a time waster. Some gatherings meet needs other than task accomplishment—they provide a time to vent feelings, work on relationships, or just get away from the pressures of the job for a short time. These needs are important, so it is a good idea to analyze the value of a group meeting before dismissing it as worthless.

Much paperwork is also duplicative or unnecessary altogether. You may find, for example, that certain nursing interventions must be charted in two or three different places on the patient record. Most of the time duplications can be eliminated. Each setting will have its own rituals and duplications, well-established but unnecessary routines. It requires a critical eye to spot these and a persistent questioning of their purpose to eliminate them.

Social chatter in the hallways, nurses' lounge, cafeterias, and refreshment areas takes up a lot of time during the day. Some of this seemingly useless talk really has a purpose. If you recall the leadership theories that emphasize both the task and relationship aspects of work, you will recognize this purpose. You might compare it to the need for the oil that greases a machine so that it runs smoothly. Some of this talk, then, serves a very useful purpose and meets important human needs. However, you must use your judgment as to how much is good for working relationships and when it begins to reduce productivity. In time of crisis or heightened tensions, more attention to relationships will be needed; at other times, you can cut it shorter and return to the task, leading others to do the same by saying, "Let's get back to work."

You may also have created additional work for yourself without realizing it. Do you rewrite assignment sheets every day when they could be duplicated and have recent changes written in? Do you write long answers to memos when a brief note could be written right on the memo that was sent to you? Do you do work that you could delegate to other people? Do you drive to client's home or walk down the hall to a patient's room when you could use the telephone or intercom system? Are you ritualistic in your care, doing procedures as you originally learned them, or do you modify them according to the principles behind them to eliminate unnecessary steps? Is your staff still collecting vital signs at preset intervals instead of making informed judgments regarding individual patients' needs for monitoring? Or are they giving medications to rehabilitation patients who should be learning how to do it themselves before they go home? These are just a few examples of the kind of work that takes a great deal of time but may not need to be done at all (Huey, 1986).

Keeping Goals Reasonable

Do you plan to do more than it is reasonable to expect of one person? Many people's time management problems stem from their failure to keep their goals reasonable. Only the rare superhuman individual can accept every challenge and excell in every endeavor. For the rest of us, we need to limit our goals to those that are likely to be attainable and then to be satisfied with what we are able to do.

Delegating

As you move up the organizational ladder, it will become more and more necessary for you to delegate work to other people, a major responsibility of most managers. But even at the staff-nurse level, there are many opportunities to delegate work to the unit secretary, auxiliary nursing personnel, housekeeping, dietary, and other support departments, and to gain some time for yourself. In many jobs, you cannot do all of the work yourself. Yet a good many people try to do this with the result that they are severely overloaded. Why do they do it? Out of perfectionism, insecurity, a desire for power and control, lack of leadership ability, or, sometimes, enjoyment of the tasks that could be delegated. Occasionally, the perfectionistic demands of their supervisors make it difficult to delegate (Dorney, 1988; Haynes, 1985) even when they want to.

There are several important points to consider in delegating work to others to save time:

1. ***Delegate Work but Do Not Dump It.*** Delegation is assigning work with the assurance of the necessary training, supervision, and authority to get it done; dumping is just getting rid of work in any way possible. Also, it would quickly become obvious if you attempt to get rid of all the unpleasant or boring tasks and keep all of the interesting, challenging work for yourself.
2. ***Select the Appropriate Level of Delegation.*** The amount of supervision and control you maintain should be appropriate to the task and to the skills of the staff member. Delegation can range from telling the staff member exactly what needs to be done and how to do it and following the work closely (level 1) to allowing some freedom to decide how to do it (level 2) to telling the staff members what has to be done and letting them decide how to best get it done (level 3) (Haynes, 1985). For example:

> If you delegate the task of ambulating an orthopedic patient to a new nurse aide, you have to give explicit directions and observe how well they are carried out (level 1). If the aide is

more experienced, you only have to remind the aide of particularly important points such as limitations on weight bearing or prevention of falls (level 2). With a well-trained rehabilitation aide, however, you may just give the assignment and confirm that the aide is familiar with the patient's needs (level 3).

3. *Maintain Control and Responsibility.* Even when you have delegated work, you are still ultimately responsible for the outcome. It is important to communicate your expectations clearly about quality of care and to ensure that performance standards are met.

STREAMLINING YOUR WORK

Many tasks can be neither eliminated nor delegated but can be done more efficiently. There are many axioms that reflect the principle of streamlining your work. "Work smarter, not harder," is a favorite that should appeal to nurses facing increasing demands on their time. "Never handle a piece of paper more than once," is a more specific one that reflects the need to avoid disorganization and procrastination. "A stitch in time saves nine," reflects the degree to which preventive action saves time in the long run. "Time is money," reflects the organization's interest in streamlining work.

How can you streamline your work? A few general suggestions follow, but the first one, a time log, can assist you in developing more specific ones for your particular job. If you do it correctly, a few surprises about how you really spend your time are almost guaranteed.

Keeping a Time Log

Our perception of time is elastic. People do not accurately estimate the time they spend on any particular task, so we cannot rely on our memories for accurate information about how we have been spending our time. The time log is an objective source of information. Most people spend a much smaller percentage of their time on productive activities than they would estimate. Once you see how large amounts of your time are spent, you will be able to eliminate or reduce the time spent on nonproductive or minimally productive activities (Drucker 1967; Robichaud, 1986).

Figure 12–3 illustrates a general format for a time log in which you enter your activities every half hour. This means that you will have to pay careful attention to what you are doing so that you can record it accurately every half hour. Do not postpone the recording—your memory of time is too elastic. A three-day sample may be enough for you to see a pattern emerging. It is suggested that you repeat the process in six months, both because work situations change and to see if you have made any long lasting changes in your use of time.

Reducing Interruptions

Everyone experiences interruptions. Some are welcome, others are necessary, but too many interfere with work and must be kept to a minimum. Closing the door to your office or to a patient room may reduce interrup-

Daily Time Log

Activities	Comments
6:30	
7:00	
7:30	
8:00	
8:30	
9:00	
9:30	
10:00	
10:30	
11:00	
11:30	
Noon	
12:30	
1:00	
1:30	
2:00	
2:30	
3:00	
3:30	
4:00	
4:30	
5:00	

Figure 12–3. Time log. Record your activities every half hour as accurately as possible, including time spent thinking, planning, stalling, daydreaming, worrying, talking, socializing, delegating, negotiating, networking, and so forth. Continue the log until a pattern emerges. Repeat after 6 months.

tions. You may have to ask visitors to wait a few minutes before you can answer their questions, but you must remain sensitive to their need and return to them as soon as possible. You can also ask the unit secretary to hold nonemergency telephone messages for you or to answer your beeper calls temporarily in order to have uninterrupted time in which to complete your care giving. Referring nonemergency calls to another staff member during those blocks of time you set aside to get your work done is also helpful. Unavoidable interruptions may be kept short by thanking the person for the information and saying you must get back to what you were doing. Research Example 12–1, "Interruptions in Nurse Managers' Schedules," compares the interruptions faced by lower- and higher-level nurse managers in a hospital setting and shows how difficult it is for first-line nurse managers to control interruptions.

Recurrent Crises

Recurrent crises are actually large-scale interruptions that show a pattern of recurrence (Drucker, 1967). Whether the recurrence comes daily,

---

RESEARCH EXAMPLE 12–1. Interruptions in Nursing Managers' Schedules

Do lower-level managers experience more interruptions than higher-level administrators? A group of 41 nurse managers ranging from head nurses to assistant directors was asked to break and discard a toothpick every time they were interrupted during a scheduled activity or appointment over the course of 2 days (Grantham, McKay, & Allison, 1985). Their job satisfaction and stress levels were also measured using questionnaires.

The results showed that the higher-level managers scheduled more of their time in advance, although they did not work longer days than the others. They also experienced less interruptions than the lower-level managers.

Situational stress affected job satisfaction (the origin of the stress was not identified), accounting for 27 percent of its variance. The head-nurse group experienced the highest number of interruptions in their planned time (which is already more limited), and these interruptions were related to their stress levels and job satisfaction.

The researchers recommend that more thought be given to ways in which head nurses can protect their planned time from interruptions. They suggested that head nurses be allotted adequate space that would allow them needed privacy in keeping with their position and responsibilities.

---

weekly, or annually, it is probably preventable (or at least manageable) with some planning. A crisis should be something that cannot be foreseen — if you can predict it, you should be able to prepare for it and reduce it to noncrisis proportions at least. The crisis may be a predictable staff shortage on holidays, an annual budget frenzy, or patient complaints of indigestion whenever a particular lunch menu is served. In each case, the problem can be avoided or ameliorated by preventive action.

Categorizing Activities

Clustering similar activities helps eliminate the feeling of jumping from one unrelated task to another. It also makes your managerial work and your care giving more holistic. You may, for example, find that charting takes less time if you do it immediately after seeing a patient — the information is fresh in your mind and you do not have to rely on notes or recall. Try to follow a task through to completion before beginning another whenever possible.

Finding the Fastest Way

A critical analysis of your group's work may reveal many ways to increase efficiency. Perhaps you can computerize some operations or limit the number of people who must handle an item such as a lab specimen or supply requisition. Ask your team members how their time is being wasted. Together, you can analyze your tasks and experiment with various methods to find the most efficient one.

Automating Repetitive Tasks

This method is similar to finding the fastest method, but it focuses on specific tasks that are repeated again and again. These are not necessarily simple tasks but ones that can be automated in some way. For example, a series of classes for families with infants requiring apnea monitors may contain enough standard material that this content can be filmed, video-taped, or printed and repeated automatically each time it is needed by a family. The nurse would then discuss the content, family concerns, and individual adaptations with each family. The nurse's time could be reduced by half without reducing the effectiveness of the teaching.

ENHANCING PRODUCTIVITY THROUGH LEADERSHIP

A careful analysis of your goals, priorities, personal work habits, and the characteristics of your job has been emphasized in this chapter on time management. Effective time management also requires analysis of the characteristics of the work and individual work habits of your team members and intervention where a nonproductive use of time is found. This strategy requires a great deal of leadership on your part, first, in initiating the analysis; second, in involving team members and gaining their interested cooperation; and third, in guiding the work to its conclusion and successful implementation.

Sometimes major blocks to effective use of time come from higher up in the organizational hierarchy rather than from your level or below. Your supervisor may not delegate responsibility effectively or may not allow you sufficient authority to implement more efficient work methods. This situation requires confrontation on your part and negotiation of the problem with the supervisor.

As you recall, one component of effective leadership is self-awareness. Keeping this in mind, you should also look for any personal blocks to effective time management such as fear of failure, fear of success, or personal crises that drain your energy and interfere with your effectiveness. You may have unconsciously developed time-consuming rituals or work habits that unnecessarily fill your work day. An analysis of each task or project to find the shortest route to its completion is usually worth the effort.

Most general of all is the suggestion to apply the most effective leadership possible. Your leadership will make the work flow more smoothly for all around you, enhancing productivity through the elimination of time-wasting frustrations and frictions that divert energy and reduce satisfaction when leadership is absent.

A set of questions posed by Drucker in 1967 are still worth keeping in mind as you try to manage your time more effectively:

▷ What would happen if this was not done at all?
▷ Which tasks could be done by someone else?
▷ What do you do that wastes your time and other people's time?

SUMMARY

Time can be a tyrant if we do not learn how to manage it effectively. Time management is accomplished through identifying and concentrating on your most important goals, and making them your priorities for time allotment. More specifically, time management is accomplished by organizing your work through lists, tickler files, time lines, and scheduling; by setting limits on the number of requests, interruptions, and assignments you will accept; by delegating work appropriately to others; and by streamlining your work after you have kept a time log to see where most of your time is spent. Effective leadership in general also leads to increased productivity.

REFERENCES*

*Barkas, J.L. (1984). *Creative time management.* Englewood Cliffs, New Jersey: Prentice-Hall.

Bech, A.C. (1988). A manager's time shock. *Management World,* 17 (2), 7–8.

Chapple, E.D. (1970). *Culture and Biological Man: Explorations in Behavioral Anthropology.* New York: Holt, Rinehart and Winston. (Reprinted as *The Biological Foundations of Individuality and Culture.* Huntington, New York: Robert Krieger, 1979.)

Davis, M. (1982). *Interaction Rhythms: Periodicity in Communicative Behavior.* New York: Human Sciences Press.

*Dorney, R.C. (1988). Making time to manage. *Harvard Business Review,* 88 (1), 38–40.

Drucker, P.F. (1967). *The Effective Executive.* New York: Harper and Row.

Grantham, M.A., McKay, R.C., & Allison, C.M. (1985). Job satisfaction and interruptions in planned time of nursing managers. *Journal of Nursing Administration,* 15 (5), 7,10.

*Haynes, M.E. (1985). *Practical Time Management.* Tulsa: PennWell Books.

*Huey, F.L. (1986). Working smart. *American Journal of Nursing,* 86, 679–684.

Kluckhohn, F.R. (1976). Dominant and variant value orientations. In Brink, P.J. *Transcultural Nursing: A Book of Readings.* Englewood Cliffs, New Jersey: Prentice-Hall.

Lakein, A. (1973). *How to Get Control of Your Life and Time.* New York: New American Library.

Matejka, J.K. & Dunsing, R.J. (1988). Time management: Changing some traditions. *Management World,* 17(2), 6–7.

Robichaud, A.M. (1986). Time documentation of clinical nurse specialist activities. *Journal of Nursing Administration,* 16 (1), 31–36.

Webber, R.A. (1972). *Time and Management.* New York: Moffat Publishers (reprinted in 1982).

*Webber, R.A. (1980). *Time Is Money: The Key to Managerial Success.* New York: The Free Press.

*References marked with an asterisk are recommended for further reading.

Chapter 13

COMPUTER APPLICATIONS

Chapter 13

OUTLINE

Computer Hardware and Software
Equipment
Programs

Applications to Nursing Practice and Management
Clerical and Secretarial Support
Patient Records
Patient Assessment and Monitoring
Education and Information Resource
Administration
Billing
Budgeting
Planning
Evaluating
Scheduling
Research

Selection of Equipment and Programs
Purpose of the System
Expectations
Comprehensive Plan
Compatibility and Coordination
Use of Consultants
Training of Personnel
Adequacy of the System
Finding the Right Program

Issues in Computer Usage
Depersonalization
Privacy and Security
Overdependence
Cost Versus Benefit

Summary

LEARNING OBJECTIVES

Upon completion of this chapter, the reader will be able to:

▷ Define the most basic computer terms.

▷ Describe the various ways in which the computer can be used in nursing practice, management, and research.

▷ Participate intelligently in the selection of a computer system to be used by nursing service.

▷ Discuss the issues of depersonalization, rights to privacy, overdependence, and cost versus benefit in computer use in health care organizations.

━━━ *COMPUTER APPLICATIONS*

U se of the computer is a relatively recent addition to management techniques. The computer can organize, analyze, and store various kinds of information in a fast, accurate, and easily retrievable manner, if used properly. The uses, or *applications*, of a computer in nursing management are quite varied and rapidly increasing. Following a brief introduction to basic terms and types of computers, their use in clerical and secretarial chores, patient assessment and monitoring, record keeping, education, administration and research, and some of the issues surrounding its use in these various areas will be described.

The purpose of this chapter is to help you become acquainted with computer applications so that you can appreciate the broad range of computer applications and use this knowledge to work intelligently with computer experts in planning the computer needs of your nursing unit or facility.

COMPUTER HARDWARE AND SOFTWARE ━━━━━━━

Equipment

Although intermediate sizes do exist and are becoming increasingly popular, it is easiest at first to think of computer hardware (the equipment or machines themselves) as coming in two major types: the large *mainframe computer*, which can fill an entire room, and the small *personal computer*, a self-contained unit that fits on the top of a desk (Fig. 13–1).

The mainframe computer usually serves a large number of people in many different departments. Communication is done through terminals within the departments using the computer. The terminals usually resemble a television-type of screen (*monitor*) and a typewriter-like keyboard.

People in different departments communicate with the same mainframe computer at the same time. Usually the computer is so fast in accepting and responding to communications that you do not even notice that it is working with several different terminals at the same time. However, no matter how large and fast computers are, each one has its ultimate limits. If the computer is overloaded, you will notice that its response is very slow or even that you cannot get *on line* (i.e., initiate communication with the computer) at all until other people's work is done. It is also possible to be connected with a mainframe computer in a different building, even a different city, through the use of special telephone lines or other equipment. A *modem* is a device that allows you to connect your terminal or computer to a remote computer via telephone lines.

The smaller personal computer can either be completely self-contained or connected to larger computers. The components typically include the

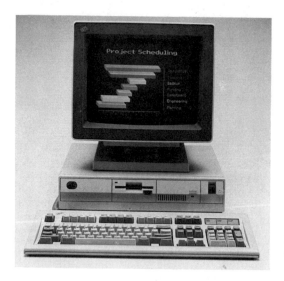

Figure 13-1. An IBM Personal System/2 Model 30 computer. (Courtesy of IBM Corporation.)

computer itself, a keyboard, screen, and a printer. These instruments come in a variety of styles, sizes and, most important, capacity to do work for you. Communication with the personal computer is most often done through typing on the keyboard but may also be done by using a light pen that "writes" directly on the screen or through voice commands. The computer responds with messages on the screen or types out information on paper through the printer (*hard copy*). Any work that is on the screen can be saved in the computer's permanent memory, which stores information for later use. If the work is not saved, however, it can be lost when you leave (*exit*) the program or turn off the computer.

Although computers can store a great deal of information (especially the large ones) over time, the long-term memory can eventually be filled so that no more can be put in and retained at which point other storage space is required. To acquire more space, information is stored on hard disks; removable, exchangeable diskettes (which look somewhat like 45-rpm records); or on larger tapes. These disks or tapes can be read by the computer and their information temporarily stored in the computer while it is being updated or analyzed. When you are done with this information, it is put back on the disk or tape in its new form, removed from the computer, and stored separately until it is needed again. It is up to you, the user, to decide which information will be used occasionally and should be stored on tapes or disks and which will be used constantly and must be available in the computer's active files for immediate retrieval.

Programs

The computer is a machine that uses a very simple language quite different from our complex written and spoken languages. Communication between the computer and its user is done through intermediaries or translators called *programs* (*software* in contrast to the equipment or hardware).

It is through these programs that we communicate with the computer, telling it what we want done and receiving the results. These programs can be very high level and seem to speak to us in our own language. Some, for example, have been designed to simulate a therapist's mode of communication, and actual therapy sessions have been conducted between an individual and a computer using them.

In other cases, however, the program uses a much more simplified language, and it is necessary to learn the meaning of the basic terms before being able to communicate with the computer. The term *DIR*, for example, may be used in one program to ask the computer to list all of the patient records already put into the computer while the word *LIST* or *FILES* or *RECORDS* may be used in other programs for the same thing. The computer cannot *interpret* your commands and will appear quite stupid or even inoperable if your message has any misspellings or extraneous letters or numbers in it. Typing *DIRR*, for example, could be easily interpreted by another person as meaning that you want a list of the records. However, the computer will not understand it unless it has been specifically programmed to accept this alteration.

Computer programs also guide your work with the computer. They can, for example, prompt you in completing a patient assessment record by listing the various categories (cognition, nutrition, elimination) in which you should be entering information on a care plan or by listing a number of possible observations or diagnoses to consider within each of these categories. Other programs can be used to check for spelling errors and can suggest alternate words if they contain a thesaurus, in which you search for a word with similar meaning much as you would in a dictionary. Some programs even can help you write new programs.

Many programs also have "Help" messages that you can use to call for assistance if you are having difficulty with the program. In many instances, however, the information in accompanying manuals is far more complete than the information that appears on the screen. You can easily be too lost, especially at first, to know what Help message to request. You may find it is more useful to ask another person familiar with the program to assist you. As you can see, the selection of the right program is important because it can either limit or expand your ability to use your computer.

APPLICATIONS TO NURSING PRACTICE AND MANAGEMENT

Clerical and Secretarial Support

The computer can keep track of many details for you. It can, for instance, provide you with a list of people scheduled for surgery when you come in to work in the morning or tell you what families are scheduled to be visited that day. It can tell you when supplies are running low and need to be reordered or list the new referrals or transfers received since you last checked the list. All of these functions, of course, require that the information be communicated to the computer and that the computer be programmed to sort and categorize the information. Either it must be connected to the source of the data (for example, via telephone lines to other hospitals who frequently refer patients) or someone must enter the information correctly.

Computers can also function as word processors, organizing and printing labels, letters, forms, and reports. Once typed into the computer, these letters or forms can be combined, altered, modified, or typed repeatedly with variations as needed. You could, for example, have last year's budget retrieved and last year's figures replaced with this year's figures without typing a whole new form. Or, you can compose one letter to all of your clients explaining a change in Medicare reimbursement and have a letter typed for each one with his or her own name and address on it instead of the impersonal "to whom it may concern" format.

Even with these relatively simple tasks, the computer can be very helpful in saving time, keeping track of details and producing professional-looking documents. If you use it with some imagination and creativity, you can do far more than is suggested here.

Patient Records

Given a sufficient number of accessible terminals (some are portable and can be carried into a patient's room) and adequate programming, most record keeping can be computerized. Although the degree to which patient or client charting is standardized varies from one institution to another, most have uniform procedures by which information about patients is recorded and stored for later reference. A similar procedure can be stored as a program in the computer's memory and used as an outline for entering information about a specific client.

The computerized recording system may be very simple, merely listing categories under which information is classified, or it may be comprehensive and very detailed. The latter would include an entire nursing assessment form providing options under each item (for example, the degree to which the patient can manage the activities of daily living on his own), followed by a set of nursing diagnoses from which to select the appropriate ones, and then modifiable goals and plans for care, including recommended interventions and descriptions of possible outcomes. Once the care plan has been entered for each patient or client, the computer can also be programmed to produce daily work lists (Hudgings, 1987). As you can see, the design of such a system could become very complex and time consuming, but there are existing programs that can be used as models or adapted to the needs of your organization.

The advantages of computerizing patient or client information should be weighed against the cost of the equipment and program development as well as the cost of staff training. One advantage of the computer system is that it becomes an electronic reminder to staff of what information should be recorded and where gaps in information exist. If properly formatted, the information should be retrievable for chart audits and other measures of quality control.

In addition, the patient record contains much valuable information that, if we could tap into it more easily, would provide data for nursing research. It can also provide information to the nurse manager on changes in levels of care needed by various groups of patients served by the facility. These data can be of great value in determining staff levels, in supporting the need for additional staff, and in meeting the information demands of various regulatory agencies. A computerized system also lends itself to multidisciplinary use, merging data from the many health-related disciplines and services within one comprehensive record.

Patient Assessment and Monitoring

An entire health history can be collected from a capable, literate client on a computer terminal using an interactive program. The computer can only ask or answer questions for which it has been programmed, however, so that any unusual circumstances or responses must be referred to the nurse in much the same way that the computer in the lab refers unidentifiable blood cells to the technician. The advantages are that the client is given as much time as he or she needs to think about the answers to the questions and that none of the questions is forgotten or skipped by a person in a hurry. On the other hand, this method permits no human interaction, no opportunity to observe the client's response to the interview, and no mechanism for answering the client's questions until the computerized interview is followed up by the caregiver.

It should be evident by now that the computer can do only what it has been told to do and can respond only to information that is received. It cannot seek information for itself or make decisions unless parameters are set ahead of time by its human programmers. When these parameters can be clearly and precisely defined, the computer can be a constantly alert and accurate monitor of patient condition. It can, for example, alert staff to potential drug interactions or set off alarms when vital signs change too quickly or drastically (Johnson & Ranzenberger, 1981; Saba & McCormick, 1986). It can warn the unit manager when assigned tasks have not been completed or recorded on time. It can alert staff to laboratory results that are not within normal limits. It can alert the health department when the number of reported cases of a particular illness or a hospital's reported mortality is greater than anticipated, serving as an early warning device signalling the need for preventive action to protect the public's health.

Education and Information Resource

The computer's ability to store and recall large amounts of information quickly makes it potentially useful in both patient and staff education. It is possible, for example, to store all policies and procedures within the computer so that you can call them up as needed. The particular procedure can then appear on the screen for you to read or printed on a tear-off sheet that you can take with you to a patient's home or bedside. The same can be done with standardized care plans.

Computer-assisted instruction has become quite common. It is possible to purchase programs that allow the learner to respond to simulated or taped clinical situations, to practice drug calculations, or to review material for a test or even to take a test. The computer's infinite patience and capacity to respond quickly are of particular value to people who want to work at their own pace, whether faster or slower than others. It can also be made available at any time of day or evening, and advantage to staff on the evening or night shifts. On the other hand, the computer cannot answer questions unless it has been programmed to do so. It also cannot discuss the ramifications of a particularly important or interesting point or share its own experience with the learner, limitations to keep in mind when considering its use for patients, families, or staff.

You can exercise a great deal of creativity in developing computerized educational programs. Imagine having a daily health tip as the introductory message when the computer terminal is turned on anywhere in your facility, or providing staff with the schedule of inservice programs for the week on their unit's computer terminals. You could also count the number of times that someone calls up the schedule if you want to evaluate its use and use the computer to accept and keep track of registrations (Buisson, 1985).

Many of the same principles are true of computerized patient education. Even if having terminals available to patients is not feasible, must patient education material can be stored on the computer to be called up and printed out when needed. Such information could be updated and individualized as necessary. This is an important consideration to keep in mind when planning for educational uses of the computer.

Administration

A computerized system usually is first considered for an administrative purpose in an organization, especially for bookkeeping and billing. The system is later expanded into other areas such as budgeting, planning, scheduling, and evaluation.

BILLING. Computerization has become an integral part of charging for services in all but the very smallest health care organizations. The type and duration of service for each individual or family is entered, the charges automatically calculated, and a bill printed out. Client names, addresses, telephone numbers, and so forth are all standard information stored within a billing program. Sliding scale fees can be entered and used to determine charges. The totals from this part of the system then become the basis for calculating the revenues or income produced by a particular department and by the organization as a whole.

BUDGETING. Another program would be used to compute the costs (salaries, supplies, building maintenance) of running the organization. Both sets of data are then used in evaluating the financial health of the organization and in planning future budgets.

Budget revision is also facilitated by computerization. If you have ever produced a budget by hand, you know that changing just one figure means that many other figures must be changed. This frequently leads to errors in calculation that can be prevented by automatic recalculation done within a computer program called an *electronic spreadsheet*. The program cannot make your budgeting decisions for you, but it can assist you in evaluating alternatives and in keeping individual figures and totals accurate as you try out various budgetary allocations (Finkler, 1985). It can also format the completed budget for presentation.

PLANNING. Budgeting can be thought of as just one part of the long-range planning done by the health care organization. Such planning can become very complex when all of the multiple factors affecting the future growth of a particular health care organization are considered: federal policies, local regulations, changes in the health care market, increase in competition, changing availability of insurance coverage, preferences of referral sources, preferences of clients, and so forth.

The prediction of future trends has become an important concern of health care organizations. Nurse managers are increasingly being asked to forecast the effects of these trends on the availability and demand for nursing staff and nursing services. There are sophisticated computer programs that can be used to assist you in making these decisions (McHugh, 1986). They are very complex and not necessarily designed to account for the special characteristics of the nursing profession but can be an aid to the important administrative function of planning and forecasting future trends.

Simpler programs that produce graphs, charts, and other pictorial representations of statistical information can also be very helpful. They can illustrate important trends such as an increase in the proportion of older people in the patient population of a particular hospital or the increase in the number of AIDS patients coming to a particular clinic (Christensen & Stearns, 1984).

EVALUATING. The amount of income produced by a particular department is only one indicator of its potential health. Others include the cost of running the department, low absenteeism, low staff turnover rates, low morbidity (infection rate or incidence of decubiti, for example) and mortality, number of patient complaints, number of incident reports, and so forth. Results of chart audits and other quality-control measures are another important source of evaluative data that can be gathered and analyzed by means of the computer. All of the information must, however, be evaluated on the basis of the situation in which the unit or department operated just as an individual staff member's success in achieving his or her objectives must be evaluated in terms of the factors that helped or hindered achievement.

SCHEDULING. Staff scheduling has long been a tedious task, one that requires sensitivity to individual needs as well as the needs of the organization. While there will always be some decisions that call for the judgment of the nurse manager, most of the work of preparing a weekly or monthly staffing schedule can be computerized. Changes made necessary by emergencies or special requests can be added later or can be made as part of the computer program. In either case, the objectivity of the computerized program eliminates the problems of favoritism and people who regularly ask for special consideration, but it should not be allowed to become the final authority on scheduling. This still rests with the managers who implement the schedule.

Research

Whether the research is of a clinical, educational or administrative nature and a small or large part of your work, the computer is an essential support mechanism for all but the very smallest studies. Its functions in research have been mentioned before: sorting and organizing data, analyzing the data, and then printing out the results. It can also manage the data from qualitative studies.

Many statistical computations are so lengthy and complex that a computer is virtually required to complete them in a reasonable amount of time. Some programs that do statistical analysis are quite simple but do only a limited number of statistics and are unable to handle large amounts of data. Those that do handle large amounts of data may require use of the mainframe computer or a powerful personal computer. The programs available in health care organizations for clerical and budgetary purposes unfortunately are often inadequate for research. However, sophisticated evaluation requires the use of similar statistics, and you may find that the same programs can be used for both administrative evaluation and for research.

SELECTION OF EQUIPMENT AND PROGRAMS

As with other types of planning, the introduction or expansion of computerization should begin with careful consideration of purposes and all potential uses or the system that results will very likely be inappropriate, inadequate, incompatible, or all of these. People's expectations of the degree to which computers can make work more efficient and effective may be quite unrealistic. On the other hand, with adequate planning, a system can be designed and installed that allows you to do things that simply were not possible without it.

Often an organization-wide committee is set up to plan for computerization. It is important that nursing be well represented on such a committee. Among the factors that are particularly important to consider in planning for computerization are the purpose of the system, people's expectations, development of a comprehensive plan for its use, coordination between departments and disciplines within the organization, and training of personnel to use the system. The ultimate goal is a system designed to be both adequate and compatible with other operations of the organization.

Purpose of the System

Why are computers being purchased? Is it because everyone else is putting them into their facilities? Because they will give a modern, technological appearance to the facility? Or is it because they can improve the efficiency and effectiveness of the services being provided there? As with other planning, clarification and agreement on the purpose is an early and important step.

Expectations

When the benefits of computerization are also oversold, expectations can become even more unrealistic. Often people expect the computer system to work smoothly from the beginning and to save them a great deal of time with little effort on their part.

In reality, the system will probably not work smoothly in the beginning. Both equipment and programs must be checked for any flaws in production or installation. Secondly, a smooth transition from the old manual system to the new one must be carried out. This requires time, patience, much coordination and adaptation of the system. Thirdly, with the possible exception of very simple tasks, it takes some time and practice to learn how to use these systems, even if you have had previous experience.

The first time that you use a computer to do a task, it will probably take you *longer* than it did to do it manually. With some practice, however, it should quickly become faster to use the computer. If it does not, the problem may be with the system or with the way in which it was planned.

Comprehensive Plan

Often a health care organization begins computerization of its operations with the installation of a computerized billing system. However, billing is only one potential use as we have seen. A comprehensive hospital information system (HIS) would include patient monitoring, computerized history taking, patient classification, staff scheduling, communication between departments, and so forth, but a system designed to do only billing usually cannot be used for these additional purposes. Therefore, it should be designed with the information management needs of the entire organization in mind. Without a comprehensive plan, staff become frustrated with the limits of a system when it is too late to change it without a substantial new investment or even without rendering the current system completely useless because of the incompatibility of programs between departments.

Compatibility and Coordination

Different equipment and different programs cannot necessarily communicate with each other. Again, planning is important in avoiding this difficulty. Without planning, for example, the laboratory may install a computer system that is incompatible with the nursing department's system. In other words, the systems cannot "talk" to each other. Imagine the frustration and loss of efficiency resulting from this incompatibility! Cooperation and communication between departments and between professional disciplines is clearly necessary in the planning phase so that a coordinated system is developed in which information can be shared with other departments and brought together into one file. Developing a graphic representation of the way information will move through the system while still in the planning stages is one way to promote the development of a compatible and coordinated system (Rosenberger & Kaiser, 1985).

Use of Consultants

It is necessary to have some basic knowledge of computers to understand and use the experts. These experts will know far more about computers and about how to develop an appropriate and adequate system. However, it is also very important to know the needs of the organization, and this cannot be expected of the outside consultants. It is important, therefore, not to abdicate your responsibility, allowing consultants to tell you what is needed, but to use their expertise in making the final decision within the organization (Ball & Hannah, 1984; Lenkman, 1985).

Training of Personnel

Even computer experts need time to learn a new system. Computers are still new, strange, and somewhat frightening to some people, and those who are not yet computer literate will require extra time to become familiar with a new system. Time must be allowed for learning. Without adequate training of staff, expensive equipment will go unused or be used poorly.

Adequacy of the System

Even a large system can eventually become overloaded with too much information and too many users. Unfortunately, adequate systems are expensive and the temptation to cut corners to save money is great. When limited budgets prevent the purchase of a complete system, it is particularly important to ensure that what is purchased now can later be expanded. It is also important to ensure that methods are available to remove repetitious information or to compress it and that plans are made to stagger use of the system (hospital systems tend to have predictable peak-use times) to make the best use of the available capacity.

Finding the Right Program

Even this brief survey suggested the availability of a wide variety of software and hardware and has urged careful selection of both. The use of outside consultants has also been discussed, but these generally are not available all of the time. What other sources of assistance can you find? Within larger health care organizations with extensive computer systems, you will find computer experts who can share their expertise and their information with you. They can also customize programs to suit the needs of your particular nursing unit or team (Roberts, 1986). In addition, a number of journals and books recently have been published that provide evaluations of the cost and quality of various programs and equipment. Finally, you may want to talk with other people in positions similar to yours who have been using a program or piece of equipment that your facility is considering. Their experience may help you predict its usefulness in your organization.

ISSUES IN COMPUTER USAGE

A number of issues have been raised about using computers in health care. One is the patient's right to privacy and concern over security, that is, who has access to patient information that has been put into a computer. Other concerns include the depersonalizing effects of using electronic interviewers, schedule makers, and evaluators and the cost of computerization versus the benefits and overdependence on the computer.

Depersonalization

Is it depersonalizing to talk with a computer about your personal problems or to type your health history into a computer terminal instead of telling it to a nurse or physician? Is it less depersonalizing to talk with a person who is typing your information into a terminal (Computers and Medicine, 1986)? Is it depersonalizing to have a computer schedule your days off? Or is it fairer and more objective than having to depend on the personal biases and idiosyncrasies of your supervisor or the supervisor's secretary? These are just a few of the questions raised about the computer's possible dehumanizing effects.

Part of this concern probably stems from the fact that we realize one cannot cajole, persuade, flatter, or reason with a computer to change its mind. In this sense, it is truly not human, unable to respond with a genuinely felt sympathy for one's unique situation or problems. On the other hand, it also is not subject to the unfair influence of a particularly persuasive individual who often gets preferential treatment. It also cannot be surprised, shocked or embarrassed by personal revelations. The computer lacks feelings, and in some instances, this seems to be an advantage; in others, it is a characteristic to be avoided.

Privacy and Security

It is easy to imagine the scenario by which a patient or client's right to privacy is violated when records are computerized. A large hospital with a comprehensive computer system has terminals distributed throughout the facility. These terminals are accessible to most employees, including the curious volunteer or accounting clerk who has no need for information about a patient's psychiatric consultation or pathology report. Actually such a violation of privacy is possible with written charts as well.

Computerized records can be safeguarded to some extent through the use of identification numbers. These numbers indicate a person's status in the facility and determine the information to which that person may have access. In other words, it is possible to allow access to only certain specified parts of a record on a "need-to-know" basis. For example, laboratory personnel would be able to access the patient's identifying data and lab results but would not be able to access the progress notes that are available to nursing personnel using their assigned identification numbers.

Overdependence

Can we become too dependent on the computer? Will they be responsible for our losing some of our manual skills or not being able to remember what an assessment should include without referring to a screen? Do we assume that the computer is always right and that our mental calculations are wrong even when the computer produces questionable results?

Serious disruptions in work flow can occur when the central computer is "down," that is, temporarily out of service, for any length of time. Tapes or disks can be damaged or inadvertently erased and the data irretrievably lost unless backup copies were made. A backup system is essential and should be automatic rather than dependent on human intervention. It is also important to have people who do any essential procedures, such as patient monitoring, continue to maintain their manual skills for times when the machines are down. The existence of alternate methods for any essential operation should be planned in advance. They cannot be created quickly enough at the time that they are needed.

A much more subtle problem is the assumption that when there is a discrepancy between expected outcome and the computer's output, the computer must be right. This is a dangerous assumption. The well-known *GIGO* ("garbage in, garbage out") maxim about computers is true and explains one reason why output from a computer can be as wrong as it appears to be. In other words, if you put garbage (erroneous data) in, the results you get will also be garbage (erroneous results). The occasional extreme result may be correct, but it must be verified before accepting it.

Cost Versus Benefit

Is computerization cost-effective? Both the hardware and software are very expensive, as is the time and energy needed to install, learn, and maintain the system. Is it worth it? The degree to which computerization is of benefit in health care organizations must be considered in relation to the characteristics of both the organization and its clients and the computer system. A very small organization, for example, may decide that it needs computer assistance only in accounting and budgeting and therefore needs a relatively simple system. A large health department or hospital, on the other hand, may find a large, comprehensive system most effective in coordinating the vast amounts of information and complex analyses required by these organizations.

The quality of the system itself is very important: its adequacy in terms of capacity, appropriateness, maintenance, and support for staff who will use it are are just a few of the considerations. When the system is properly planned and designed, it is a fast, efficient, and accurate way to handle large amounts of information — information needed to manage health care effectively. The health care organization can and should expect that a good part of the expense will be offset through such savings as decreased time spent by professionals in doing clerical work, fewer forms to fill out and less duplication of forms and records, improved communication between departments, more effective quality assurance programs, and fewer errors or omissions in charging for supplies and services (Ginsberg & Brown, 1985).

SUMMARY

Both the hardware (equipment) and software (programs) of a computer system are important components and must be selected with thought given to their adequacy, compatibility, cost, and purpose. The applications or uses of computerization in nursing practice and management cover a wide range from assisting with secretarial and clerical work to patient assessment, monitoring, and record keeping; education; administration (including billing, budgeting, planning, scheduling, and evaluation); and research. Important issues in computerization include the development of too much dependence on the computer, maintenance of privacy, avoiding depersonalization, and balancing cost with benefit.

REFERENCES*

Ball, M.J. & Hannah, K.J. (1984). *Using computers in nursing.* Reston, Virginia: Reston Pub. Co.

Buisson, C.J. (1985). Computer applications in nursing continuing education. *The Nursing Clinics of North America. 20,* 505–516.

Christensen, W.W. & Stearns, E.I. (1984). *Microcomputers in Health Care Management.* Rockville, Maryland: Aspen Systems.

———(1986). MDs' testing habits yield to computer persuasion. *Computers and Medicine. 15* (4), 1–2.

Finkler, S.A. (1985). Microcomputers in nursing administration: A software overview. *Journal of Nursing Administration. 15* (4), 18–22.

*Ginsberg, D.A. & Browning, S.J. (1985). Selecting automated patient care systems. *Journal of Nursing Administration. 15* (12). 16–21.

Hudgings, C. (1987). Challenges in information management for nursing practice. *Nursing Administration Quarterly, 11* (2), 44–48.

*Johnson, D.S. & Ranzenberger, J.A. (1981). A computer-based system for hospital-wide patient monitoring. In Werley, H.H. & Grier, M.R. Eds. *Nursing Information Systems.* New York: Springer.

Lenkman, S. (1985). Management information systems and the role of the nurse vendor. *The Nursing Clinics of North America. 20,* 529–547.

McHugh, M.L. (1986). Information access: A basis for strategic planning and control of operations. *Nursing Administration Quarterly. 10,* 10–20.

Roberts, N. (1986). Hospital Information System Analyst, University Hospital, New York. Personal Communication.

Rosenberger, H.R. & Kaiser, K.M. (1985). Strategic planning for health care management information systems. *Health Care Management Review. 10,* 7–17.

*Saba, V.K. & McCormick, K.A.: (1986). *Essentials of Computers for Nurses.* Philadelphia: J.B. Lippincott.

*References marked with an asterisk are suggested for further reading.

Chapter 14 ━━━━━━━━━━

OUTLINE ━━━━━━━━━━━━━━━━━━━━━━━━━━━━━━

Collective Bargaining Defined

Purposes of Collective Bargaining

Issues Arising from Collective
    Bargaining
Unprofessional
Unethical
Divisive
Endangering Job Security

Collective Bargaining from the
    Employee's Viewpoint
Organizing
    The Organizing Council
    Elections
Negotiating a Contract
    Negotiations

Stalemates
Ratification
Contract Administration
Grievances
Binding Arbitration

Collective Bargaining from the
    Management Viewpoint
Preventing Unionization
    The Positive Approach
    The Aggressive Approach
Supervision and Management Under a
    Collective Bargaining Agreement
    First-Line Management Under a Contract
    Handling Grievances

Summary

LEARNING OBJECTIVES ━━━━━━━━━━━━━━━━━━━━━━

Upon completion of this chapter, the reader will be able to:

▷ Debate the advantages and disadvantages of collective bargaining from both labor's and management's points of view.

▷ Describe the activities of labor and management during the development of a collective bargaining agreement.

▷ Compare and contrast the rights and responsibilities of labor and management in a grievance procedure.

▷ Discuss the ways in which unionization can be prevented using both proactive and aggressive strategies.

━━━━━━ *COLLECTIVE BARGAINING*

$\mathbf{T}$he terms *labor relations* and *collective bargaining* still conjure up images of coal miner, steelworker, and truck driver unions in people's minds. This image reflects only half of the people who have joined organizations that represent them collectively at work. Administrators, college faculties, physical therapists, interns and residents, nurses, and other professionals in many parts of the country are also engaged in collective bargaining for reasons that we will consider in this chapter.

We will also look at the other side of this interesting phenomenon: the manager's point of view. From the manager's point of view, collective bargaining changes and regulates the staff member–manager relationship. It imposes, at the very least, an additional set of rules governing this relationship. At its worst, it can be a source of constant tension and serious conflicts between managers and their staffs. Regardless of one's opinion of collective bargaining, it is an influential factor in many health care organizations and a subject of concern in the health care field, where it has continued to grow in contrast to the weakening trend in industry (Fossum, 1979; Lockhart, 1980; Numerof & Abrams, 1984; O'Rourke, 1981; Willis, 1988).

COLLECTIVE BARGAINING DEFINED ━━━━━━━━━━━━

Collective bargaining is the joining together of employees for the purpose of increasing their ability to influence their employer and improve working conditions. In labor relations parlance, the employer is referred to as *management* and the employees are referred to as *labor*, even if they are professionals.

Anyone involved in the hiring, firing, scheduling, disciplining, or evaluating of employees is considered part of management and cannot be included in a collective bargaining unit. People in management can form their own groups but are not protected by the collective bargaining laws discussed here. There are often too small a number of management people in one organization to benefit from the same kind of collective action. This definition of management includes directors of nursing, assistant directors, and supervisors but not always head nurses. Some organizations deliberately include head nurses in the hiring and firing process to keep them out of collective bargaining units.

The National Labor Relations Act and its amendments are the primary laws that protect an employee's right to engage in collective bargaining. This act also established the National Labor Relations Board (NLRB), which has two major functions. The first is to ensure that employees are able to choose freely whether they want to be represented by a particular bargaining agent —for nurses, usually the professional association or an affiliate of a local or national labor union. The American Nurses' Association and its state associations have been the major representative of nurses, along with 22 different unions that have been attempting to attract nurses to their ranks (Numerof & Abrams, 1984). The second function of the NLRB is to prevent or remedy any violations of the labor laws, called *unfair labor practices.*

Nonprofit health care organizations—including hospitals, nursing homes, visiting nurse associations, clinics, and other health care organizations—have been subject to these labor laws only since 1974, making them relative newcomers to collective bargaining. Special rules designed to safeguard the welfare of patients apply to health care organizations. Proprietary (for-profit) organizations are also covered by these laws, but government-operated health care facilities are subject to an entirely different set of rules that generally affords less protection of the employee's collective bargaining rights (strikes are generally forbidden, but benefits are more generous than in nongovernmental organizations).

PURPOSES OF COLLECTIVE BARGAINING

Collective bargaining is a power strategy based on the principle that there is increased strength in numbers. Its fundamental purpose is to equalize the power distribution between labor and management. If you think back to the organizational hierarchy discussed in Chapter 10, the desire for equalization of power becomes more understandable. The majority of employees in most organizations are at or near the bottom of the hierarchy, a position with very little authority. People higher up in the hierarchy (the "management") appear far more powerful to people below them in the hierarchy.

The distribution of power is not actually as unequal as it appears to be, however. The organization depends on these employees lower in the hierarchy to carry on its work; they are vital to the growth and development—even the survival—of the organization and far outnumber the people higher up in the hierarchy. Collective bargaining takes advantages of both of these factors. A single employee who attempts to bargain with an employer is far more vulnerable to potential threats or reprisals from the employer than is an entire group of employees.

Basic economic issues such as salaries are usually the first concern of people joining a collective bargaining unit. Despite the continuing need for nurses, hospitals in many areas have managed to keep nurses' salaries artificially low, often by setting up agreements with other area institutions to keep the wages low. Some nurses have found that other employees in their organization who have the same or less education and responsibility are making better salaries.

Other economic concerns covered by collective bargaining include shift differentials, overtime pay, holidays, personal days, the length of the workday, sick leave, maternity and paternity leaves, payment for uniforms, lunch and rest periods (breaks), health insurance, pension plans, and severance pay. People often assume that these are provided by any employer, but, in fact, some vital and costly ones are not provided by every employer (The Nation's Health, 1986).

Unfair or arbitrary treatment can be anything from being the only one who has to work three weekends in a row to being passed over for a promotion without explanation to being fired because a physician thought your assertion of a patient's rights was "insubordinate." Other bargainable issues include staffing and scheduling policies governing days off, rotating shifts, being on call, promotion policies, transfers, layoffs, seniority rights, and the posting of job openings.

Perhaps the most important protection against arbitrary treatment is the inclusion of a grievance procedure in the collective bargaining agreement. This enables an employee to bring a complaint to management without having to fear later reprisals for his or her assertiveness.

Maintenance and promotion of professional practice is a third strategy often underestimated by management (see Research Example 14–1). Proponents of collective bargaining believe that it is one means by which nurses and other health care professionals can increase and maintain control over their practice (Riffer, 1986). For example, some nurses' bargaining units

---

RESEARCH EXAMPLE 14–1. Nurses' Purposes Versus Management's Perceptions in Collective Bargaining

Are nurses primarily concerned with economic issues or with professional issues when they bargain collectively? Do managers know what issues are actually important to their staff members?

Bloom, Parlette, and O'Reilly (1980) interviewed 78 public health and registered nurses and 11 supervisory nurses from three large community health care agencies in California for this study. Two of the agencies had recently settled work stoppages. These nurses had worked an average of 7.5 years for the county, and all county employees were represented by an international labor union. The nurses were asked to rate the importance of 17 different issues on a four-point scale from *not a factor at all* to a *major factor* in the decision to strike. Ten top management people, including the director of nursing, three assistant directors of nursing, the director of public health, and the county manager were also asked to rate the same 17 issues.

Little relationship was found between the ratings of the nurses and people in management over what issues were important (the correlation was a low 0.17). The nurses considered support for nurses in their unit, difficulty communicating with management, management's authoritarian behavior, a belief in collective bargaining as a way to balance the power between management and employees, and the need for more nursing positions (the only economic issue) to be most important. In contrast, the people in top management positions thought that the most important factors in the strike decision were a pay increase, allowing two nurses to share a full-time position, a union attempt to gain power, and pressure from other nurses to go on strike. None of the four issues rated important by management were actually important to the nurses.

In their discussion, the researchers asked why people in management fail to use principles of effective communication and the basic concepts of the well-known motivational theories when dealing with collective bargaining. They concluded that management thought that the industrial type of bargaining issues such as wages and job security were the critical issues, but that the nurses were actually more concerned about professional issues, especially with improving communication with management and increased participation in organizational decision making.

have succeeded in putting the entire American Nurses' Association Code of Ethics into the contractual agreement with their employers. Adequate staffing, acceptable standards of care, and other quality-of-care issues also can be negotiated with employers. Research Examples 14–1 and 14–2 describe some sources of dissatisfaction experienced by hospital employees.

ISSUES ARISING FROM COLLECTIVE BARGAINING

Most issues and objections to collective bargaining center on the conviction that it is an unprofessional activity damaging to the professional image and that some of the related activities are unethical. A different concern is that, paradoxically, it may endanger job security.

Unprofessional

Many people associate unions with blue-collar workers and believe that it is unprofessional for nurses to engage in such an activity. Collective bargaining does not fit their image of the nurse as a professional, and they emphasize that other means can be found to achieve the purposes of collective bargaining.

Organizers of collective bargaining units, on the other hand, argue that other professionals (pharmacists, engineers, college professors, and even some employed physicians) are members of unions and that the NLRB defines nurses as professionals because their work requires advanced specialized training and making critical judgments. The NLRB allows nurses and physicians to have separate bargaining units because of their unique characteristics. Another favorite response of union organizers is that it is unprofessional to accept low salaries and poor working conditions. Control over one's practice, they would say, is the essence of professionalism (Luttman, 1982).

Unethical

Most health care professionals have a strong set of values emphasizing the priority of the patient's health and welfare over their own personal needs and gain. These values conflict with some collective bargaining strategies, especially any type of work slow down or stoppage. Many health care professionals think that they could not abandon their patients during a strike under any circumstances and that it would be unprofessional and unethical to do so.

The opposing argument is that the poor, sometimes intolerable, conditions under which many nurses work are also a threat to patients' welfare. The threat of a strike is needed to improve these conditions. The law requires giving 10 days' notice before striking and has other provisions that reduce the possibility of a strike or the possibility of harm to patients if a strike does occur. This allows time for management to make preparations for the patients' safety, such as reducing elective surgeries and admissions or transferring patients to other facilities.

When the American Nurses' Association had a no-strike policy (prior to 1968), nurses who tried to bargain collectively with their employers found that they had little or no success. Their employers ignored them, refused to bargain with them, or gave them platitudes about how important they were while raising other people's salaries. Without the clout of a potential strike, nurses could not get their employers to listen to them or to respond to their requests.

Divisive

Collective bargaining has a potentially divisive effect on the profession. State nurses' associations have acted as bargaining agents for many groups of nurses, yet many supervisors and directors of nursing are members of these associations and hold offices in them. For these management nurses, there is a potential conflict of interest in being a member of an association that supports strikes, perhaps even a strike against their own institution. On the other hand, there is also a potential legal conflict of having management people attempting to influence the association in its function as a labor organization, although most have taken steps to separate these functions.

These conflicts have evoked strong emotions and led to many debates about the role of the professional association, even threatening a split into management and nonmanagement factions. Some nurse administrators feel torn between representing management and supporting their professional association. Others feel angry and bitter about the collective bargaining efforts of their fellow nurses. Collective bargaining does draw a clear line between management and labor and tends to treat their relationship as an adversarial one, which is not the most productive working relationship. On the other hand, it has enabled staff nurses to bring about some of the same changes that nursing administrators have been trying unsuccessfully to implement through persuasive means for years. The adversarial nature of the relationship is one that often can be prevented or ameliorated.

Endangering Job Security

Because one of the major purposes of collective bargaining is to improve working conditions and protect workers from unfair treatment, it is somewhat ironic that collective bargaining is also seen as a potential threat to job security in two ways. The first is that those people who actively engage in collective bargaining and become well known to management may become targets for reprisals, particularly if the collective bargaining effort fails. The second is that a union that is too successful in gaining concessions from management can actually drain too much of the organization's resources and inhibit the organization's growth or even endanger its survival.

Some risk is always involved in taking action, particularly action against those who have the authority to remove you from your position. For this reason, most collective bargaining activities begin when working conditions become so difficult that people believe it is worth the risk. Initial attempts at organizing the people are usually done outside the organization, and representatives of the nurses' association or the union act as spokespersons for the employees, shielding the employees somewhat from management's anger.

Pro	Con
Equalization of power between labor and management	Unprofessional conduct
Prevents unfair treatment of employees	Leads to unethical actions affecting patient welfare
Promotes professionalism and increased control of practice	Interferes with management of the organization
Economic security	Inhibits organizational growth
Improves the quality of care	Endangers job security of employees active in collective bargaining

Figure 14–1. A summary of the pros and cons of collective bargaining.

Although there are few examples from the health care industry, there are organizations in other fields that have become so restricted by union rules and so inefficient because of high union wages that they have failed to keep up with their competitors. Some unions' actions have been compared to those of a parasite that lives off the organization and eventually kills it. Obviously, it is not in the union's best interest to destroy the organization that employs its members. A fair distribution of resources between the management and owners of the organization and its employees can benefit both labor and management. However, in a conflict between two opposing groups, it is often difficult to achieve this delicate balance of competing interests. Figure 14–1 summarizes the pros and cons of engaging in collective bargaining.

COLLECTIVE BARGAINING FROM THE EMPLOYEE'S VIEWPOINT

Organizing

In this first phase of the collective bargaining process, a labor organization is formed, and that organization seeks recognition as the employees' bargaining agent. While it is possible to form an independent group and be protected by the same laws, the professional associations and unions have already established themselves as bargaining agents and have developed the expertise on the applicable laws and in the multiple strategies needed to bargain effectively with management. Health care organizations frequently hire consultants to help them fight unionization and sometimes pool their resources with other area institutions to improve their own expertise and bargaining position. Their access to this expertise would put an independent group at a disadvantage.

THE ORGANIZING COUNCIL.   The movement toward unionization begins when a group of interested employees forms an informal organizing council. This council becomes the core group that gets other nurses interested in joining a union by pointing out the need for one. The need for collective bargaining is usually based on a combination of some or all of the items listed under the purposes of collective bargaining in which management failed to meet the needs of the employees. The council can ask for assistance from the professional association or a union, or it can attempt to form an independent bargaining unit. Sometimes the initiative to organize comes from a union or competing unions, but the core group of committed employees is essential to the success of an organizing effort.

The organizing council usually meets outside of working hours in a nonwork setting to plan its organizing strategies. As they persuade other nurses that collective action is needed, core group members ask them to sign authorization cards. These cards indicate their desire to be represented by a particular labor organization. The cards are checked by a neutral third party; management does not see the signatures at any time. When a majority of the nurses employed in the organization have signed these cards, the employer is asked to voluntarily recognize the union or nurses' association as the bargaining agent. Most of the time, the employer will not do this and so an election supervised by the NLRB is held.

ELECTIONS. The pre-election campaigning on both sides can become intense. Management often plays on nurses' feelings of guilt, implying that they are planning to abandon the patients who depend on them or that they are betraying the director who has worked so hard on their behalf. Other tactics may be aimed at stirring fear of reprisals (such as being fired); but actual threats or coercion, or even promises of benefits for those who vote against the union, are illegal.

An entirely different strategy used by management is to take a positive approach. Suddenly, the pay scale for nurses is raised, and supervisors become very attentive to the needs of individual employees. This attentiveness fades quickly, however, if the organizing effort ends.

The union side has its own strategies. Unions often mount an educational campaign explaining what a union is and what it can do for employees. These campaigns often include responses to criticisms that collective bargaining is unprofessional or unethical. Unions also use fear by pointing out how vulnerable an employee is without the protection of a union. The unsatisfactory conditions that led to the interest in collective bargaining are emphasized, and individual incidents may be exaggerated to stir anger against management. Any threats or coercion from the union are also illegal.

All full-time and most part-time nurses who are employed by health care organizations but not in management positions are eligible to vote for or against the proposed bargaining agent. The bargaining agent that wins the election is certified by the NLRB, and the employer must bargain with this designated representative of its employees.

Negotiating a Contract

Once a bargaining agent has been certified by the NLRB, collective bargaining enters the second phase, in which an agreement on a contract is reached. This contract is a legal document that both management and labor must abide by after it is signed. All of the items listed earlier under the purposes of collective bargaining can be included in this agreement as well as items about union membership and payment of dues (called *union security items*).

Negotiations. Both management and labor groups form negotiating teams and designate one member of the team as their spokesperson. Before negotiations begin, each team meets separately to decide what their priorities are and what items they are willing to compromise on at the bargaining table. As with other types of negotiations, they begin by asking for everything they might possibly want but avoid making completely unreasonable demands. When an expiring contract is being renegotiated, either side may ask for something that they lost at the last contract negotiation.

As a rule, management is very reluctant to give up any of its power or to spend more money; the union, conversely, attempts to equalize the power balance between labor and management and to gain benefits for its members. These recitations of who-wants-what can go back and forth for many meetings, but they do have some purpose. During this time, the negotiating teams find out what the key issues are and where compromise is possible.

Much of what happens in these early rounds are demonstrations by each team aimed at gaining public support for its side. There is often a great deal of posturing and showmanship during these early talks, and the serious bargaining is done later behind closed doors. Then the really difficult issues are dealt with and necessary compromises are made to reach an agreement.

In this particular type of negotiation, each side is *obliged by law* to bargain in good faith. *Good faith* means that both parties must agree to meet at reasonable times, to send representatives with the authority to negotiate to the bargaining table, and to bargain with the other side. Presenting a take-it-or-leave-it package of demands and refusing to negotiate any changes in that package is not bargaining in good faith.

STALEMATES. Despite good faith bargaining by both sides, negotiations may reach a stalemate in which the two teams are unable to reach an agreement. If this happens, both sides must notify the Federal Mediation and Conciliation Service, a government agency. Several actions may then be taken to break a stalemate: mediation, fact finding, binding arbitration, and work stoppages.

Mediation. A neutral party provided by the Federal Mediation and Conciliation Service may meet with each of the negotiating teams to explore the nature of the stalemate and then bring the two sides together to try to work out a settlement of the dispute. Both sides must cooperate with this federal mediator, but they do not have to accept the mediator's recommendations.

Fact Finding. The Federal Mediation and Conciliation Service may also appoint a fact-finding board of inquiry to investigate the situation and make recommendations. This board's report and recommendations are made public and can be used to pressure one or both sides to move toward an agreement.

Binding Arbitration. Like the mediator and fact-finding board, the arbitrator is a neutral party who thoroughly investigates the situation, meets with each side, and makes a decision regarding a settlement between the two. However, both sides must accept the arbitrator's decision, so both management and labor are reluctant to voluntarily limit their bargaining power by submitting the dispute to binding arbitration unless no better alternative exists.

One of the risks of binding arbitration is that either side may lose something gained during previous negotiations. For example, the arbitrator could reverse a hard-won agreement to reduce the probation time of new employees from six to two months. This change would be a victory for management because benefits do not have to be paid for these first six months, and pay raises for new employees are pushed back.

Work Stoppages.   When talks reach an impasse, employees have a fourth alternative: They can slow down or stop working. Employers can also lock employees out. Although they are usually reluctant to do this, the number of lockouts by management have increased in recent years (Williams, 1986). The union must give 10 days' notice before striking unless management has committed an unfair labor practice.

At this point, the tension builds rapidly. In fact, the prospect of a strike usually leads to more intense negotiation and often to a last-minute settlement. Generally speaking, no one really wants a strike, and the decision is preceded by a great deal of discussion between the union and the membership of the bargaining unit. Unions do not want to strike unless their members are solidly in support of the action.

While management is preparing (often frantically) for the loss of the nurses' services, the union has to organize the strike; set up strike headquarters; and build support from its members, the public, and other unions for its strike. Once begun, strikes usually continue until some kind of settlement is reached.

RATIFICATION.   When an agreement is finally reached, the union negotiators take it back to the membership for their approval. A vote is taken, and, if approved, the agreement becomes a legally binding contract under which management and labor now have to work.

Contract Administration

Collective bargaining does not end with the signing of the agreement. The hard-won agreement now has to be enforced.

GRIEVANCES.   Almost every collective bargaining agreement includes provisions for a grievance procedure to deal with any dispute or complaint from either the employer or any employee in the bargaining unit regarding implementation of the contract. The contract usually specifies certain steps to be taken and the time limits for each of these steps. For example, employees may be given a limit of five days after an incident occurs to file a grievance with their immediate supervisors, and the supervisors must respond within another given number of days.

If the problem is not resolved at this first step, it proceeds through further steps. The grievance may be brought next to the director of personnel and then to the administrator of the organization. If the grievance is still not resolved at the end of these steps, it can then be taken to arbitration (Collective Bargaining Agreement, 1984–1986; Thomas & Murray, 1976).

A typical grievance begins when an employee feels mistreated and contacts the union delegate (a fellow employee who represents a particular work group) or association representative to find out if this perceived mistreatment is a violation of the contract. The delegate then discusses the situation with the employee and decides how to handle the complaint. The following is an example:

An employee informed the delegate about not receiving a raise that was due. The delegate spoke to the employee's manager, who said it was just an oversight, and the problem was quickly resolved.

If the problem affects other employees too, the delegate will also speak to them before deciding how to handle it. Here is an example:

The supervisor of the intensive care units told the day-shift nurses that they would have to work an extra weekend for the next 3 months. One of the nurses informed their delegate. The delegate spoke with several other nurses, who confirmed that they had been told the same thing. The delegate then went to the supervisor, told the supervisor that this was a violation of the contract, and showed the supervisor the relevant clause in the contract. The extra weekend work was removed from the schedule before it was posted and was not mentioned again.

Often the delegate needs to use his or her understanding of human behavior and effective communication techniques in dealing with grievances because supervisors may take a grievance personally and become defensive about having made a mistake, or they may feel threatened by the power that the delegate represents. The following is an example of a situation that the delegate handled tactfully to avoid making the supervisor defensive:

At the end of an unusually busy week, during which the staff could not get all their work done on time and everyone was becoming tired and short tempered, an irritable supervisor decided that staff members were spending too much time in the lavatories and tried to limit them to one trip a day. Most of the staff ignored the order, but a few became angry, and one threatened to use the supply room sink. The delegate approached the supervisor privately and told the supervisor that staff members could not obey the rule and that it could not be enforced. The supervisor realized that the head of the department would not approve of the absurd rule and dropped the whole matter after the conversation with the delegate.

As you can see, many grievances are minor and can be resolved in an informal manner by the employee, immediate supervisor, and delegate at the first steps of the grievance procedure.

Any disputes more serious or complex than the examples given above are usually brought to a union employee, called an *organizer* or *association representative*. These individuals have more experience in resolving grievances and are in a less vulnerable position than the delegate, who is an employee of the organization. The organizer is not emotionally involved in the situation, cannot be harassed by management, and can be more objective than the others involved. This is an instance in which it is an advantage to be represented by a large union or active professional association that has locally based organizers available to represent employees throughout the steps of the grievance procedure.

The organizer is likely to confront supervisors or administrators more directly than a delegate would. The following are two examples in which the problem was resolved at the first step of the grievance procedure.

A nursing assistant, Miss M., thought that she was being treated unfairly by her head nurse, who often criticized her, never praised her, and never granted her requests for a particular assignment or day off. The aide brought her problem to the delegate, who referred it to the organizer. The organizer was direct with the head nurse. The organizer told the head nurse, ''You don't have any respect for this nursing assistant as a person. She's a human being.'' The head nurse responded somewhat defensively but did begin to treat the nursing assistant more like a human being after the confrontation.

A nurse, Mr. P., requested a particular day off to take care of some important personal business that had to be done during work hours, but his supervisor denied the request. The organizer accompanied the nurse to meet with the supervisor to repeat his request. The supervisor said that he could have the day off only if he found someone to work his shift. The organizer said, ''Are you asking Mr. P. to do your job for you?'' The supervisor backed down, rearranged the schedule and allowed the nurse to take the day off.

The organizer plays the same roles of mediator and defender of the employee's rights if the grievance is not resolved at the first step. The next steps involve management higher up in the hierarchy of the organization. If the grievance is a very serious matter, such as the firing of an employee, it may be taken directly to the administrator of the organization.

BINDING ARBITRATION. When the previously mentioned steps of the grievance procedure fail to resolve the dispute, the problem can be taken to binding arbitration. This kind of arbitration is much the same as the arbitration used during contract negotiations except that, in this case, it is done to resolve a disagreement over implementation of the contract.

The contract usually specifies the way in which an arbitrator is selected, most often from a list supplied by the American Arbitration Association, which acts like a clearing house. Both sides must agree with the choice.

Again, there is some reluctance to go to arbitration because the decision is binding on both parties and the arbitrator's fees, which are paid by both sides, can be substantial. If the employee has been offered a reasonable settlement at an earlier stage and does not have a strong case, the organizer will encourage the person privately to accept the offer. If the employee is completely in the wrong in the dispute, the organizer may refuse to proceed with the arbitration. This refusal can be appealed to the union board.

The arbitrator acts very much like a judge in hearing the case, except that the rules of evidence are not as strict as they are in a courtroom. The arbitrator's duty is to decide whether the contract was violated and what action is to be taken. The following are two examples in which the firing of a hospital employee was taken to arbitration:

A shipment of perishable materials was due some time during the day, and a pharmacy aide was assigned to unpack and store the materials. The shipment arrived just before quitting time, and the pharmacist said that the aide had to stay. The aide refused, saying, ''I would have stayed if I had been asked earlier in the day.'' Because the aide had received disciplinary warnings in the past, the aide was fired for insubordination.

Because this was a serious case, the union organizer began the grievance procedure at the second step with the personnel department. Eventually, the case was brought to arbitration. The contract stipulated that management could ask employees to work overtime and that this employee had been warned about insubordination in the past. The employee lost the arbitration procedure and remained fired.

In another case, a new technician in a training program suffered a convulsion, fell down a flight of stairs, and broke several bones. The technician was fired by the hospital for excessive absenteeism while out of work on disability. The hospital claimed that the technician was incapable of completing the training program or doing the job for which he was hired. The technician said, ''I just forgot to take my Dilantin that day,'' but the hospital would not reinstate the employee.

> The union brought this case to arbitration and the arbitrator ruled in favor of the employee, noting that it was an accident, that anyone could make that kind of mistake. The employee got the job back.

The grievance procedure provides employees with two safeguards not always available to employees who have not organized to bargain collectively. The first is a guarantee of a fair hearing and a response within a given time. The second is that employees have someone to represent and defend them and do not have to face an authority figure alone.

COLLECTIVE BARGAINING FROM THE MANAGEMENT VIEWPOINT

Preventing Unionization

From the management point of view, the nonunionized organization's goal in regard to collective bargaining is to remain nonunionized. It would be extremely unusual to find management anywhere that wanted unionization.

We will look at two approaches to preventing unionization: a general, positive approach to management that generates a climate in which most of the work force is satisfied and has little interest in unions and collective bargaining, and a more aggressive approach in which the organization takes deliberate steps to prevent unionization.

THE POSITIVE APPROACH. It is generally agreed that widespread job dissatisfaction within an organization makes that organization vulnerable to unionization (Hunter, Bamberg, Castaglia, & McCausland, 1986). In fact, union organizers will say that in many organizations management has done their work for them, that "management is our best advertisement." What they mean is that poor leadership and management practices in the organization have led to a strongly felt need for collective bargaining to equalize the power relationship between labor and management and to improve working conditions. Research Example 14–2 describes some typical areas of employee dissatisfaction in hospitals, many of which could be eliminated by effective leadership and management.

The solution, then, is responsive, proactive leadership and management throughout the organization. Certainly, the first-line manager to whom this book is primarily addressed cannot do this alone. However, upper-level administration depends on first-line managers to implement this approach, and so we will look at the most common and generally effective approaches.

In analyzing why a strike took place at a Michigan hospital, Simms and Dalston (1984) divided the factors into those specific to collective bargaining and those of a more general nature. The more specific factors included economic issues; overtime; rotating shifts; working weekends; recruitment; retention; morale; appreciation and valuing of nurses; provision for adequate input into the quality of care, scope; and autonomy of nursing practice; relationships with other disciplines; lines of accountability; and other general working conditions. The general factors included the influence of a general reorganization within the institution; a restructuring of the chief of nursing role; and the effect of many outside parties including politicians,

RESEARCH EXAMPLE 14 – 2. Hospital Employees' Opinions About Their Work

What do hospital employees like and dislike about their jobs? Holloway (1976) reported the results of a survey of the attitudes of 21,748 employees of 29 voluntary (nonprofit) community hospitals. These hospitals were located in New England, California, and the Midwest. Holloway points out that, although the sample was large, it was not a random sample and therefore may not be representative of all hospital employees in the United States. The size of the hospital had no relation to employee satisfaction with the work environment in this sample.

Employees were asked to rate their satisfaction with many different aspects of the work environment. Their responses were reported in terms of percentages of the sample that were satisfied with each factor. Some examples from the different categories:

Work Productivity. Fifty-five percent rated the amount of job pressure as unsatisfactory.

Coordination of Work. Fifty-five percent rated teamwork satisfactory; 42 percent rated interdepartmental cooperation as satisfactory.

Administrative Procedures. Seventy-five percent rated the procedure fair, but only 55 percent rated the handling of complaints as satisfactory.

Salary and Benefits. These areas were found generally satisfactory, but only 40 percent thought that the promotion incentives were satisfactory.

Communications. Most employees rated their hospitals highly on communication of hospital policies and fire and disaster procedures. However, only 30 percent rated communication between departments and grievance procedures as satisfactory.

Organizational Orientation. Again, grievance procedures were the lowest-rated factor (only 20 percent found them satisfactory). First impressions of the institution, cleanliness, and job security were rated high by 80 percent of the sample.

Staff Relationships. Acceptance of new staff was highly rated (80 percent), but only 20 percent were satisfied with physician-staff relationships.

Job Enrichment. Education and training were rated satisfactory by 60 percent; 65 percent thought that good use was made of their talents.

Staff Appraisal and Development. Career planning and the availability of career ladders for advancement within the organization were not highly rated (35 and 40 percent, respectively) nor was the amount of praise given (40 percent). The fairness of the appraisals and resultant corrective actions taken were rated higher— 65 percent found them satisfactory.

Even the survey itself was rated. Seventy-five percent of those responding trusted that the results would be kept anonymous.

On the basis of these findings, grievance procedures; lack of administrative response to complaints; and lack of mutual respect among managers, professionals, and other staff seemed to be of major concern to employees according to Holloway. Job pressures and staffing patterns were also serious problems, as were a lack of recognition for performance, lack of a career ladder, and lack of communications between departments and with administration. Holloway suggests that many of these concerns are due to management problems and the lack of effective leadership, listing the following examples: using the old trait approach in evaluation procedures; inconsistency in enforcing personnel policies; inadequate career planning and mobility for employees; supervisors and department heads who perform tasks instead of managing; rapid change and turnover so that supervisors cannot explain policies to employees; and the failure to develop an open, participative organizational climate.

other organizations, and the news media. These factors may vary from one situation to another, but they give you a good idea of how complex and far-reaching the influences can be.

Although all-round high-quality, effective leadership and management are needed to create a positive organization climate resistant to unionization, there are some specific areas on which to focus attention in preventing unionization:

1. *Provide real opportunities for participation in organization decision making.* We are going back to a very basic principle in leadership and management here in saying that the participative approach is most effective. However, the participative approach also requires more effort and openness to suggestions for change, particularly when implemented at the organization-wide level. On the other hand, the professionals who work within the organization have a great deal to contribute, and much of this is lost in an organization with autocratic leadership. Staff members should, at the very least, have input into scheduling, quality assurance, and patient care procedures. They should also be consulted on budgetary matters and long-range planning goals of the organization.

2. *Treat professionals as professionals.* This sounds so obvious, but many nurses are not accorded all of the respect, value, and authority they are due. Staff members generally live up to your expectations, but when little is expected of them, they often will not display as much professionalism as they could. This leads to a vicious circle in which administration believes that their poor treatment is justified. Just a few small examples will be mentioned here. Timing coffee breaks taken by professional staff, for example, or monitoring mileage for community nurses is insulting. Professionals skip their breaks when the need arises and should be able to judge for themselves when they can extend a break. Expecting nurses to yield to physician demands is demeaning. In some organizations, nurses also find themselves acceding to the demands of housekeeping, dietary, pharmacy, and so forth. The relationship should be one of equals, of colleagues working together toward a common goal of good patient care. A narrow, limited view of nursing practice on the part of administration leads to a dissatisfied nursing staff more easily convinced to bargain collectively.

3. *Pay salaries in keeping with the education required and the responsibility given.* This is an effective way to demonstrate the degree to which nurses are valued by the organization. It also helps to reduce staff turnover.

4. *Develop a procedure for handling grievances.* One of the most appealing aspects of collective bargaining is the opportunity to appeal a decision made by your boss if you think that the decision is unfair. A management-initiated grievance policy should be well defined and administration supported, and should include safeguards for the employee who decides to use it. An "open-door" policy that allows staff members to approach higher-level management people if they believe that they need a hearing is one component of such a policy. Another would be the organization of an appeals committee composed of both staff and management to hear any grievances that were not satisfactorily resolved through other means.

5. *Regular staff surveys.* One of the best ways to communicate administrative concern and to provide a channel of communication for all staff members is to institute a regular survey of staff opinions, asking questions such as those listed in Research Example 14–2. Such a survey is useless or worse, however, if management does not do anything about the problems that are uncovered through the survey.

THE AGGRESSIVE APPROACH.   Some organizations go even further and are quite aggressive in their efforts to prevent unionization. The following are some more specific actions that can be taken on an organization-wide basis to prevent unionization:

1. *Keep salaries and benefits at rates equal to or greater than those offered by unionized organizations.* The organization regularly surveys the salaries and benefits offered at neighboring institutions and agencies and deliberately sets its salaries to keep up with the other organizations.
2. *Control communications.* Company newsletters, bulletin boards, and other means of communication with employees are controlled by a designated department or individual. Employees would not be permitted to post or distribute any kinds of advertisements or flyers, for example, without their manager's permission.
3. *Negotiate with individuals, never with groups.* If a group of employees approaches their manager together, requesting a clarification of promotion policies or some other matter, the manager is advised to agree to speak with them but only on an individual basis. This is an application of the power tactic of "divide and conquer." It prevents employees from using one of their major sources of power, their greater number within the organization.
4. *Prohibit prounion speakers.* This is related to the control of communication mentioned above. An organization has the right to determine who is allowed to speak to its employees on work time in areas that are designated as work areas. The organization does not have the right, of course, to determine what its employees do outside of work on their own time in this regard.

One last comment on the subject of preventing unionization. All of the approaches mentioned above are generally effective and allowed under the labor laws. Some of the very aggressive tactics that management may try to use when threatened by unionization can be illegal or unfair labor practices. In general, management is not allowed to spy on its employees, to make any promises to employees to influence union elections, or to attempt to influence or threaten employees.

Supervision and Management Under a Collective Bargaining Agreement

In the past, much of the management literature spoke of collective bargaining as an evil thing that interfered with their work, tied their hands, and threatened to destroy their companies. That attitude has changed a great deal as unions in general have become weaker in the United States and as management has realized that they both share a very important goal:

survival of the institution that employs them. The current attitude seems to be leaning toward the feeling that it is possible to work effectively under a collective bargaining agreement and that it is not always management that ends up making concessions when a disagreement arises (Fay & Morrill, 1985; Katz, 1988; Williams, 1986).

First-Line Management Under a Contract. To manage effectively under a collective bargaining agreement, it may be necessary first to deal with your feelings about the agreement. It would not be unusual to feel as if the necessity for the contract implied that even first-line managers were the enemy of the staff members and that your staff had to be protected from the enemy, you. Working under a legal contract also makes some managers anxious about being confronted by the delegate about a mistake or having a particular action brought up in a grievance. Either of these concerns is, of course, possible, but careful management can prevent them.

The most important point in managing under a contract is to know and understand that contract very well. The contract is a legal document, and violations of that contract are unfair labor practices that can be opposed, usually successfully, by the union. A thorough knowledge of the contract, including such details as scheduling overtime or granting time off can prevent most grievances. But you cannot expect to prevent all grievances because some people will grieve almost anything, even the smallest infraction, and it is important not to feel that the occurrence of a grievance is a sign that you have been an ineffective manager.

Following the contract stipulations for people who are working under a collective bargaining contract may lead you inadvertently to be less considerate of noncontract people on your staff. This would lead to accusations of favoritism and a sense among your noncontract staff that they were not being treated fairly. A high level of morale among all staff members requires equal consideration for all employees.

When a problem does arise, it is important to react in as nondefensive a manner as possible. Most problems can be dealt with at the manager-delegate-employee level as was shown in the examples in the previous section. Working with both the delegate or union organizer and staff member on an adult-to-adult level will facilitate the resolution of most problems. It is particularly important to avoid getting caught up in the Karpman Triangle of victim-persecutor-rescuer or in other organizational games.

The practice of effective leadership and management with everyone involved, including the union people, and a thorough knowledge of the contract are your most important safeguards against a high-tension, conflict-ridden management-labor relationship. When a conflict does arise that cannot be immediately resolved using these approaches, it should be brought to the attention of higher level management or the personnel department, depending on the way it is handled in your particular institution or agency.

Handling Grievances.   Despite all efforts to prevent them, grievances will arise. When it appears that a problem will be grieved, you need to immediately seek support from upper-level management to handle the situation. The grievance procedure itself has already been described in some detail from the employee's point of view, so we will just consider some of the major points in handling a grievance from the management's point of view.

If informal counseling with the dissatisfied employee does not lead to resolution of the problem, the first-line manager should bring the problem to the attention of the next higher level manager. Together they conduct an investigation of the situation and the specific policy as stated in the collective bargaining agreement and bring their results to the director of nursing or vice-president for nursing. At this point, the analysis should include consideration of the accuracy and completeness of the facts presented, whether or not the particular policy was appropriately interpreted and applied, and whether or not the policy has been applied in the same way in other situations. If all of these questions are answered satisfactorily, the administrator will generally support the first-line manager's decision.

This support of the first-line manager's decision may lead the employee to decide to file a grievance. As described earlier, the steps within the grievance process usually are spelled out clearly in the contract. This second step often consists of an evaluation of the situation by the head of the personnel department. If personnel supports the manager, the employee may, in consultation with the union or representative, decide to take the grievance further, usually to arbitration.

The following list of questions has been suggested by Fay and Morrill (1985) for review of the strength of management's case before deciding to proceed to arbitration:

1. Regarding the policy or practice itself (a requirement that all staff work rotating shifts or that promotions are based on merit ratings, for example): Is the policy itself clearly stated? Have the consequences of violating that policy been communicated clearly? Has the policy been applied uniformly in the past?
2. Regarding management's decision to pursue arbitration: Does administration support continuing the action? Is the cost worthwhile in terms of the money, time, effort, and potential outcome? How will this action affect staff morale?
3. What is the likelihood of management winning the case at arbitration?

The organization's legal counsel and other experts in collective bargaining will probably be called in for consultation. All pertinent facts will be reviewed again, and such questions as were listed above will be debated. If management decides to continue to arbitration (rather than attempting to settle with the employee), a team will be assigned to handle the case. A "dress rehearsal" for the arbitration hearing is very helpful, especially for those who have never been to an arbitration hearing. It reduces anxiety and provides a final check on whether everyone is prepared for the real hearing.

The seriousness of the matter usually leads to some self-questioning as to whether the initial decision was correct and if all this further effort is worthwhile. However, not every grievance is justified, and failure to defend a fair decision made by a first-line manager can have a deleterious effect on the morale of all first-line managers and leave employees with the impression that the policy in question does not have to be taken seriously. Seen from this point of view, proceeding to arbitration can be a positive step in management under a collective bargaining agreement.

SUMMARY

Collective bargaining is the joint action taken by employees to gain economic benefits, improved staffing and scheduling, equitable treatment, and improved standards of care from their employer. Opponents of collective bargaining by health care professionals say that it is unprofessional, unethical, divisive, a threat to both job security and organizational health, and unnecessary.

From the employee's point of view, collective bargaining begins with the formation of an organizing council and recognition of a bargaining agent (the professional association or a national union) by the employer. Then contract negotiations begin. If there is a stalemate, mediation, fact finding, binding arbitration, or work stoppages may be used to bring about an agreement. Once a contract is signed, it must be enforced. When a problem arises, the grievance procedure is used to work out the problem as specified in the contract.

From the management's point of view, action can be taken to prevent unionization. These activities include regular surveys of employee opinions, adequate compensation and benefits, an effective grievance procedure, opportunities for participation in decision making, and treating professionals like professionals. More specific measures include controlling communication within the organization and refusing to negotiate with employees in groups. If the organization is unionized, good leadership and management and a thorough knowledge of the contract are the most important components of an effective management strategy for dealing with unionized employees.

REFERENCES*

Bloom, J.R., Parlette, G.N. & O'Reilly, C. (1980). Collective bargaining by nurses: A comparative analysis of management and employee perceptions. *Health Care Management Review*, 5, 25.

Collective Bargaining Agreement Between League of Voluntary Hospitals and Homes of New York and District 1199 Nation Union of Hospital and Health Care Employees, RWDSU/AFL-CIO, 1984–1986.

*Fay, M.S. & Morrill, A. K. (1985). The grievance-arbitration process: The experience of one nursing administration. *Journal of Nursing Administration*, 15 (6), 11–16.

Fossum, J.A. (1979). *Labor Relations: Development, Structure and Process*. Dallas: Business Publications.

Holloway, R.G. (1976). Management can reverse declining employee work attitudes. *Journal of the American Hospital Association*, 50, 71.

Hunter, J.K., Bamberg, D. & Castaglia, P.T. (1986). Job satisfaction: Is collective bargaining the answer? *Nursing Management*, 17 (3), 56–60.

Katz, H.C. (1988). 'Adversarial', not the right word. *Management Review*, 77(2), 21.

*Lockhart, C.A. & Werther, W.B. (1980). *Labor Relations in Nursing*. Wakefield, Massachusetts: Nursing Resources.

*Luttman, P.A. (1982). Collective bargaining and professionalism: Incompatible ideologies? *Nursing Administration Quarterly*, 6 (2), 21.

*Numerof, R. & Abram, M.N. (1984). Collective bargaining among nurses: Current issues and future prospects. *Health Care Management Review*, 9 (2) 61–67.

*O'Rourke, K. & Barton, S.R. (1981). *Nurse power: Unions and the Law*. Bowie, Maryland: Brady Publishing.

Riffer, J. (1986). Physician unions fight loss of control. *Hospitals*, January 20, 82.

Simms, L.M. & Dalston, J.W. (1984). A professional imperative. *Health and Health Services Administration*, 29 (6), 115–123.

The Nation's Health. (1987). Push aimed at reducing numbers of uninsured. *The Nation's Health*, XVII (1), 1, 13.

Thomas, A.W.J. & Murray, V.V. (1976). *Grievance Procedures*. Westmead, England: Saxon House, DC.

Williams, W. (1986) Business brings back the lockout. *The New York Times*, October 5, 1986.

Willis, R. (1988). Can American unions transform themselves? *Management Review*, 77(2), 14–21.

*References marked with an asterisk are suggested for further reading.

UNIT III LEARNING ACTIVITIES ⎯⎯⎯⎯⎯⎯⎯⎯⎯⎯⎯

▷ Obtain a copy of your organization's (or clinical agency's) Table of Organization. Using this as a model for the *formal* level of operation, observe how decisions are made and redraw the Table of Organization to represent the *informal* level of operation. The same can be done with the organization's stated goals and philosophy in comparison with the informal level of operations.

▷ Draw up a table that lists the advantages and disadvantages of each model for delivering nursing care. Discuss the relative importance of each of these and decide which one best suits your philosophy of nursing care and which best suits the organization in which you are working.

▷ Interview a union delegate, union organizer and/or the representative of either the state or local nurses' association regarding the pros and cons of collective bargaining. Compare their answers with the responses of first-line managers, supervisors, and nursing administrators. Whose argument do you find most convincing? Apply the questions from critical analysis to their arguments in reaching your conclusion.

▷ Using the tables in Chapter 12, draw up a set of personal and professional goals, and explain how you plan to achieve them. In particular, consider how you currently spend your time and what modifications you would have to make to achieve your goals.

▷ Either through a literature search or by browsing in the periodical section of your library, find out what new computer programs (software) are available that would be useful to the nurse manager. Try to locate both those that are for general managerial purposes and those that are specifically designed for use in health care.

Unit IV

LEADERSHIP AND MOTIVATION

Chapter 15. Communication
Chapter 16. Understanding Groups
Chapter 17. Leading Meetings and Conferences
Chapter 18. Teamwork and Motivation
Chapter 19. Strategies for Planned Changed
Chapter 20. Leadership in the Community
Unit IV Learning Activities

Chapter 15

OUTLINE

Communication as an Exchange
Elements of the Exchange
Nonverbal Communication
Interpretation

Basic Communication Skills
Attending
Responding
Encouraging Communication with
    Open-ended Questions
Focusing
Clarifying and Checking Out Your
    Perceptions
Personalizing
Giving Information
Support

Confrontation Techniques
Confrontation Defined
Avoiding Confrontation
Confrontation Through Information
Calling the Other's Game
Tape Recordings
Processing
The Confrontation Meeting

Negotiation
Setting the Stage
The Opening Move
Continuing the Negotiation Process
Strategies to Influence the Process

Summary

LEARNING OBJECTIVES

Upon completion of this chapter, the reader will be able to:

▷ Define *communication*, *nonverbal communication*, and *metacommunication*.

▷ Use attending, responding, open-ended questions, focusing, clarifying, personalizing, and giving information to increase the effectiveness of communication.

▷ Describe the type of leadership and management situations in which confrontation and negotiation are appropriate and helpful.

▷ Discuss several precautions to take in confronting others.

▷ Confront and negotiate appropriately and effectively in work situations.

COMMUNICATION

T his chapter is concerned with the whole range of communication skills, from simple listening to asserting your leadership through confrontation and negotiation. The focus is on improving working relationships by improving communications. Effective communication skills are used to establish and maintain productive working relationships, to handle problems that may arise, and to encourage progress toward self-actualization for everyone involved.

The importance of using good communication techniques cannot be overstated. It is one of the hallmarks of effective leadership and management. Research has shown repeatedly that open communication is a major characteristic of successful organizations. Communication affects all aspects of our work, from effective patient care to successful collective bargaining. It is a key element worthy of careful study (Donnellon, Gray, & Bougon, 1986; Wolf, 1986).

COMMUNICATION AS AN EXCHANGE

Communication involves an interaction between at least two people who coact or affect each other. It is not unidirectional. You will recall from the components of effective leadership that you cannot *not* communicate, which means that communication between two people always flows in both directions. Neither person can be left totally unaffected by the exchange. This statement is in accord with the basic principles of systems theory that life is dynamic, not static, and that an interaction between two people is mutual and simultaneous. Everyone involved in the exchange is somehow affected by the exchange and has some effect on it. Consider an example that shows how this happens:

> If you greet a friend with the ritual greeting, "Hi, how are you?" and instead of the ritual response of, "Fine, how are you?" your friend turns away, your friend has clearly communicated that something is wrong even though your friend did not answer you verbally.

This exchange could be diagrammed as a feedback loop as shown in Figure 1–2. in Chapter 1.

When you send a message to someone, that person's response is influenced by the message (both verbal and nonverbal) that you sent as well as by that person's own values, beliefs, present mood, and usual patterns of responding. You, in turn, will be influenced by the way in which the person responds as well as by your own usual patterns of response, beliefs, values, and present mood. The environment will also affect the exchange. To continue the above example:

If you and your friend are walking quickly past each other in a parking lot and you are about to be late for work, the exchange will probably end at this point. But if the two of you are sitting down for a coffee break, the exchange would continue for a while, with you asking what is bothering your friend.

Elements of the Exchange

Every message has two aspects according to Watzlawick and associates (1967). The first aspect is the *content*, or the outward, literal information, of the message. The second is the *relationship* aspect, which tells you how to interpret the message. The relationship aspect is the "information about the information," or the *metacommunication.*

Let us return to the ritual greeting example to illustrate meta-communication:

If, instead of turning away, your friend answered, "Don't ask!" the content aspect or surface message tells you not to question how your friend is feeling. You could take this literally and not ask any more questions, but this may not be what your friend wants you to do.

The metacommunication (which includes the heavy sigh that accompanied the words) will indicate what else your friend is telling you, although not clearly. The sigh has indicated that something is bothering your friend but gives no indication of whether or not your friend wants to discuss it. If your friend puts out hands as if to stop you and turns rapidly away from you, the nonverbal aspect tells you this is not the right time to press for an explanation. But if your friend stops with hand to forehead as if with a headache and looks at you expectantly, the metacommunication tells you something quite different: that your friend is hoping for encouragement from you to talk about the problem.

An interpretation of communications that focuses only on the content aspect or literal meaning of the message is clearly going to miss much of the message or even result in concluding exactly the opposite of what the sender intended to convey. *The more of the metacommunication you can pick up and interpret correctly, the better you can understand the message sent.*

Nonverbal Communication

There are several kinds of nonverbal communication, including body stance and position, sounds, gestures, and tone of voice and emphasis. The *tone of voice* and *emphasis* given to particular words in a statement are so closely related to the content that most of the time people do not consciously separate them when they interpret a message; they hear them together. For example:

"*How* did you do *that?*" asked with exasperation communicates definite disapproval of your behavior. With a different emphasis and some surprise in the tone of voice, the same question — "How did *you* do that?" — indicates there was some doubt about your ability to accomplish whatever is being discussed.

A wide variety of *sounds* (groans, giggles, laughs, sighs) convey meaning by themselves and also serve as "information about the information." *Gestures* can do the same thing. Pointing, grimacing, smiling, nodding, shaking your head, pounding the desk, and stamping your feet all convey meaning. Here is an example:

> A hospitalized stroke patient would vigorously bounce the buttocks up and down on the bed if the call light was not answered immediately. This signal for a bedpan was unmistakable from the hallway, but the patient could not at that time say a word.

Body stance and position within a room can also convey meaning. It is generally believed, for example, that people who sit back in their chairs with their arms folded across their chest are taking a defensive, self-protecting position and will be less open to the group than persons who lean forward and have their arms in a more relaxed position. People who surround themselves with piled-up books or stay behind a desk are also thought to be in a self-protective stance (Lifton, 1972). Those who stand behind a desk, sit in a higher chair, or walk around the outside of the group observing its process are generally maintaining their distance from the group. On the other hand, a group leader who wants to be seen as an equal will select a chair within the group circle to avoid taking an authoritative position. Sitting at a right angle to a person rather than directly across is said to enhance communication (Harris, 1988).

Huge desks, raised platforms, glass enclosures, and many other artifacts are signs of authority and act as distance maintainers. Such symbols are also used to designate status. In some organizations, for example, you can judge a person's rank by the size and finish of the desk:

> The person who sits at a metal desk is lower in rank than the one who sits at an imitation wood grain desk. The person with a wooden desk and a leather chair has made it to the top in such a place.

Nurses' uniforms and name tags fill a similar function. You do not have to be in the armed forces to be aware of different ranks.

Interpretation

The importance of the nonverbal aspect of a message can hardly be overestimated. Mehrabian (1971) found that facial expression has the greatest impact (55 percent) and tone of voice used is second (38 percent). The words themselves have a surprisingly weak effect (7 percent). Unless your words are backed up by a congruent facial expression and tone of voice, they will have little effect or even an unintended negative impact on the listener. With results like these, it is no wonder that therapists emphasize the importance of being genuine or authentic in your responses. Because it is easier to control your words than your nonverbal communication, knowing your real feelings and expressing them appropriately would help to ensure congruence between your verbal and nonverbal messages.

All of these meanings inferred from nonverbal communication need to be interpreted with some care and within the entire context of a situation. The group member with arms crossed might be responding to the low temperature of the room. The group leader sitting within the circle may still be exerting authority, and the nurse in uniform may simply be conforming to the regulations of the employer. A person's motives and the effect on the observer may differ substantially. The meaning of a particular position or stance may not always be the most obvious one. Checking out your perceptions can help you avoid misunderstanding. The more you are able to reduce uncertainty in your communications with others, the greater the degree of understanding will be between you and other people (Gudykunst, Yang, & Nishida, 1987).

BASIC COMMUNICATION SKILLS

This section describes the basic techniques for facilitating effective communication: attending, responding, clarifying, personalizing, and giving information. After presenting the basic communication skills, the more complex leadership skills of confrontation and negotiation are discussed in detail. Each of these increasingly complex communication techniques adds to your repertoire of leadership and management skills.

Attending

Reduced to its most basic meaning, attending is paying attention. To understand the full message being sent, you need to pay attention to all of its aspects: the tone, gestures, body language, words being spoken, and, often, what is not being said as well. This takes concentration and a well-grounded understanding of human nature. How often do people really pay attention to what someone else is saying?

> During a research study, one of the questions asked of the adults being interviewed was how often they listened to their aging mothers or fathers. Their answers show the difference between just hearing and listening with real interest and concentration. Many people said, "Well, I hear him, but I don't really listen," or, "She talks a lot, but I guess I really listen only occasionally." What they were saying is that most of the time they do not really *attend* to what their parent is saying.

This is probably true of most people most of the time. Beginning leaders need to work consciously on increasing the amount of attending they do.

Attending includes listening carefully and observing nonverbal behavior to better understand the message and to let the other person know that you are paying attention. Imagine for a moment how you would feel if you were trying to tell someone something and you get the impression that the person is not really listening (attending) to you. Attending encourages the other person to talk and to express thoughts and feelings. When you really listen, other people feel valued and begin to believe that you understand them. It conveys interest in the other person and can increase the amount of trust between the two of you or between you and a group. You can see that attending is the beginning of developing a relationship of mutual trust and understanding.

Attending can be done both verbally and nonverbally (Egan, 1976). The first way is to *position yourself so that you are facing the person*. This may seem obvious, but this simple technique is often ignored. Here are two examples:

> If you are glancing at papers on your desk or filling out a report form while your colleague is talking to you, you are not fully attending to your colleague. The nurse who turns away to straighten up the dressing tray is also not fully attending to the patient. But if you put down your papers and your pen or your sterile dressings and turn directly toward your colleague or patient, then that person will know you are ready to really listen.

Leaning toward the person speaking also indicates a desire to listen, as if you want to be sure to catch every word. An open posture indicates not only attention but receptiveness to the other person's message.

Maintaining eye contact with the other person is probably the best known of the nonverbal ways to attend. When people first try this, they may stare down the other person, their "attentive" expression frozen on their faces. A comfortable, relaxed, attentive expression and position are what you really want to achieve. If you are tense or distracted, these feelings may be communicated by the rigidity of your position or penetrating eye contact.

Silence accompanied by nonverbal attending is sometimes sufficient to encourage other people to express themselves. Some people are accustomed to doing most of the talking, others rattle on when they get nervous or to fill an uncomfortable silence. If you catch yourself doing either, make a conscious effort to pause a little longer by taking two or three deep breaths or mentally counting to 10 before you jump in to talk or repeat your question. A combination of a little patience, not filling in the silences too quickly, and genuine attentiveness encourages most people to amplify their answers and results in responses that go far beyond your original questions.

There are other times when people overwhelm you with a flood of verbalizing that you need to sort out and direct to make it more constructive and less repetitious. Here, clarifying and focusing (discussed later) are more important communication techniques to use. Somehow, though, it is the silent individual in a group or the reluctant communicator who usually seems to present the most difficulty.

Attentive silence is not always enough to encourage communication and can be overdone (Brammer, 1985). Responses like "Uh huh," "Mm, hmm," "Yes," or "I see what you mean," (if you really do) can be used to convey more interest and encourage the person to continue. You can also reflect by repeating a key word or phrase the person has used to focus on the aspect of the conversation; you can ignore the extraneous or irrelevant parts by not attending to them.

Avoid the repetition of a single phrase over and over again, especially in the same exchange. It can lose its meaning and sound mechanical, which defeats the purpose of responding. People who are just learning to use active listening often sound like prerecorded messages.

You need to listen for both information and feelings. Look for patterns and themes in what the person is saying. A person may, for example, repeat a particular point over and over again. The same situation can provoke different responses in different people. When you want to understand what a person is telling you, try to see it through that person's frame of reference rather than through your own.

You need to pay attention to the nonverbal message as well: the tone of voice, the body position, facial expression, and so on. Does the person seem depressed and slumped in a chair or rigid with pent-up anger? Are the hands shaking or is the voice quivering with emotion? Is the individual drained of energy or full of vigor and functioning well? Even poor grooming can be a sign of a low energy level, although you need to take culture and individual style into consideration (and in interpretation of communication in general). Finally, look for congruence or the lack of it between the two aspects of the communication.

Attending done with ease, warmth, and real caring can be communicated in your tone of voice, body language, and words. It will help you accomplish your goal of making the other person feel accepted, valued, and at ease talking with you. Once attending becomes a natural thing for you to do, it will be most effective. Genuineness will improve effectiveness. As Perls once said, "Our bodies do not lie (Brammer, 1985)."

Responding

Responding requires a more active kind of communication than attending. Responding is an accurate rephrasing of the message you received from the other person (Carkhuff, 1983). It is done to communicate a basic comprehension of what the other person is saying and to sustain the exchange.

You can respond to the content of the message, to the feelings communicated in the message, or to both. Two examples of responding to content are:

"In other words, schoolwork has been your major source of difficulty."

"You're saying that your team leader doesn't seem to recognize your needs as an individual."

Two examples of responding to the feelings conveyed by the other person in verbal and nonverbal communication are:

"You're worried about the outcome of this dispute."

"You feel great when someone recognizes your contribution."

Notice that you can respond to good feelings as well as bad ones, something people often forget.

There are innumerable instances in a work situation where responding is appropriate. Here are some additional examples of responding to content.

"You're saying that Deborah does not record everything she does for a patient."

"In other words, the staff does not really understand what a nursing audit involves."

The following are some examples of responding to both feelings and contents.

"You're upset about forgetting Mrs. C.'s extra sitz bath."

"You feel good about helping the L. family find a place for Suzie."

"You feel torn by the need to get the paperwork done and the need to spend time visiting Mr. D."

Responses that include feelings as well as content are more complete, although in work situations a response with just content may be appropriate, and either can be used alone.

Encouraging Communication with Open-ended Questions

Sometimes, more initiative from the leader is needed, particularly in beginning the exchange. Here, open-ended questions are very useful. They may also be used to guide an exchange and to keep it going.

An open-ended question is one that cannot be answered with a single word like "yes" or "no." A question may sound encouraging and yet not be really open-ended. For example:

If you ask, "Do you want to talk about it?" and the person responds with "No," the exchange is stopped cold, and it will be harder than ever to get a discussion underway.

Asking a truly open-ended question like, "What seems to be troubling you?" or asking the person to tell you more about something will be far more likely to initiate a productive exchange. This applies to all kinds of situations. The following illustrates the difference between an open-ended question and one that only sounds open ended.

NOT OPEN-ENDED   Do you like your new assignment?

OPEN-ENDED   Tell me, how do you feel about your new assignment?

The first question requests only a short answer, while the second encourages a much freer response and sets up expectations for a longer exchange.

You can also ask the person or group to give examples of what they mean, to elaborate, to describe, or to tell you more about the subject under discussion. For example:

If a coworker describes a relationship with another staff member as "poor," you can ask the coworker to tell you what it is about the relationship that makes it poor.

These open-ended questions also encourage the other person to give more thought to the subject and to develop a greater awareness of the complexities involved in a situation. When a problem arises, it is often important to seek elaboration and explanations such as, "What do you mean by . . ." or even just, "Tell me what happened," in order to encourage discussion and to increase understanding.

Focusing

A leader may need to use several other communication techniques to make the exchange most helpful for all concerned. The exchange may be vague and need more focus or it may be confusing and need clarification. When you do not understand what the problem is, you may need to do more exploration of the subject.

If you have had the experience of allowing others to ventilate their feelings without making any attempt to direct the flow of words, you will know why there are times when you need to bring more focus into an exchange.

Several ways are available to bring focus to an interaction. You can focus on the most pressing problem, the main point of an exchange, who owns the problem, the dominant theme that runs through a person's rambling, or the aspect of a problem for which a solution can be found. A focus on feelings may be needed in some instances. For example:

A discussion may be centering on the problems your staff expect to face in implementing a new procedure, but you suspect that the main difficulty is related to the anxieties aroused by the change from a familiar routine. To deal with the feelings aroused by the change, you need to refocus the discussion. One way you could do this would be to say, "You've all indicated in one way or another that this new procedure is going to be difficult to do. How do you feel about this?"

Focusing helps to pull seemingly unconnected statements together and to direct attention to the most important or solvable problems, or both.

To focus on the main point, you can repeat key words or phrases as questions or use open-ended questions. For example:

> Erratic behavior?
>
> Can you tell me more about Delia's behavior, specifically here on the unit?
>
> You've been talking about several things that are on your mind. Which of them concerns you the most?

Personal crises and conflicts among staff members are not at all uncommon. When dealing with a crisis situation, you may often find it helpful to focus on the part of the problem that can be solved. This would usually be done after allowing ventilation of feelings through active listening. For example, once an accident has occurred, a focus on minimizing its effects is more productive than a focus on placing blame.

Sometimes, the difficulty lies in identifying who owns the problem. For example:

> Is Delia's behavior Delia's problem, or is it Jose's problem because it irritates him so much? Does the problem also belong to you, the nurse manager, because your team cannot function effectively with the constant friction between Delia and Jose?

Open-ended questions can be useful in bringing some focus to a discussion as well as in getting it started.

Clarifying and Checking Out Your Perceptions

If you keep on nodding your head in agreement when you really don't know what others are talking about, it will be difficult to respond when they ask, "What do you think about this?" Pretending to understand undermines trust and discourage further exchanges.

If you get lost and cannot follow what the person is saying, then you can say, "I lost you there," or, "I'm not sure what you mean." You can also use the focusing kinds of open-ended questions to clarify. For example:

> When a coworker is upset and repeating a description of being continually harassed by the administration, you could ask, "Would you give me an example of what you mean by 'harassment'?"

When your main purpose is to check out your perceptions, rather than to reduce confusion, what you say will give more of an indication of what you understood the other person to be saying. This usually includes a rephrasing in your own words. For example:

> Did you mean that Delia's gum chewing and joke cracking irritates the patients?
>
> Are you saying that my observing your work upsets you?

Personalizing

As the exchange progresses, you may find it necessary to pull together what has been said and add some meaning to it, a technique termed *personalizing* (Carkhuff, 1983). This technique has two purposes. The first is to facilitate increased self-awareness and exploration of the many human factors involved in any situation. The second purpose is to facilitate progress toward a clear identification of the problem (problem solving).

Personalizing does involve some interpretation, more than the preceding actions did in most cases. It involves a response to the individual that includes a summary of the situation, a description of the meaning it has to that person, and the ways in which that person has and has not been able to cope with it. It is really an extension of responding. The main difference is found in the added meanings you are offering. Here are some examples of personalizing.

> You feel torn by the need to do your paperwork and to visit longer with Mr. D. because you cannot find the time to do both and yet believe both are important.

> Delia's behavior upsets you because it seems to make the patients irritable. As a result, it is harder to keep them comfortable and satisfied with their care.

When you are not certain your interpretation is correct or if you want to avoid an "I know better than you do" posture, you can put your personalizing comments in the form of a question.

Giving Information

Once a problem or need has been identified, a lack of information is often found to be the culprit. A professional is frequently called on to share expertise, and this sharing of knowledge is an expected part of the leader's and manager's roles. The following are two examples of situations in which information giving is appropriate:

> Patients frequently are not given adequate information about their problems, about procedures that are going to be done, or about regimens they are expected to follow at home.

> Staff members are often faced with a similar lack of information about work expectations, procedures, and so forth that create unnecessary frustration and difficulties.

Information giving and advice are *not* the same thing. Brammer (1985) thinks that advice is appropriate only if the final decision is left up to the person receiving it. It may also be appropriate in times of crisis when people cannot make a decision by themselves or in a relatively inconsequential decision where the outcome is not very important. Any kind of advice giving has its disadvantages: the danger of fostering dependency, the possibility that your advice may be wrong for that individual, and, finally, the fact that most people won't follow it anyway.

Support

Being a trustworthy, available listener is a very effective way to provide support.

Assistance in a time of crisis can be very supportive and will help the person get through the crisis intact and better able to function without encouraging long-term dependence. Finding transportation, making that difficult telephone call, or filling out that impossible form are all examples of concrete help you can offer a client or coworker when the individual is overloaded or under severe stress.

Reassurance, on the other hand, should be given only in small doses, if at all, because it seems to minimize the problem or encourage dependency

(Brammer, 1985). Reassuring phrases such as, "It will all work out" sound false to the person who is desperately worried. Agreeing with the other person's statements or plans and telling that person that others have had the same problems are actually forms of reassurance also and should be used in small doses.

When a very difficult situation exists, these basic communication techniques are only the beginning of the intervention process. They can be used to increase readiness to negotiate and solve problems and will be useful throughout the relationship to keep the negotiation or problem-solving process going.

CONFRONTATION TECHNIQUES

There are times when people—staff members, colleagues, or supervisors—will not readily participate in free and open communications. This can happen for any number of reasons: conflicts arise, defensiveness is high, trust or empathy is limited, the problem-solving process gets bogged down, and so forth. As the leader or manager, you will face these situations. They are difficult to handle, but a group of communication skills known as *confrontation techniques* (Tappen, 1978) can help you break up these common interpersonal log jams.

Confrontation Defined

Confrontation is a direct approach to a problem or conflict. It is an act that challenges others, pulls them up short, directs them to reflect on their behavior and, as a result, change that behavior. People often do not realize how their behavior affects others until they are confronted with these effects.

Walton (1969) defines confrontation as the "process in which the parties directly engage each other and focus on the conflict between them." It is not just "telling someone off." Correctly done, it is *not* a hostile attack on another person.

Anyone in a group or organization can confront an individual or a whole group. The nursing staff of one unit can confront the pharmacy over medication distribution problems or the dietary department about the adequacy of nutrition education for their patients. Aides may confront nurses, the medical staff may confront administration, and so on. One organization may confront another organization. For example, a state nurse's association may confront a hospital on employment issues or another professional organization on encroachment into nursing functions. The special logistics of organizational confrontation are often political strategies or collective bargaining (see Chapters 14 and 20). These groups may designate representatives to confront and then negotiate with one another.

Avoiding Confrontation

The leader should move quickly to intervene when progress toward a goal ceases. Avoidance of problems is usually unproductive because they tend to grow larger if left unmanaged. People often think, "If I leave it alone,

maybe it will resolve itself." While sometimes true, more often minor disagreements become major conflicts and small misunderstandings become
serious communication blocks when they are not resolved.

Former Secretary of State Henry Kissinger noted for his negotiation
skills, expressed the same idea this way: "Competing pressures tempt one to
believe that an issue deferred is a problem avoided; more often it is a crisis
invited" (Kissinger, 1979). Delaying a confrontation also increases the likelihood that by the time you finally do confront the issue, you and the other
party involved are so frustrated and angry that your effectiveness in carrying
out that confrontation is reduced.

Your silence in the face of a conflict can be interpreted as acceptance of
the status quo. If you fail to confront a problem, you will lose opportunities
to open communication and promote growth. Stereotypes will prevail and
misunderstandings continue unless you confront what is happening. The
following story is an illustration of what can be lost if you fail to confront a
problem when this action is needed:

> A student in a community health nursing course visited a young mother (about 15 years old)
> every week to see how she and her infant were progressing. Every week the mother
> undressed the baby, and every week the student did a complete physical assessment of
> the infant's condition. At the end of the semester, the student would no longer be visiting the
> young mother and informed her of this. The mother then asked if the student had found her
> care of the infant satisfactory. This question led to a more open discussion than had
> occurred before and some surprising discoveries.
>
> The young mother thought the student was coming to check the infant for signs of
> neglect and abuse because the student had been sent by a government agency, the public
> health department. The student had thought that the mother wanted the infant checked
> every week to see if the infant was all right. The mother feared that any negative evaluation
> from the student would result in the baby's being taken away from her. The student had
> been aware of the fact that there was little trust between them but had failed to confront
> the problem until the client did so at this last meeting. What a loss for both of them that the
> misperception of each other's motives was not dealt with sooner.

Many writers have been critical of nurses' tendency to avoid confrontation. Nurses, they say, lack assertiveness. They nurture and protect people
when they should confront and challenge them. This tendency is attributed
to a caring, humanitarian set of values and also to the habit of overclassify-
ing people as "sick" and in need of help rather than as well and able to
handle a confrontation (Smoyak, 1974). This situation is changing rapidly
for some nurses and gradually for others. Many nurses are becoming more
assertive and confronting.

Your colleagues can handle an objective and appropriate confrontation.
So can your employer. In fact, when you are too protective of them, you
violate your own rights. The following is an example of how this can happen.

> Imagine that your employer has refused to consider your request for a salary increase and
> tells you how much the agency would like to give you a raise but cannot because of its
> terrible financial troubles. If you are prone to using the unassertive approach, you can find
> yourself reassuring your employer that it's all right and you understand the problem. This is
> an inappropriate use of reassurance; you are trying to help your employer feel better
> when, in fact, by doing so, you will feel worse, or at least poorer. A more appropriate
> initial response would be to describe your accomplishments and your value to the
> organization.

Some people avoid confrontation because they fear retaliation. This fear is not always unreasonable; in fact, it may be realistic in some instances. Bennis (1976) provides an example of a situation where retaliation is a possibility:

Samuel Goldwyn (the movie producer), a notorious martinet, called his top staff together after a particularly bad box-office flop and said, "Look, you guys, I want you to tell me exactly what's wrong with this operation and my leadership—even if it means losing your jobs."

If you are unfortunate enough to work for a "notorious martinet," you should consider retaliation a possibility. However, in most cases, a confrontation done well is much more likely to improve your work situation than remove you from it.

There are several confrontation strategies that differ in content, method, and strength. We will begin with the most common strategy, confrontation through information, and then look at several useful variations of it.

Confrontation Through Information

Confrontation through information is one of several strategies suggested by Egan (1973). This type of confrontation is frequently delivered as an "I" message, to use Gordon's (1970) term. It is the honest, open, and direct communication of the way you are experiencing a situation. Its purpose is to foster openness in the relationship, especially to stimulate a reciprocal open response to you in order to improve the interpersonal relationship involved. Indirectly, it is a challenge to the other person. The following are examples of confrontation through information.

I was embarrassed that the lounge was dirty when our visitors came through today.

I have been assigned the last-minute tasks every day this week.

I'm afraid that we're not going to get done on time.

Confrontation through information is a powerful form of communication that should be used with respect for its force (Walton, 1969). *Do confront*—and do it with care for the other person or persons. Several cautions are important to keep in mind. First, *do not make the confrontation message a statement of blame*. Messages that begin with "you" instead of "I" tend to put all the blame on the other person. For example:

You didn't clean up the lounge after your break.

You've been picking on me, giving me all the last-minute tasks every day this week.

You're running late again today.

These "you" messages usually provoke defensive responses such as:

If it's so important, why didn't *you* clean it up?

I couldn't help it.

No, I'm not!

The fact that a message begins with "I" is not enough if a put-down or blaming message is hidden in the confrontation. For example, "I am really disappointed in you," is full of blame even though it looks like an "I" message. A little more subtle but still negative is, "I feel that you have been careless." You can be sure that these lightly disguised blaming messages will be recognized for what they are by the person receiving them. Instead, put the emphasis on your feelings in these messages and avoid blaming the other person.

A second important point is *do not use confrontation to make blanket negative statements about the other person* or group such as, "You are so lazy," or, "You never get your work done." It is also important to avoid psychoanalyzing, which is almost guaranteed to provoke a defensive response. Some example of psychoanalyzing statements:

> You have trouble relating to patients because you're always on an ego trip.
>
> Your insecurity is at the root of all your problems here.
>
> Your hostility is showing.

How would you feel if someone said those things to you? How would you react?

Direct challenges to shape up also provoke more defensive than honest attempts to improve. Some direct challenges are:

> Why don't you pay more attention?
>
> Pull yourself together.

The inappropriate confrontations often contain a ready-made solution devised by the confronter. All the nonrecommended forms of confrontation show more concern for the confronter than for the confronted and a lack of faith in the confronted person's or group's ability to make constructive decisions to change. Direct challenges are usually stronger than they need to be.

Confrontations have impact. The importance of the contents of the message can vary from person to person. A particular message could stir a painful memory or strike an Achilles heel (a particularly vulnerable spot). For example, the joking comment to a colleague who forgot a meeting— "You're getting so forgetful; it must be hardening of the arteries"—might sound funny to a younger colleague but hurt an older one who is fighting a mandatory retirement.

Inappropriate confrontations are often done in anger. Gordon (1970) believes that anger is a secondary response following the earlier primary reaction of fright, embarrassment, or disappointment. For example, anger at a coworker's rough handling of a patient with multiple myeloma is the secondary result of your fear that the patient will be hurt. Anger at a friend who reveals a confidence may be secondary to the embarrassment you feel. It is the primary reaction you should express in a confrontation, not the secondary anger, which may carry a blaming message with it.

This caution applies only to anger and other negative feelings such as wanting to get revenge on someone. Ordinarily, you do not want to minimize your feelings. If you are very disturbed about a particular situation, then say so rather than minimizing it so much that no one recognizes your concern.

The inappropriate confrontations are so labeled for some very specific reasons. They provoke defensive or angry responses, imply a lack of trust in others' abilities to find their own solutions, reinforce feelings of inadequacy, or emphasize your needs at the expense of the other person or group. In other words, they are not constructive.

It is possible for a confrontation through information to be ignored. Usually this happens when you have understated your own feelings regarding the situation. If this does happen, you can tell the other person how you feel about being ignored—this usually gets through to the other person (Gordon, 1970).

When you confront someone, be prepared to be confronted in return. In fact, a whole lot of issues may arise as a result of a confrontation, issues that had not been confronted in the past and so were left to develop and grow more serious. This multiplication of issues is called *issue proliferation* and will be discussed later, in the section on confrontation meetings. Frequent confrontations through information and the fostering of an open climate prevent issue proliferation.

When you are confronted in return, use attending, responding, and other communication skills to identify clearly the problems that exist in the relationship between you and the other person or group you confronted. The return confrontation may be in the form of "you" messages and direct challenges, so try to avoid the defensiveness that could turn the confrontation into an angry exchange.

Calling the Other's Game

We often find ourselves getting caught up in "games" with other people such as, "Let's keep talking about the weather and avoid the problems we face," or, "I won't mention any of your shortcomings if you won't mention any of mine," or, "If you yell, I'll yell louder," and many others (Egan, 1973). There is a whole series of these games given humorous titles in transactional analysis (Berne, 1964, 1972). People can get caught up in these games without realizing it.

The leader-manager with a heightened consciousness of these games will be able to spot them and take action to break them up. To do this, the effective leader makes an unexpected response that breaks up the game by refusing to play it. For example, social chatter is sometimes used to avoid getting down to work or facing the unpleasant decision. The following demonstrates how the leader can call such a game:

SOCIAL CHATTER: Staff 1: Did you hear that M. got a new sports car?

                          Staff 2: No, where did you hear that?"

                          Staff 1: Well, I was down in the cafeteria getting some coffee and Danish when. . . .

BREAKING UP THE GAME: Leader: Let's get started on that report.

While this game is a time waster, it is otherwise harmless. Others are far more destructive but are still broken up by simply refusing to play them.

A game that is peculiarly appealing to members of the helping professions is called the Karpman Triangle (Karpman, 1968). Nurses are expert players of this game. There are three roles to choose from in the triangle: victim, persecutor, and rescuer (Fig. 15–1). Participants switch from one role to another around the triangle. To break up the game, participants must refuse to play *any* of these roles and instead give a nondefensive and non-hostile adult response.

To illustrate the Karpman Triangle, we can return to the earlier example about asking for a raise.

> Saying "no" to you makes your employer feel like a persecutor, so your employer switches into the victim role by telling you of all the budgetary woes and saying that it is impossible to give you a raise. If you respond by telling your employer you understand the trouble, you've been sucked into the game in the rescuer role. Responding in a nondefensive, adult manner by describing your contributions to the organization is one way to avoid getting trapped in the game.

Nurses can get caught in this particular game with their patients or clients too. For example:

> Let's say you have a patient who has missed three important appointments in a row. When you visit the patient at home to find out what the problem is, she tells you she is really sorry but she has to babysit her sister's children all day so she cannot get out to the clinic. Your patient has moved into the victim role. You have several choices for a response, all common responses from caregivers:
>
> 1. You could scold her for missing the appointment and tell her not to miss the next one.
> 2. You could offer to babysit the children while she goes to the clinic.

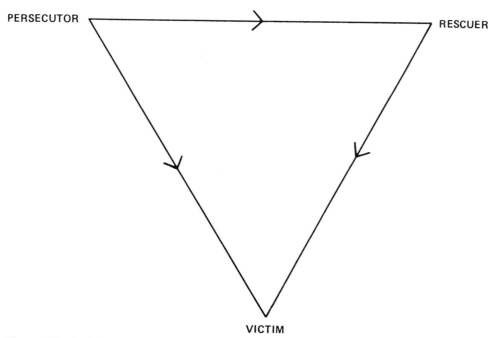

Figure 15–1. The Karpman triangle. A game in which players frequently switch roles. (From Karpman, SB: Fairy Tales and Script Drama Analysis. Transactional Analysis Bulletin [now TA Journal] 7:26 [April 1968] p 39.)

3. You could ask her how she is going to solve her problem.

Which one of these options would you choose?

1. If you chose the first, you would have moved right into the persecutor role in response to her victim role, giving her a good excuse not to go to the clinic where those *heartless* people are who want her to leave her sister's babies alone or take them out with her in this cold weather.

2. If you chose the second, you would be rushing into the rescuer role and leave her expecting to have you babysit the next time she has to go to the clinic. If you do this, you have also lost the opportunity to help her problem solve, a skill many people have not learned very well.

3. The third choice speaks to the responsible adult your patient is and gives her credit for being able to handle everyday problems herself or at least to make her own choices among the alternatives that you can help her come up with.

Breaking up the game with a client is in keeping with the notion that clients should be treated as partners in their care and as responsible adults capable of varying amounts of self-care.

Tape Recordings

Videotapes and audio recordings are objective confrontations in which an individual or group can see themselves almost in the same way that others see and hear them. Tapes are a "clean" confrontation (Egan, 1973) because they are not filtered through another person's perceptions of a situation.

These recordings create a permanent record that can be analyzed objectively to improve performance. So much goes on at one time in a group that you frequently see things on the videotape that you did not even realize were happening in the midst of the interaction. Videotapes can also be used to evaluate nurse-patient interactions and the correctness of technical procedures as well as interviews, staff conferences, and the like.

They are also useful in analyzing the effectiveness of a leader, the responses of a group to its leader and the responses of individual members to one another.

Knowing that they are being taped increases self-consciousness in some people. Making the recorder unobtrusive helps to keep them focused on their purpose as does the use of tapes only for self-improvement rather than for grading or job evaluation purposes. Tapes should be used only with the knowledge and consent of those who are being recorded.

Processing

This is another form of confrontation described by Egan (1973). Processing is a direct commentary on the group process. The degree of directness can vary. To illustrate this, imagine that you are working with a group of parents and not making any progress at all:

One way to get the group moving is to stop the group interaction and ask the group to evaluate what has been happening within it. In a more direct way, you can point out that the group seems to be getting nowhere and ask group members if they agree, why they think this is happening, or both. Most directly, you can point out the hidden agenda that is blocking the group's process and say, "None of you really wants a sex education program and that's why we're not getting anywhere."

This last, very direct type of processing is a direct challenge. However, there will be times when this much directness is the only way to break up a real stalemate. While you risk having people becoming defensive, you might also get a direct response in return such as:

"You're right. We have been dragging our feet on this. Let's get going."

Rogers (1970) says that he does not like to use direct processing because it makes the group too self-conscious and slows down its processes, all of which destroy spontaneity. If comments are needed, it is best to have them come from the group. He tends to avoid probing into what is behind behavior (interpreting or psychoanalyzing) because it can never be more than an educated guess in any circumstances.

Despite these limitations, processing has some real benefits. Rogers's groups generally had more time to deal with a situation than the work groups that a nurse leader encounters every day. While open communication and increased group awareness are important goals for work groups, too, you cannot always wait for the group to achieve them spontaneously. The less directive kind of processing strategy in which you verbalize your observations of group process without interpreting the reasons for the behavior can be very useful in stimulating group awareness and in getting the process going, both of which are part of the leader's role.

An *indirect* way to confront a group or individual through processing is to change some aspect of their routine function. Both individuals and groups get into routines that they find hard to break. Just rearranging the chairs into a circle so that no one can hide in the back can change group interaction (and indirectly confronts those who were hiding in the back). Did you ever wonder how a class would react if a professor began to lecture standing in the back of the room? You can also introduce new members into a group to change the dynamics—for example, staff from other units or from other disciplines. Including patients and their families in a patient-centered conference makes it much harder to talk about the patient as a nonperson when the patient is sitting right there (although some care givers manage to do so anyway, especially on rounds in a hospital). Any strategy that points out or changes the status quo will confront the individual or group with the way in which they have been behaving.

The Confrontation Meeting

The confrontation meeting (Beckhard, 1969) is a strong, dynamic form of confrontation. A large number of people can be involved. The leader may confront the group or vice versa, or an individual member of the group may initiate the confrontation. It can be an effective way to bring about change if you can handle it. It can also happen spontaneously, usually as the result of an accumulation of unexpressed feelings or unresolved conflicts.

In a productive confrontation meeting, the group as a whole quickly assesses its own conflicts and within hours negotiates a plan for resolving them. A confrontation meeting usually has a high degree of open communication and mutual confrontation. The information exchanged during the meeting is current and subject to validation by those present. The release of unexpressed feelings and expression of unresolved conflicts means that emotions will be high, even intense. This sharing of feelings and information increases the level of trust within the group if communications are kept on a mature, constructive level. During a confrontation, a skilled leader is needed to:

1. Make sure everybody is heard.
2. List or at least keep track of everything that is said. (This task can be delegated to a responsible individual.)
3. Guide the group toward using "I" messages and constructive criticism rather than direct challenges and blaming, destructive kinds of criticism.
4. Use attending and responding skills to keep communication flowing, and use focusing, clarifying, and sometimes informing skills to set the stage for negotiating a settlement of the differences.

During the meeting, intentions and procedures are clarified, issues needing attention are brought out, and plans are made for resolving the conflicts. Negotiation is usually needed to devise a plan agreeable to all and to bring the meeting to a satisfying conclusion.

Before reaching the negotiation stage, attitudes and feelings need to be explored. Participants describe how they see themselves and how they see the other party during a confrontation. This brings out the misunderstandings and misinterpretations of each other's behavior that have been operating. Explanations of the real motivations behind the behavior and increased ability to see each other as individuals, rather than in stereotyped roles, can resolve the conflict that led to the confrontation (Filley, 1975).

A whole host of issues may arise in addition to the one that sparked the confrontation meeting in the first place. This is called *issue proliferation* (Walton, 1969). It can be an attempt to save face on the part of the confronted person or group, it can be a counterattack, or it can be the result of the unleashing of pent-up emotions and frustrations.

If these new issues are symptoms of the basic conflict and fairly easy to resolve, you may want to deal with them first in order to interrupt the continuing build-up of negative feelings and to demonstrate the possibility of constructive action. If they are not easily resolved or sidetrack the group from the basic conflict, you will find it more productive to lead the discussion back to the main issues. Sometimes, they indicate that a far more basic conflict is operating than the one that had begun the confrontation meeting. If this happens, the more basic conflict should become the major focus of the discussion and of the negotiations that follow.

An increase in tensions usually accompanies issue proliferation. When this happens you will find it necessary to set some limits in order to reduce and control the tension. Walton compares this to the use of boxing gloves in a fight: it softens the blows (Walton, 1969). Openness should be encouraged; power plays should be discouraged. Putting all the blame on one person should not be allowed; destructive criticism and name calling also should not be allowed. Allow only constructive criticism and suggestions for improvement that are both specific and concrete ways to improve whatever is criticized.

A moderate level of tension sustains the confrontation, although too much will increase hostility and may become intolerable to some people. Humor is an excellent tension reliever. Occasionally, a cooling-off period or premeetings with individuals can be used to reduce tensions, but they should not be used to avoid confrontation.

Listing the issues that are in conflict helps to keep the confrontation in focus and under control. This can be followed by asking for alternative solutions, which usually succeeds in creating a more cooperative atmosphere. However, you do not want to cut short the discussion of the problems by doing this too soon.

A confrontation meeting is an efficient, effective way for you to determine the sources and extent of a serious conflict and to come up with ways to resolve the problems involved. If you plan such a meeting, it is essential to approach it with a willingness to be confronted as well as to confront, to handle the intense feelings, to listen, to change yourself as well as others, and, perhaps most important in the long run, to follow up on the resulting plans made. Failure to follow through on the plans made will negate the entire process, close off communication again (probably more than before), and reduce trust dramatically. But if you are prepared to do all these things, a group of people can accomplish more in one intensive confrontation meeting than they ordinarily would do in a month otherwise.

NEGOTIATION

Negotiation is a give-and-take situation between individuals or groups during which the parties involved try to come up with a resolution of their problems that is acceptable to all concerned. It is needed to resolve complex problems, especially conflicts, once they have been identified and explored. Much more has been written about facilitating open communication and confronting problems than about negotiation, as if it is assumed that once you have an agreement with the other person or group on what the problem is, you will also agree on the solution. Such an assumption is false.

A lot of questions can arise during the negotiation. Should you compromise? If you're willing to concede something, should you do it immediately or wait until the negotiations get bogged down? Should you start out tough or try to sound reasonable? Who wins? Most of the literature concerns union–management relations, but negotiation can be necessary in any interpersonal relationship. It is discussed in this more general sense of resolving interpersonal conflicts.

Setting the Stage

Several conditions set the stage for negotiation (Lax & Sebenius, 1986; Rubin & Brown, 1975). First, of course, there must be a *recognized conflict of interest or incompatibility* between the people or groups involved. Those involved in the negotiation must be prepared (usually by using some form of confrontation) to enter into the exchange of offers and counteroffers that constitute the negotiation process.

Another condition that is often overlooked is that the *relationship must be voluntary*. This means that the people involved must want the relationship to continue but have the option to withdraw from the relationship. In fact, it is the existence of this option to withdraw that motivates both sides to seek a resolution that will allow the relationship to continue. In an employment relationship, for example, as an employee, you have the option (however reluctantly you might exercise it) to quit, and your employer has the option (however reluctantly) to fire you.

Negotiations should end in an agreement that satisfies everyone involved. It should be a win-win proposition, not win-lose. Ideally, both sides should feel as if they had won; neither should feel as if it had lost or even had to compromise something important to it. Realistically, however, some negotiations will turn out to be win-lose situations in which at least one party has to compromise, usually when the distribution of power is unequal. Telbert King, an expert union negotiator, recommends that you try hard *not* to compromise your fundamental position in any negotiation (King, 1982).

The *key issues* must be identified at the beginning of negotiation. These are the issues that are of primary concern to the people involved in the negotiation. You need to find out as much as possible about the other side's position on the key issues and any underlying emotional issues that may be disguised as disagreements over policies during the confrontation and the discussions that follow. Your knowledge of human motivation and behavior is very useful in doing this.

The key issues may be divided into two categories: emotional issues and substantive issues. *Emotional issues* may revolve around feelings such as desire for recognition or status, fear of rejection, anxiety, or personal need deprivation. *Substantive issues* are concerned with such things as policies, rules and regulations, differing concepts of roles, role invasion, salary, and other questions about the work being done and the way it is organized (Walton, 1969). Any situation that has created enough conflict to require negotiation usually has a mixture of both the emotional and substantive issues. Actually, considering the holistic nature of human beings, both cognitive and affective needs will be operating at any given time. But separating the issues into emotional and substantive helps you to identify all the major issues and decide which is primary in a given situation.

The Opening Move

The opening move in a negotiation is considered a decisive point by most negotiators because it sets the climate or tone for the rest of the negotiation. "Extreme but not ridiculous," seems to be the best description of the general rule for making your opening move. In other words, you should begin the negotiation phase by informing the other person or group of the full extent, unmodified, of what it is that you want. Here is an example:

> Let's say that you are negotiating for a new position. If you think $25,000 is a reasonable beginning salary but really want $29,000, then begin the negotiations by asking for the upper limit of your expectations, which in this instance is $29,000. If you begin by asking for $25,000, you really have very little chance of getting $29,000, and in the negotiating, you are likely to come down a little in your demands.

Beginning with the upper limit of your wishes makes you more likely to get what you think is reasonable. Do not worry too much about seeming unreasonable—you will have an opportunity to demonstrate your reasonableness later in the negotiation. To reiterate, avoid the absurd demand, but inform the other party of the upper limit of what you want from the negotiation in the crucial opening move.

It is far harder to escalate your demands later than to moderate them. Moderating your demands in a later move makes you seem more cooperative. The extreme (but within reason) opening move sets the tone of the negotiation. It allows you room to negotiate without having to compromise your needs and gives you time and space within which to move and to find out more about the other person's or group's preferences and intentions. It also communicates that you will not allow yourself to be exploited, which may be even more important. It is an assertive position that has proved to be the most effective way to begin negotiations. At least one research study indicated that it is by far the most influential factor deciding the outcome of negotiations. The extreme opening move followed by gradual concessions results in far more satisfaction with the outcome than a moderate stance held firmly (Rubin, 1975).

The recommended pattern for a negotiation, then, is a tough opening move followed by willingness to make some concessions but not to give in on the basic needs that led you into the negotiation process in the first place. The effect of a strong opening move in collective bargaining was tested in the experiment described in Research Example 15–1.

Continuing the Negotiation Process

Following the opening moves from both sides, the rest of the negotiation is a series of offers, counteroffers, and elaborations of each side's position until an agreement is reached. Too many concessions made too quickly will weaken your ability to get any concessions from the other side. Since negotiations proceed most effectively under conditions of relatively equal power, making concessions too quickly could be giving too much of your power away to the other side. It is more effective to pace your concessions in order to appear cooperative but firm.

As the negotiation process proceeds, each side is trying to do several things. They will still be seeking to find out the real preferences of the other side. They will also be attempting to communicate their own positions more clearly. Most important, each side will be trying to influence the outcome of the negotiation. To show how events lead up to this point and then proceed to a series of offers, counteroffers, and elaborations, an example of a common staffing problem will be used.

> A group of staff nurses has confronted their head nurse because they are dissatisfied with the organization of nursing care on their unit. As a result of their confrontation meeting with the head nurse, the group concludes that the main conflict is over the way in which each nurse is assigned a different set of patients daily. The result of this assignment procedure is that continuity of care on the unit is minimal; the satisfactions that result from continuity have been drastically reduced; the staff nurses believe that they have no autonomy; and the head nurse thinks that the staff has been uncooperative.
>
> In their opening move, the staff nurses declare that they should be allowed to choose their own patients and be assigned the same patients every day. The head nurse responds

RESEARCH EXAMPLE 15–1. A Simulated Negotiation

Is a tough initial stance more effective than a soft one in the opening move of a negotiation? What effect does mediation or arbitration have on the course and the outcome of negotiations?

A simulated collective bargaining game was used by Bigoness (1976) to compare the effects of taking a hard or soft initial position and the effects of anticipating mediation, voluntary arbitration, or compulsory arbitration on a negotiation. To provide some incentive to bargain seriously, game players were paid on the basis of their success in bargaining for wages, fringe benefits, and cost-of-living increases.

Game players were divided into pairs: one of the pair represented management, the other represented the union. Each was instructed to take a hard or soft initial position. For example, a soft management position was to offer a 6-cent increase, while the tough position was to offer a 2-cent increase. On the other side, the soft union position was to demand 10 cents more and the tough position was an opening demand for a 20-cent increase. Pairs of players who were assigned to mediation or arbitration were told to accept a 12-cent increase for either if they had not reached an agreement on their own after 15 minutes of play.

When analyzed, the results showed that the total amount eventually conceded by management was significantly less under a tough initial stance than under a soft one. The difference was not significant for the union side. However, fewer issues were left unresolved at the end of the game when management began with a soft stance.

The least number of issues was left unresolved when straight bargaining without mediation or arbitration was done. Compulsory arbitration left fewer issues unresolved than mediation or voluntary arbitration. Mediation usually was not successful. The researcher found that the players were most likely to reach a successful agreement when they could not anticipate having any outside assistance. Straight bargaining was the most successful when management took a tough initial stance, but arbitration was more effective when a soft stance was taken. Parties who entered into negotiations with less distance between their initial positions were most successful in reaching an agreement. It was concluded that the threat of outside intervention may facilitate agreement under low-conflict conditions but may be detrimental under high-conflict conditions.

that this is impossible. Suppose some patients were not chosen? How will they provide for continuity on their days off?

Elaborations of positions follow.

The head nurse must ensure that the patients receive the best nursing care possible and be responsible for the care given to all patients. The staff nurses agree but point out that the present system is not doing this well.

At this point, if a competitive or hostile atmosphere prevails, both sides can become entrenched in their positions. Both sides can refuse to budge, and the negotiations would then be likely to be concluded with a power play from either side:

The head nurse could declare the staff nurses' plan unworkable, assert managerial authority, and insist that they continue with the old assignment method. The staff nurses, on the other hand, can refuse to work until their proposal is accepted.

However, if a cooperative mood prevails, either side can suggest a workable alternative.

> Either the head nurse or staff nurses can suggest that they find a workable way to provide better continuity of care and increased satisfaction for the staff while ensuring quality care for all patients over the whole week. The group can then proceed with suggestions from both sides and further elaborations of what exactly each one wants and why certain conditions are particularly important to them.
>
> For instance, a set of criteria to be used by the head nurse in making patient assignments could be agreed upon by the whole group so that it would satisfy everyone (including the patients). The head nurse would retain authority to assign staff and gain by increasing continuity and staff cooperativeness. The staff would gain increased continuity and satisfaction in their work as well as satisfaction from having had input into the way they are assigned.

A poor compromise leads to one or both sides feeling they have lost in the negotiation. A good agreement results when both sides believe they have gained something important to them and has the added benefit of leading to increased cooperation in the future.

Strategies to Influence the Process

A number of factors will influence the negotiation process and the outcome (Bigoness, 1976). Most contain elements of change strategies, and some are power tactics.

Most of the research studies done on the subject indicate that a *cooperative orientation* will result in more satisfactory outcomes than a competitive orientation. It would seem, then, that it is worth the effort to try to establish a cooperative climate and to encourage cooperative efforts. This does not mean, however, that you should make a lot of concessions or compromises.

One strategy for influencing the negotiation process is by *emphasizing the similarity* between your demands and theirs, pointing out that you really want the same thing or have the same need (as occurred in the example of the staff nurses above) or that you have a common enemy. The latter is a popular political strategy, by the way. You can also *supply information* that supports your proposal as the head nurse in the example did by pointing out the need to account for days off in making patient assignments.

Appeals to fair play are often persuasive. For example, the head nurse in the example could point out the responsibility they all had to provide quality care to every patient, not just those selected by individual staff members, while the staff nurses could point out that an arbitrary method of making assignments does not divide the work fairly.

Promising some kind of *reward* is another way to influence the outcome. This depends, of course, on your ability actually to provide one. In the example given, neither side had much capability for providing tangible rewards. However, the head nurse could write favorable evaluations or grant time off, and the staff nurses could make the work climate more agreeable when they are satisfied with the work assignments. Both could provide general satisfaction for each other from a job well done, but this is really an outcome of the process, not a specific reward that one side could promise the other.

If overdone, promises can make you seem too anxious to concede. They can seem like bribes, in which case the other side may begin to demand bribes in all subsequent negotiations. Used sparingly, promises can increase the cooperative climate of the negotiation. If they are used too much or too often, they will weaken your position.

Threats do just the opposite of rewards: they increase the competitive climate of the negotiating process. If the threat is too small, it can be seen as an insult. If it is too large, the threat will increase hostility to the point where effective negotiation is not possible. To return once more to the example given, the head nurse could have threatened to fire the nurses and the nurses could have threatened to walk off the job, either of which would have increased the tensions tremendously.

Even if left unspoken, both sides are aware that the other has these ultimate weapons, such as the ability to quit or fire. Any statement regarding this kind of ultimate weapon is going to be perceived as a threat. When the problem is solvable by other means, the threat is better left unstated. Threats are out of place in a cooperative negotiation process, but they can be very subtly implied if the process has stalled or become hostile.

Some occasions will arise in which a person or group refuses to enter into cooperative negotiations despite your confrontations and attempts to influence the negotiation process. If this happens, you have two choices: you can concede, or you can use the more powerful political strategies that will be discussed in Chapter 20 (DeTurck, 1987).

SUMMARY

Communication is a mutual and simultaneous exchange of information. There are two aspects of a communication, both of which need to be considered in interpreting the message. The first is the content aspect, which is the literal message. The second is the relationship aspect or metacommunication, which tells you how to interpret a message. Interpretation is frequently done through nonverbal types of communication that can include tone of voice and emphasis, gestures, body position and stance, sounds, and facial expressions.

Attending, responding, encouraging, focusing, clarifying, personalizing, and informing are techniques you can use to establish open, productive relationships with others as individuals and in groups. These techniques not only encourage a free exchange of ideas and feelings, but also help the participants in the exchange increase their self-awareness, encourage personal growth, and facilitate problem-solving.

The different types of confrontations, confrontation through information, calling the other's game, taped recordings, processing, and confrontation meetings, are appropriately used to resolve various kinds of conflicts and communication blockages. When embarking on a confrontation, you need to evaluate the strength of the confrontation in terms of the need for confrontation, the quality of your relationship with the person or group, and the psychological state of the confronted individual or group of people. You also need to be aware of your motives for confronting: getting back at the other person is not an acceptable motive, but resolving conflicts, improving relationships, and furthering individual and group growth are valid reasons to confront another. Finally, you need to be aware of your individual capabilities for carrying out a confrontation and the subsequent negotiation.

Negotiation is a give-and-take situation between individuals or groups that is aimed at coming up with a solution acceptable to everyone involved. The opening move is considered to be a crucial point in the negotiation and should be used as an opportunity to inform the other party of the upper limits of your demands. This is then followed by a series of offers, counter-offers, and elaborations of each side's positions. A cooperative atmosphere, emphasizing the similarity of each side's demands, supplying information, and appealing to fair play influence the negotiation process positively. Threats and competitiveness generally have a negative influence.

REFERENCES*

Bennis, W.G. (1976). Post-bureaucratic leadership. In Lassey, W.P. & Fernandez, R.R. *Leadership and Social Change*. La Jolla, California: University Associates.

*Beckhard, R. (1969). The confrontation meeting. In Bennis, W.G., Benne, K.D. & Chin, R: *Dynamics of Planned Change*. (2nd ed). New York: Holt, Rinehart & Winston.

Berne, E. (1964). *Games People Play*. New York: Grove Press.

Berne, E. (1972). *What Do You Say After You Say Hello?* New York: Grove Press.

Bigoness, W. (1980). The impact of initial bargaining position and alternative modes of third party intervention in resolving bargaining impasses. In Katz, D., Kahn, R.L. & Adams, J.S. *The Study of Organizations*. San Francisco: Jossey-Bass. (Reprinted from *Organizational Behavior and Human Performance, 17,* 1976, p. 185.)

Brammer, L.M. (1985). *The Helping Relationship: Process and Skills*. Englewood Cliffs, New Jersey: Prentice Hall.

Carkhuff, R.R. (1983). *The Art of Helping*. Amherst, Massachusetts: Development Press.

DeTurck, M.A., (1987). When communication fails: Physical aggression as a compliance-gaining strategy. *Communication Monographs, 54,* 106–111.

Donnellon, A., Gray, B. & Bougon, M.G. (1986). Communication, meaning and organized action. *Administrative Science Quarterly, 31,* 43–55.

*Egan, G. (1973). *The Small Group Experience and Interpersonal Growth*. Monterey, California: Brooks/Cole.

Egan, G. (1976). *Interpersonal Living*. Monterey, California: Brooks/Cole.

*Egan, G. (1985). *The Skilled Helper: Model Skills and Methods for Effective Helping*. Monterey, California: Brooks/Cole.

*Filley, A.C. (1975). *Interpersonal Conflict Resolution*. Glenview, Illinois: Scott Foresman & Co.

Gordon, T. (1970). *Parent Effectiveness Training*. New York: New American Library.

Gordon T. (1980). *Leader Effectiveness Training*. New York: Bantam Books.

Gudykunst, W.B., Yang, S-M, & Nishida, T. (1987). Cultural differences in self-consciousness and self-monitoring. *Communication Research, 14* (1), 7–34.

Harris, T.E. (1988). Mastering the art of talking back. *Management World, 17* (3), 9–11.

Karpman, S.P. (1968). Fairy tales and script drama analysis. *Transactional Analysis Bulletin, 7,* 39.

King, T. (1982). Personal communication.

Kissinger, H. (1979). Crisis and confrontation. *Time* (October, 15) p. 82. (Excerpted from his book *White House Years*. Boston: Little, Brown & Company.)

Lax, D.A. & Sebenius, J.K. (1986). *The Manager as Negotiator: Bargaining for Cooperation and Competitive Gain*. New York: Free Press.

Lifton, W.M. (1972). *Groups: Facilitating Individual Growth and Societal Change*. New York: John Wiley & Sons.

Mehrabian, A. (1971). *Silent Messages*. New York: Wadsworth.

Rogers, C.R. (1970). *Carl Rogers on Encounter Groups*. New York: Harper & Row.

*Rubin, J.Z. & Brown, B.R. (1975). *The Social Psychology of Bargaining and Negotiation*. New York: Academic Press.

Smoyak, S.A. (1975). The confrontation process. *American Journal of Nursing, 74,* 1632

Tappen, R.M. (1978). Strategies for dealing with conflict: Using confrontation. *Journal of Nursing Education, 17,* 47.

Walton, R.F. (1969). *Interpersonal Peacemaking: Confrontation and Third-Party Consultation*. Reading, Massachusetts: Addison-Wesley.

*Watzlawick, P., Beavin, J.H. & Jackson, D.D. (1967). *Pragmatics of Human Communication*. New York: W.W. Norton.

Wolf, G.A. (1986). Communication: Key contributor to effectiveness. *Journal of Nursing Administration, 16* (9), 26–28.

*References marked with an asterisk are suggested for further reading.

Chapter 16 ▬▬▬▬▬▬▬

OUTLINE ─────────────────────────────────────

Small Groups
Common Bonds
The Group as an Open System

Stages of Group Development
Forming
Individual Tasks
Group Tasks
Climate and Behavior
Leader Action
Storming
Individual Tasks
Group Tasks
Climate and Behavior
Leader Action
Norming
Individual Tasks
Group Tasks
Climate and Behavior
Leader Action
Performing
Individual Tasks
Group Tasks
Climate and Behavior
Leader Action

Adjourning
Individual Tasks
Group Tasks
Climate and Behavior
Leader Action

Patterns of Interaction
Group Roles
Functional Task Roles
Functional Group-Building Roles
Nonfunctional Roles
Communication Patterns
One Way
Stilted
Limited
Open
Chaotic
Public and Hidden Agendas
Sources
Leader Action
Dominant Synchronizers
Types of Synchronizers
Leader Action

Summary

LEARNING OBJECTIVES ────────────────────────────

Upon completion of this chapter, the reader will be able to:

▷ Describe the small group as an open system.

▷ Name the five stages in group development and describe their characteristic group climate, individual and group tasks, and appropriate leader action for that stage.

▷ Assess the stage of development of small groups in actual work situations.

▷ Distinguish between functional and nonfunctional group roles played by various group members.

▷ Identify the group communication pattern, hidden agendas, and dominant synchronizers of small groups in actual work situations.

UNDERSTANDING GROUPS

T his chapter deals with the basic dynamics of the small group in general, whether the group is an ad hoc committee, a working team, a community group, a patient group, or any other type of group in which you may be involved in a professional capacity. In particular, we will consider the growth and the development of a group, common patterns of interaction within a group, and common blocks to group interaction and growth. The following two chapters will then look at specific kinds of groups—teams and conference groups—and how the leader-manager can facilitate their development and function.

SMALL GROUPS

A group is an open system composed of three or more people held together by a common bond or interest. The individuals who make up the group are its subsystems.

The number *three* was used deliberately as the minimum to constitute a group because it is only when there are three or more in the system that the complex set of relationships develops that characterizes a group. When there are three or more people in a group, an interaction is affected by the presence of other people, and there is a group climate or state in which the exchange takes place (Sapir, 1973).

Common Bonds

The common bond or interest mentioned in the definition is the relationship that holds people together as a group. This bond may be physical proximity, a shared purpose or goal, a special meaning that has been attached to the group, or a combination of these factors.

Sharing the same physical space is a bond that can bring people together into a group. For example, five people who get caught in a sudden rain shower and huddle together under the same awning to keep dry form a temporary group. If they had not been caught by the rain, they most likely would not have become a group but remained an aggregate with nothing to hold them together, even temporarily. An aggregate is a number of people without a common bond. People in a group have developed some kind of connection with one another; people in an aggregate have not.

Living or working in the same physical space increases the number of contacts between people and the likelihood of their developing a common bond. People who live near one another form social groups such as neighborhood clubs or block associations. People who attend school in the same class or work together in the same office often form groups because they spend so much time together in the same place and share many common experiences.

Many groups are formed primarily to accomplish a specific goal or purpose. For example, people may form groups to plan a health fair, to analyze budget cuts, to preserve the environment, to fight crime in their neighborhood, or for any number of other reasons.

For most groups in the work setting, a shared purpose or goal is the strongest bond. The shared purpose of a work group or team could be to survey the needs of people living in a designated geographical area or to provide nursing care for a given number of patients. Other work groups, such as task forces and committees, are formed to accomplish more limited goals. Committees may, for example, be formed to develop a new protocol for hyperalimentation, evaluate research utilization, or to carry out a peer review procedure. The variety of purposes for which a group can be formed is almost endless.

Some groups are formed primarily because of the special meaning they have for their members. This kind of group holds some special significance or meets some basic need of its members. Community groups often begin this way. They may be formed on the basis of shared beliefs, a common ethnic background, a shared concern, or a community need such as groups of bereaved parents or families of AIDS patients. Groups originally formed to accomplish a specific purpose may develop a shared meaning over time. For example:

> Membership on the peer review committee may become a desirable position because of the power of the committee and the qualifications for membership. The committee then becomes a symbol of power and prestige to its members.

> A team that was formed to provide rehabilitative services may become a source of satisfaction and support for its members. It may also develop social significance if team members find that they enjoy spending time together during and after work.

The Group as an Open System

Like other open systems, groups evidence wholeness, pattern, growth, individuality, and sentience. Groups also exchange energy with their environment and are continually affecting and being affected by their environment.

The group as a whole has its own unique characteristics that are different from the characteristics of the individual members. A group has its own identity, its own rhythms, growth patterns, and interactions with the environment. You cannot accurately predict the behavior of a group from an assessment of the individual members (Burggraf & Sillars, 1987; Glisson, 1986). One group theorist pointed out that a group can act completely irrationally even though its members are rational people (Bion, 1961). It is also interesting to note that people act differently in different groups.

In leadership and management, we are interested in both the group and the individual. The patterns of interaction that characterize the group as a whole and the patterns exhibited by people when they are acting as members of a group are important. An assessment of only one or the other would be inadequate. For many people, this is a different focus, one that requires a change in perspective.

There is a regular and predictable sequence to the development of a group. Although not every group completes this sequence successfully, those that are able to do so will proceed through identifiable stages in their evolution. There are very evident differences between an immature group in the early stages of development and the mature group that has progressed to the later stages of development.

Groups exchange energy in the form of information and matter with their environment. There is an ebb and flow of energy both within the group and in its exchange with the environment.

A group may take action to change its environment, or it may make a decision based on the demands of people outside the system. Environmental influences may be as subtle as the effects of spatial arrangements or as obvious as a directive from the administration. This influence is not a one-way exchange—the group may also make demands of the administrator, and its very existence can subtly affect those who are not members and see themselves as "outsiders."

Groups have common patterns of behavior that can be identified, analyzed, and influenced by the leader. Certain patterns of interaction are likely to appear in groups and tend to change as groups mature. The way in which a group responds to its members, makes decisions, and handles conflicts are just a few examples of these patterns. Some of them promote group development, but others are indications of group disharmony and immaturity.

Individual members of the group also have common patterns of behavior that can be identified, analyzed, and influenced by the leader or manager of the group. Some are functional within the group; others tend to disrupt the group and delay group progress. These patterns will be discussed later.

STAGES OF GROUP DEVELOPMENT _____

Years of observation by group theorists as well as a number of research studies indicate that groups go through predictable developmental stages in the course of their existence. Groups evolve over time from an immature to a mature stage of development.

Of course, not every group achieves maturity, just as not every individual successfully fulfills the developmental tasks of each stage of life. Also, like individuals, groups may proceed to the next stage without completely accomplishing the tasks of the earlier ones and may need to go back to complete them later or may terminate before progressing through all of these stages.

Tuckman and Jensen (1977) call these five stages of group development *forming, storming, norming, performing,* and *adjourning.* While a number of different terms are used to describe the stages, there is agreement on a general pattern and order to the evolution of these stages.

Groups first go through a formation stage characterized by the uncertainty felt by group members about their place in the group. This stage is followed by a stormy period in which there is a great deal of conflict and emotions are high. The group must find a way to deal with these conflicts and develop a functional pattern of interaction. If it succeeds, the group then matures into a highly functional system abundantly able to perform its tasks and meet the relationship needs of its members as well. At some point, the group finishes its task or is no longer of use to its members or to the organization and thus ceases to exist. The course of the group's development will be affected by the purpose of the group and the setting in which it functions as well as by the internal dynamics of the group.

Each of these five stages is described in more detail below. The tasks of the group as a whole and of the individual members will be mentioned as well as the characteristic group climate, behavior during the stage, and leader action to facilitate group development (Brill, 1984; Lacoursiere, 1980; Hill, Lippitt & Serkownek, 1979; Bradford, 1978; Bennis & Shepard, 1978; Neilsen, 1978; Braaten, 1974–75).

Forming

This is the stage in which the group forms and begins to develop an identity. By the end of this stage, the group will have developed a sufficient sense of self that it can at least define a boundary between itself and the environment. People in the group will be able to say who is and who is not a member of the group but will not yet know exactly what being a member entails.

In this first stage, the group is very immature. In fact, it can barely be called a group because its members have just begun to identify their common bonds and have not yet formed any relationships within the group. Group members will also have differing perceptions of the purpose and goals of the group and will be uncertain about their position within the group.

INDIVIDUAL TASKS. Members of a new group do not know yet what the group will be like or what will be expected of them. The first individual task, then, is to learn about the group and to find out what roles and responsibilities they will be fulfilling in this particular group.

Individual members also need to deal with individual feelings about entering a new group. These feelings can include uncertainty, curiosity, high hopes, mistrust, or anxiety related to the unknowns of the group. A certain amount of stress can be expected to accompany the change in pattern required when entering a new group. The amount can vary a great deal according to the demands of the situation and individual response to these demands. For example, joining a group similar to one you have enjoyed working in before would be less stressful than joining a group in which you will be asked to carry out an entirely new task for which you feel unprepared.

GROUP TASKS. The group as a whole has two tasks to accomplish in the forming stage. The first is to establish its identity as a group. This is done in several ways. One way is by defining who is and who is not a member of the group. Another is to define and to talk about what members of the group have in common with one another (for example, went to the same school, are all new in their jobs, have the same problem, have the same goal). This discussion will eventually lead to a definition of group expectations. A third way is to give the group a name and to decide on a time and place to meet again. This last activity also extends the existence of the group beyond the initial encounter.

The second group task is to provide support for those individual mem-

bers who are experiencing some discomfort. This is difficult for the immature group to achieve. Introductions and discussion of common bonds provide some support. Avoiding conflict and direct confrontation at this time
are also temporary means of providing support. As the group matures, it is
more capable of meeting its members' basic needs and can therefore allow
more open communication and confrontation.

CLIMATE AND BEHAVIOR.   Uncertainty and insecurity characterize
the forming stage of a group. Members' basic needs for security and belonging have not yet been met within the group, and, therefore, much of their
behavior is aimed at meeting these needs. More specifically, behavior in the
group at this time is aimed at assuring acceptance, avoiding rejection, increasing feelings of comfort, reducing anxiety, reducing ambiguity, and
attempting to clarify roles and expectations.

Members of a forming group do not know whether or not they will be
accepted by the group and so are cautious in their behavior. For some
people, this uncertainty and anxiety can become so intolerable that they
literally flee from the group.

From what was just said about acceptance and rejection, it is clear that
the level of trust within the group is low at this stage (Gibb & Gibb, 1978).
Coupled with unmet needs for security and belonging, this situation results
in numerous attempts to bring some order and structure to the group and in
guarded, nonconfronting, nonrevealing communications. Typically, conversation is somewhat formal and very polite. People will talk about safe,
familiar subjects (the weather, the traffic, or a current item of general
interest) and try to conceal their feelings and personal concerns. These
maneuvers keep other people at a safe distance and prevent open confrontation, retaliation, or rejection.

A new group lacks form and organization; it hasn't had time yet to
develop regular patterns of interaction and so is quite unpredictable, even to
its members. The politeness and formality used for self-concealment also
serve to structure and pattern communication.

Another way the group can increase structure and predictability is to set
limits on each other's behavior. For example, members will control participation by having each one take a turn to speak or by interrupting those who
stray beyond the limits, saying, "Let's stick to the subject." Other ways to
set limits are by setting up an agenda for the meeting and by designating not
only a specific time and place for the next meeting but also a specific
duration and restrictions on who is welcome to attend.

Several other behaviors are common at this stage. One is a concentration on the task of the group to avoid dealing with feelings. Another common occurrence is for the group to get stuck on a minor point and spend the
whole meeting squabbling about it, so that the group does not have to deal
with its major task. A forming group may take a different approach and try
to rush through too many decisions at the first meeting in order to reduce
tension. However the group first approaches these issues, it usually has to
return to them later and resolve them in a more mature manner.

Despite these limitations and ambiguities, and the concentration of
energy on dealing with them, an underlying tone of optimism usually prevails. People who enter a new group tend to bring with them the expectation
that the group will somehow be able to accomplish its purpose. While it does

need to be kept within realistic bounds, this optimism helps to keep the group together through its difficult early stages.

LEADER ACTION. A newly formed group needs a leader. In fact, the group can easily become too dependent on the direction of a strong leader, which hinders group development over the long term. The leader's actions should be aimed at providing support and structure without encouraging dependence (Ettling & Jago, 1988).

As the leader of a forming group, you will experience some of the same feelings of ambiguity and insecurity that the rest of the group does. Recognizing that these feelings are related to the formation of the group can help you deal with them constructively. One way is by helping the group to accomplish its developmental tasks and complete this stage successfully.

It is important to be alert to the individual needs of group members. For example, some people prefer to remain silent at this stage, and the leader can encourage the group to allow them to "skip their turn for now." Other people may need recognition to feel comfortable in the group. The leader can supply some of this recognition.

As leader, you can also be a role model for more mature group behavior by engaging in more open communication than the rest of the group. This encourages others to speak more freely. You can reinforce mature group behavior, but only indirect, low-pressure kinds of confrontation should be used at this stage. You can also help the group develop the needed group identity and structure and begin to clarify its purpose. Simply using the word *we* in referring to the group helps to promote a group identity. Giving the group a name, using this name, and distinguishing it from other groups also reinforces the group's identity.

While some structure is needed, it should be flexible to allow growth. A rigid structure will retard further development. The following is an example of the difference:

Flexible: Encourage the group to discuss when they want to meet next time and to decide what they want to do or discuss.

Rigid: Ask the group to make a list of each separate item to be discussed at the next meeting and allow no deviation from that list no matter what comes up.

The group leader can suggest constructive approaches and encourage the group to keep things flexible yet predictable enough for comfort.

A real clarification of the group's goals is not a realistic expectation for most groups in the forming stage. Firmly set goals would be premature and probably have to be renegotiated later on, which frustrates and discourages those who are very task oriented. A general statement about the reason why people are getting together as a group would be appropriate, however, and reduces ambiguity to a more manageable level. Group members can also be assigned to some general responsibilities, such as taking minutes or thinking about the group's goals and bringing some information or ideas with them to the next meeting.

The leader's function in a forming group is to encourage optimism, flexibility, and open communication and to provide support, some clarification of purpose, and some guidance to promote accomplishment of the individual and group tasks of the forming stage. Failure to complete these tasks means that the group either remains at this low level of function or that it will have to return to them and deal with them later.

Example. There is no substitute for real group experience in which you can actually be involved in the complex interactions and changes that take place and feel the tensions rise and fall as the group moves through the stages of development. The example illustrates the way in which a group changes from stage to stage but cannot do justice to the complexities of group dynamics.

> An outbreak of meningitis in a grade school upset many parents in the district. Three parents, two from the affected grade school and one from the middle school, met with the school superintendent to express their concern and demand that action be taken to improve school health services. The superintendent suggested that they meet with the district coordinator of special services, who is responsible for health services in that district.
>
> The following evening, the three parents and the coordinator met at the grade school. The coordinator expected that the blame for inadequate health services would fall on the coordinator and was apprehensive about the meeting. Each of the parents was very anxious to see some action taken and had a list of suggested actions. Each list was different from the others.
>
> After everyone arrived and had been introduced to everyone else, the coordinator read a long report (which the coordinator had written for the school board) to the parents. When the coordinator finally finished, the parents took turns asking questions about the way the outbreak had been discovered and handled. They gradually realized that the person who had been most actively dealing with the outbreak was a nurse from the health department. Someone suggested they speak with the nurse. The parent whose children attended the middle school offered to call the nurse and ask the nurse to meet the group at the same time next week. Because it was very late by then, the meeting broke up after this.

Not a single item on any of the three parents' lists was accomplished at this meeting. The coordinator was expected to attend another meeting despite the coordinator's hope that the parents would be satisfied by the report and drop the whole thing. You may have noted that only the coordinator felt any real anxiety and insecurity about the formation of the group in this particular example. The maneuver of reading the long report succeeded in protecting the coordinator from attack but did not help the group make any progress toward a goal. A real leader has not yet emerged in this group. The example will be continued in the discussion of the second stage, storming.

Storming

It would seem that, after the relative uneasiness of the first stage, the group should move into a calmer phase next, but it does not. Although group members usually feel a little more comfortable by the end of the first stage, the group then moves into the second stage, which is characterized by an increase in tension and conflict. This stage is a difficult, stormy one. It is probably the most stressful and unpleasant for everyone in the group. This tension has some value, however, because it eventually pushes the group to work on resolving the problems and issues that were evaded in the first stage.

INDIVIDUAL TASKS. As the group rearranges and reorganizes itself throughout this stage, the main task of the individual member is to find a position in the group. This includes defining what one is able to contribute to the group, the degree to which one can fulfill group expectations, and the decision whether or not to remain a part of the group.

To do these things, the group member needs to develop more connections with other group members and some idea of the purpose of the group and its probable objectives. Group members often test several different roles and options available to them before the conclusion of this stage.

GROUP TASKS.   The group's tasks in this second stage are to resolve the conflicts that emerge and to begin reorganizing itself into a more functional whole. Conflicts were avoided in the first stage but now emerge and demand most of the energy of the group to resolve them.

In order to reorganize successfully, the group must develop more common bonds between its members and further develop its identity. The minimal structure developed in the first stage is usually challenged and often reworked. While the purpose of the group becomes clearer, specific objectives are usually established in the next (Norming) stage.

CLIMATE AND BEHAVIOR.   As the name *storming* implies, the climate of the group is unstable and emotional. When previously hidden conflicts emerge, the tension level rises rapidly. Trust is still low and the group is clearly still immature, although it is struggling to mature.

People who are not familiar with group dynamics are often surprised that decisions made in the first stage are either ignored or completely changed in the second stage. This seemingly irrational behavior is necessary if the decisions were made hastily or based on a superficial consensus that concealed serious disagreement.

Communication may become openly hostile and attacking in the second stage. Angry individuals may stomp out of a meeting when they do not get their way. The noise level can rise dramatically, and shouting matches may occur. In other groups, the hostility may be more restrained and covert but still evident to the alert observer and still felt by members of the group. People who fear open hostility may withdraw from the group, temporarily or permanently, physically or emotionally.

The conflicts that arise in the group may stem from such trivial matters as the way to pay for refreshments or where minutes of the meetings should be kept, or from more serious issues such as the purpose of the group. Personal conflicts are also common. For example, one group member may become irritated by another's mannerisms; another may become upset or sulky when criticized. When a group focuses too long on a trivial disagreement, despite attempts to get moving again, it is usually because it is avoiding or unable to deal with more substantial issues such as the group's purpose or its inability to meet members' individual needs.

Why would a work group with an assigned task have difficulty defining its purpose? There are several theories about this. Some propose that organized action can take place only if there is a *consensus* within the group. Another point of view is that working together leads to the development of common goals and shared meanings (Donnellon, Gray & Bougon, 1986). In either case, the purpose is clarified, modified, and redefined as the group evolves.

Differences between individual members become much more apparent than they were in the first stage. As these differences appear, individual members begin to develop affiliations with other members who seem to agree with them or share their interests. *Subgroups* or factions may form out of these affiliations. Within the subgroups, members begin to show more interest and concern for one another than had been shown earlier. Any sharing of personal concerns is usually still superficial, but subgroup members do begin to listen to each other more than they had before.

As these subgroups form, people begin to take sides on issues and to support those who agree with them. Sometimes, the conflicts between these subgroups can escalate into serious battles. To an observer, they may seem to be literally at war with each other. The group may seem ready to split into two or more separate groups, and this does occasionally happen.

Those members who do not join the subgroups or will not commit themselves on a hot issue may be pressured to choose sides. Sometimes, a member is singled out for criticism and blamed, often unfairly, for the problems of the group. This occurrence is called *scapegoating.* The leader of the group is often the target.

Power struggles may erupt as people try to maneuver themselves into favorable positions within the group. For example, two or more people may try to designate themselves as leaders of the group, or they may try to remove the already-designated leader by calling for a vote, constantly challenging the leader's actions, or simply taking over. These power struggles often develop over control of group functions. For example, one group member might try to impose a set of rules on the group and, in response, a second member will demand that the group accept his or her own completely different rules. The struggle over whose rules will be accepted can quickly turn into a shouting match or become an endless argument unless someone intervenes.

LEADER ACTION.   The group leader can do much to channel the energies released during this stage into constructive activity. These actions include the use of confrontation and negotiation, linking, testing for consensus, encouragement, and reinforcement.

Confrontation is an appropriate kind of communication at this stage. It can be used, for example, to get things moving again when the group gets stuck on a trivial matter and is avoiding more substantial issues. *Confrontation and negotiation* together (see Chapter 15) are useful in the resolution of the many conflicts and power struggles that emerge in this stage.

Along with using confrontation, however, it is very important to lay down ground rules for confronting issues such as using "I" messages and not attacking the person. These ground rules may need to be repeated and violations pointed out until the group becomes accustomed to following the rules. The purpose of emphasizing these rules is not to suppress open expression of feelings but to keep these expressions from feeding the tension that already exists, to avoid provoking more hostility, and to avoid driving anxious or angry members away from the group, that is, to keep emotions and tensions within reasonable bounds.

As the leader of a group in the second stage, you can also point out the commonalities that exist and can be further developed between individuals and subgroups. This is the linking function that you may recall from the components of effective leadership (Chapter 3). *Linking* can help strengthen group identity, assist people in making connections with each other and clarify the purpose of the group.

Also important is encouraging free discussion and the *testing for consensus.* Once some commonalities have been found, the leader can ask, "Do we all agree that . . . ?" When it seems that the group has reached some agreement on purpose, the leader then can test for agreement. When there has been much disagreement, testing for consensus may be used to identify what commonalities do exist.

During the second stage, the group may not be ready to come to consensus on every question that is raised and may have to vote on some issues. The problem with voting is that some people (the minority) will lose to the majority, and this can polarize the group even further. Voting is preferable, however, to autocratic decisions by the leader or another member of the group. On some points, it may be necessary for group members to agree to disagree to avoid splitting the group permanently.

There are several different ways in which the leader can *encourage and reinforce* positive group action. Encouragement of open discussion of issues has already been mentioned. The leader can also point out to the group that it usually takes a long time for a group to get organized and to reach the planning stage. This observation can restore flagging optimism. The leader can also reinforce positive action by recognizing contributions and pointing out ways in which individual members have been helpful to the group.

Many of the leader actions from the first stage are still helpful here. The leader can continue to use open communication and to provide support for individual members when others in the group do not. You can also continue to use *we* to refer to the group and to point out features indicating group identity. At the same time, however, it is important to allow the group to grapple with its own problems and to resist trying to impose your own solutions in an autocratic fashion. It has been said that we have such a strong cultural belief that the leader *must* provide direction to the group that we often ignore the contribution of group members (Gemmill, 1986).

Example. Let us return to the group of three concerned parents and the coordinator of special services as they come together for their second meeting and the second stage — storming.

> As the group members sat down around a table, the parent who had offered to call the nurse was asked when the nurse was coming. ''The nurse couldn't come this week because of a previously scheduled conference. The nurse will be here next week,'' the parent replied. The other group members looked annoyed and said, ''Why didn't you tell us! We wasted our time coming tonight.'' The first parent responded that they could use the time to decide what questions to ask the nurse.
>
> Although everyone thought they had agreed on the questions, when people began bringing up questions, each one was different. One parent wanted to ask how meningitis spread, but another one said they knew that already. When the third parent suggested that they ask the nurse how the problem could be handled better next time, the coordinator took offense and said, ''No one said it was badly handled this time.'' Almost in a chorus, three parents said, ''But that's why we're here! Our children were dangerously exposed.'' Again, the coordinator said that everything possible had been done and, anyway, the coordinator didn't think that parents should get involved in administrative decisions. While saying this, the coordinator started to put papers away as if getting ready to leave.
>
> As the coordinator finished packing up the papers, a parent said coldly, ''If you don't want to cooperate, we'll be glad to tell that to the superintendent,'' and the other parents nodded in agreement. The coordinator backed down from the aggressive stance and said, ''Well, I do want to be cooperative.'' The first parent said, ''I know the coordinator is concerned, and we all want the children to be healthy.''
>
> The group then decided that each person could ask the nurse questions, but should try to keep to the subject. Everyone agreed to return the next week.

The first parent (who called the nurse) is emerging as the leader of the group. At one point, the parents sided together against the coordinator and the group nearly split apart. But the meeting ended with the positive, although vague, agreement that they were all concerned about the children's health. The group now has a defined purpose, even though it still has no specific objectives.

Norming

In the norming stage, the group experiences some relief from the anxieties and tensions of the first two stages. Conflicts are resolved, positions and responsibilities are defined, and plans are made. Confrontations become less hostile and actions are more productive. The group begins to establish more predictable patterns that will be carried over into the next stage.

The group is more relaxed, and participation in the group is less stressful than it was in the first two stages. By the end of this stage, group members are beginning to feel a sense of belonging to the group and of making some progress. The group is clearly maturing.

INDIVIDUAL TASKS.   The main tasks of the individual group members at this stage are to clarify positions in the group and to develop their ability to be fully functional group members. By this stage, the individual has made a decision to remain a member of the group and has begun the task of defining a position for himself or herself in the group. In the norming stage, the members can test and refine their positions and begin functioning as an integral part of the group as a whole.

Interactions with others in the group are more purposeful and constructive now. The individual member can practice such actions as confronting, disagreeing, and collaborating within this more predictable group. He or she should be contributing to accomplishment of the group's task and offering support to other group members.

GROUP TASKS.   A major task of the group is to decide on the specific goals or objectives to carry out in the next stage. If the purpose was not clearly defined during the second stage, it will need to be defined now in order to develop objectives. After developing its objectives, the group also needs to decide what has to be done and who will do it (select and assign tasks).

Two other tasks are to develop cohesiveness as a group and to establish functional patterns of behavior. The group also needs to complete the tasks of working out its own constructive ways to resolve conflicts and to meet individual members' needs.

CLIMATE AND BEHAVIOR.   This third stage is characterized by a gradually increasing feeling of progress, openness, and relatedness among group members. Both group members and the leader feel a sense of relief after having made it through the storms of the second stage.

This change in group climate is not quite as radical as it may seem. Although unnoticed because of the tension and conflict of the second stage, some positive steps were being taken then that finally bear fruit. For example, you will recall that there were instances of mutual support and developing connections between subgroup members in the second stage. These are now extended to the rest of the group as the conflicts are resolved and the hostilities decrease.

Also, as connections develop, group members feel less isolated, which contributes to the development of cohesiveness. Finally, as group members take more active roles in the group, they usually become more comfortable with communicating openly. All of these gradual changes assist the group in completing the third-stage tasks.

Exchanges between group members are freer and more open in the third stage. People are more likely to share their personal concerns than they were before. When they do, the group is more likely to respond with support and helpful suggestions.

Responses from the group are now more predictable. This does not mean that people do or say the same thing over and over again. It means that if a group member offers a constructive suggestion, someone will at least acknowledge the contribution. Or, if someone makes an insulting remark, this violation of the ground rules will be pointed out in some way, usually constructively. In neither case will the people be ignored or attacked as they might have been in the storming stage.

Discussion turns away from conflicts over trivial matters to the sharing of ideas and suggestions. As the discussion proceeds, the group finally is able to agree on its purpose and begin planning how it will carry out this purpose. By the end of this stage, the plan should include objectives, activities to carry out the objectives, and decisions on how the work will be shared by the group. When this is done, everyone will know what will be expected of each group member.

Decisions are made more democratically now. Reaching consensus on an issue is not only possible but happens more frequently. Voting is much less common, and autocratic decisions are no longer acceptable to the group.

Cautious optimism about the outcome of the group replaces frustration and discouragement. The group has finally proved that it can get something done, but it has not yet proved its ability to carry out the plan to completion.

The group becomes more autonomous and less likely to look to the leader for assistance. In fact, you could say that as each member of the group learns more about effectively influencing other group members, the leader becomes more like just another member of the group.

LEADER ACTION. As the leader, you can help to guide the group through the planning process by doing such things as keeping the group from getting sidetracked, testing the feasibility of suggestions, and encouraging the use of consensus in making decisions. At the same time, it is important to avoid the temptation to give advice. When the group assumes responsibility for planning, it will believe that it owns the final plan and be more committed to it. It is still helpful to encourage debate on issues that arise, to test for consensus, and to use confrontation and negotiation when needed. There should be less need to provide support or to enforce the ground rules for confrontation except for an occasional reminder.

Example. At the third meeting, the three parents and the coordinator met with the nurse from the health department to discuss the meningitis outbreak.

> Each group member brought a new list of questions to ask the nurse and was surprised that
> the others had done so as well. Most of the questions were about the handling of the

meningitis outbreak. The discussion flowed freely. The coordinator seemed less defensive and more relaxed than at the second meeting. The parents were attentive and impressed with the nurse's thorough knowledge of the situation and the way the nurse had dealt with the problem.

As they neared the end of their questions, one of the parents said, "I guess we were fortunate to have you on hand when this happened." "Yes, it was very fortunate because I only visit the school once a month," said the nurse. The parents gasped and asked the nurse to explain. The nurse described the way in which nurses were assigned to schools in the district. The nurse was able to provide only minimal services to the school because that was all the district contracted for.

Another parent asked the nurse what services should be available, and the discussion of this subject took up the rest of the meeting time. When it was time to end the meeting, the first parent thanked the nurse for coming and said some notes were taken and that the nurse had given them something to think about. The others agreed and asked if the nurse could return to consult with their committee in the future. The nurse agreed. The group left after agreeing to meet the next week.

At the next meeting, the group discussed the nurse's suggestions for a comprehensive health service. The coordinator pointed out that such services would be expensive. The parents agreed but said it would be worth the cost.

By the end of the meeting, the group had decided to propose an improved health service for the district but also agreed that they needed much more information first. The Coordinator was asked to look into the costs and feasibility of improved services. The first parent volunteered to speak with other health department officials and the other two parents offered to do some library research. Each member would bring their information back to the group in 2 weeks.

Not every group progresses as rapidly through the stages of development as this one. It may take many weeks for some groups to even enter the second stage. The group in the example has matured substantially; note how differently the coordinator's disagreement was handled in this stage.

Performing

This is the most productive and enjoyable stage in the life cycle of a group. By this stage, the group has clearly defined its purpose and agreed on its objectives and a plan to achieve them. Each member also feels a part of the group, knows what behaviors are expected of individual members in the group, and knows what one can expect from other members of the group. In other words, the group has finally reached maturity and is ready to perform at a fully functional level.

INDIVIDUAL TASKS. Individual members now carry out the roles and responsibilities that were defined gradually over the last three stages. The two developmental tasks of the individual member can be described in terms of those two familiar aspects of leadership style — task and relationships. The first task of every individual member is to carry out their part of the work. Attempts to do this are usually made during earlier stages, but it is not until this stage that group members have sufficient energy free to concentrate on performing the work of the group.

The second task is to relate to both the group as a whole and to individual members. Group members now address their messages to the group as a whole as well as to the other individuals. For example, a characteristic of the mature group is the degree to which a group member who is unhappy about a group action discusses that displeasure with the group (mature group behavior) rather than with another person outside the group (immature group behavior). In a mature group, there should be few barriers to communications between individual members. While there may still be a need to have subgroups in order to divide up complex tasks, communication between them should flow freely and openly.

GROUP TASKS. The tasks of the group at this stage are to move toward its goals by engaging in productive behavior and to maintain relationships within the group and with the environment. These tasks are closely related to those of the individual group member because the needs and goals of the group as a whole are much more congruent with those of the individual members now.

To fulfill these tasks, the group must now function as a whole whose members are functionally interrelated. The following is a description of a group exercise to illustrate this interrelatedness.

> Six or seven volunteers are asked to stand together in a group and link arms with one another. Then, each person is asked to select a point somewhere in the room. After each person indicates that they have decided on a point in the room, they are told to move toward that point.
>
> Of course, with their arms linked, everyone finds themselves pulling against the others and the group goes nowhere. The people in the group become frustrated. Finally, they realize that they cannot all reach their different points at once and begin to move together from point to point in the room until each point has been reached. As this is done, the people in the group usually begin to smile and laugh with pleasure at their accomplishment.

You can see how the climate changed as the group moved from unproductive to functional behavior.

CLIMATE AND BEHAVIOR. The climate of the group at this stage is generally open, pleasant, and relaxed. Most behavior is purposeful and constructive. The level of trust among group members is high, and each member has a sense of involvement in the group. Cooperation has replaced conflict. Participation in a mature group is usually a satisfying experience.

The pleasant, cooperative climate does not mean that differences no longer exist. The differences do exist but are handled in a different manner in a mature group. In fact, the leader should be suspicious of a group that claims it never has to deal with differences or disagreements among its members. When a group presents a totally harmonious, unanimous front, it may mean that it has set up rigid norms that prohibit disagreement. Beneath this surface agreement, members may be concealing their concerns and opinions for fear of rejection by the group. The harmony is an illusion, and those members who believe in it are deceiving themselves.

In contrast, the mature group recognizes that each member is a unique individual who is likely to disagree with some of the things that are said or done in the group. The mature group can tolerate individuality and disagreement. It is capable of openly confronting conflicts that may arise from disagreements and of negotiating a resolution. Each member's abilities are recognized and used, and individuality is appreciated rather than suppressed.

Because group maturity is finally achieved in this performing stage, it seems appropriate to summarize the characteristics of the mature group here (Bion, 1961). Table 16–1 compares the characteristics of mature and immature groups.

TABLE 16–1. Characteristics of Mature and Immature Groups

Mature	Immature
Definite boundary	Indefinite, shifting boundary
Defined purpose	Vague purpose
Common, shared goals	Conflicting or absence of goals
Strong identity as a whole	Uncertain identity threatened by gain or loss of members
Relaxed, informal	Rigid and formal or chaotic
Open, confronting communications	Closed, concealing communications
Accepting	Rejecting, indifferent, hostile
Tolerates differences	Suppresses or is disrupted by differences
Flexible, predictable norms	Rigid or inconsistent norms
Cohesiveness	Few connections between members
Deals with both tasks and relationships	Ignores relationship concerns, focuses on tasks
Recognizes and responds to member's input and needs	Often fails to recognize or respond to its members
Feedback is constructive	Feedback is minimal or destructive or both

The group that has achieved all of the characteristics of maturity listed above may not be perfect, but it is far more functional and effective than the immature group.

LEADER ACTION. The effective leader acts as a group facilitator in the performing stage. Group members, even more than in the last stage, can assume many leadership functions but still benefit from guidance during this stage.

The leader is a valuable resource for the group. The group still needs feedback on its progress; to be refocused on objectives when sidetracked; support when facing a particularly difficult task; and guidance for such things as how to delegate responsibility, make assignments, and revise plans when necessary.

It is important to avoid being overprotective during this stage because it is not only unnecessary but counterproductive with a group able to confront and resolve its own problems. At this stage, the activities involved in working out a problem contribute to the cohesiveness of the group and to its general development. The overly helpful leader can inhibit the group's continued development.

Example. The school health committee, composed of three parents and the coordinator of special services, met again after gathering some data needed to develop a proposal.

Committee members shared their findings with the rest of the group. As they discussed their proposal for improving health services again, they began to realize how many people would be affected by this change and decided that they needed more input. They decided to survey not only school and health department officials but also the students, parents, and teachers in the entire school system.

At the same time, they also planned to find out how other school systems designed and financed their health services. To do these tasks, they formed two subcommittees. During the survey, two more parents and a school principal joined the committee and became involved in the surveys.

The group as a whole met regularly to discuss their progress and share the results. Some ideas presented to the committee by the members were too ambitious; others were too limited. Many disagreements arose as discussions of the proposal progressed. Finally, the committee worked out a realistic proposal that satisfied each member and was feasible financially.

The survey activities had generated much community support for the proposal by the time the committee presented it to the school board. The school board conducted public hearings on the proposal and finally approved it after making some minor changes in it.

The group in this example completed its work successfully, but not every group is able to do this. Some fail to progress this far in their development as a group and either abandon their objectives or work ineffectively on them. Even those groups that do reach this stage may find that their project cannot be completed or will not be accepted for some reason that wasn't apparent when they began their work. If this happens, the group has to decide whether to give up its objectives or revise its work plan and continue on.

Adjourning

In this fifth and last stage, the group reaches closure and ends. Closure should include a summary of events that took place over the life of the group and an evaluation of both the group process and the degree to which the group fulfilled its purpose and met its objectives. The evaluation part of this stage, especially evaluation of the relationship aspects of the group process, is often overlooked or avoided. Some of this behavior is due to avoidance of a potentially threatening situation. Some of it is also due to a failure to appreciate its value in terms of learning and increased self-awareness. When a group fails to complete closure, its members are left with an unsatisfied, unfinished feeling.

INDIVIDUAL TASKS. The task of the individual member is to evaluate both the process and the outcome of the group. All members give and receive feedback on their own roles, other members' roles, and on the group as a whole. Group process, achievement of the group objectives, individual members' contributions, productive and unproductive behaviors, and ways in which all these could have been improved should be included in the evaluation.

GROUP TASKS. Two group tasks are to support a thorough evaluation of the group's processes and outcome and to continue to foster an open climate in which the evaluation can take place. Without this support, individual members will not be able to engage in objective, worthwhile evaluations.

A third task of the group in this last stage is to obtain or provide some recognition of the group's work and achievements. This recognition can be in the form of an announcement of the group's success, a recounting of what has been attempted and accomplished, or a celebration of some kind.

CLIMATE AND BEHAVIOR.   This stage is characterized by mixed emotions: relief that the work is done, satisfaction from the job well done, sadness that the group is coming to an end. Of course, not every group succeeds, but even if it does not, its members can get some satisfaction from having at least attempted to reach their objective. They can also evaluate how they worked together and how they planned their work.

Evaluation promotes learning and awareness in several ways. It can make the group more aware of how it has changed since its first meeting, which is something people may not realize unless it is pointed out to them. It also raises awareness as people receive feedback on how they have influenced others.

LEADER ACTION.   As a member of the group, the leader should expect to both give and receive feedback. An important function of the leader at this stage is to encourage this sharing. Because many are reluctant to do this, the leader can initiate the process by asking the others to evaluate the leader's role. Another way is to ask group members to fill out questionnaires or checklists and then share the results with the group. For example, you could give group members the list of characteristics of the mature and immature group and ask them to rate the maturity of the group on each characteristic. As was done with other confrontations, the leader can also set ground rules for constructive rather than destructive evaluation. Independence can be encouraged by the leader's refusal to do all of the evaluation even if the group requests this decision.

The leader can also challenge the group to face the reality that it is coming to an end. You can encourage the group to recognize and validate members' contributions to the process and achievement of goals. It is also important to ensure some expression of appreciation of the group's efforts and a celebration of the group's accomplishments so that its members can leave the group with some feeling of satisfaction from having completed what they and their fellow group members set out to do.

Example.   With the acceptance of their proposal by the school board, the school health committee had met its primary objective.

All seven members of the committee gathered after the school board meeting, and a reporter took a picture for the local newspaper. They decided to celebrate their success by meeting for lunch at a favorite restaurant the next day.

Over lunch the next day, committee members reminisced about all the meetings they had had and the work they had done. The newer members expressed surprise over the difficulties the committee had in getting started. One of the parents from the original group said to the coordinator, "You seemed to think we were out to get you at first." The coordinator responded, "Yes, it did seem that way. None of you realized how little money we had to work with. I thought I was doing the best I could." The other parents agreed and shared how angry they had felt at first about the poor health services and how their feelings changed as they began to work on ways to improve the services offered.

At the end of lunch, one of the newer members expressed some regret that the committee would no longer meet. "We could meet once in a while to check on the progress of the proposal," said another parent. "No, it's up to the school board now, and it's our job as individual citizens and parents to check on their progress," said the parent who had been the informal leader of the group. The others agreed somewhat reluctantly, congratulated each other on a job well done, and left the restaurant.

PATTERNS OF INTERACTION _____

A number of different patterns can be found in the interactions of a group. Some of these, such as the roles played by group members, are primarily patterns of individual behavior. Others, such as the communication patterns, hidden agendas, and dominant synchronizers, are patterns of the group as a whole.

Group Roles

Group roles are descriptions of the behavior of individual group members in terms of their effect on the group. With this definition in mind, the various roles can be divided into two categories: *functional* and *nonfunctional* roles. Behaviors that contribute to the completion of a group task are called *task roles;* those that encourage or support group function are called *group-building roles.* Both task and group-building roles are functional roles within a group.

Roles that meet the needs of the individual member but not the group are called *individual* roles. Usually, these are nonfunctional or at best neutral in terms of group progress.

Each time a person interacts with the group, that member is playing at least one and sometimes several different roles. Some members restrict themselves to one or two roles, while others may play many different roles.

People may play different roles in different kinds of groups, but there is usually an identifiable pattern of roles within the same group over a series of meetings. While there is some relationship between personality and the roles a person is likely to play in a group, it is important to remember that when you describe the roles played, you are not describing the person or the person's intent but rather the effect the person's behavior is having on the group process (Trujillo, 1986). For example, a person's objections to a decision may be blocking group progress, but this does not mean this person is always a blocker or even deliberately being a blocker.

The functional task roles, the group building roles, and the nonfunctional roles are listed below (Bradford, 1978). Examples are given in Chapter 17 within the analysis of a problem discussion.

FUNCTIONAL TASK ROLES. The following roles contribute to the completion of a group task:

Initiator/Contributor. Makes suggestions, proposes new ideas to the group. The suggestions may be a way to solve a problem, a new way to approach a problem, or a new way for the group to proceed in its work.

Information Giver. Offers pertinent facts from personal knowledge or experience that might help a group in its deliberations.

Information Seeker. Asks for pertinent information or clarification of facts or suggestions.

Opinion Giver. Offers opinions, judgments, or feelings about suggestions. May comment on their appropriateness in terms of a particular set of values.

Opinion Seeker. Asks for opinions, judgments, or feelings of other group members; seeks clarification of values.

Disagreer.   Points out errors in information given or takes a different point of view.

Coordinator (Linker).   Points out relationships between different suggestions or statements that have been made.

Elaborator.   Expands on suggestions or ideas made and gives examples or rationales.

Energizer.   Stimulates the group; encourages activity and movement toward group goals.

Summarizer.   Pulls together all the ideas or suggestions from the group; briefly restates or outlines what the group has accomplished.

Procedural Technician.   Performs needed mechanical tasks such as setting up chairs, running the video camera, passing out papers, or serving refreshments.

Recorder.   Writes down ideas, suggestions, or decisions made by the group; may also diagram group interactions.

FUNCTIONAL GROUP-BUILDING ROLES.   The following roles encourage and support group development and function.

Encourager.   Responds to others warmly; accepts and sometimes praises contributions of others.

Standard Setter.   Expresses standards or guidelines for the group to use in its deliberations.

Gatekeeper.   Elicits contributions from other members; sometimes suggests limits or ways to make sure everyone has a chance to speak.

Consensus Taker.   Tests group opinions and decisions by stating them and asking whether members agree.

Diagnoser.   Determines and points out blocks to group progress.

Expresser.   Describes feelings, reactions, and responses of self and others; expresses feelings of the group.

Tension Reliever.   Provides an outlet for tensions built up in the group through use of humor, conciliation, and mediation.

Follower.   Accepts group decisions; goes along with the group without initiating or taking other active role.

NONFUNCTIONAL ROLES.   The following roles are played to satisfy individual needs rather than to promote group development or progress toward a goal.

Aggressor.   Makes hostile, attacking remarks, criticizes others; is overly assertive.

Recognition Seeker.   Does things to call attention to himself or herself; uses the group as personal audience.

Monopolizer.   Talks so often or so long that others do not get a chance to speak.

Dominator/Usurper.   Tries to take over leadership of the group; wants to have his or her own way and tells the group what to do.

Blocker.   Obstructs progress of the group by making unconstructive contributions, being negative, and resisting beyond a reasonable point.

Playboy.   Makes irrelevant and silly comments; whispers, plays around, and does not take the group task seriously.

Zipper-Mouth.   Does not participate even in nonverbal manner; demonstrates no acceptance of the group (as follower does); may sulk.

Identifying the group roles played by individual members is a useful way to describe what is going on within the group. When you can quickly recognize the effect certain behaviors are having on the group, you can take action to encourage the productive behaviors and to redirect or discourage the nonfunctional behaviors. You can also analyze your own behavior within a group in terms of the functional and nonfunctional roles you play.

An analysis of group roles can point out the need for further diagnosis and intervention. A high proportion of nonfunctional individual roles in comparison to task and group building roles indicates either group immaturity or a more specific problem (low morale, lack of cohesion or agreement on group objectives, poorly defined tasks, or an inappropriate leadership style).

Communication Patterns

While there will be some unique characteristics about the communications in each group, the overall patterns of verbal communication can usually be compared to one of five patterns commonly found.

These patterns are best identified by observing and recording who speaks to whom during a group meeting. While casual observation will pick up the extreme patterns of communication, written, audiotape, and videotape records are more complete and pick up the less extreme patterns more accurately and objectively.

The five common patterns range from very formal, one-way communication to the chaotic patterns found in some disorganized groups. Between these extremes are the stilted, limited, and open patterns of verbal communication (Bion, 1961). Diagrams showing the flow of communications in these five different patterns are shown in Figure 16–1.

ONE WAY. Verbal communication moves in only one direction in this pattern: from the speaker (or leader) to the rest of the group. The formal lecture is the best-known example of this pattern but it can also be found in other situations. The one-way pattern can be compared to a live performance in a theater in the sense that the speaker is performing and the rest of the group acts as the audience.

The one-way pattern is a highly organized form of communication controlled by the leader or speaker. Although the leader seems to have total control in this kind of group, the group has actually allowed this control or at least not tried to take it away from the leader.

The extreme form of one-way communication allows no verbal feedback from the group, but the leader is still influenced by the nonverbal responses of the group, which can be surprisingly powerful. Boos, hisses, laughter, and clapping from an audience tell the performer how well the performer is doing. The more subtle smiles and nods of agreement from a group listening to a lecture positively reinforce the speaker, while frowns, yawns, or restlessness can discourage the speaker. Despite the highly controlled nature of this communication pattern, the principle that you cannot *not* communicate still holds true.

In less extreme forms, the speaker will recognize people in the group and let them ask questions or make comments. The speaker responds, but retains control of participation. This allows for some clarification and disagreement, which the extreme form does not.

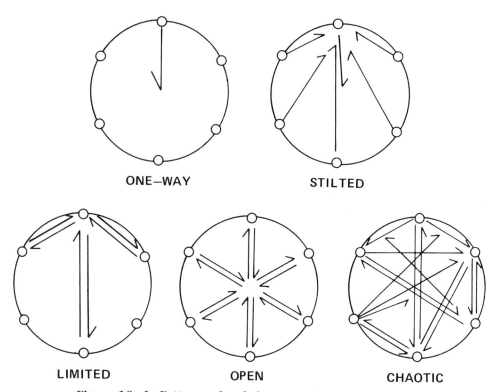

ONE—WAY   STILTED

LIMITED   OPEN   CHAOTIC

Figure 16–1. Patterns of verbal communication in groups.

The one-way pattern is appropriate for a performance or for rapidly transmitting information to a group. It is an efficient way to communicate information to a large number of people in a short time but not necessarily the best way to facilitate communication or learning. It is an authoritarian approach that sets the leader apart from the group and allows little or no group interaction. It is not an appropriate pattern for group problem solving, decision making, sharing of feelings, confrontation, evaluation, and other processes in which people need to reflect upon and respond to one another's input. A group cannot mature when a one-way pattern is continued.

STILTED. Verbal communication flows in both directions, but the stilted pattern is still somewhat formal. The most common type is one in which each member takes a turn to speak, usually going around the circle or up and down rows. In the most stilted version, all communication is directed at the leader. In the less formal form, communication may also be addressed to the group as a whole.

Although less controlling than the one-way pattern, the stilted pattern still imposes a great deal of structure on the group's interaction. Discussion is not likely to be lively or animated so long as it continues.

The stilted pattern is very common in new groups and can be helpful as a temporary way to impose some order or to make sure that everyone has a chance to speak. Insistence on continuing this pattern would retard the development of the group. It is also used for introductions and for "show-and-tell" presentations, even with adults. It may be used because of the authoritarian style of the leader or because group members are not yet comfortable with one another. Members can simply be asked to talk to the whole group to make the pattern less stilted, but it usually takes more than this for them to relax enough to move into a more open pattern of communication.

LIMITED. In the limited pattern of communication, some group members communicate with both the leader and one another, but others do not. When these interactions are animated, it may seem that the group has an open pattern of communication but careful observation or recording of the interaction reveals that the communications are limited to some members of the group and that others are not taking part.

This limited pattern can be the result of increasing dominance of a subgroup. It may also be due to the leader's and group's inability to prevent some members from monopolizing the discussion. Monopolizers are not always seeking dominance—some people mask anxiety by hyperactivity, while others may withdraw and become isolated.

The silent members in the group must also be considered. Their silence may indicate disapproval of the group's actions or feelings of discomfort. They may be interested followers who simply need some encouragement or an opportunity to participate more actively. Or they may be zipper-mouths whose negative feelings about the group need to be dealt with by the group. Leader intervention should be directed at diagnosing and acting on the reasons for the pattern and at promoting group progress toward maturity.

OPEN. This pattern is characterized by free and easy exchange between all members of the group, including the leader; it is usually found in mature groups. Each member of the group has an opportunity to speak, to be heard, and to receive some kind of response. The leadership style is usually democratic, but it could be laissez-faire in a mature group.

An open pattern of communication is flexibly organized but predictable in the sense that members know what they can expect of one another. This underlying order may be hard for an observer to detect in a very open pattern.

Open communication is appropriate for most group interactions. However, it is not the most efficient pattern for completing a simple task or the fastest way to make a decision. It is effective, however, for meeting most other leadership goals.

CHAOTIC. The chaotic pattern goes beyond the free and easy exchange of the open pattern to disorganized, unpredictable, and uncontrollable interactions. Side conversations between two members are common. Group members interrupt one another, ignore each other, or talk at the same time, sometimes shouting to be heard. The group may be as relaxed as people at a party, or it may be tense with openly warring factions. The leadership is usually laissez-faire and almost completely lacking in control.

The open pattern may seem to approach chaos at times, but careful analysis of its interactions reveals the predictability and organization that the chaotic pattern lacks, somewhat like the difference between a three-ring circus and a rioting mob.

Anything accomplished by a group with a chaotic pattern of communication has happened by accident. The chaotic pattern is not appropriate for any group that has a task to accomplish. Leader intervention should be aimed first at bringing some order into the communication pattern and then at increasing group maturity.

Public and Hidden Agendas

As they form, groups develop some kind of stated, evident reason, goal, or objective for meeting. This is called the *public or official agenda,* somewhat like an organization's official goals. Below the surface, however, other goals usually are operating that influence the group process even though they are not openly acknowledged; these goals are called the *hidden agenda* (Bradford, 1978).

Unless called to the group's attention, hidden agendas operate below the surface of the group's awareness. Although their existence is not recognized, they can be strongly felt by group members and greatly influence the outcome of the group process. The following is an example:

> A task force was formed to develop a peer review procedure for a community health agency. However, the caregivers appointed to the task force found peer review threatening. As a result of their feelings about peer review, a hidden agenda of avoiding the implementation of peer review developed and operated below the surface of this group.
>
> While this hidden agenda operated, the task force employed an astonishing variety of delay tactics in the course of its discussion of peer review. At the end of a year of meetings, the task force was still unable to find or develop a working definition of peer review that satisfied everyone in the group.

The leader-manager should have intervened with this group long before a year had passed. You can see from this example that nonproductive hidden agendas can prevent a group from making any progress at all if they are not dealt with in some way. Groups will react the same way to a goal they do not accept (such as staffing changes) or to a goal they believe is not worthwhile.

SOURCES. The sources of a hidden agenda are varied: an individual group member, several group members together, the leader or the group as a whole can have a hidden agenda. Sometimes the group is aware of having a hidden agenda, but often it is outside the awareness even of those who are its source.

Some hidden agendas arise from individual needs that are not met within the group. For example, individual group members may believe that their position is threatened by something that is happening in the group and may act to reduce this threat. Others may have feelings of dependency or hostility toward the leader. Some people try to dominate the group while others are very passive.

Preconceived ideas about how the group should function are often the source of hidden agendas. People may come to the group with a ready-made solution to the problem the group is trying to solve. Their hidden agenda would be to convince the group to accept their solution and to block acceptance of any other solution.

A similar kind of hidden agenda occurs when one or more group members have a special interest or a strong loyalty to another group. Either of these can influence behavior in the group. For example:

Two nurses were appointed to an interdisciplinary committee that was responsible for screening research studies proposed in their institution. Both nurses worked on the unstated goal (hidden agenda) of ensuring that all proposals submitted by nurses would be approved.

The leader may also bring hidden agendas to the group. Leaders also have individual needs and conflicting loyalties. More often, they find themselves wanting to present the group with ready-made solutions to the group's problems. Even if they resist this temptation, it can be difficult to keep it from operating as a hidden agenda. Some enjoy being dominant or having others dependent on them and unwittingly encourage dependence, even though they say publicly that they want group members to be independent and assertive.

Groups often give lip service to a goal that they do not genuinely accept. This lack of acceptance may be due to the fact that the goal was imposed on the group by the leader or by an outside authority; the group may have chosen a goal that sounded good, but really was not important to the group; or the group may be working on a goal that is no longer relevant to it.

Another common hidden agenda found in groups is the unspoken agreement to behave in a certain way. You may recall that immature groups frequently have an unspoken agreement that members will be polite and nonconfrontational. This is not discussed but is understood by group members. Groups may also have an unspoken agreement to ignore certain behavior (such as the acting out of a particular member) or they may agree to attack certain behaviors. Other hidden agendas may be to avoid discussing certain subjects or to slow down work deliberately on stated (public) goals.

LEADER ACTION. The purpose of leader intervention when hidden agendas arise is to help the group work out the conflicts between goals so that the group's and members' goals are congruent and genuinely accepted. Although they do not always conflict with the stated goals, hidden agendas often impede the group's progress. Because they are hidden, their existence tends to restrict open communication and to support immature rather than mature group behavior.

The first and most important leader action is to recognize the existence of a hidden agenda. Self-awareness is needed to recognize one's own hidden agendas. Some are easy to recognize, but others are much more subtle and are detected only when the group fails to make progress.

Once the hidden agenda has been identified, the leader must decide how to deal with it. Hidden agendas are not entirely negative. Some of them reflect attempts to meet real needs that have been ignored in the public agenda. Others provide a needed defense against a perceived threat. When these situations exist, finding a more direct way to meet these needs is generally preferable to confronting the individual or group about the hidden agenda. When the hidden agenda seems to reflect the real goals of the group or to be a sign that the group cannot or will not work on the publicly stated goal, an open discussion of both public and hidden goals is usually appropriate.

The leader needs to judge how much confrontation the group is ready to handle. A mature group that is accustomed to evaluating its process would be able to handle a confrontation with information about the hidden agenda. However, making a direct statement that a hidden agenda is operating is offering a diagnosis or interpretation and is likely to provoke a defensive response even from a mature group. A more acceptable form of confrontation would be to present the information without the interpretation. For example, if the group is avoiding dealing with staffing changes that have to be made, you could say either of the following:

We have been talking more about problems on units than about staffing changes.

What kinds of problems do you think these staffing changes will cause on your units?

When dealing with hidden agendas, you will also find that it is helpful to recognize the legitimacy of the needs or problems reflected by the hidden agendas and to avoid implying that anyone should feel guilty about their existence. The achievement of congruent, acceptable goals can have a dramatic effect on the group's ability to progress toward maturity and work on fulfilling its objectives.

Dominant Synchronizers

Dominant synchronizers are the primary forces affecting the group at a given time. These forces may be within the group or in the environment of the group.

As with other open, living systems, there are identifiable rhythms and patterns in the behavior of a group. *Synchronizers* are any forces that influence the rate, character, or recurrence of these patterns. The degree to which the synchronizer influences a pattern depends on both the strength of the force and how sensitive the group is to that particular force. Those that have a major influence, of course, are the *dominant synchronizers.*

You may find the concept of a dominant synchronizer difficult to understand at first, partly because the manner in which these forces influence the group cannot be observed directly and because the concept has not yet been fully developed in regard to its application to groups. More research is needed on this subject.

Although the concept may be hard to grasp in its present stage of development, it has some value in the analysis of group dynamics. There is so much happening in a group at one time—and so much needs analysis—that if the leader can identify the primary or major forces affecting the group, he or she can concentrate on influencing these forces rather than on trying to influence every aspect of the group's functioning, which may be too complex a task.

If you would like to see how a group behavior pattern can become synchronized, you might want to try the following experiment (Buck & Buck, 1976).

A fairly large group is best for this experiment, but a minimum of six or seven people may be enough to demonstrate the effect.

Everyone in the group needs a large coin (such as a quarter) and a hard surface on which to tap the coin (such as a table). When everyone is ready, ask them to close their eyes and begin tapping the coin on the hard surface.

At first, the tapping noises made will seem random or out of synch but as the group continues to rap their quarters on the table, the tapping noises begin to come closer together until the whole group is rapping their coins in unison.

Groups differ in the rhythm that results. Some rhythms are slow; others are loud and insistent. They may even be more complex or syncopated in some groups. The character of the rhythm seems to reflect the climate of the group at the time of the experiment.

The pattern of behavior in the example given was the eventual rhythmic tapping of coins. The dominant synchronizer in this case was the actual noise made by tapping the coin, not the behavior itself, as group members had their eyes closed. Hearing when others tapped their coins influenced the timing of the next coin tap by each group member.

Chapple's (1979) description of the way in which synchronization occurs in a group helps to explain how the noise of the tapping quarters set up a new pattern of behavior within the group.

> If one person initiates and several others respond, in *that* interaction sequence their interaction rhythms have become synchronized with one another, even though there may not be perfect synchronization with the initiator. So doing, their *orientation system* is no longer random. . . . When set (group) events become repetitive and the group initiated to responds in unison, they share a common rhythm. . . . It is well known from practical experience that once such group response patterns are established, they generate a powerful influence on the emotional states of the individuals participating (p. 225).

Although Chapple is describing a situation in which there is a single initiator, the noise of the coins worked the same way to synchronize the group's behavior. Other dominant synchronizers are more subtle in their influence and harder to detect, but the way in which they influence the flow of the group is the same.

TYPES OF SYNCHRONIZERS. A number of physical and interactional forces originate in the group or in the group's environment and can be identified as potential dominant synchronizers. Because each group's situation is unique, it is possible only to provide a sampling of the most common ones.

A group can be strongly influenced by the amount of heat, light, or humidity in its immediate environment. For example, it is very difficult to concentrate on a lecture if you're sitting in a near-freezing classroom. A darkened room may evoke a feeling of intimacy, as it does in a candlelit restaurant, but it could also inspire fear or put people to sleep under different circumstances and in combination with other forces. In either case, however, the darkness can have a real effect on the group and can be a dominant synchronizer of that group.

The time of day, noises in a room or outside, colors, textures, and furnishings may also influence the group. For example, a formal arrangement of hard chairs in straight rows creates an air of formality and can reinforce polite, formal behavior, while soft couches and chairs evoke a casual feeling and encourage more casual behavior. Serving refreshments can have the same effect.

Each of the physical forces mentioned so far may be strong enough to influence the group, but the character of the interpersonal relations often outweighs their influence. For example:

> A group that is exhilarated over the successful completion of a long campaign is likely to respond enthusiastically to a suggestion for a new project despite fatigue or a physically uncomfortable environment. The force of the emotion of exhilaration can predominate over the fatigue or the environment, at least temporarily.

Another common example of social interaction as a dominant synchronizer is the effect of the hidden agenda. A strong hidden agenda that everyone must be serious and formally polite to one another can overcome the informality of a setting and the serving of refreshments.

Social interactions within the group's environment can also become dominant synchronizers. For example, if a large number of people are fired in an apparently indiscriminant manner when a new administration comes into an organization, the resulting climate of fear and tension is felt within the group and will affect the group's ability to function.

LEADER ACTION. The main reason for identifying the dominant synchronizers of a group is to bring some focus to the analysis of the group's dynamics. This does not mean that less dominant forces influencing the group should be completely ignored. However, because it is difficult or impossible to deal with all these forces at once, the leader can identify those that predominate and concentrate efforts on them.

The specific action taken by the leader is dependent on the types of forces predominating. For example, if a physical force dominates, the appropriate action may be to change the temperature or lighting in the meeting room. If a hidden agenda is operating, the appropriate action may be to confront the hidden agenda that is influencing the group's behavior.

Those dominant synchronizers that have a positive effect on the group should be continued. If a new seating arrangement seems to encourage participation in discussions, the leader would want to continue or perhaps improve on it.

When the force is outside the control or influence of the leader, the major action would be to increase the development of relevant coping skills. For example, if the organizational climate is tense and fearful, the leader-manager would work on keeping the fear and tension in the group limited and within bounds. You would also want to avoid actions that may escalate the tension and encourage the use of the group as a support system for individual group members and perhaps as a force to change the climate of the organization.

SUMMARY

A group is an open system consisting of three or more people joined together by either physical proximity, a shared purpose, a special meaning, or a combination of these common bonds. As an open system, groups have their own characteristics and identifiable patterns, are open to and exchange energy with their environments, and may grow and evolve over time.

The evolution of a group can be divided into five stages: forming, storming, norming, performing, and adjourning. Each of these stages has a characteristic emotional climate, group behaviors, and specific group and individual developmental tasks. Different leader actions are appropriate for each of these stages. The group reaches maturity by the fourth, or performing, stage and is a far more functional and effective system at this point than it was in the earlier stages, during which it was likely to be disorganized, inflexible, unresponsive, and uncertain of its purpose or goals. During the fifth stage, the group reaches closure by reviewing prior events, evaluating both the process and achievements, and celebrating its achievements.

Several patterns of interaction were discussed. On the individual level, group members may play functional or nonfunctional roles. Functional task roles include initiator/contributor, information giver, information seeker, opinion giver, opinion seeker, disagreer, coordinator, elaborator, energizer, summarizer, procedural technician, and recorder. Functional group-building roles are encourager, standard setter, gatekeeper, consensus taker, diagnoser, expresser, tension reliever, and follower. Nonfunctional roles are aggressor, recognition seeker, monopolizer, dominator/usurper, blocker, playboy, and zipper mouth.

On the group level, patterns of communication may be one-way, stilted, limited, open, or chaotic, Hidden agendas are unacknowledged goals that operate below the surface but exert a great deal of influence on the group. Dominant synchronizers are the primary forces affecting the behavior patterns of the group. These forces may come from within the group or from the environment and may be physical or interactional in nature.

REFERENCES*

Bennis, W.G. & Shepard, H. (1978). A theory of group development. In Bradford, L.P. *Group Development.* La Jolla, California: University Associates.

*Bion, W.R. (1961). *Experiences in Groups and Others Papers.* New York: Basic Books.

Braaten, L.J. (1974–5). Developmental phases of encounter groups and related intensive groups: A critical review of models and a new proposal. *Interpersonal Development.* 5, 112–129.

*Bradford, L.P. (1978). *Group Development.* La Jolla, California: University Associates.

Bradford, L.P. (1978). The case of the hidden agenda. In Bradford, L.P. *Group development.* La Jolla, California: University Associates.

Brill, N: (1984). *Teamwork: Working Together in the Human Services.* Philadelphia: J.B. Lippincott.

Buck, J. & Buck, E. (1976). Synchronous fireflies. *Scientific American.* 234, 5, 74.

Burggraf, C.S. & Sillars, A.L. (1987). A critical examination of sex differences in marital communication. *Communication monographs,* 54 (3), 276–294.

Chapple, E.D. (1970). *Culture and Biological Man: Explorations in Behavioral Anthropology.* New York: Holt, Rinehart & Winston. (Reprinted 1979 as *The Biological Foundations of Individuality and Culture.* Huntington, New York: Robert Krieger.)

Donnellon, A., Gray, B. & Bougon, M.G. (1986). Communication, meaning and organized action. *Administrative Science Quarterly,* 31, 43–55.

Ettling, J.T. & Jago, A.G. (1988). Participation under conditions of conflict: More on the validity of the Vroom-Yetton Model. *Journal of Management Studies,* 25 (2), 73–85.

Gemmill, G. (1986). The mythology of the leader role in small groups. *Small Group Behavior,* 17 (1), 41–50.

Gibb, J.R. & Gibb, L.M. (1978). The group as a growing organism, In Bradford, L.P. *Group Development.* La Jolla, California: University Associates.

Glisson, C. (1986). The group versus the individual as the unit of analysis in small group research. *Social Work with Groups,* 9 (13), 15–30.

Hill, B., Lippitt, L. & Serkownek, K. (1979). The emotional dimensions of the problem-solving process. *Group and Organization Studies.* 4, 1, 93.

Lacoursiere, R.B. (1980). *The Life Cycle of Groups: Group Developmental Stage Theory.* New York: Human Sciences Press.

Nielsen, E.H. (1978). Applying a group development model to managing a class. In Bradford, L.P. *Group Development.* La Jolla, California: University Associates.

*Sapir, E. (1973). Group. *Group Process.* 5 (2), 105.

Trujillo, N. (1986). Toward a taxonomy of small group interaction-coding systems. *Small Group Behavior,* 17 (4), 371–390.

*Tuckman, B.W. & Jensen, M.A.C. (1977). Stages of small group development revisited. *Group and Organization Studies.* 2 (4), 419.

*References marked with an asterisk are suggested for further reading.

Chapter 17

LEADING MEETINGS AND CONFERENCES

Chapter 17 ▬▬▬▬▬

OUTLINE

Problem Discussion Meetings
Preparation
Purpose
Plan the Presentation
Choose a Date
Choose a Place
Set the Time
Publicize the Meeting
Provide Coverage
Provide Refreshments
Reduce Threats
Implementation
Opening the Meeting
Guiding the Meeting
Summarizing
Scripts
Analysis of the Script
Sociogram
Seating Arrangement
Communication Pattern
Roles Played by Group Members

Maturity of the Group
Course of the Discussion, Decision
Making, and Outcome
Dominant Synchronizers
Leadership Style and Effectiveness

Problem-Solving Conferences
Preparation
Purpose
Plan the Presentation
Reduce Threats
Implementation
Opening the Meeting
Guiding the Meeting
Summarizing
Follow-up
Analysis
Decision Making
Outcomes

Summary

LEARNING OBJECTIVES

Upon completion of this chapter, the reader will be able to:

▷ Plan and lead a problem-discussion meeting.

▷ Plan and lead a problem-solving conference.

▷ Analyze the dynamics of a conference.

▷ Evaluate his or her leadership of a meeting or conference.

▷ Evaluate the outcomes of a problem discussion or problem-solving conference.

LEADING MEETINGS AND CONFERENCES*

T his chapter continues our study of groups. It focuses on the types of meetings and small group conferences in which health care professionals are most often involved. This includes meetings to discuss problems and ventilate feelings and conferences designed to solve problems, especially those concerned with the delivery of care.

PROBLEM DISCUSSION MEETINGS

It is often necessary to bring people together for a meeting to find out what is bothering them and to provide an opportunity for them to express their feelings (Douglas & Bevis, 1983). This kind of meeting is a problem discussion.

There is no universally accepted term for this type of meeting. It has been called a feelings conference, a confrontation meeting, a feedback meeting, and a discussion of issues. The problem discussion meeting bears some resemblance to encounter and sensitivity groups because they all deal with feelings. The primary purpose of a problem discussion, however, is to deal with a work-related problem, while encounter and sensitivity groups are formed primarily to explore the self and emotions in depth. This is not appropriate for a work group meeting in which everyone is expected to participate.

A meeting to discuss problems is frequently necessary before problem solving can be accomplished. Feelings can be so strong on an issue that they block group progress until they are dealt with in some way. Also, when emotions are high it is often not clear exactly what the problem is. Different group members can have very different perceptions of the problem. When this happens, the problem discussion is an effective way to confront the issue and clarify it before it can be resolved.

Preparing for this type of meeting will be discussed as well as points to consider in conducting a problem discussion and analyzing it afterward. The script of an entire problem discussion is included in this chapter so that you can see how a meeting like this could actually be conducted. You will see that there are flaws in the way the meeting proceeded — these are to be expected in any real meeting.

Preparation

Thorough preparation results in a more effective meeting and better use of everyone's time. There are many things to consider in preparing to lead a

---

*Co-authored by Ruth M. Tappen, R.N., Ed.D. and Cynthia Daubman, R.N., M.S.

meeting, including your purpose; the presentation; the date, the place, and time of the meeting; publicity; refreshments; providing staff coverage; and reducing any possible threat the meeting may be to those who attend.

PURPOSE. You need to think about why you are having the meeting and to decide whether a problem discussion is the right approach. If your purpose is to encourage more open communication between group members and ventilation of feelings and opinions in order to confront an unresolved conflict or identify the problem, a problem discussion is appropriate. However, if the sharing of information or the solving of a known problem is your primary purpose, a problem discussion is not appropriate.

As usual, you need to assess the situation thoroughly. A good way to do this is to write down what you have observed. Because your interpretation may differ from those of the group, be sure to separate your interpretation from your observations. You will be sharing some of these observations with the group in your opening statement and throughout the meeting. Your observations will also be the basis on which you decide who should be invited to the meeting and what needs to be accomplished at the meeting.

Usually, only one subject or problem is dealt with in the meeting. This is done to limit the meeting to a reasonable length of time, to keep it focused, and to deal with the subject of concern adequately. For example, the problem discussion script presented later in this chapter is taken from a meeting of nursing staff that was held to encourage the staff to express their feelings about caring for a particular patient and to evaluate critically the care they gave in order to improve it in the future.

> The subject of the meeting was how the staff felt about caring for patients like Mr. C. Mr. C. was an older man who had been on the unit several months before he died (his death occurred 1 week before the meeting). Mr. C. had had an extensively gangrenous foot that was hideously decayed but could not be treated surgically because he was an extremely poor surgical risk.
>
> Mr. C. also had many decubiti, was contracted into a fetal position, and was unable to care for himself at all. He did not respond verbally to the staff, and his level of awareness fluctuated. Most members of the staff found it extremely distasteful to care for him because of the odor and horrible condition of his foot and his complete dependence. The leader had observed several staff members express their distaste in Mr. C.'s presence. The leader also noticed that they spent as little time as possible in his room, although he had been there a long time and had few visitors.

When Mr. C. died, the staff felt a mixture of relief from the horror of his physical condition and guilt for the feelings they had had about caring for him. The meeting could have focused on the staff's feelings about his death, but the leader who planned it believed that it was more important to deal with their feelings about giving care to patients in this condition in the future.

PLAN THE PRESENTATION. It is important to have a design for the meeting, one that is flexible enough to accommodate the needs of the group but structured enough to guide the group toward the accomplishment of the meeting's purpose. There are two major aspects to consider: your opening remarks and prepared comments and questions to guide the group through the rest of the discussion.

The leader or manager's presentation at the beginning of the conference should be brief. A few words of welcome and comments designed to help people feel at ease are included. The purpose of the conference, the subject to be discussed, and the ground rules for the discussion (like those for confrontation) are included in the opening remarks.

If you have looked ahead at the script, you may have noticed that the leader of the meeting about Mr. C. did not directly confront the staff with their specific behavior toward this patient. Based on the leader's knowledge of the staff, the leader judged that such a strong confrontation would have been difficult for some to handle: it might have provoked anger, denials, and defensiveness, which would not have been productive. Instead, the leader took a less direct approach and encouraged the staff to discuss their experiences with Mr. C. and how they felt about caring for him. If the members of the group had not brought up some of these behaviors, however, the leader would have had to introduce them to achieve the purpose of the meeting.

It is also helpful to write down some questions, preferably open ended ones, and some additional points or observations that would help to move the group along during the discussion. For example: the leader of the problem discussion about Mr. C. prepared and used the following list of questions and points to bring out during the meeting:

1. How did you feel about him? How did you feel about caring for him? About the condition he was in?
2. Do you think that he was suffering?
3. Toward the end, was he conscious of anything?
4. When caring for a patient like Mr. C., put yourself in the patient's place. How would you feel?
5. How do you deal with suffering? Is it difficult?
6. Can nurses become desensitized to others' pain? How can the desensitization be counteracted?
7. Was it worthwhile to speak to him?
8. What was the likelihood that Mr. C. could still hear you and understood how you felt about him?
9. How should we deal with patients who are suffering, someone like Mr. C. who is comatose part of the time and aware some of the time?
10. How well did we take care of Mr. C.? What could we have done better? What can we do in the future to give better care to patients like Mr. C.?

CHOOSE A DATE.   Each situation must be assessed separately to decide the best time for the conference. Do you want to allow time for people to think about a problem before they discuss it in the group, or do you want them to share their thoughts and feelings immediately after something has happened? If a patient on the unit commits suicide during the morning, the head nurse may call a meeting just after lunchtime that same day. This allows time for the commotion surrounding the actual suicide to settle, but it does not allow much time for unexpressed feelings of guilt, grief, and anger to build up in the staff. In this case, the conference needs to be held quickly to deal with the emotions aroused by the traumatic event.

On the other hand, if the administrator announces that the agency will be changing over to management by objectives (explained in Chapter 7), the supervisor may wait until staff members have attended some inservice programs on management by objectives before calling a meeting. This could provide staff members with an opportunity to acquire some knowledge of the subject before the meeting is held. In this second instance, staff members are not as likely to have strong feelings on the subject and can discuss it more intelligently after they read about it.

Two other considerations in choosing a time are avoiding conflicts with other scheduled events and selecting a day when most staff members are able to attend.

CHOOSE A PLACE. Convenience, comfort, and an agreeable atmosphere should be considered when deciding where to hold a meeting. The place you choose should be convenient so that a minimum of time and effort are required to get there. This is true whether or not members of the group are all from the same organization. Most health care professionals are quite busy, and consideration of their need to make the best use of their time is usually appreciated.

The room you select should be comfortable. It is important to avoid any discomfort great enough to distract group members from the discussion: too hot, too cold, chairs too hard, or insufficient seating so that some have to stand. Lighting that is too harsh or too dim is also distracting; so are loud noises and harsh echoes in a room.

The atmosphere or climate of the room also affects the group. For example, the meeting room used by the board of directors may be too formal or forbidding for some people in your group, while sitting outside under a tree may be to much like a picnic to keep others serious. The size of the room can also affect the group. A small group feels lost and uncomfortable in an auditorium, while a room that is too small and crowded makes people feel constrained from moving freely because they might bump into someone. Between these extremes, the size, color, and style of a room will have a more subtle effect on the group. The personal and cultural preferences of people in the group will also affect people's response to the place selected.

The arrangement of furniture in the room is another consideration. For most small meetings, it is preferable to arrange the seating so that everyone can see each other and so that there are no obviously designated status positions in the group. An auditorium or a classroom with desks that are bolted to the floor would not meet these criteria as well as a circular table with chairs around it. It is more difficult to achieve this seating arrangement for a large group.

SET THE TIME. The time for which the conference is set should also be as convenient as possible for both the leader and the members of the group. For example, staff working the day shift often find a relative lull in the day's activities just before and just after lunch. On the other hand, people who have to travel to a meting often prefer to have it either at the beginning of the day or late in the afternoon to reduce the degree to which it interrupts their day.

PUBLICIZE THE MEETING. The people who are invited to the meeting should receive adequate notice of the time, place, and purpose. This allows them to arrange their work schedules so that they can attend the meeting and also gives them some time to think about the subject of the meeting. Reminders are also a good idea. They reduce the possibility of a busy person's forgetting the meeting, communicate the importance of that person's attendance, and eliminate that familiar excuse for absence from a meeting —"I forgot".

PROVIDE COVERAGE. Unless meetings are held before or after the usual work day, staff members must be assured that their responsibilities are being taken care of while they attend the meeting. This may necessitate having someone take telephone messages or having several staff members remain on the unit in order to provide adequate care. Unless this coverage is provided, staff members will not be able to focus their full attention on the subject of the meeting and may have to run in and out of the meeting to attend to other responsibilities, which is very distracting.

PROVIDE REFRESHMENTS. Refreshments are not necessary, but they can have a positive effect on the climate of the group. They add a feeling of warmth, sociability, and informality to the meeting, which is often desirable. The activities surrounding the distribution of refreshments help to relieve tension. Sometimes the refreshments themselves are welcome because staff have not taken time out for meals (a pattern that should be discouraged because it affects people's ability to function). Refreshments should not be so elaborate, however, that they draw the attention of either the leader or the group away from the purpose of the meeting.

REDUCE THREATS. Unless you know the individuals and the group as a whole, it is difficult to estimate how much of a threat a particular problem discussion poses for them. The meeting can be perceived as a welcome break from work or a dreaded source of tension and anxiety. Because people differ in their responses, each situation and individual will have to be assessed separately to reduce the threatening nature of a problem discussion.

The unknown is often a source of anxiety. People unfamiliar with this type of meeting will wonder what is going to happen during the meeting and what they will be asked to do. Some may feel threatened by the anticipation of any kind of confrontation. Others may be worried about being criticized or embarrassed in front of the group. An explanation of the meeting and its ground rules and prior positive experiences in problem discussions will help to reduce this threat.

People who are not accustomed to expressing any kind of feelings in a group may need extra support before they are comfortable in a problem discussion meeting. Those who are uncomfortable with being the center of attention need to be treated differently from those who feel threatened when they are not the center of attention. As leader, you need to adjust your actions and expectations accordingly.

People who hold low status positions (such as aides or orderlies) may feel uncomfortable when asked to give their opinions in front of the professionals on a health care team. Other people with higher status may see the meeting as a threat to their authority when they are not leading it. For example, in the meeting about Mr. C., the leader asked Mr. C.'s primary nurse to describe his condition to the group to prevent the primary nurse from feeling that her leadership had been usurped.

Implementation

OPENING THE MEETING. There are several things you can do to get the meeting off to a smooth start. The furniture can be arranged ahead of time, and any equipment, such as a tape recorder, can be in place and ready to use. If refreshments are being served, they should be ready and offered to people as they arrive. Greeting each person by name as they arrive makes people feel welcome and important.

It is important to start on time. Some people may have left work incomplete in order to get to the meeting on time and will resent being kept waiting. Also, if you start late, people will arrive even later for your next meeting. Those who have time to socialize can do so at the end of the meeting, so do not hesitate to break into social chatter that is going on before the meeting.

The leader opens the meeting by welcoming the group and briefly stating the purpose of the meeting. A short description of the problem to be discussed and the ground rules for the discussion is followed by an open-ended question that opens up the discussion to the rest of the group. The first page of the script is an example of the way one leader opened a meeting.

GUIDING THE MEETING. One of the leader's primary responsibilities during the rest of the meeting is to foster open communication within a nonthreatening environment. A statement at the beginning of the meeting that all group members should recognize and respect the personal and subjective nature of the opinions expressed will help to establish an accepting climate within the group. If necessary, the leader can stress that no contribution should be attacked or labeled as a "wrong" feeling or "wrong" thought. Any contribution should be accepted as stated and not judged by the group, but it may be further explored and discussed.

As the discussion proceeds, the leader can remind the group of the ground rules if it is necessary. The leader should also cut off any personal attacks and point out the differences between constructive and destructive statements and confrontations.

The leader can confront any nonfunctional behavior. For example, you can ask someone who is monopolizing the conversation to give someone else a chance to speak. Confrontation is also appropriate if the group evades the issue or denies having any problem when it is evident that a problem exists.

When the group is not sufficiently mature to recognize the needs of group members, the leader can meet some of the need for support and recognition. Nonverbal nods, smiles, positive voice tones, and eye contact, as well as verbal expressions can be used. It may also be necessary to encourage contributions from the silent members either verbally or nonverbally by looking in their direction when asking a question.

Another responsibility of the leader is to keep the discussion focused on the subject of the meeting. This is done by asking pertinent questions. Sometimes it is necessary to remind the group of the problem under consideration or to point out that the discussion is getting off the track. The leader's evident interest and concern about the problem also acts as a stimulus to keep the discussion going. Once group members become actively involved in the discussion, they too can act as energizers.

The prepared questions and comments of the leader have two other purposes. They can be used as a stimulus for discussion and to guide the group toward some kind of closure at the end of the meeting. The kind of closure needed depends on the purpose of the meeting: it may be agreement on what the problem actually is, resolution of a conflict, or simply a sense of having shared feelings and supported one another. In the example (the meeting about Mr. C.), the leader tried to guide the group toward an evaluation of the care it was giving and a commitment to improve it in the future.

SUMMARIZING. At the end of the discussion, the leader summarizes the points of view offered and identifies any closure that has been achieved by the group. It is often helpful to take notes during the conference or ask someone else to do this to be able to summarize quickly and accurately the results at the end of the meeting. Meetings that end abruptly, without a summarizing statement about the resolution of differences or consensus on how a situation can be improved, are apt to leave people feeling that nothing has been accomplished.

Scripts

The following script presents a discussion by nursing staff that took place at an actual conference. The script shows the leader carrying out many of the actions discussed above but omitting others. Comments about the leader's actions and roles played by various group members are given alongside the script. An analysis follows the script.

Problem Discussion Script

Script	Comments and Roles Played
Leader: I'm really happy that you're all taking time out to do this today, 'cause I know it's time out of your really busy schedules. We've been talking a little about what a problem discussion is. A problem discussion is when you take a subject and examine your own feelings about it and share with others your feelings and perhaps things that influence your thoughts — maybe something in your background, your past experience, or your training that influences your feelings about a certain person or a disease — something to do with nursing. And hopefully, the goal of this is to understand your fellow team members, and to promote communication. The end result is better patient care.	*Role: Initiator* The leader sounds uncertain about staff members' interest in attending the meeting. The leader could have been more positive and assertive about the value of spending time at the meeting.
This is the ideal. Would you like to try this for the next 15 minutes? (pause) Okay. I would like to talk about Mr. C. Even though he passed away about a week ago, I thought we might still discuss him because we might have patients now who are like him. Or in the future, you'll most likely run into patients like him again.	The words by themselves do not convey the nonverbal interest in the meeting evident in the leader's voice, which had staff members nodding their heads at this point.

Problem Discussion Script—*Continued*

Script	Comments and Roles Played
Would someone briefly like to run over his problems—what his condition was?	Here, the leader looked at the primary nurse, encouraging this individual's participation and showed a willingness to share leadership of the meeting.
Primary Nurse: Mr. C. was a cardiac patient. His problem was that he was such a poor surgical risk that he was not operated on. He had gangrene of the foot, and it got worse. He had contractures of both arms and legs; in fact, he was almost in the fetal position. At first, he was unable to speak to us.	*Roles: Information Giver, Contributor*
Leader: How many people here came in contact with him or cared for him?	*Role: Information Seeker*
Nurse 2: I think all of us did at one time or another.	*Role: Information Giver*
Leader: How did you feel about him? About caring for him? About the condition he was in?	Note how every other sentence is spoken by the leader here. The interaction has a stilted pattern that gradually changes as the conference progresses.
Primary Nurse: Sorry for him. So sorry that someone would have to suffer like that.	*Role: Expresser*
Leader: Do you feel that he was suffering?	
LPN 2: Oh yes, because he knew what was going on for a long time. Like, when you were doing anything to him, when he'd had enough, he'd pat you on the arm. That was for a long time. Well, toward the end it was like he wasn't a person. I mean, he was a person, but it was like he was already dead but still alive.	*Roles: Information Giver, Expresser*
Leader: So, toward the end, do you think he was conscious of anything?	Not an open-ended question. Note the response.
LPN 2: Yes.	

Problem Discussion Script—*Continued*

Script	Comments and Roles Played
Leader: Why do you think so?	
LPN 2: Because I still think Mr. C. responded to pain. When you did his dressing, he certainly indicated his discomfort. When you spoke to him and managed to get through his subconscious, I think he sort of acknowledged the fact that you were there. The response of his eyes. But even the last days it seemed he was aware.	*Roles: Information Giver, Opinion Giver*
Leader: How did you feel when you cared for him? Was it something you liked doing because he was suffering, or was it distasteful to you?	
LPN 2: I found it unpleasant. With Mr. C., I just felt like I could pick him up and hold him. You just felt empathy and I never minded being assigned Mr. C. I mean it was distasteful, *yes*. But he was just so dear. When he was himself, he used to squeeze your hand and his eyes would just twinkle. And I think when you remember these things about a patient . . . when you had a patient for so many weeks, I don't think anybody could enjoy doing the dressings because it was an almost insurmountable task. Sometimes, we ended up with the dressing looking less than desirable. It was a difficult chore. Speaking for myself, I never minded doing Mr. C. I just thought he was the sweetest thing.	*Role: Expresser*
Nurse 3: I feel pretty much the way LPN 2 did. I have my own personal problem with odors. I had to leave the room many times and come back because I really got kind of nauseated at times. I'd walk away for a minute, but I came back. But I just felt he was a patient who needed a	*Roles: Expresser, Elaborator, Contributor* This group member is openly sharing a reaction to the patient, which is what the leader had hoped to elicit from the group.

Problem Discussion Script—*Continued*

Script	Comments and Roles Played
lot of care, the basic needs. I think he was very much aware that you were taking care of him—that we did care, that we'd do anything we could to keep him comfortable. I do feel he had pain, and more could have been done in that area. We could have stressed that he should have had something for pain, which he did not have. He was a real challenge to do, but I think he was very much aware of what was happening in his room and of who came and went.	
Leader: How do you deal with a patient who's suffering?—Someone like Mr. C. who is semicomatose some of the time, aware some of the time.	*Roles: Information Seeker, Gatekeeper*
LPN 2: I don't think Mr. C. was ever what you'd call "comatose." He was, I think, deep in sleep quite a bit, but we could always manage to reach his subconscious.	At this point, the leader had to decide whether to clarify these terms for the LPN or to continue the focus on feelings—a difficult decision.
Leader: Do you think it was worthwhile to speak with him, to him?	*Role: Opinion Seeker* Again, not an open-ended question. Could have stifled discussion but it did not.
LPN 2: To him, yes.	
Nurse 3: Oh, definitely, yes. Because he was aware that we were in the room. They don't have T.V.s, they don't have radios, and I think a lot of the patients really look forward to whatever reason we come in. That's a couple of minutes they can talk to somebody. Because I think it's extremely lonesome for these patients and I really think that's a very important part of our nursing care, that you do talk about the weather or what's in the headlines. To talk to them—some kind of interaction— it keeps them in touch with reality.	*Roles: Elaborator, Contributor*

Problem Discussion Script—*Continued*

Script	Comments and Roles Played
LPN 2: I know in orientation classes, they tell us that we are to keep a patient in contact with time and place and even though the patient is unable to respond to you, you should still treat the patient as somebody with a mind that is still functioning whether we're aware of it or not. No matter how comatose a patient is, that's always the proper thing to do.	*Role: Information Giver*
Nurse 2: I had what would be termed, I suppose, a real awakening. I know when I was at another hospital we had a young man, not Mr. C., but I think it is a good simile. This young man had been in a motorcycle accident. He was only married about 3 months. I think he was about age 25. He was on a Stryker frame, fully paralyzed, totally unresponsive, with a tracheostomy tube, Foley catheter, and the whole bit. And yet his wife—it was almost eerie, and it sent shudders up and down your spine to walk past the room and hear her, day after day, reciting her marriage vows, for richer and poorer, in sickness and health. She and his whole family came in and would tell him what happened in church today, and do you know that boy came around. He walked out of that hospital and went home. And I think it's because his family kept his brain alive. As a matter of fact, even when he had the tracheostomy, we had to caution his wife against feeding him whole pieces of turkey that she had prepared at home and we'd end up suctioning him. But I mean, they would not give up on him. And I'm glad they didn't. I'm not going to say that his mind was as healthy as we would	*Roles: Elaborator, Recognition Seeker* The example given here generally supports the idea that it's important to give good care to a comatose patient but is getting off the track and could divert the group from the subject of the meeting.

Problem Discussion Script—*Continued*

Script	Comments and Roles Played
have liked it to have been; he was rather juvenile. But at least he was a functional human being. So we can't ever say that they don't hear you and that it's not going to be worth the effort.	
Leader: So you feel even if they can't respond to you in some big way that they still can hear you and understand you and get your vibes and feel how you're feeling.	Role: *Consensus Taker* The leader is bringing the discussion back to the subject.
Nurse 2: Hearing is supposed to be one of the very last senses to leave the body. And this is something we have to caution our visitors about repeatedly. Visitors will come in, and they'll even talk about funeral arrangements right over a patient. And we always have to caution them, "You know, the patient may not be talking to you but he is listening to us."	Role: *Information Giver*
LPN 3: Some things, even to say, "Gee, he must be so uncomfortable" —at least that person may hear what you're saying and at least know that you're trying to understand he's uncomfortable. Those things, I feel are right to be said. It's a real situation to them, it's a real situation to us. And I think we should be factual, and if he's uncomfortable, let's do something about it.	Role: *Opinion Giver*
Leader: When you're caring for a patient who is in very sad condition, like Mr. C., or someone who really wins your heart, do you feel sorry for those patients, do you ever put yourself in their place?	Role: *Opinion Seeker*
LPN 2: I think that's a good idea, to put yourself in another's place, because then you would be gentler with them. And you wouldn't want somebody to be rough with you if you were a patient.	Roles: *Encourager (accepting another's idea), Opinion Giver*

Problem Discussion Script—*Continued*

Script	Comments and Roles Played
Leader: Is it difficult to deal with suffering?	Again, this question could have elicited a discussion-stopping *yes* or *no* answer, but the group is moving along well enough that it did not have this effect.
LPN 2: Yes, it always is if you have compassion for someone. We had a nursing arts instructor who told us whenever we enter a room we are to consider a patient's age. And if the patient is 25 years old and you are 24, you consider this your husband, brother, sister, or whatever the case may be. If the patient's twice your age you can say, "This could well be my father or mother, and I intend to take care of the patient as I would care for my own parents, and so forth." I think this is something everybody should do. Aside from putting yourself in that person's position, just to think in terms of this person belonging to you in some relationship.	*Roles: Information Giver, Contributor*
LPN 3: Just in terms of interaction between one human being and another. If you were very ill, and some stranger came in to care for you, you'd hope that that stranger would treat you like a human being. The family concept I was also taught —person to person, stranger to stranger. You walk into that room and consider how you'd like to be cared for by a stranger.	*Role: Elaborator*
Leader: Do you feel that a nurse can be desensitized to pain? Can you be bombarded with people who are suffering so much that you might forget?	*Role: Consensus Taker*
Nurse 3: I think you can be too busy sometimes, for the moment, to stop and think, but I don't think you could ever be really desensitized.	*Role: Opinion Giver*

Problem Discussion Script—*Continued*

Script	Comments and Roles Played
Nurse 2: You build up certain protections for yourself, because you are around them so much. You have to protect yourself—we'd be drained, thoroughly drained, if we didn't. But myself, no, I would never be completely desensitized.	*Roles: Elaborator, Opinion Giver*
Leader: So, summing up, if we were to walk into a patient's room who couldn't communicate with us or whose communication was minimal, and it was evident that the patient was suffering a great deal—and needed total care—and you had to give the patient a bed bath, what kinds of things would you consider or should do or think of while you were caring for the patient, knowing that the patient is suffering?	*Role: Coordinator and Information Seeker, not Summarizer* The leader is not really summarizing as stated here but is guiding the group toward moving on to the second purpose of the conference which was to critically evaluate the care they give.
LPN 3: Be gentle, don't take too long, just straighten the patient out —wash, turn, and position the patient. Just remember the patient's a human being. Every patient's different and you see so much suffering. And I really felt terrible for Mr. C.— it was terrible to see someone have to die like that, and see that gangrene every day. And then we had a Mr. H. here and I found that very bad. That was enough to break your heart, watching that man suffer.	*Roles: Contributor, Expresser*
LPN 2: They both had the problem, too, of loose bowels. I know I will certainly admit to being guilty of saying, just after getting Mr. C. repositioned and dressed, "Oh, no, not again!" I would voice what crossed my mind because all of a sudden it was running all over and we had to begin from scratch again.	*Roles: Information Giver, Expresser*
LPN 3: What could you talk to the patient about when you were going to give the patient a bath? If you had to move him into the portatub?	*Roles: Information Seeker, Gatekeeper* Nonverbally, the LPN looked around the group while saying this.

Problem Discussion Script—*Continued*

Script	Comments and Roles Played
Nurse 2: You're supposed to tell your patient, "Now, Mr. C., we have to move you, and pick you up. It's going to hurt." Let them know what's being done. You're not supposed to pick the patient up and just suddenly put the patient in the middle of the air even though they're supported by strong arms. They should know where they're going and why.	*Roles: Information Giver, Opinion Giver*
LPN 2: I don't think any of us do that. We all talk to them—we all say, "Okay, you're going to get a bath and have to roll over." We all talk to them. That would be scary. . . .	You can see that the meeting has become much less stilted here. This is a common pattern as people relax and become more involved in the discussion.
Nurse 3: Even a patient that you're not sure what they're hearing and seeing or how much they're aware of, if we say our name to them, "I'm S.T., and I'm going to take care of you and give you a bath," a voice and a name. They remember good things and bad things, so, if they're waiting for that one person, it must drive them crazy when we don't say our name! Even though they can't say, "Good morning, I'm Mr. C.," we should still say, "Good morning, I'm S.T."	*Role: Elaborator*
LPN 1: He didn't want to be touched. He just wanted you to leave him alone and let him die.	*Role: Blocker* The tone of voice and body language strongly communicated negative feelings from this group member, who only spoke once. If it were not for the nonverbal negativism, the role would have been disagreer.
LPN 2: I know, especially when you were doing his mouth and suctioning, and so forth, he just sort of looked up annoyed. I think sometimes they just wish you wouldn't show up on the scene when they're bubbling froth and so forth. I got that impression.	*Role: Elaborator*

Problem Discussion Script—*Continued*

Script	Comments and Roles Played
Nurse 2: I think we were with him the last day, and, LPN 2, you were doing him up and we rolled him over. He ceased breathing. We suctioned him and he went on for another 12 hours.	*Role: Information Giver* This group member is getting off the track again.
Leader: But you felt he communicated with his eyes.	Again, the leader is bringing the group back on the track by restating what LPN 2 had said. This is also a good way to support what people have said.
Nurse 2: I think he certainly did, and with his hand, too. There would be pressure from his hand. When I spoke to him and asked if he could hear me, it was like he was really trying to communicate. The reason we knew he was in pain, too, because when you were dressing him, and he was turned to his side, his arms were extremely long and he had 7-inch fingers, and he'd be doing this, trying to grasp your bottom or your waist or your back, just to let you know that you were hurting him. I mean I don't think it was any other sense, it was just his way of reacting. You don't often see, thank goodness, challenges quite like Mr. C. Most of them never get to that stage. He was an elderly man, but he had an extremely strong heart. He had pneumonia three times while he was here.	*Roles: Expresser, Information Giver, Opinion Giver* Note that this response is back on the track.
Leader: Is there anything else anyone would like to say?	*Role: Gatekeeper*
Leader: Well, thank you all very much for taking time out. I really am very appreciative of it.	The summary belongs here but was omitted by the leader.
LPN 2: Thanks a lot. I learned a lot from you.	*Role: Encourager.*

ANALYSIS OF THE SCRIPT. The number of factors that can be included in the analysis of a conference is almost endless. For the most part, the ones included here are those that have been emphasized before: the seating arrangement, communication patterns, roles played by each group member, maturity of the group, course of the discussion, the decision-making process and outcomes of the conference, dominant synchronizers, and the leader's style and effectiveness. In addition to these, a sociogram that illustrates the pattern of the group interaction has been included.

SOCIOGRAM. A sociogram (Beal, Bohlen, & Raudabaugh, 1962) is simply a diagram that illustrates the seating arrangement of the group, the number of contributions and side comments each member made, and to whom they were directed: the leader, a group member, or the group as a whole (Fig. 17–1). It can be drawn during the meeting, or it can be made afterward from a videotape of the meeting. The leader of the group is usually too involved in other activities to make a sociogram during the meeting. To draw a sociogram:

> Begin with an outline of the room and a schematic representation of the furniture arrangement. As people take their seats their names are placed on the diagram. When the meeting begins, the recorder draws a line from one group member to another to indicate who

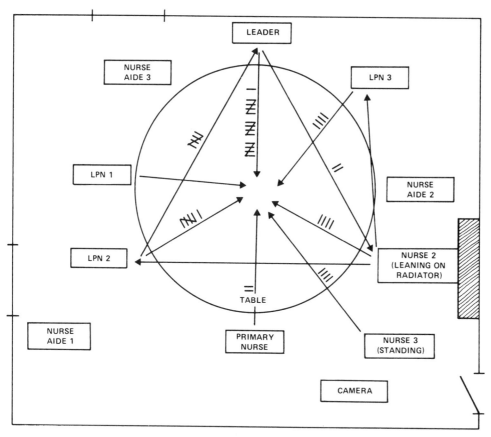

Figure 17–1. Sociogram drawn during a problem discussion.

spoke to whom. An arrow to the center of the diagram indicates a comment made to the group as a whole. The slashes on these lines indicate how many times a message was sent in this same direction.

When it is done, the sociogram indicates who the most active contributors were, who was the recipient of most of the comments, and who did not participate. The pattern of interaction can be seen from the lines and direction of the arrows. It may also show how the seating arrangement influenced the interaction. The sociogram cannot tell you what the climate of the group was, what roles were played by group members, or the value of the contributions made. For example:

Figure 17–1 shows the sociogram drawn for the problem discussion relating to Mr. C.'s care. You can see that the leader spoke much more often than anyone else and that none of the nurses aides spoke at all. Note also that Nurse Aide 1 was voluntarily positioned outside the group. LPN 1 spoke only once, but the other two LPNs were more active contributors. Nurse 2 directed comments to several different people as well as to the group, and this active role would lead you to look at the script to see if Nurse 2 dominated the group or tried to usurp the leadership of the group, which was not done in this case.

SEATING ARRANGEMENT. The number of chairs available was inadequate, leaving two people standing throughout the meeting. One of the people began shifting from foot to foot as though getting tired of standing. The arrangement of the chairs was an informal circle that allowed each member to make eye contact with everyone else who sat in a circle. Those who stood and the aide who moved to sit in the corner could not make eye contact as well as the others.

COMMUNICATION PATTERN. You can see from both the sociogram and the script that the overall communication pattern was somewhat stilted. This is especially true for the beginning of the meeting, when every other contribution came from the leader. Later in the meeting, the spontaneity of the group increased considerably.

ROLES PLAYED BY GROUP MEMBERS. Most of the roles played by group members were functional ones, as you will see in the following review. You will also notice that nonverbal behavior, which cannot be communicated well in either the script or in the sociogram, is an important component of the role played.

1. The PRIMARY NURSE played the roles of *information giver, contributor, expresser, and follower.* At the beginning of the conference, the primary nurse reviewed Mr. C.'s condition, and the information this group member gave served as the basis for further discussion. Throughout the rest of the meeting, the primary nurse sat in silence, not a disinterested or sulky silence, but one that communicated an attentive attitude, as this member looked at each speaker with an expression of interest. The primary nurse also indirectly encouraged others to feel free to say what they felt by having done so early in the conference.
2. NURSE 2 played the roles of *information giver, recognition seeker, elaborator, and opinion giver.* Nurse 2 also played a nonfunctional role once. Twice this group member's contributions tended to get off the track, but Nurse 2's overall contribution to the group was not really negative because this member generally supported the purpose of the meeting and other people's comments. Owing to the lack of chairs, this

group member stood leaning against the radiator through the whole meting.

3. NURSE 3 played only functional roles. Nurse 3 shared feelings near the beginning of the meeting about caring for Mr. C. and about how odors were offensive to Nurse 3. Nurse 3 acted as an *elaborator, contributor, opinion giver, and expresser* several times. This member's overall contribution was very positive, and, with frequent participation, Nurse 3 helped to keep the discussion moving along. This group member also stood through the whole meeting and seemed to get tired and restless near the end.

4. LPN 1, in contrast, played only nonfunctional roles. LPN 1 was a *blocker and a zipper mouth.* Except for one comment, which was negative, this member sat silently throughout the conference, looking around the room, not making eye contact with any of the speakers. A slight scowl and peeved expression were evident on this member's face.

   Apparently, LPN 1 came to the meeting because this member felt pressured to attend by both the leader and the primary nurse, not because of a desire to attend. Before the meeting, LPN 1 said, "I can't be in two places at one time. Someone has to stay on the floor!" in an angry voice. During the meeting, LPN 1 sulked and LPN 1's overall contribution was negative because this member's behavior had a dampening effect on the group.

5. LPN 2 was an *information giver, opinion giver, expresser, contributor, elaborator, and encourager.* The roles LPN 2 played were as functional and positive as those played by Nurse 3, except that some of what LPN 2 said was not entirely accurate. LPN 2 sat at the table actively listening and making eye contact with each speaker, sometimes frowning with concern when Mr. C.'s suffering was mentioned. LPN 2's contributions and voice were warm and friendly in tone, indicating this member's willingness to support the stated purpose of the meetings.

6. LPN 3 played the roles of *opinion giver, elaborator, contributor, expresser, information seeker, and gatekeeper.* LPN 3 responded positively to other people's contributions and expressed some feelings about Mr. C. This group member sat at the table and remained silent at the beginning of the meeting, seeming to need time to warm up.

7. NURSE AIDE 1 played only the role of the *zipper mouth.* Nurse Aide 1 did not say one word during the conference but sat in a corner, removed from the group physically as well as socially. Nurse Aide 1 was inattentive, looked down frequently, and had a bored facial expression. This member's yawns seemed to indicate a lack of interest. Nurse Aide 1 enjoyed the provided refreshments and seemed to regard the conference as a chance to sit down and get away from the unit for a while.

   This group member's effect was primarily neutral. Nurse Aide 1 neither added nor detracted, this member's presence was barely felt. This member was like an object that was simply present, similar to one of the lockers.

8. NURSE AIDE 2 acted as a *follower.* Although Nurse Aide 2 did not say a single word, this group member sat up straight and made eye contact with each speaker, occasionally nodding in agreement. Nurse Aide 2's contribution to the group was positive in the sense that this member nonverbally supported others when they spoke.

9. NURSE AIDE 3 was also a *follower*. Nurse Aide 3 sat at the table near the leader and watched with wide-eyed curiosity. This group member had never attended a problem discussion before and was attentive throughout the meeting. Nurse Aide 3's contribution was positive in the sense that this member acted as an attentive audience.

MATURITY OF THE GROUP. The somewhat stilted communication pattern is one indication that the group had not achieved maturity. Much of the discussion had an air of politeness and restraint (noted also nonverbally), and there were no group-generated confrontations. Several group members were quite open about their reactions to Mr. C., but others seemed to hold back. Still others contributed nothing, and the group made no attempt to include them, which would have been another sign of a mature group.

This group was composed of people from the same patient care unit. They work together on a regular basis but evidently have not developed into a mature group. They certainly have not completed the performing stage of group development and are probably working on some of the tasks of the norming stage of group development.

COURSE OF THE DISCUSSION, DECISION MAKING, AND OUTCOME. There were only two minor instances in which members of the group began to get off the track. With these exceptions, the discussion remained focused on the subject introduced by the leader.

Although the discussion became less stilted and more relaxed as it continued, there was little change in the way group members dealt with the subject. In fact, there wasn't much more sharing at the end of the meeting than at the beginning nor was there any increase in the depth or strength of the feelings shared or of the emotions aroused during the meeting. This indicates that an unspoken agreement—that no group member would confront another member about their feelings or about the care they gave to Mr. C.—was probably operating as a hidden agenda. In spite of this hidden agenda, there was some discussion of the ways in which patients such as Mr. C. should be cared for, which was something the leader had hoped to accomplish.

It is interesting to note that all of the nurses and most of the LPNs participated verbally in the discussion, but the aides did not. The reasons for their lack of verbal participation need to be explored before the next problem discussion to increase their involvement in the group. The aides could have been uncomfortable with the subject of the meeting, with expressing negative feelings in a group that contains people who have some authority over them, or both. Because the aides did not participate verbally, any decision made by this group would have come from the nurses and two of the LPNs and would not have been a true consensus of the group.

Actually, the design of the meeting was not meant to lead to any specific decisions about actions that the group would take in the future. These decisions would probably have been premature at this point and so probably would not be carried out later. The group did come to some agreement on the fact that a patient such as Mr. C. can suffer terribly, can understand and respond to their communications, and is greatly in need of good nursing care. Also, the meeting did increase the staff's awareness of the needs of patients such as Mr. C. and supported those who tried to give them good care. However, they did not directly confront the fact that their care of Mr. C. had been lacking in several respects or that they needed to improve the standard of care in the future for patients with similar conditions, which was the leader's hoped-for outcome of the meeting. Additional meetings with a deeper exploration of the issues could eventually lead to such a commitment from the entire group.

To summarize the outcomes, the first purpose of this meeting, to encourage a sharing of feelings about caring for Mr. C., was fairly well accomplished, although the depth of the sharing could have been greater. The second purpose, to critically evaluate the care they gave, was partially met. The hoped-for commitment to improve care in the future was not achieved.

DOMINANT SYNCHRONIZERS.   The hidden agenda to avoid confrontation was the most apparent dominant synchronizer of this group, from the beginning of the meeting right to the end. The leader's evident concern for the needs of patients such as Mr. C. was a second influence throughout the discussion, but it did not overcome the force of the hidden agenda.

LEADERSHIP STYLE AND EFFECTIVENESS.   The leader's style during the meeting was clearly participative, but the leader was more directive (authoritarian) in the preparation of the meeting, having chosen the subject without input from the group. However, the choice itself was appropriate and based on the leader's observations.

The leader's preparation for the meeting was thorough in some respects but not in others. Everyone invited to the meeting was given adequate notice of the date, time, and place, and all knew what the subject of the meeting would be. Everyone who was invited attended, although one did so under protest. This member's needs were clearly not met by the leader or the group. The meeting started and ended on time. The refreshments were simple and ready when people began to arrive. The seating was inadequate, and this could and should have been avoided. The leader prepared some helpful questions and comments ahead of time, but the opening remarks did not explain the ground rules clearly. Apparently, the leader did not take notes or have anyone record comments during the meeting to use as a summary at the end.

Comments have already been made about the effectiveness of most of the leader's actions during the meeting so they will be only summarized here. The leader's questions, although not always open ended, were pertinent and helped to keep the discussion moving along in the right direction. The group was kept on track most of the time (which is not always easy to do) and did share some thoughts and feelings. The leader's verbal and nonverbal behavior was supportive, encouraging, and nonjudgmental throughout the meeting, which is especially important during a problem discussion.

No meeting or conference is perfect. The flaws that are pointed out in this analysis do not reflect any serious errors in judgment or failure to take action on the part of the leader. Instead, they reflect the ordinary ups and downs of leading meetings and conferences that you can expect to encounter in your practice of leadership and management.

PROBLEM-SOLVING CONFERENCES ————————————

Problem-solving conferences are meetings held for the purpose of finding solutions to the numerous problems encountered by people at work.

Although many problems can be solved by an individual, group problem solving has several advantages. Group problem solving brings together the expertise and diverse viewpoints of several people. Combining the energies of group members can have a synergistic effect and result in more inventive, creative solutions to problems. In addition, people who are actively involved in the whole process are far more likely to be committed to carrying out the solution than are people who have been handed a ready-made solution.

Many different types of problems can be raised and dealt with in a problem-solving conference, including procedural problems, difficulties in relationships within the team or with other departments and agencies, and problems encountered in working with patients or clients. Patient-centered, client-centered, and family-centered conferences are all different types of problem-solving conferences concerned with working out better ways to deliver care.

The term *problem* is used in the broad sense here to mean any kind of difficulty, dilemma, or complex situation in which careful and thorough planning is needed to work out the best way to approach the situation. The problems can be minor ones that are dealt with in a few minutes, or they can be major ones that require a series of meetings for their resolution.

A format for problem-solving conferences is described in this section. It is a suggested format that can be adapted to one's own particular situation. Many of the considerations in preparing, implementing, and analyzing the problem-solving conference are the same as those for leading a problem discussion, so only the areas in which there are differences are discussed.

Preparation

PURPOSE.   A problem-solving conference is held for the purpose of proposing alternative actions that can be taken in a particular situation, weighing each of these alternatives, and deciding which ones to implement after the conference. It is a group approach to the problem-solving process.

The problem discussion is held primarily to allow the ventilation of feelings and to clarify issues. Once this is done, problem solving can take place. It is not always necessary to hold a problem discussion first. When the subject is not an emotional one and the problem can be readily identified and agreed upon, you can proceed directly to problem solving with the group.

Problem-solving conferences are most effective when they are an integral part of your team's or department's regular functions. They are designed to bring together the knowledge and skills of all team members to deal with the regularly occurring perplexities of providing high-quality health care services. They are not meant to be held only when something has gone wrong or when students are assigned to the team.

When problem-solving conferences are regularly scheduled, team members can anticipate them and plan their work schedules accordingly. These conferences can also increase the team's cohesiveness by providing opportunities to share ideas and experiences. When staff members are accustomed to the conferences, they are more likely to suggest subjects to be dealt with and less likely to be threatened—provided, of course, that the conferences are conducted in a nonthreatening manner.

PLAN THE PRESENTATION. Problems are identified and clarified before the conference so that the group can move quickly into generating solutions. The extent to which group members need to be involved in this part of the presentation depends on how difficult it is to clarify the problem.

To set the stage for problem solving, it is important to gather all information available on the subject and to present a clear picture of the problem to the group. This preparation usually requires more extensive fact gathering than is necessary for a problem discussion. If preparation is not done well, the group will spend too much time adding information or disagreeing with your initial presentation of the problem, and little problem solving will be done.

Usually there are several sources of information that can be tapped for the needed data, including the people who will be invited to the conference. For example, if you were planning a family-centered conference, you would use your own observations, agency records, other agencies who were involved with the family, the family itself, and each participant in the conference as sources of information. Consulting with conference participants not only supplies information but also gives you an opportunity to find out their opinions, identify potential blockers, and reinforce the importance of each group member's participation.

When your data gathering has been completed, the information is summarized in a brief but complete description of the situation and statement of the problem. The emphasis should be on the most pertinent facts and the current picture rather than on the history except when it influences the current problem. This is especially important when preparing a summary about a client with a long and complicated health history. You may want to share this summary with group members ahead of time.

When the problem concerns a client, it can be stated in terms of a theoretical framework. For example, if the conference is about a family about to be evicted from their apartment, the problem can be stated as a threat to the family's basic physical need for shelter, using Maslow's hierarchy of needs as the theoretical framework. The use of a theoretical framework may help to prevent participants from restating the problem in terms of their own framework, especially in an interdisciplinary conference where people from different professions often use different terms and concepts to describe the same problems.

REDUCE THREATS. Because current situations and alternative actions are discussed more than personal feelings during a problem-solving conference, the meeting itself is not likely to be threatening, even to those who are not accustomed to attending them. However, the unfamiliar is always potentially threatening to some people, so be alert to this potential response.

A problem-solving conference may pose a threat to people in several other ways. Some people are uncomfortable about having their work discussed in a group and may be anxious about the possibility of being criticized or embarrassed during the meeting. Others, especially ancillary personnel, may be afraid of saying something stupid or of not having anything to contribute. Most of the time, these feelings are not strong enough to keep people from attending the conference. Although this can and does happen, you can take action so that people feel comfortable enough to attend and participate in the meeting.

Implementation

A problem-solving conference begins with opening remarks, a description of the problem, and a statement of the problem. This is followed by discussion of alternative solutions to the problem and a decision on which actions will be taken. Finally, the conference is summarized and the decisions that were made are carried out.

The leader of the conference makes the opening remarks, describes the problem, and then turns over the discussion to the group. The leader guides the discussion, summarizes the results of the meeting, and ensures that the decisions are followed up after the meeting.

OPENING THE MEETING.   A few words of welcome from the leader are a good way to begin any meeting. Greetings are followed by a brief explanation of the purpose of the meeting. Reminding people about the ground rules for confrontation is not always necessary as it was for the problem discussion, but it is helpful to remind the group that time is limited, ask them to keep to the subject, and encourage contributions. In some situations, it may be a good idea also to remind the group of the difference between constructive and destructive criticism.

The description of the problem is probably the most important part of your opening remarks because it sets the stage for the rest of the meeting. After describing the problem (a useful rule of thumb is to limit yourself to 5 minutes for doing this), you open the floor for suggestions from the group. For example, you can say, "How can we as a group [or team] help the family meet their need for adequate shelter?" This statement, or one similar, serves to summarize the problem and encourage contributions. It also fosters group feelings and emphasizes the responsibility of the group members rather than the leader to generate suggestions for solving the problem.

Once the leader has asked this question, the leader remains silent in order to allow group members to get involved in the discussion. Remaining silent can be difficult to do if you are anxious to have the meeting go well. While the period of silence may seem like an eternity, it is usually only a matter of seconds before someone in the group begins the problem solving.

GUIDING THE MEETING.   There are two goals to accomplish during the meeting: Generate alternative solutions to the problem, and decide which will actually be implemented after the conference.

Most of the suggestions should come from the group. The leader's primary role is to encourage and recognize these contributions and keep the group focused on the subject of the meeting. You can list suggestions on a blackboard if one is available. If the group gets stuck, you can suggest that they try brainstorming to come up with a solution. At other times during the meeting, it may be necessary to restate the problem if the group gets off the track. If restating the problem does not help, you can point out to group members that they are getting off the subject.

A climate of acceptance encourages creative suggestions, so you also need to ensure that people are not criticized or attacked for making a contribution. Verbal or nonverbal attention from the leader also stimulates contributions. Every suggestion should be responded to in some way so that people are not discouraged from making further suggestions. The suggestions should also be recorded so that none are forgotten and all are recognized.

When the group has finished generating alternatives, the leader guides the discussion into the decision-making phase of the conference. Both a selection from among the alternatives and a commitment to carrying out the actions are needed to fulfill the purpose of the conference.

While the suggestions were being made, there may have been some spontaneous evaluative comments, and some mature groups will progress to a consensus without guidance. Most groups, however, will need some direction from the leader in order to reach a consensus. If the group comes to a decision too quickly, it may be necessary to test and challenge their commitment to the decisions made because a superficial agreement will quickly fall apart after the conference.

There are several common problems with group members that you are likely to encounter when leading problem-solving conferences (Bradford, 1976; Haiman, 1951): group members who talk too much, who do not talk at all, or who try to take over the leadership of the group. These nonfunctional behaviors usually reflect an unmet need of some kind. For example, aggressive and monopolizing behavior can be the result of frustration from not being able to achieve a desired goal. Feelings of insecurity may also be manifested by aggressive behavior. When these needs cannot be met within the group or by other actions of the leader, other measures must be taken to reduce their disruptive effects on the group. In this case, the leader can encourage contributions from others and avoid making eye contact with the monopolizer. A person who continually monopolizes the discussion can also be asked to give someone else a chance to speak. Direct statements about expected behavior in the group may be necessary in dealing with a person who attacks others. Group pressure also effectively restrains attacking behavior. Occasionally, it is necessary to speak with the person before or after the meeting if the behavior is sufficiently disruptive and/or part of a long-term pattern.

Lack of participation may be the result of fears of being ridiculed, hurt, or embarrassed by the group. It may also be the result of disinterest, sulking, or simply having nothing to say. Although the nonparticipant is usually not disruptive, this member's silence does affect the group. Just imagine leading an entire group of zipper mouths and you will understand why.

Assertive behavior on the part of the leader is necessary when faced with attempts to usurp that leadership. The participative leader shares leadership with the group but does not abdicate the leadership role. Weak, unassertive leaders leave a leadership gap that others will try to fill. People who are accustomed to the leadership role may find it difficult or uncomfortable to allow someone else to act as the leader of a conference in which they are participating. When the usurping of leadership is a conscious power play, the leader needs to confront this behavior or counter it with a stronger power play. It can actually become necessary to use power tactics to overcome an attempt to take over your leadership in some instances.

SUMMARIZING. Summarizing the results at the end of a meeting reviews the conference, ensures that everyone agrees with the results, and reminds everyone of what they have agreed on during the conference. Every suggestion offered should be mentioned in order to provide recognition for participation and to avoid anyone's feeling that their contribution was worthless. This listing is followed by a statement of the actions that the group has decided to take to resolve the problem.

FOLLOW-UP. Unless the actions chosen by the group are actually implemented, there is little reason to hold the conference. For this reason, the leader-manager's responsibility extends beyond the end of the conference to following up and ensuring that these actions are actually carried out. Even when the group seems to be highly motivated to carry out its decisions, you cannot assume that all decisions will be implemented. If the decisions are not carried out, the time and energy spent on planning and attending the meeting are wasted, and future problem-solving conferences are likely to be viewed with disinterest, or even resistance.

Analysis

DECISION MAKING. A participative, democratic decision-making process is vital to the successful outcome of a problem-solving conference. The active participation of every member of the group is sought because each participant will be expected to carry out the decisions made by the group. Decisions made by the leader or by only a few group members will not get as much support from the rest of the group as would decisions based on a true consensus of the group. When the leader or a subgroup dominates the decision making during the meeting, the rest of the group may simply ignore the decisions after the conference (see Research Example 18-1).

OUTCOMES. The decision made should effectively resolve the original problem as well as represent a consensus from the group. For example, if the group decides to continue an action that has not been helpful in the past, the meeting probably did not accomplish anything, even if a consensus was achieved. On the other hand, if the group has come up with a well-conceived, creative solution and is committed to carrying out the solution, the meeting was worthwhile.

With the exception of the decision-making process and the outcomes discussed above, the analysis of a problem-solving conference should look for the same elements as the analysis of a problem discussion: the sociogram, seating arrangements, pattern of interaction, group roles, course of the discussion, dominant synchronizers, and leader style and effectiveness, all discussed in the previous section on problem discussions.

SUMMARY ─────────────────────────────────

Problem discussions are a type of meeting designed to allow ventilation of feelings, confrontation, and clarification of issues before problem solving can be accomplished. Preparation for such a meeting involves consideration of the purpose and the potentially threatening nature of the meeting, the leader's presentation, and coverage for the staff as well as deciding on the date, time, place, seating arrangements, and refreshments. The opening remarks by the leader should include greetings, the purpose of the meeting, the ground rules, and a brief description of the problem. The main responsibilities of the leader during the rest of the meeting are to enforce the group rules, keep the discussion focused on the subject, provide support, encourage participation, confront when needed, guide the group toward closure, and summarize accomplishments at the end of the meeting. The script of an actual problem-discussion meeting was included with a detailed analysis of the group dynamics and leader's actions.

Problem-solving conferences are meetings held to work out ways to resolve the many procedural, interpersonal, and nursing care problems encountered by work groups. The preparation, implementation, and analysis is similar to the problem discussion except that a more complete presentation of the problem is made. The purpose of the meeting is to generate a list of alternative solutions and to obtain a commitment from the group to carry out the selected actions after the conference. A successful conference results in action that will effectively resolve the original problem.

REFERENCES

Beal, G.M., Bohlen, J.M., & Raudabaugh, J.N. (1962). *Leadership and dynamic group action.* The Iowa State University Press, Ames, Iowa.

Bradford, L.P. (1976). *Making Meetings Work: A Guide for Leaders and Group Members.* University Associates, La Jolla, California.

Douglass, L.M. & Bevis, E.O. (1983). *Nursing Management and Leadership in Action.* 3d ed. C.V. Mosby, St. Louis.

Haiman, F.S. (1951). *Group Leadership and Democratic Action.* Houghton Mifflin, New York.

Chapter 18

OUTLINE

Motivating the Individual Employee
Five Basic Needs as Motivators
  Economic Security
  Control
  Recognition
  Personal Self-Worth
  Belonging
A Goal-Based Model

Facilitating Teamwork
Teams
  Composition
  Purpose
  Leadership
  Function
Advantages and Disadvantages Of
  Teamwork
  Advantages
  Disadvantages
Team Building
  Select Team Members
  Set Goals

Define Roles
Develop Team Identity and
  Cohesiveness
Guide Decision Making
Influence Group Norms
Encourage Open Communication
Manage Conflicts

**Staffing Decisions: Delegating
Responsibility**
Criteria for Making Assignments
  Task-Related Factors
  Relationship Factors
Communicating Assignments
Issues and Problems in Delegation
  Difficulty Delegating
  Manager or Specialist or Both?
  Inadequate Staff
  Assigning Undesirable Work

Summary

LEARNING OBJECTIVES

Upon completion of this chapter, the reader will be able to:

▷ Compare and contrast the goal-based and needs-based models for motivating employees.

▷ Discuss the advantages and disadvantages of team versus individual work assignments.

▷ Make appropriate and fair staffing decisions on a nursing unit.

▷ Build an effective nursing or interdisciplinary team in a health care setting.

TEAMWORK AND MOTIVATION

How can I get people to do their work? How can I get them to work well together? These two fundamental questions have plagued and bewildered leader-managers for years, if not centuries.

Certainly there are no simple answers to these two important questions, but in this chapter we will attempt to find some solutions. We will begin by looking at the major factors thought to motivate individuals at work and at a goal-based model to explain motivation. We will also consider how people work together as a team. The advantages and disadvantages of teamwork, ways in which the leader-manager can facilitate teamwork, direct efforts at team building, and appropriate ways to divide and delegate responsibility among team members are then explored.

MOTIVATING THE INDIVIDUAL EMPLOYEE

A look back at the leadership and management theories of Chapter 3 (especially those of Herzberg, McGregor, and Ouchi) will show you how many possible answers there are to the question of how to motivate people. "Participative management," would be one theorist's answer to this question. "No, the efficient design of the job is most important," would be another theorist's response. "You must provide adequate monetary rewards," cries a third theorist. "No, you must do all of these things and more!" shouts the fourth theorist.

As a leader or manager you cannot actually motivate other people, but you can stimulate and encourage motivation. Motivation is intrinsic, an internal drive that cannot be applied from the outside. What you *can* do is to stimulate that motivation, to draw it out and nurture it where the potential exists.

Five Basic Needs as Motivators

Kafka (1986) identified five basic motivators that can be influenced by the leader-manager. These basic motivators are as follows.

ECONOMIC SECURITY. Money in the form of good salary, pay raises, bonuses, and so forth. Example: Bonuses for the unit that submitted the best cost-saving suggestion; merit payraises.

CONTROL. Ability and opportunity to influence the situation. Example: Staff participation in scheduling days off.

RECOGNITION. Attention and visibility. Example: Announcement of accomplishments at team meetings.

PERSONAL SELF-WORTH. The feeling of being appreciated. Example: Thanking a staff member for a job well done.

BELONGING. The feeling of being accepted. Example: Being included in an invitation to lunch or an after-work celebration of someone's birthday.

Every staff member has these basic needs, but each person has them to a different degree. People also differ in their perception of whether or not a need is fulfilled. For example, one employee might see two tickets to a football game as an adequate reward for working overtime during the past month, while another would not be satisfied with anything less than time and a half for each extra hour worked.

According to Maslow's theory (see Chapter 1), there is a hierarchy of needs, beginning with the physiologic need, progressing to safety and security, and so on until the person whose other more basic needs are met will strive for selfactualization. Based on this hierarchy, it would be assumed that the employee's more basic needs had to be met before the employee would be motivated to meet his or her need for recognition or self-actualization.

However, not everyone agrees with the concept of a hierarchy of needs. Some research has shown, for example, that men and women differ somewhat in their needs. For both men and women, control or the ability to influence a situation is the most important motivator; however, economic security is the second most important motivator for men, while it is third most important for women (following personal self-worth). The point is that *employees cannot all be treated alike* if you wish to stimulate each one's motivation (Kafka, 1986; Matejka & Dunsing, 1988).

A Goal-Based Model

A different approach to motivation is based on an analysis of the goals that are set and responses to the degree to which they are met (Evans, 1986). This model is quite complicated, but it does suggest some leader actions to increase motivation.

In the first stage (Fig. 18–1), the employee faces a new task and accepts a goal that has been set by the manager, by the employee, or by both. Accepting the goal has several effects. It directs attention to the task, mobilizes and sustains effort, and stimulates thinking about ways to meet the goal. A difficult goal is generally thought to increase motivation unless it is considered unrealistic or impossible to achieve. The effort to reach the goal occurs in the second or performance stage of the cycle.

At the third stage of this cyclical process, both the employee and manager evaluate the degree to which the original goal was met, measuring it in terms of degrees of success or failure. In the fourth stage, the reasons for success or failure are analyzed. These include the amount of effort put into meeting the goal, the difficulty level of the task, the employee's skill level, and how much luck was involved in achieving success.

If luck is considered the major reason for success, the employee's satisfaction and feelings of self-efficacy (effectiveness) will not increase as much as when effort and ability are thought to be the cause of success (Stage V). At this point, the cycle is complete and the employee faces a new goal. The cycle begins all over again; but it may be with increased satisfaction, self-confidence, and motivation or with the same or less motivation, depending on the results of the previous experience.

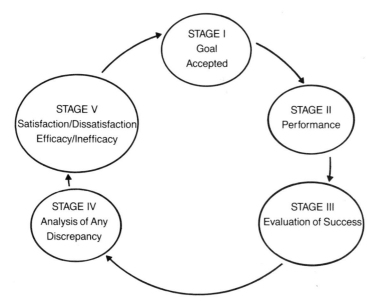

Figure 18–1. Goal-based model of motivation. (Adapted from Evans, M.A. (1986) Organizational Behavior: The Central Role of Motivation.)

This model suggests that there are many different actions that can be taken by the leader-manager at different points in the cycle to increase motivation. The following is a listing of some of these actions (Evans, 1986):

▷ Communicate a vision and a sense of purpose.
▷ Provide intellectual stimulation.
▷ Set challenging goals.
▷ Encourage employee participation in goal setting.
▷ Give individual attention to each staff member.
▷ Boost self-confidence.
▷ Provide assistance and encouragement in reaching goals.
▷ Remove any organizational barriers to success if possible.
▷ Give feedback during performance phase as well as at the conclusion of the cycle.
▷ Provide rewards and punishments according to success or failure in achieving goals.
▷ If possible, attribute failure to lack of effort or bad luck (rather than incompetence) to encourage persistence in the next cycle.
▷ Reward success due to effort and ability.
▷ Punish failure resulting from lack of effort.
▷ Recognize small gains as well as large ones.

Punishment may seem a very harsh word to the reader, but it is the clearest term for the appropriate consequences of continued lack of effort and failure to achieve reasonable, attainable goals. Typical forms of punishment are poor evaluations, failure to achieve recognition or promotion, withholding raises, and demotion or termination of employment.

The importance of taking an active role in providing evaluative feedback is evident in this model. Goal setting combined with feedback on performance leads to enhanced performance (Stall, 1986). You can see that you need to tailor your approach to the needs of the particular employee and the particular situation to be most effective in stimulating and nurturing the motivation of each individual employee.

We turn our attention away from the individual employee now to the larger group for which the leader-manager is responsible. While the group may not actually be called a *team* (other common words are *department*, *unit*, or *group*), in essence the task of motivating this group of people is the task of facilitating teamwork.

FACILITATING TEAMWORK

Teams

Teams are working groups. To be considered a team, a group must have some stability of membership and a common purpose. The people who are members of the team work interdependently; they function as interrelated parts of the whole team. People who work independently of one another—with little communication, coordination, or shared responsibility—are not working as a team.

Teams can be classified according to their composition, purpose, leadership, and function. These categories are not mutually exclusive; teams can be described according to any or all of these categories.

COMPOSITION. The skill and experience of the people who make up the team are important characteristics of any team. Some, such as the medical team, are made up of people in only one profession, even though members often have different specialities. Others—such as the nursing team consisting of registered nurses, practical nurses, aides, and orderlies—are made up of people at different levels within a particular health profession. Another example is the dental health team, which includes the dentist, dental hygienist, dental assistant, and sometimes a dental health educator.

Another type of increasing importance in health care is the interdisciplinary team made up of people from two or more different professions. The various combinations are almost endless. The following is one example:

> A team formed to design a cardiac rehabilitation program could include a physician cardiologist, an exercise physiologist, a physical therapist, nurses specializing in cardiology and rehabilitation, a patient educator, a community health nurse, a dietitian, a social worker, and a psychologist specializing in stress reduction and biofeedback. In addition, the team would probably consult with others including administrators of the organization supporting the program, community health educators, public relation experts, and other specialists in cardiology, rehabilitation, and health education.

These combinations create some difficulties and challenges to effective team functioning because of the addition of differences in professional background.

PURPOSE.   The purpose of the team or the kind of work it does is often indicated by its name. There are surgical teams, IV teams, primary care teams, and cardiac care teams. There are also teams with vague names such as project teams or management teams. Having a purposeful name, however, does not guarantee that the team's purpose and goals are clearly defined or even that it really does the type of work implied by its name in some cases. You can find project teams that never complete a project and primary care teams that rarely give primary health care.

LEADERSHIP.   The leadership of most teams can be divided into three categories, according to the way in which a person became the leader of the team: designated, emergent, or situational leaders (Brill, 1976). One or more such leaders can exist at any one time on a team.

The *designated leader* is one who has been deliberately chosen by the team, by an administrator, or by someone else with some authority over the team. The leader chosen by the team itself is more likely to have the respect and support of the rest of the team but may not have as much delegated authority as the one imposed on the team by an administrator. The designated leader has clearer roles and responsibilities and usually a more permanent position as leader of the team than does the emergent or situational leader. Most immature groups seem to need and prefer having a designated leader because it offers some structure to the group.

The *emergent leader* is one who evolves from the group by acting as the leader consistently enough to become the actual leader of the team. Emergent leaders arise when the designated leader is weak and ineffective or when the team has no designated leader.

The *situational leader* emerges from the group in response to a particular situation or need. This leader is far more temporary than either the emergent or designated leader. The situational leader's role is limited to situations in which that person has the best skills or experience to guide the teams' work. This switching of people in and out of the leadership role allows a great deal of flexibility as the team responds to different demands, but it can create some difficulties with continuity and coordination. The exception is mature teams whose members can handle the frequent changes and are able to move in and out of the leadership position without friction or power struggles.

Teams can also be described in terms of their predominant style of leadership. Some have a strong preference for the participative (democratic) style of leadership and will resist any attempts on the part of their leader to be too directive (autocratic). This is especially true of mature groups. Others have a nondirective or laissez-faire style, which can characterize both members and leader. Still others are very task-oriented and have leaders who are controlling, allowing team members little or no say in the decisions made. Conflicts within teams often arise from a mismatch between the leader's style and the needs and developmental level of the team.

FUNCTION.   Teams can also be categorized according to the way in which they function. Teams evolve and develop in identifiable stages just as other groups do. They can be classified according to their stage of development (forming, storming, norming, performing, or adjourning) or degree of maturity as described in Chapter 16.

Another classification of teams closely related to the style of leadership concerns the way members of the team relate to one another. When the relationships are collegial, every member is accorded equal worth as an individual and recognition is based on contribution to the team, rather than on status and position within the team, larger organization, or community. In other words, all team members treat one another as equal and worthy colleagues.

In contrast to the collegial type of relationships, hierarchical relationships are based on each team member's status and position. Individual team members are not accorded equal worth. Recognition is based on their status rather than on their ability to contribute to the team. For example, on a team with a hierarchical pattern of relationships, the recommendations of a social worker would automatically take precedence over the recommendations of a home health aide. When strictly adhered to, the hierarchical pattern of relationships discourages free exchanges between team members of different status and results in team meetings dominated by higher status members. At team meetings, the lower status members would typically remain silent or go unheard when they try to contribute their ideas.

Advantages and Disadvantages of Teamwork

Leading teams and working as a member of a team presents a number of difficulties and challenges as well as benefits (Francis & Young, 1979; Parker, 1972; Wise, Beckhard, Rubin & Kyte, 1974). Although they can't actually work in total isolation from other people in any health care setting, some people prefer to work independently rather than interdependently on teams. Some of the reasons for the preference will be mentioned in the listing of the disadvantages of teamwork. However, many types of health care can be delivered effectively only by well-functioning teams.

ADVANTAGES. The following are some of the advantages of using teamwork.

Best Use of Skills. When people with complementary skills are brought together on a team, each is able to contribute his or her own special skill, experience, and viewpoint to the task at hand. With the right combination, a highly functional team can manage more complex situations, provide more comprehensive care, and produce more creative ideas than any individual could do alone. Teams also allow greater use of paraprofessionals by providing close supervision from the professionals on the team.

Coordination. Teamwork demands that team members communicate with one another about the work they are doing. It reduces duplication of effort and the possibility that people are working at cross purposes. For example, clients may be given conflicting advice from their caregivers: one advises more rest, another advises more exercise, and the clients do not know what change to make in their activities.

Synergy. Combining energies to complete a task has a synergistic effect in which each team member stimulates and reinforces the others. This contributes to the development of a highly motivated group of people committed to producing high-quality work.

Flexibility. A team with its combination of talents and skills is able to handle a greater variety of situations competently. Team members are also able to help one another and to substitute for each other in an emergency so that the team is more flexible and responsive than individual workers can be.

Support.   Team members can also provide emotional support for one another. Effective teams can help manage the anxieties and tensions that build up in many health care organizations. They also provide collective strength, supplying a small power base and political support when needed.

Increased Commitment.   When team members have been involved in setting the team's objectives and deciding how they will be met, they are usually more committed to the successful completion of these objectives. Team synergy and support reinforce this commitment.

Evaluative Feedback.   When people work together on a team, the quality of their performance is more apparent and their colleagues can serve as sources of helpful feedback.

Opportunity for Growth.   In addition to being a valuable source of feedback, the team provides other opportunities for growth, especially for the development of interpersonal and leadership skills. Because people work more closely together and share more of their experiences with others, team members can expand their knowledge and skills in areas outside their specialities.

Disadvantages.   The advantages of teamwork occur only when the team functions well. Likewise, many but not all of the disadvantages arise when the team functions poorly.

Demands Interpersonal Skills.   It is often assumed that you can simply put people together and they will function as a team. Of course, this does not happen. Effective teamwork requires a considerable amount of interpersonal skill from team members as well as the leader. Without this skill, teamwork can be a frustrating, discouraging, energy-consuming experience. People who prefer to work by themselves may find the continued interaction and demands for sharing among team members quite uncomfortable.

Conflicts.   Differences in personality, culture, professional experience, norms, education, skills, status, and pay are all potential sources of conflict among team members. If you consider the fact that they work together 8 hours a day, you can see why tensions can build up to an intolerable level if not dealt with effectively. Conflicts also arise when the team's goals are not well defined or when roles and responsibilities of individual team members are not clearly differentiated.

Time Demands.   Even the most ardent supporters of participative management cannot claim that it is a faster way to make decisions. An autocratic leader can make an instantaneous decision and communicate it to the group later. It takes more time to bring team members together and ask for their input or decision.

Reduced Autonomy.   The person who values independence and autonomy over opportunities for feedback, support, and sharing of experiences may feel a sense of loss when assigned to a team. Some care givers find it difficult to ''share'' their clients with others and prefer to think of themselves as able to provide all the care needed. Others find it difficult to compromise or to get along with the team's decision when it is not in agreement with their own.

Conformity.   An overly cohesive, authoritarian group may prohibit disagreement and pressure its members to adhere to group norms. This can have serious consequences when complex health care demands flexibility and a great deal of professional judgment.

Increased Scrutiny. A person who works alone can hide mistakes and inadequacies better than one who works on a team. Being put in a position where these flaws will be revealed can be threatening to many people, especially to professionals who think they should be perfect.

Diffusion of Responsibility. Because of the differences and uniqueness of each team member, teamwork demands flexibility and tolerance about the way work will be done by different team members. This requirement can frustrate people who have a great need for structure and predictability. Also, when responsibility for patient care outcomes is shared by all team members, each member has to be able to trust the skill and judgment of other team members (Goddard, 1988).

Team Building

Effective teams do not just happen. Team building requires specific knowledge, skill, and work (Fry, Lech, & Rubin, 1974; Scherer, 1979). In this section, the steps to building a team into an effective functioning unit and some problems encountered in this process are discussed.

SELECT TEAM MEMBERS. Although you will not always be free to choose the people on your team, you will often have an opportunity to influence the selection. Ability to contribute to the work of the team (task) and to work as a member of the team (relationship), or at least the potential, are important considerations in selecting team members. It is important to consider both task and relationship functions; neither one alone is a sufficient qualification to be a valuable team member or leader.

A third consideration in selecting team members is having appropriate people and skills on the team. For example, some nurses are especially good at responding quickly but calmly in emergencies while others have more skill in gaining the trust of a new client. Or, you might find that your team needs a bilingual member to communicate more effectively with some clients served by the team.

SET GOALS. The need to define clearly your purpose and objectives or goals is a component of effective leadership and a common theme throughout this book.

Many teams are formed with only the vaguest idea of what they are actually expected to do. In fact, they are often formed to deal with a problem that has not been effectively handled in the past and for which there is no clear solution. Unfortunately, this is often not clearly spelled out, and the team flounders trying to resolve a problem before it has been analyzed and the solution has been worked out.

Even when the purpose is self-evident, as would be the case with a surgical team or a home care team, there often is a lack of agreement on specific objectives or on the way to meet these objectives. The following is an example:

> The home care team has obviously been formed to provide health care in the client's home. However, many questions about the team's specific objectives can arise. Is the purpose of the home visit to enable the person to stay in the home rather than be hospitalized or is it to encourage hospitalization for a serious illness? Will the team meet

only physical needs or will it also provide psychosocial support and counseling? Will the team help a client with housework and repairs and make referrals to meet these needs or not deal with them at all?

You can imagine the inefficiency and potential for conflicts if these and similar questions are not answered before the team begins to provide home care.

DEFINE ROLES. As with the purpose and objectives of the team, the roles of individual team members often are not clearly defined. This ambiguity can also lead to conflicts, especially on an interdisciplinary team, where there are even more opportunities for confusion and misunderstandings about others' roles than on a single discipline team.

Role clarification is essential to smooth team function. Definition of roles is related to what best meets the team's purpose and objectives. For example:

A question arose at a planning meeting for the home care team: Will the physician and dentist on the team visit people in their homes or will the team's clients have to travel to the hospital for medical and dental care? Because most physicians and dentists do not make home visits, some team members assumed that their clients would travel to the hospital for these services. However, if two of the team's objectives are to avoid hospitalization and to reduce the necessity of travel as much as possible for their homebound clients, the physician and dentist would be expected to provide as many of their services as possible in the home.

It is difficult to overstate the importance of clarifying such role expectations. Conflicts over differing expectations can immobilize the team and even contribute to its demise.

Even when the team's objectives are clearly spelled out, role negotiation among team members may be necessary because often more than one team member can and wants to do a specific task or fill a certain role. Many overlaps exist between the usual functions of people in different health care professions. Nurses, social workers, psychologists, psychiatrists, and chaplains may all see themselves as counselors or group therapists. Physicians, physician's assistants, pharmacists, and nurses are all likely to consider themselves prepared to develop and dispense information about medications to their patients. When this overlap occurs, a decision must be made whether to share the task, divide it, or designate who will do it. This decision needs to be made in such a way that it does not turn into a power struggle and that each person's ability is recognized by the team.

DEVELOP TEAM IDENTITY AND COHESIVENESS. To mature as a group and foster cooperative effort, people must first identify with the team. The team needs to develop a sense of itself as a functioning whole. To develop commitment to the goals of the team and the willingness of team members to engage in the sharing and support functions of the team, cohesiveness is also needed. There are a number of actions the leader can take from the beginning of the team's formation to develop cohesiveness.

Definition. The team first needs to be defined. The more team members know about their team and its functions, the more they can identify with the team. They need to know who is a member of the team and who is not and what its purpose and objectives are. If the team has not been given a name, you can do this or encourage team members to come up with one that reflects the purpose of the team. Using *we* to refer to team members and yourself emphasizes the unity of the team as a functioning whole.

Territory.   A new team needs to stake out its territory; an established team holds and often expands its territory. This territory is not only geographical but also functional and psychological.

The influence of geographical territory should not be underestimated. The team needs a place to meet, one that is sufficiently quiet, comfortable, and private so that team matters can be discussed freely. If the work spaces of team members (such as offices, examining rooms, patients rooms) are physically close together, there are more opportunities for informal exchanges during the course of the work day. When the team has acquired work space, its territory can be identified and personalized by signs, arrangement of furnishings, and verbal statements of ownership, such as, "This is our team's conference room, but you may use it for your meeting tomorrow."

The team also needs to acquire a functional and psychological space in the organization or community within which it functions. This means that, in addition to team members' having a clear conception of its identity and purpose, other health care givers must also recognize and accept the functions and purposes of the team. To maintain its identity and cohesiveness, it is important to have people outside the team respect its territory. Here is an example:

> If you were the director of the inservice education department, you would want your team (department) to be involved in the development of all the inservice programs given within your organization. You would not necessarily insist that members of your team actually conduct every inservice but if you are to hold on to your territory, you would want all inservice programs to be coordinated through your department.

Maintaining your functional and psychological territory within the organization is necessary in team building.

Connections.   Cohesiveness is developed by increasing the number of connections among team members. Simply holding team meetings increases these connections. Every time people interact with one another as members of the same team, their sense of being part of the team can be strengthened.

There are many other ways to develop cohesiveness. Whenever something exciting happens, the leader can make sure the experience is shared with the rest of the team. When someone on the team needs help solving a problem or getting work done on time, the leader can ask another team member to offer help. When a job is done well by the team, the leader can point out how cooperation between team members contributed to its successful completion. Each of these and similar actions build positive connections among team members and increase team cohesiveness.

Esprit de Corps.   Esprit de corps is a shared spirit, a feeling of enthusiasm that characterizes the team as a whole. The leader's own energy and enthusiasm can suffuse the entire team. It is also developed when members' needs are met within the team.

Setting some worthwhile but fairly easy goals helps to develop esprit de corps. Even failure can be used by the resourceful leader to show how team members need to work together to overcome the failure along the lines of that famous saying, "We must hang together or we will all hang separately." Healthy competition between teams can be used the same way. The power tactic of identifying a common enemy can also be used if needed. However, competition and working against an enemy must be used with care because they tend to set the team up in win-lose situations.

GUIDE DECISION MAKING. The different ways in which decisions are made by a group include default, authority, minority, majority vote, consensus, and unanimous consent (Schein, 1969).

Default. A decision by default is the result of nondecision by the group. Silence or lack of response from the team is taken to mean consent.

An idea is proposed to the group. When no opposition to the idea is expressed, it is assumed that everyone accepts it. This assumption is often false — team members may actually be strongly opposed to the ideas but, for some reason, have not expressed their opinion. A lack of response is usually a sign of withdrawal or apathy on the part of team members, often a symptom of some serious problems in team relationships and a threat to team function.

Authority. A decision made by authority is made by a single person with authority in the group, usually the leader. This method is faster than having the whole team make the decision but fails to use the expertise of other team members. It also fails to encourage the professional growth of individual team members or the maturing of the team as a group and may reduce the team's motivation to carry out the decision.

At times, however, decision by authority is the most appropriate method. For example, in an emergency situation, the speed and accuracy with which the decision is made is more important than either the team's growth or motivation. Administrative decisions, such as the firing of an employee, are also usually done by someone in authority rather than by a team, even a top-management team.

Minority. Decisions made by a minority are those made by a small number of people on the team, often a dominant subgroup. This occurs when the rest of the team either feels powerless to oppose the subgroup or when withdrawal, passivity, and apathy on the part of the majority of the team results in decision making by a minority. When a decision is "railroaded" by a small number of people, it is often resented by the rest of the group. An effective leader-manager tries to prevent this.

There are occasions when the team may decide to designate a subgroup to make certain decisions. This would be appropriate when only the people in the subgroup are affected by the decisions or when they are the only ones with sufficient information to make the decision. When the decision affects the whole team, it is preferable to present a summary of the information with recommendations to the team and ask for a final decision from the whole team.

Majority Vote. Decisions made by taking a poll of the entire team are acceptable to most people. This has the advantage of soliciting everyone's opinion and of recognizing the desires of the majority of the group. However, decisions made by majority vote often leave those who voted for the losing side feeling somewhat dissatisfied, even though they usually accept the decision.

While voting has the advantage of fairness, it sets up a win–lose situation in which the majority wins but the minority loses. It can lead to some serious battles to gain the majority vote, which can be divisive and even disruptive if opponents begin attacking each other. Voting is particularly appropriate in a large group, where it is difficult to give everyone a chance to speak on every issue, or in a immature group that is not ready to reach consensus on an issue.

Consensus. Decisions made by consensus are those in which the team seeks to gain every member's agreement on an issue. Decision by consensus is based on the prior understanding that everyone will go along with the final decision even if they are not completely satisfied with it. Members of a mature group are willing to do this because it is also understood that the team will attempt to resolve any differences of opinion in order to come as close as possible to a decision that satisfies every team member.

Decision by consensus recognizes both the right to disagree and the necessity of having some basic agreements to work well together. It avoids setting up a win–lose situation and makes the achievement of a win–win situation possible. True consensus decisions demand that all members be willing to express their opinions openly and to negotiate their positions when disagreement exists. Although other groups can try doing this, a true consensus on a difficult issue requires substantial maturity on the part of the group.

Unanimous Consent. Unanimous consent is the genuine agreement of every team member on an issue. Although usually a sign of a mature group, it can be reached on noncontroversial questions even by immature groups. However, when unanimous consent is reached too easily, the agreement may be superficial, concealing an underlying disagreement. For this reason, the leader should test the unanimity of a decision, particularly in an immature group or when consensus is reached too quickly. Unanimity is not always possible on an issue. It is preferable to agree to disagree and to try to resolve these differences enough to work together, rather than to press for unanimous consent and force team members into hiding their disagreement.

Selection of a Decision-making Mode. The type of decision, the maturity of the group, and the effect on the team of the particular mode of decision making should all be considered when guiding your team toward a decision-making method. Most teams will not actually discuss their choice of decision-making method unless the leader brings up the subject, so you will probably have to initiate the discussion when a decision needs to be made. The positive effects of including team members in decision making are described in Research Example 18–1.

While each of these six ways is used by teams, some are more appropriate than others. Consensus and unanimity on a difficult issue require more maturity than does voting. Decisions by authority may be necessary, but decisions by default should be avoided as much as possible. Minority decisions are occasionally appropriate but often cause problems when the decisions affect the team as a whole.

INFLUENCE GROUP NORMS. Norms are those unwritten rules that prescribe acceptable behavior in the group. Because they are often unspoken as well, they can develop virtually unnoticed, yet their influence on what happens within the group is significant. Norms that support creativity and flexibility over rigidity and resistance would affect the way the team responds to a new assignment. Norms supporting open communication over the suppression of feelings and disagreements would affect the way conflicts are handled. Norms can support arriving at work on time, working at a

RESEARCH EXAMPLE 18–1. A Case Study of Participative Decision Making

Bragg and Andrews (1973) reported the results of an 18-month study of the implementation of participative decision making in a hospital laundry. They compared the outcomes with two control hospital laundries. They defined participative decision making as an approach in which the decisions about the way work is to be done are made by the same people who will carry out those decisions.

The administrator of the experimental hospital was in favor of participative decision making, but the laundry supervisor used an effective authoritarian style of leadership and was doubtful about the experiment at first, although the supervisor did agree to try it. The union also approved but provided no active support.

The 32 workers in the laundry who would be affected by this change were told that the goal was to make their work more interesting, not to increase their already high level of productivity. To implement participative decision making, a total of 28 meetings were held in which the employees made suggestions for change. The supervisor changed roles, from direction giver and overseer to one of being available, being a good listener, and sharing expertise with others.

At one of the early meetings, the employees suggested beginning and ending work 2 hours earlier. This suggestion was implemented in less than 2 weeks, as was the case with other suggestions when it was possible to act quickly. By the fifth meeting, the supervisor was no longer an active moderator for the group but did continue to schedule the meetings, set the agenda, assist in the implementation of suggested changes. As the group's climate became more cooperative and supportive, even the most reticent members began suggesting changes. Although the researchers anticipated that the older workers would resist the most, it was actually three younger employees who strongly resisted for a long time.

The implementation of participative decision making resulted in increased employee satisfaction, increased productivity, and a total of 147 suggested changes. Eleven of these changes involved working conditions (such as the change in working hours), 44 involved equipment changes, 90 involved work methods, and 2 were concerned with safety. The score on an employee attitude scale rose from 62 percent at the beginning of the project to 90 percent near the end. The already low absentee rate improved even more during the experiment (from 1791 hours to 1194 hours of sick time), and productivity increased significantly, resulting in a cost saving to the hospital of about $1000 a year per employee. These results did not occur immediately but happened gradually over the 18-month implementation period, and they did not occur in the control groups. One of the reasons that productivity increased over an already high level was that most of the employees' suggestions were technical and measurably improved the work flow of the laundry. The researchers concluded that the employees had begun to adopt the organization's goals (for example, increased productivity) as their own when they were included in the decision-making process.

POSTSCRIPT

After the success of this experiment, participative decision making was also implemented in the hospital's medical records department with a resulting decrease in a high employee turnover and in the number of union grievances. However, implementation of participative decision making on a nursing unit was a failure because of a lack of administrative support and the strong resistance of the head nurse. The appointment of a supportive head nurse helped considerably, but continued resistance from the medical personnel kept the experiment from doing as well as it had in other departments.

steady pace, and getting finished on time or arriving late, doing the least amount of work possible, and leaving early.

Once a norm is established within the team, it can be difficult to change. The following is an example:

> When the IV team was first established, team members often finished their work early and were allowed to leave at 3:00 although their work day actually ended at 3:30. Over the next year, their workload increased gradually, but team members were still able to finish by 3:00. The team coordinator (leader-manager) usually stayed until 3:30 to provide coverage until the evening shift came in but rarely experienced any trouble doing this and thought that the team would appreciate the coordinator's allowing them to leave early. The coordinator had not actually verbalized any of this to the team.
>
> The team's work increased more rapidly the next summer, and team members worked harder to be finished by 3:00. One Friday, the team had a particularly heavy workload and had twice the usual number of emergency calls. By 3:00, the emergencies were over, but much of the routine work had not been finished. When team members begin putting on their coats at 2:55, the coordinator asked them what they were doing and they responded that it was time for them to leave. The coordinator pointed out that there was a lot of work left, and a team member said, "Well, you usually do the leftover work because you work later than we do." The coordinator told them it was too much for one person to finish and that they would have to stay. The same team member said, "Sorry, but we leave at 3:00," and the entire team walked out, leaving an angry coordinator with several hours of work to complete since the evening shift team was a small group that could barely handle their own work.
>
> In this example, the norm had developed to the point that team members actually believed they had the right to leave at 3:00 and thought that the coordinator's request was unreasonable. As you can imagine, there was a great deal of tension between the coordinator and the team the following week until the differences in expectations were clarified and the norm was changed.

The leader-manager who is alert to the development of norms within the team can reinforce those that support effective working relationships and challenge those that reduce effectiveness, preferably before they become well established. You can support effective norms by pointing out their positive effects; by encouraging and rewarding their use; and by being a role model for effective working relationships. If these actions fail to change an established norm that is interfering with team function, stronger measures including confrontation, negotiation, and change strategies would be needed.

ENCOURAGE OPEN COMMUNICATION WITHIN THE TEAM. Open communication is essential to the development of effective working relationships within the team and with outside groups. Open communication leads to the kind of understanding that promotes positive relationships. It is the means by which purposes and objectives are clarified, roles defined and negotiated, conflicts dealt with, and decisions made.

Written communications are also important, especially when team members are not in frequent personal contact with each other. They need to be direct, clear, concise, and free of jargon and abbreviations that are likely to be misunderstood by people with different backgrounds, education, and experience. Also, if they are to serve any purpose, they must actually be read by other team members, and this cannot be assumed.

Communication With Other Teams. Although the focus here has been on what happens within the team, teams operate within a given environment and have to deal with other individuals and groups within that environment.

Relationships between teams can be cooperative and productive or unproductive, full of conflict, and even hostile. Teams often share areas of common interest, such as having similar objectives, experiencing the same problems within the organization and community, or having overlapping work responsibilities. When these concerns are discussed openly, the potential for understanding each other and developing cordial working relationships is increased. The team needs to know what type of work is being done by other teams to prevent duplication of effort and working at cross purposes, which are even more likely to occur between teams than within a single team. Even teams with similar or overlapping functions can be widely separated and isolated from each other, so the leader may have to plan meetings between the teams. Stronger measures may also be necessary when conflicts with other teams arise.

MANAGE CONFLICTS. Conflicts within a team are inevitable and sometimes necessary. While they raise tensions and disrupt team functioning to some degree, they are not necessarily harmful. In fact, they can stimulate creativity and provide opportunities to improve interpersonal and leadership skills and to develop a deeper understanding of other people (Brill, 1976).

As a general rule, conflict is neither to be avoided nor stimulated, but managed. Too much conflict or unresolved conflict reduces the team's effectiveness and eventually immobilizes the team. On the other hand, suppressed conflict continues to grow underground and is more difficult to resolve when it eventually surfaces because people have had time to harden their position on issues and to become increasingly bitter or angry about the continuing conflict. Too many conflicts at once can overstress team members however, so it is sometimes necessary to wait until the most immediate problems are taken care of so that enough energy is available to deal with the remaining conflicts facing the team.

Sources of Conflict. The conflicts experienced by a team can arise from any number of sources, including incompatible differences, a dispute over the allocation of resources, or a perceived threat to an individual member or to the team itself. Incompatible differences may be due to culture, values, beliefs, language, education, experience, skills, professional values and norms, behavior patterns, status, pay differentials, and many other reasons. Cultural differences, for example, can be related to d^{iffe}ring concepts of work, change, and openness. Work may be seen as a mea end or as satisfying in itself. Change may be seen as progress or an nate disruption in the present order of things. Some cultural gro individuality and autonomy, while others place a higher value and other social groups. Revealing personal feelings may seer some people but inappropriate to others. Some of these diffe profound. Adaptation is slow and may be resisted as a diluti cultural heritage. These differences are often resolved by ag and live with each other's differences.

The resources over which conflicts can arise are e These include work space, budgetary allocations, promo higher authority, salaries, equipment and supplies, ar administration or from the community. When resources are plentiful, equitable sharing and negotiation for highly prized resources usually resolves the conflict. When resources are scarce or inequitably distributed, those with a greater share are very resistant to reducing their share, and conflicts can be long and acrimonious.

In many instances, an individual team member or the team as a whole becomes involved in a conflict in an attempt to reduce or remove a perceived threat. For example, some people perceive teamwork as a threat to their professional identity and to the territorial rights of their profession. There can be conflicts over who can change treatment orders, who tells the patient the diagnosis, who teaches the patient how to manage problems, who counsels the patient, who orders the lab tests needed, and so forth. Role clarification and role negotiation may help resolve this type of conflict.

Conflict Resolution.   Conflict resolution begins with preventive measures to reduce the number of conflicts facing the team. It proceeds through accepting the existence of the conflict, identifying the source of the conflict, seeking areas of agreement, and generating a solution.

Even before a conflict arises, a leader can take certain actions to prepare for conflict resolution. It is especially helpful to create a climate in which individual differences are considered natural and acceptable. Although this does not sound difficult, there are often strong pressures for conformity to counteract in establishing this climate, especially in immature groups. Encouraging open communication and developing skills in confrontation and negotiation prepares the team to handle conflict constructively. Leader and group efforts to meet the needs of team members before a conflict arises help to reduce the occurrence of the type of conflicts that are perceived to be threatening.

The existence of a conflict within the team should not be interpreted as a symptom of serious malfunction but rather as a sign of a problem that needs to be resolved. It is helpful to maintain a realistically optimistic attitude that the conflict can be resolved. When team members refuse to accept the fact that a conflict exists, either because they cannot handle it or because of accepted norms for ignoring and suppressing conflict, you may stay at this stage of conflict resolution for a considerable time.

Once the team has accepted the existence of the conflict, it is analyzed to determine its source and who is involved. If the source is not clear or emotions are too high to move into problem solving, a problem-discussion type of meeting devoted to ventilation of feelings and clarification of the problem is needed. During this whole process, a high level of leadership skill is needed to keep the conflict from escalating.

The next step is to discuss areas of agreement. This discussion helps to reduce the gap between the opposing sides in the conflict and also serves to make the conflict appear a lot smaller and more manageable than it did when the focus was on the areas of disagreement. When the areas of agreement have been mapped out, the core conflict is more apparent and may actually be different from what is first appeared to be. Once the core of the conflict is evident, the team can generate alternate solutions. It may take a great deal of confrontation and negotiation finally to arrive at an acceptable solution of the conflict.

STAFFING DECISIONS:
DELEGATING RESPONSIBILITY _____

The delegation of responsibility and assignment of work is a basic leader-manager function that may be more complicated in the health care field than it is in some other fields. This complexity is due to the great number and diversity of care givers; the vast amount of knowledge from a number of different fields needed to provide comprehensive care; and the numerous interrelationships between staff members, clients, and the environment that must be considered (Brown, 1980).

In this section, the many factors that need to be considered will be listed, followed by a discussion of ways to communicate assignments and some problems and issues faced by the health care team leader.

Criteria for Making Assignments

As you read about these criteria — and especially when you try to fulfill them — you will find that it is not always possible to satisfy every one of them. This means that a great deal of judgment on the part of the leader is required to make assignments that are as appropriate and fair as possible in a given set of circumstances.

Two criteria are of paramount importance in the delegation of responsibility, one primarily related to the task, the other to team relationships: the individual must have the *ability* to carry out the task, and the assignment must be *fair* not only for the individual but also for the team as a whole. Effective delegation requires that both of these criteria be met as well as all or at least most of the others listed.

TASK-RELATED FACTORS.   The primary task-related concern is that the person assigned to the job has the ability to carry it out. It is also important that you have chosen the best person available for the job; and that priorities, efficiency, and continuity have been considered.

Ability.   To make appropriate assignments, you need to know the customary knowledge and skills, legal definition, and job description for each health care discipline represented on your team. It is also necessary to be able to differentiate between the different levels of care givers within each discipline, because the amount of education and ability to assume responsibility can differ widely. In addition to being accountable for your own work, you are also accountable for work that is delegated to others.

Not only are there many different kinds of caregivers, there are also many individual variations in work-related abilities. Every individual has his or her own particular strengths and weaknesses. A careful assessment of these characteristics is needed before making individual assignments. The emphasis should be a positive one, however, rather than a negative one that focuses on weaknesses or deficits. "Assign from strength, not weakness," is a useful rule of thumb that emphasizes the positive. The difference is subtle but important.

Individuals should not be assigned a task they cannot do, regardless of their professional level. At any level there are people who are reluctant to admit that they cannot do something. Instead of telling you that the assignment is inappropriate, they may avoid doing it, delay getting started, try to look as if they've begun the task but not actually get any work done, or, perhaps most dangerous, try to bluff their way through the task.

Orientation is necessary before assignment to a new task. It may be a brief explanation, a short demonstration and return demonstration, a referral to written information or to someone who has done the task well, or a formal educational program — the choice depends on the need. While this is especially true for the new employee, you cannot assume that current employees necessarily have the needed education, skill, or experience to complete a task correctly either.

Priorities. Although ideally the team would be able to complete all of its work in a given time, the reality is that there is often less staff than needed and that the course of most work is rarely so predictable that it is always done exactly as planned. With this in mind, certain tasks or projects are given priority over others.

The priority rating is based on client needs, team needs, and organizational and community demands. Counseling an anxious parent would take priority over completing paperwork. An immunization clinic may be set up before a parent's group is started because both meet equally important client needs, but the community is more interested in obtaining the clinic.

Determining priorities can be very difficult, because the values of the client, care givers, organization, and community may be quite different, even diametrically opposed. These differences should be discussed with team members so that they can participate in making a knowledgeable decision on the team's priorities.

Efficiency. Although other care-giving values may take precedence over efficiency, the cost of health care in terms of time and money must be considered. The time and money available for health care are often limited resources that need to be allocated wisely. For example:

> You would avoid having two nurses travel to the same distant location if one could handle both of the tasks well. Or, if a telephone consultation can meet a client's needs as well as a home visit, the telephone consultation is the better choice because it is far more efficient. If the travel time saved is used for giving care to someone else, then more health care has been offered at the same cost by using the more efficient method.

Another example:

> If two professionals can perform physical examinations equally well, efficiency dictates the use of the lower-paid team member for doing physical examinations. Attention to the comparable costs of different work methods and assignments can sometimes appreciably increase the team's efficiency without reducing the quality of the care given.

Continuity. Continuity is related to efficiency, quality of care, and client and staff satisfaction. Every time a new person takes over a task from an experienced person, some time must be spent in familiarization before the task can be done efficiently; this can be costly. Clients appreciate having the same caregiver: it reduces the number of times they have to repeat the same information; it increases the opportunities to develop a personal, trusting relationship with caregivers; and it makes the health care experience more predictable, increasing their feelings of security. Continuity also makes a more holistic approach to care possible and gives caregivers an opportunity to see the client's progress over time.

There are, however, some drawbacks to an emphasis on continuity. Some tasks are monotonous, and if repeatedly assigned to the same person, they lead to too much routinization and boredom. There are times when either the caregiver or the client wants a change from the same people. Also, it is helpful to have more than one person on the team able to carry out a task so that adequate substitutes are available during absences or vacations. Continuity has to be balanced against the problem of monotony, desire for change, and need for prepared substitutes.

RELATIONSHIP FACTORS. Fairness is the second major concern in delegation. It includes an evenly distributed work load, equal consideration for each team member, avoidance of favoritism, opportunities for learning, health needs, compatibility, and staff preferences.

Fairness. There is probably no faster way to alienate team members than by making assignments that are either not fair or seem to be unfair. Fairness means distributing the work load evenly so that no one has substantially more or less work than the others. Because the workload is not completely predictable, what began as a fair assignment may have to be adjusted to balance the changing work load.

Fairness also means distributing the work so that no one gets all the enjoyable tasks or all the unpleasant ones. For example, if one aide is always cleaning the supply rooms or bathing all the incontinent patients, the aide may begin to wonder about being singled out for punishment even if the aide has no more work to do than anyone else.

Fairness also means an equitable amount of consideration for each team member, including consideration of requests for special assignments or vacation time, adequate recognition for the contribution of each team member, and an equal sharing of rewards as well as of the hard work.

When special consideration or an assignment that could be interpreted as favoritism is given to a team member, it is a good idea to discuss this action with team members so that they understand your reasons for doing it. Misunderstandings and resentments are likely to build up if this is not done. When team members actively participate in making the decisions regarding distribution of assignments, they are more likely to cooperate when the assignments are difficult.

Learning Opportunities. Although the assignments given must be within the capability of the individual, another factor to consider is that challenging assignments stimulate motivation and learning. Carefully planned assignments can promote the professional growth of individual team members and the team as a whole. The effective leader also seeks stimulating new tasks and projects for the team to provide additional opportunities for challenge and learning.

Health. The health and well-being of team members are other factors to consider. Certain jobs are very stressful, and while it may be preferable to learn how to reduce this stress, team members may need to be rotated through these assignments to keep stress at a tolerable level. Another concern in hospitals is the effect of rotating shifts and frequent overtime, which disrupts body rhythms and increases fatigue. There may also be individual health needs such as a family crisis for which additional time off is needed or special physical problems (such as back problems) which must be considered in making assignments.

Compatibility. Even when every effort is made to develop an effective team, there may still be some individuals who do not work well together. For example, the highly task-oriented nurse may have a great deal of difficulty working alongside an empathic colleague who spends much more time interacting with both clients and staff. An experienced, aggressive, and impatient physician would not be an appropriate partner for an inexperienced, timid technician. Given sufficient time and effort, these people can learn to work together. However, there may be instances, especially when the team is new or in the midst of a crisis, when the frictions of incompatible work relationships are better avoided.

This does not mean that you should try to put people who are alike together. A complementary blend of skills, talents, and personalities is desirable. Mixing people on this basis creates opportunities for sharing and learning from others and can increase the overall effectiveness of the team.

Preferences. When they do not conflict with the other criteria for delegating responsibility, the preferences of individual team members should also be considered. Often these preferences will reflect the ability and learning or health needs of the individual and so will be congruent with other criteria. Considering preferences demonstrates a respect for the team member as a unique individual.

Communicating Assignments

Even when team members participate in deciding how to delegate responsibility, the leader still needs to make sure that each team member knows what to do. Assignments and directions must be clear and concise so that all individuals know exactly what is expected of them and so they can plan their work schedules accordingly. The assignment and accompanying directions also need to be complete so that team members have all the information they need to begin the assigned task (Douglass & Bevis, 1983).

To ensure that team members understand and remember their assignments, both written and verbal means of communication are used. The written form can be used for later reference and evaluation as well as for a reminder. Long-term assignments are often written in the form of objectives to facilitate later evaluation. Verbal communication of the assignment is done to encourage comments about the assignment; to verify that it is understood by asking to have it repeated, if necessary; to add further explanation when needed; and to answer any questions the team members may have about the assignment.

Issues and Problems in Delegation

When you have adequate staff and satisfying work to delegate, assigning people to different tasks is usually not too difficult, but when the staffing is inadequate or the work is difficult and unpleasant, the decisions are much harder to make.

DIFFICULTY DELEGATING. The reasons people have difficulty delegating responsibility are varied but the outcome is generally predictable. The following is an example:

Leaders who cannot delegate responsibility to their team members are always very busy. They usually need to be in three places at once and are often seen rushing from one crisis to another because they do not have time to deal with a problem before it becomes a crisis. Perhaps because they have so much practice, they are very good at dealing with crises, but they do not do much planning.

These leaders are frequently heard saying how busy they are, and it is hard to make an appointment with them. When they are away from work for more than a day or two, the team falls apart because no one else knows how to handle many of the team's regular functions. Team members don't know anything about these ordinary routines because the leader always does them.

Leaders who have difficulty delegating responsibility end up taking on most of the team's responsibilities themselves. This limits the amount of work that can be done by the team, decreases team members' contributions to the team, and reduces opportunities for growth.

Why do some leaders have this difficulty? First, some do not even realize that this is what they are doing. They believe that they are hard-working, dedicated people (which they are) and do not realize how much they limit the effective functioning of the team. Others simply do not trust their team members and firmly believe the old saying "If you want a job well done, you have to do it yourself." For others, the need to retain control or to dominate others is so strong that they cannot let other team members share the leadership role or even become proficient in too many team tasks. Consciously or unconsciously, they withhold needed information from team members as a means of control.

If you see yourself in the description of the leader who does not delegate responsibility, you need to begin working on sharing responsibility with others. It may be easier for both you and the rest of the team to do this a little at a time so that things do not become chaotic in the transition, reinforcing your desire to maintain control. Team members can help by assuming more responsibility and reducing their dependency on the leader, at the same time offering support to the leader who may feel threatened by the loss of control. Team members' actions to assume more responsibility may lead to a power struggle with the leader if the team moves too quickly or if the leader refuses to share control.

MANAGER OR SPECIALIST OR BOTH?   This problem in defining the role of the leader-manager is common on health care teams and in other fields too. The manager-versus-specialist problem is essentially a role conflict that arises from conflicting expectations of the leader-manager, the team, the administration, or all three. The following is an example:

When the new chief administrator reorganized the administrative structure of the hospital, the head nurses were told that they were now expected to be the managers of their units. They were given courses on communication skills, group dynamics, and evaluation procedures. They were also given additional responsibility for doing their own budgets and staffing schedules, and told that they were now "part of the management team." Although some head nurses resisted the change, most liked the feeling of having a higher status and more management responsibility and so they assumed their new roles willingly.

About a year later, the director of nursing decided to expand primary nursing from three demonstration units to the entire hospital. Although some of the head nurses thought that their staffs were inadequate for full implementation of primary nursing, most supported the concept. However, after they accepted the plan, they were informed that head nurses would now become the clinical specialists on their units and their major functions would be to act as expert consultants to the primary nurses and to provide highly skilled care to patients with particularly complex problems. The title *head nurse* would be eliminated and those head nurses who did not qualify as clinical specialists (and many did not) would be able to apply for any primary nurse positions that were open. No mention was made of budgeting, staffing, or evaluation, and it was not clear who would perform these functions.

The head nurses rebelled. They refused to implement primary nursing until their roles were renegotiated. Most of the staff nurses and ancillary personnel supported the head nurses, primarily because they felt the need for the kind of leadership the head nurses had been providing. The director of nursing finally agreed to suspend the plans to implement primary nursing until the head nurse role was redefined. Eventually, the *head nurse* title was changed to *nurse manager*, and a separate clinical specialist position was created. Head nurses were expected to be well qualified in their field of nursing and also to fulfill a reasonable number of management functions, but they were not required to be clinical specialists nor were they expected to be administrators. The council of head nurses and supervisors was reorganized and given more influence over future decisions affecting their units, including the implementation of primary nursing and the evolution of the head nurse role on primary nursing units.

Expectations regarding the manager-versus-specialist roles will differ according to the policies and norms of various health care organizations. However, if you recall the components of effective leadership and management, you will see that an emphasis on either role to the complete exclusion of the other is less effective. The effective leader-manager needs both adequate expertise in the team's work and the ability to communicate, delegate, energize, support, and evaluate this work. While in some situations a greater emphasis on one or the other skills may be needed, both are necessary for the most effective leadership of the team.

INADEQUATE STAFF. Inadequate staff is a common and often chronic problem in the health care professions. It may involve the total number of staff; staff members' level of education, skills, and experience; and the mix of disciplines represented on the team. While some of these may be more serious than others and each has a slightly different effect, they all have the same general result — the team cannot fulfill its responsibilities effectively if staffing is inadequate.

Providing adequate staff for each team is primarily an administrative responsibility, but the first-line manager can take several actions to encourage administrators to fulfill their responsibility to provide adequate staff. The leader-manager can ensure that the people in administration are aware of the inadequacy and of the effects of this inadequacy in detail. You can point out the losses to the organization in terms of lower quality care, reduced efficiency, poor public relations, failure to meet legal requirements or accreditation standards, and inability to expand operations that result. The more specific, emphatic, and persistent you are, the more likely you are to be heard. If the administration does not respond, it may be necessary to make the appropriate regulatory agencies and the public aware of the problem. Although recruitment is primarily an administrative responsibility, you can be alert to opportunities to attract potential team members with the needed qualifications.

When staff deficiencies are minor, careful consideration of priorities and use of staff to their optimum level can make up for the deficiency temporarily. However, when there are major staff deficiencies, it becomes necessary to reduce the team's workload to a safe level and to refuse to take on any additional responsibilities. For example, you might have to refuse new admissions to your unit or to stop opening new cases in your agency because the team cannot deliver safe care to any more clients. The extremity of these measures may be necessary to call attention to the staff inadequacies and elicit a helpful response from your supervisors and administrators.

ASSIGNING UNDESIRABLE WORK. There are always some tasks that are more desirable than others. It usually isn't too difficult to distribute these pleasant tasks equitably, but it can be difficult for leaders to decide how to distribute the unpleasant tasks that teams also have to complete. Some leaders succumb to the temptation to give these jobs to the willing team member who rarely complains, but this method violates the criterion of fairness and inadvertently rewards the less cooperative team members who avoid doing their share of the unpleasant work.

Essentially, the leader just has to resist this temptation and distribute the undesirable work fairly. A few strategies can make this task a little easier. Often, the undesirable task has some kind of advantage that you can point out to reduce team members' resistance to doing it. For example, although unpleasant, the task may be vital to team function or vital to the client. (If you cannot say that it is necessary to do this work, you need to reconsider why you are asking someone to do it.) Occasionally, it is also an opportunity to learn something new or to upgrade a skill to improve a future evaluation rating. However, pretending the job is desirable when it obviously is not will only promote resentment.

A mature group can probably handle the responsibility to decide how undesirable tasks will be distributed among team members. With an immature group, the leader will probably find it necessary either to make the decision or to provide guidelines for making the decision to ensure that the criteria of appropriateness and fairness are met.

SUMMARY

Motivation is an intrinsic drive that can be stimulated by certain leadership actions. One approach is to meet the individual's basic needs, including control, personal self worth, economic security, recognition, and belonging. A different approach is to intervene at strategic points within the work cycle of goal setting, goal acceptance, performance, evaluation of success or failure, analysis of discrepancy between the goal and actual outcome and resultant increase or decrease in job satisfaction and perception of self-efficacy.

Teams are groups of people who work together for a common purpose over a given time. The different types can be described by their composition, purpose, leadership style, manner in which the leader evolves, degree of maturity, and pattern of relationships within the team. Advantages of teamwork include the best use of skills, improved coordination, synergy, flexibility, support for members, increased commitment, availability of evaluative feedback, and opportunities for growth. Disadvantages include the increased demand for interpersonal skills, conflicts, time demands, reduced autonomy, increased scrutiny, and increased uncertainty and diffusion of responsibility.

Team building involves many actions to develop effective working relationships. Team members are selected on the basis of their ability to contribute to the team. The purposes, objectives, and team members' roles need to be clearly defined and often negotiated. The team needs to define itself, stake out its territory, develop connections, and build a team spirit to achieve identity and cohesiveness. The leader also guides the team in decision making, influences the establishment of norms, encourages effective communication, and manages the resolution of conflicts within the team and with other teams.

The two major criteria to consider when delegating responsibility are the appropriateness and the fairness of the assignment. Additional criteria include priority, efficiency, continuity, compatibility, learning, health, and staff preferences. Assignments should be clear, concise, complete, and written and explained verbally. Common problems encountered are difficulty delegating responsibility, achieving a satisfactory balance between specialist and managerial roles, inadequate staffing, and delegating undesirable work.

REFERENCES*

Bragg, J.E. & Andrews, I.R. (1973). Participative decision making: An experimental study in a hospital. *Journal of Applied Behavioral Science*, 9(6), 727.

*Brill, N: (1976). *Teamwork: Working Together in the Human Services*. Philadelphia: J.B. Lippincott.

*Brown, B.J. (1980). *Nurse Staffing: A Practical Guide*. Germantown, Maryland: Aspen Systems.

Douglass, L.M. & Bevis, E.O. (1983). *Nursing Management and Leadership in Action*. St Louis: C.V. Mosby.

*Evans, M.G. (1986). Organizational behavior: The central role of motivation. In Hunt, J.G. & Blair, J.D. (eds): *1986 Yearly Review of Management*, 12 (2):203–222.

Francis, D. & Young, D. (1979). *Improving Work Groups: A Practical Manual for Team Building*. La Jolla, California: University Associates.

*Fry, R.E., Lech, B.A. & Rubin, I. (1974). Working with the primary care team: The first intervention. In Wise, H., Beckhard, R., Rubin, I. & Kyte, A.L. *Making Health Teams Work*. Cambridge, Massachusetts: Ballinger Publishing.

*Goddard, R.W. (1988). Gathering a great team. *Management World*, 17 (4), 20–23.

Kafka, V.W. (1986). A new look at motivation. *Supervisory Management*, 31 (4), 19–24.

Matejka, J.K. & Dunsing, R.J. (1988). Time management: Changing some traditions. *Management World*, 17 (2), 6–7.

Parker, A.W. (1972). *The Team Approach to Primary Health Care*. University of California, Berkeley: University Extension.

Schein, J.E. (1969). *Process Consultation*. Reading, Massachusetts: Addison-Wesley.

Scherer, J.J. Can team building increase productivity or can something that feels so good not be worthwhile? *Group and Organizational Studies*, 4 (3), 335.

Stull, M.K. (1986). Staff nurse performance: Effects of goal-setting and performance feedback. *Journal of Nursing Administration*, 16, 7–8.

Wise, H., Beckhard, R., Rubin, I. & Kyte, A.L. (1974). *Making Health Teams Work*. Cambridge, Massachusetts: Ballinger Publishing.

*References marked with an asterisk are suggested for further reading.

Chapter 19

STRATEGIES FOR PLANNED CHANGE

Chapter 19

OUTLINE

Dynamics of Change
Potential for Change
System Response to Change
Myths About Change
Multifactorial Influences
Rate of Change

Rational Model
Assumptions
Step 1. Invention
Step 2. Diffusion
Using Mass Media
Estimating Diffusibility
Step 3. Consequences
Discussion of the Rational Model

Normative Model
Assumptions of the Normative Models
Types of Normative Models
Lewin's Phases of Change
Driving and Restraining Forces
Unfreezing
Changing
Refreezing
Havelock and Lippitt's Steps in the
Change Process
Assumptions of the Change Agent
Model
Discussion

Paradoxical Model
First-Order Change

The Paradoxes
Nothing Changes
Be Spontaneous
Second-Order Change
Reframing
Comments on the Paradoxical Model

Power-Coercive Model
Assumptions
Power
Sources of Power
Physical Strength
Ability to Harm
Positional Power
Money
Legal Power
Public Recognition and Support
Expert Power
Power of an Idea
Strength in Numbers
Control of Access to Resources
Basic Steps of the Power-coercive Model
Step 1. Define the Issue and Identify
the Opponent
Step 2. Organize a Following
Step 3. Build a Power Base
Step 4. Begin Action Phase
Step 5. Keep the Pressure On
Step 6. The Final Struggle

Summary

LEARNING OBJECTIVES

Upon completion of this chapter, the reader will be able to:

▷ Discuss and refute myths about change.

▷ Apply the rational model for change appropriately and effectively.

▷ Apply the normative models for change appropriately and effectively.

▷ Apply the paradoxical model effectively to appropriate situations.

▷ Apply the power-coercive model effectively to appropriate situations.

▷ Evaluate the relative appropriateness and effectiveness of the various models for change in a given leadership-management situation.

STRATEGIES FOR PLANNED CHANGE

Planned change is a deliberate, conscious application of your knowledge and skills to guide and influence the direction of change (Bennis, et al., 1976). The opposite approach would be to let change occur spontaneously, to go along with whatever happens. This would not be an effective approach in most cases.

This chapter is organized around four major models or approaches to change. They can be thought of as a continuum from the low-key rational model to the midpoint normative and sometimes humorous paradoxical model to the high-pressure power-coercive model (Fig. 19–1).

All of these models for change can be used with open systems of various sizes, from individuals to entire communities, even to the profession as a whole. There are times when these models are appropriate for work with clients as well as with colleagues, with the exception of the power-coercive model. Each model and the strategies that accompany it is based on different assumptions about people and their behavior. The models help to explain the puzzling and sometimes contradictory ways that people react to change.

Attention will be given to the selection of the most appropriate approach for a given situation. Each model is particularly appropriate for certain types of situations.

The following is an example of how selecting the best model for the job can improve your effectiveness.

> After applying the normative model to a situation that had frustrated a community health nurse for a long time, the nurse said, ''Now I understand why I couldn't get my team members to allow their clients more autonomy before. I had thoroughly assessed the need for this change and planned a smooth implementation of this new approach to case management. But I didn't analyze the sources of resistance because I had assumed that every health care giver would naturally support a change in procedure that improved his or her clients' ability to care for themselves.''

As you read about the different models, you may find that some of your past attempts to bring about change did not work because you were not using the most appropriate model.

To engage yourself actively in learning about the application of the four models and the differences between them, it would be helpful for you to think of a particular change you desire and imagine using each model to bring about that change. Some examples of changes you could use:

▷ Helping a client to stop smoking.
▷ Starting a support group for families of cancer patients.
▷ Implementing an employee wellness program.
▷ Increasing communication between nurses and social workers.

Model	Anticipated Resistance to Change	Amount of Force Behind Change Approach	Major Approach of Model
Rational	Low	Low	Education and Communication
Normative	Moderate	Moderate	Persuasion and Participation
Paradoxical	Moderate	Moderate	Rethinking
Power-coercive	High	High	Force

Figure 19–1. Four models for planned change.

▷ Developing guidelines for the care of AIDS patients.
▷ Implementing an improved triage system in the emergency department.
▷ Improving your team's efficiency in following up on referrals.
▷ Obtaining increased funding to provide more services for older adults.
▷ Establishing a network of child care centers in your community.
▷ Getting legislation passed to support (or oppose) providing contraception services in the schools.
▷ Making changes in the Nurse Practice Act of your state.

DYNAMICS OF CHANGE

Change is essentially a repatterning of behavior. It is also a continuous process according to open systems theory. Growth and development, for example, is one kind of change that affects every human being throughout the entire life span. You may be aware of change occurring frequently and rapidly in your own life. Not every change in a system is obvious, however. It could be an imperceptible shift in the system's functioning or evolution or a large-scale alteration in the pattern and organization of the system.

Potential for Change

Remember that the potential for change is inherent in every open system. People often make remarks such as, "Nothing ever changes around here," or, "People here refuse to change," which seem to indicate that these systems have not or will not change. What they mean is that no rapid, large-scale changes have taken place or that there is a great deal of resistance to change. Some kind of change is inevitable in open systems, whether it comes primarily from within the system or from the environment.

Change in one part of a system will affect the whole system. When change occurs, it affects the system as a whole and, therefore, will also affect its relationship with the environment. Even the person who attempts to guide and influence a change in a system will in some way be affected by the process.

System Response to Change

A system can respond in several different ways to an attempt to change it. If it is neutral toward the change and does not see it as a threat, a small push can move the system in a new direction. A small force can also lead to great changes in a very unstable system. One example is how a little added force can make an angry mob turn violent and dangerous. On the other hand, if a system is very stable and considers the change a threat to its existence, it will take a strong force to change it because one of the basic needs of a system is to maintain its integrity as a system (Mathwig, n.d.). Forces both for and against change exist within the system and in the environment.

MYTHS ABOUT CHANGE. There are many myths about change that people mention and even apply to practice. The first is that people always resist change. The second is that change is always a positive occurrence, that it is always healthy for a system to change. Neither of these myths stands up under careful examination.

A system's need to maintain its integrity and identity as a unique entity does have a tendency to generate resistance to change. But systems do not always actively resist change. A mature, healthy individual, for example, seeks opportunities for further growth such as a new career challenge, learning a new sport, or meeting a person for the first time. One of the problems with bureaucracy is its built-in resistance to change, and yet even the most bureaucratic organization can and does change voluntarily over time, although it may be a slow change or just a change in some bureaucratic regulations.

Change per se is neither inherently good, as implied by the second myth, nor inherently bad. Some changes have a positive effect on a system, other changes have a negative effect. Change can be as welcome as a well-deserved holiday from work or school or as unwelcome as a speeding ticket.

Positive change is growth producing and as necessary as order and regularity are in the life of a human system. If you consider extreme sensory deprivation as an example of a system experiencing too little change, you can understand why change can be a positive occurrence.

On the other hand, not every change in a system is a productive one for that system. In fact, resistance to change can be a healthy response. The following is an example:

> A midwestern community strongly resisted attempts to locate a new dump for chemical wastes on the edge of town. Residents picketed, protested, and wrote letters to their representatives to block the dumping of potentially hazardous wastes in their community. They saw this change as a threat to themselves and to the health of their families and neighbors.

In this case, the change was seen as a threat to the integrity of the system. Resistance was a positive response in terms of the health and safety of the community.

MULTIFACTORIAL INFLUENCES. An open system's response to change is influenced by many factors. People react to change as whole persons in the same way that they react to other stimuli either from within themselves or from the environment. Their past experiences, present needs, culture, values, roles, and coping abilities may all have some influence on their responses. The same is true of groups, organizations, or communities as they respond to change. Some of the models for change take this multifactorial influence into consideration more than others do.

The apparent positive value of a proposed change is not the only factor that influences the amount of resistance that will be encountered. Health caregivers frequently fail to recognize this fact when proposing a change in lifestyle for the purpose of improving an individual's or a group's health. The following is a common example:

> Consider for a moment how difficult it is for some people to quit smoking despite overwhelming evidence regarding the health benefits of quitting. Habit, psychological craving, pleasurable handling, stimulation, tension reduction, and the physical effects of nicotine are all factors that reinforce the smoking behavior and resistance to change. Advertising and the smoking habits of friends also reinforce the habit. On the other hand, the health benefits and the fact that other friends have quit reinforce the motivation to change.

The outcome of the attempt to change smoking behavior depends on which set of forces is finally more influential, those for change or those resisting change.

RATE OF CHANGE.   Not only the type but also the degree of change that occurs within a given time affects the system's response to the change. Holmes and Rahe's Stress Scale (1967) is an example of the cumulative effect of too many changes occurring in a short time (Fig. 19–2). Some of the changes, such as "outstanding achievement," are basically positive, but too many of these occurring together can be a source of stress to the system.

Any change occurring at too rapid a rate may elicit resistance. These changes are not limited to the ones listed by Holmes and Rahe. The following is an example.

> A new director of rehabilitative services was hired for the outpatient services of a large health care center. The director thoroughly organized and modernized the entire department in 6 months, purchasing new equipment, moving the department into attractive new quarters, expanding the services offered, raising salaries, improving the therapists' roles and status within the complex, and hiring several new employees.
>
> The result? Although the changes were needed and desired, the tension level in the department rose precipitously. Several people resigned, and the rest of the employees in the department organized themselves into a bargaining unit and sought union representation for the first time. The administrator of the complex summarized the reasons for the department employee's response this way: "We tried to make too many changes too fast. They couldn't take it."

Conversely, very small or very slow changes, usually assumed to be easier to implement, may be too weak or "lost in the noise" of all the other activity going on in an organization (Lounamaa & March, 1987). The complexity of the forces within a system and in its environment makes it difficult to predict the results of the changes with any real accuracy unless you have made a thorough analysis of the change itself, that particular system, and its relationship to the environment. The four models for change are useful in doing this analysis as well as in attempting to influence the direction that change takes. Although you cannot stop change or determine its exact outcome, there is usually enough order and pattern to change to allow you to influence and predict the outcome within a range of possibilities.

EVENTS:	STRESS VALUE:
Death of a spouse	100
Divorce	73
Marital separation	65
Jail term	63
Death of a close family member	63
Personal injury, sickness	53
Marriage	50
Fired from job	47
Reconcile marriage	45
Retire	45
Illness in family	44
Pregnancy	40
Sex difficulties	39
Gain new family member	39
Change in business	39
Change in financial state	38
Death of close friend	37
Change line of work	36
Change in number of family fights	35
Mortgage over $10,000	31
Mortgage or loan foreclosed	30
Grown child leaves home	29
Change in job duties	29
In-law troubles	29
Outstanding achievement	28
Wife begins or stops work	26
Begin or end school	26
Change living conditions	25
Revise personal habits	24
Trouble with boss	23
Change work hours or conditions	20
Move to new home	20
Change schools	20
Change recreation	19
Change church activities	19
Change social activities	18
Mortgage or loan under $10,000	17
Sleeping habits change	16
Change in number of family get-togethers	15
Eating habits change	15
Vacation	13
Christmas	12
Minor violation of the law	11

Holmes and Rahe developed this scale to rate the amount of stress caused by many changes in life: major and minor, pleasant and unpleasant. To obtain your score, circle the ones that apply to you and then add up the total.
Follow-up studies show that people who accumulate more than 200 points in a year are high risks for physical or psychologic stress-related illnesses.

Figure 19–2. Holmes and Rahe's stress rating scale. (From Holmes, TH and Rahe, R: The social readjustment rating scale. Journal of Psychosomatic Research 2:213, April 1967, with permission.)

RATIONAL MODEL _____

Communication of a new idea is the focus of the rational model for change (Rogers & Shoemaker, 1971). This model is particularly concerned with assessment of the characteristics of the proposed change and how these characteristics influence the rate of adoption or rejection by the target system. (The target system is the group, organization, community, or other system in which the leader proposes to bring about change.) The original research that led to the development of this model came from such diverse sources as the study of the introduction of a new hybrid corn to farmers, research on the adoption of educational innovations (adding the kindergarten year or adopting modern math, for example), and research on the pattern and rate of adoptions of a new drug by physicians.

Assumptions

The rational model is the least power oriented of the four models on the continuum in Figure 19–1 (Bennis, 1976). It assumes a relatively passive or neutral attitude on the part of the system you want to change and, therefore, does not emphasize the use of strategies to overcome resistance to change.

A logical response is also assumed. The rational model assumes that people behave rationally, that their behavior is guided by reason and logic. This assumption implies that their behavior would be guided by rational self-interest once it is revealed to them. Once you have informed people about a better or easier way to do something, they are expected to adopt this new way.

Ignorance and superstition are seen as the main stumbling blocks in the way of change. Once people become better informed, they should adopt the new change willingly. Passing on of new information typically is accomplished through the media or other educational channels. This approach (informing the people) appeals to the American belief in the ability of science and technology to solve a wide range of problems, from curing disease to improving the quality of life.

Rogers' *diffusion of innovation* (Dutton, Rogers, & Jun, 1987; Rogers & Shoemaker, 1971), one of the best known of the rational models for change, will be used. There are three steps in the diffusion of innovation:

1. Invention of the change.
2. Diffusion (communication) of the information regarding the change.
3. Consequences (adoption or rejection) of the change.

Step 1. Invention

The leader's attention is directed toward thorough preparation of the proposed change. The change you want to implement must first be developed or invented. One way would be to develop a new method of doing something, such as distributing medications more efficiently. Or you could find a new solution to a problem through research. Another approach would be to collect all the information people would need to implement a particular change. The focus is on the change itself rather than on the target system.

EXAMPLE.   The rational model is used frequently in health education. An example from a community health program will be used to illustrate its application.

> A community health center nurse noticed that many clients with hypertension were not following their prescribed sodium-restricted diets. Most did avoid using the salt shaker but ate liberal quantities of cold cuts, cheeses, and other more hidden sources of sodium.
>
> The nurse consulted references for the latest information about sodium-restricted diets and spoke with the dietitian, who offered to assist the nurse in gathering educational materials. Together they developed an outline of the basic information needed to follow the diet correctly. They also collected and evaluated booklets from a number of sources (such as the American Heart Association) to find the best materials to give to clients with hypertension.

Step 2. Diffusion

The next step is to diffuse (communicate) the idea or information developed in the first step. Step 2 includes the selection of a way to communicate the change and an analysis of the characteristics of the change and their effect on the ease of diffusion. The goal is to ensure adequate dissemination of the information to all people in the target system. Not only does the information have to reach everyone, but it must also be presented in such a way that the people can understand it and will accept it.

USING MASS MEDIA.   The mass media are effective channels of communication for increasing people's knowledge and awareness. You are probably familiar with many of the following examples:

▷ Immunization campaigns.
▷ Food and Drug Administration warnings.
▷ Health messages during Heart Month.
▷ Antismoking posters, pamphlets, buttons, and bumper stickers.
▷ Radio and television talk show discussions of various health concerns, from infertility to relaxation exercises.
▷ Newspaper articles and health columns.
▷ Warning messages about AIDS.

While these methods are quite effective in terms of reaching large numbers of people, some experts, including Rogers, believe that a more personal communication is needed to change attitudes toward the innovation. More personal communication would include individual and small group methods.

EXAMPLE.   The next step was to consider the different ways in which information about sodium-restricted diets could be communicated to the people who need it (that is, the target system).

> The health center nurse and dietitian considered several options for disseminating the information they had put together. They could make copies of their outline for distribution, or they could have the information printed in a colorful pamphlet to give to their clients. To be sure that each person understood the information, the nurse and the dietitian could review the material with each person individually, or they could organize a class in which to do this. They decided to try the classroom approach.
>
> If the nurse and dietitian had decided to enlarge their target system to include the whole community, they could consider using mass media methods of communication. They could, for example, organize a campaign to inform the community they served by using

radio spot announcements, newspaper columns, and interviews; distributing posters and pamphlets; and so on.

ESTIMATING DIFFUSIBILITY. The degree of difficulty in diffusing a new idea or information varies considerably. Every idea has certain characteristics that make it easier or harder to diffuse successfully. These characteristics include *the relative advantage of the new idea over old methods or ideas; its compatibility; its complexity; the possibility of trying it out on a trial basis first; and the observability of the results.*

Is the proposed change in some way better than what it replaces? It is important that the change be perceived as having some advantage over the present method or information being used. There are many ways in which the innovation could be better: it may be more efficient, more satisfying, easier, more visually attractive, faster, cheaper, or safer to name just a few.

EXAMPLE.   What is the relative advantage of the sodium-restricted diet?

> The diet itself has the advantage that it can improve health and reduce serious risks (of stroke and heart attack, for example) if followed as part of a long-term treatment plan. This advantage can be noted in the printed material and in other communications.
>
> The information put together by the nurse and dietitian also has some advantages. It is more complete, more accurate, and easier to understand than the old diet instructions that the health center had been handing out with little or no explanation in the past.

To what extent is the innovation consistent with existing values and behavior patterns? Target systems that are generally open to communications from outside and have positive attitudes toward learning and change are usually more receptive to innovations. Some knowledge of the target system's culture, norms, values, and needs is necessary to evaluate the degree to which the innovation will be compatible. The system's past experiences with other changes may also affect its response. Compatibility, then, is a measure of the "fit" or congruence between the proposed change and the target system.

EXAMPLE.   Is the proposed class on sodium-restricted diets compatible with the health center clients' values and behavior patterns?

> This characteristic is a little more difficult to evaluate than was the first. If the center's clients have been making some attempts to restrict their sodium intake, the proposed change will be compatible with current behavior. If the clients have not been trying to follow the diet, the proposed change lacks compatibility in this regard, and this may be a problem area.
>
> Compatibility will also be increased if the center's clients are accustomed to seeking information on their health problems and to using health information as a guide to behavior, as well as if they feel comfortable in a classroom setting.

Is this innovation difficult to use? If the target system perceives the proposed idea as being hard to understand or difficult to use, there will be less acceptance of the change. A simple change is easier to communicate and also easier to implement.

EXAMPLE.   How complex is a sodium-restricted diet?

> One factor that increases the complexity of the sodium-restricted diet is that salt is not the only dietary source of sodium. Another related factor that increases the complexity is that foods may contain a lot of sodium and yet not taste salty at all. A sodium-restricted diet is also hard to follow when eating outside the home, in restaurants or cafeterias, for example.

If the diet could be reduced to a single, simple phrase such as, "Don't eat salt," it would be more easily communicated, but this oversimplifies the information too much. Despite this drawback, if the information is communicated in a clear, concise manner, it should not be too difficult for most people to learn.

Can the innovation be tried out on a limited basis? People are often more willing to try something new if they can do it on a trial basis first. They are more likely to be reluctant if the change requires a full-time commitment from the start.

EXAMPLE. Does a sodium-restricted diet have "trialability?"

This diet could be implemented gradually, but it is not going to be effective until it is followed on a full-time basis. Trial implementation is possible.

To what extent are the results of the change *visible*? Observable results encourage people to continue their efforts to implement the change. Seeing positive results reinforces the innovative behavior. The old saying, "Nothing succeeds like success," is another way of saying that the observability of results encourages the change activity.

EXAMPLE. How observable are the results of implementing a sodium-restricted diet?

Most people are not aware of any symptoms when they have elevated blood pressure, so they will not be able to notice that the diet has helped lower their blood pressure.

However, a lower blood pressure reading at the next visit could be one way to provide observable results. Another good substitute for observable results would be praise and encouragement from the center's staff when a client follows the diet. Keeping a food diary is another way to produce observability, but the tediousness of this activity reduces its effectiveness for all but highly motivated people.

Step 3. Consequences

The result of the effort to diffuse an innovation throughout a target system may be adoption of the change or it may be the ultimate rejection of the change. A particular change is more likely to be adopted if it has the five characteristics described in Step 2.

The adoption process usually has three phases. These phases are called *trial, installation, and institutionalization*. Each successive phase indicates an increasing degree of acceptance of the change as follows:

The change is first tried out on an experimental basis on the part of the target system. The attitude of the target system is generally one of, "Okay, we'll try it once and see how it works."

If the trial is successful, the change becomes accepted enough to make it part of the regular routine, and the attitude becomes one of, "From now on, we'll do it this way."

The third phase, institutionalization, begins when the once-new idea has become so deeply enmeshed a part of the system's behavior pattern that the attitude toward it can be described as, "We always do it this way."

EXAMPLE. The health center's clients may also go through the three phases of adoption, in the following manner:

When the clients first attend the class and try to follow the diet correctly, the change is in the *trial phase*.

If the clients accept the diet sufficiently to make it a part of their everyday routine, the change has become *installed*.

If they follow the diet so well that they don't even need to think much about it anymore, it has become *institutionalized*; the change has been successfully implemented.

Discussion of the Rational Model

When is this model a good choice? The rational model works well when there is almost universal readiness for change within the target system. For example, when the polio vaccine was developed years ago, most people were eager to obtain it because they had been very worried about outbreaks of the disease and had great faith in the ability of medical research to develop an effective vaccine. Many technologies — all kinds of mechanical inventions and new ideas — have been quickly adopted using this model.

However, the rational model's assumption that people act logically ignores the fact that, as holistic beings, they also react emotionally to attempts to change them. Any change that violates a norm, threatens a cherished tradition, or even disturbs a comfortable routine is not going to be accepted as readily as one that does not. Entire groups can react on the basis of a shared group feeling or norm that has developed.

EXAMPLE. Let's return to the sodium-restricted diet example once more to analyze the circumstances under which the rational model will be effective.

If the class consists of a highly motivated group of clients who are concerned about following their diets correctly, the rational model will probably be effective. However, food has emotional and social significance and is a part of many religious and cultural traditions. A restricted diet frequently conflicts with these other meanings.

As was mentioned before, people often experience no symptoms when they have high blood pressure and, therefore, may not be motivated even to try following a restricted diet. It is also difficult to see or feel immediate benefits from following a restricted diet, and people are easily discouraged. The change project described ignores these and other potential sources of resistance.

The rational model works best when the planned change is easy to understand, easy to implement, and provokes little resistance from the target system. It assumes readiness to change and a tendency to respond rationally; it ignores social, cultural, and emotional responses to proposed changes. The rational model is most useful when the entire situation is conducive to change. When there is more resistance to change, however, you will find that the next model, which pays more attention to the twin problems of developing readiness to change and reducing resistance, will be more effective.

NORMATIVE MODEL

The normative models of change are more holistic in their approach. Unlike the rational models, they focus on the target system and the actions of the leader as change agent as well as the characteristics of the change itself. They also recognize and deal with the influence of people's needs, feelings, attitudes, and values on their response to change.

Assumptions of the Normative Models

Normative change models are located around the midpoint of the power continuum between the rational and power-coercive models (see Fig. 19–1). Some resistance is anticipated, but it is expected that this resistance can be overcome without force. Both the leader and the target system are expected to be active, not passive, participants in the change process.

Normative models recognize the ability of the target system to resist, modify, or accept the proposed change. Therefore, they emphasize the need to include the target system and to use stronger tactics in addition to education when implementing change. These tactics are not as strong as those used in the power-coercive models.

Normative models also emphasize that needs, values, attitudes, and norms affect the target system's response to change. They do not deny rationality as a basis for behavior but correctly point out that it is only one of many factors influencing behavior.

Types of Normative Models

A number of different normative models exist, each having some variations in its approach to change. The two that will be discussed here have had a major influence on the development of change theory and its use in leadership and management. The first model originated with Lewin's 1951 work and was further developed by Schein and Bennis (1975) and many others since then. This model divides the change process into phases (unfreezing, changing, and refreezing) and emphasizes the need to first analyze the forces for and against the change, a concept of a particular value to leader-managers.

The second model combines Havelock's (1973), Havelock & Havelock's (1973), and Lippitt's (1973) steps and offers a logical sequence for implementing the change process using a democratic leadership style. This model is also the source of the widely used term *change agent*.

Lewin's Phases of Change

DRIVING AND RESTRAINING FORCES.   Lewin recommends that you begin the change process by analyzing the entire system to identify the forces for and against change. These elements are called the *driving and restraining forces*. This is quite different from beginning with the development of a new or better idea.

The forces that push the system toward change are the *driving forces*. Those that pull the system away from change are called *restraining forces* (Fig. 19–3). When the existing restraining forces are the same or stronger than the driving forces, the leader will need to use normative or power-coercive change strategies to reduce them and to increase the driving forces.

To assess these opposing forces accurately, a thorough knowledge of the target system, the environment, the characteristics of the change, and the potential responses to change is needed. The leader may have to spend some time becoming better acquainted with one or all of these elements before an accurate appraisal of the situation can be made. When this analysis is done, the forces are mapped out as shown in Figures 19–3 and 19–4.

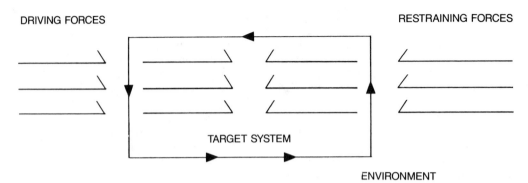

DRIVING FORCES

RESTRAINING FORCES

TARGET SYSTEM

ENVIRONMENT

Figure 19–3. Opposing change forces in a system. (Adapted from Lewin, R: *Field Theory in Social Science: Selected Theoretical Papers.* New York: Harper & Row, 1951.)

EXAMPLE. A common type of change within health care organizations will be used to illustrate the analysis of driving and restraining forces in a system and its environment.

The nurse educator of a small health care organization was asked to carry out the implementation of a new computerized patient record system. The new system has several advantages over the old one: it requires less writing, eliminates repetition, allows quicker access to stored information, combines notations from all care givers into one format that provides a total picture of the client's progress, and it can be modified for use with different kinds of health care programs. The system is also strongly supported by the administrators and executive board of the organizations.

However, none of the staff who will be using the new system have ever used it before, nor do they know how to use the new equipment. They also have not expressed any need to change the old system and seem satisfied with it. Aside from this, most staff members seem concerned about providing high quality care and believe that they are doing so.

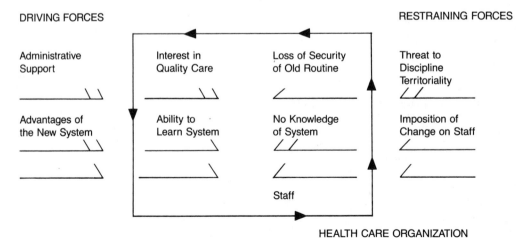

DRIVING FORCES

RESTRAINING FORCES

Administrative
Support

Interest in
Quality Care

Loss of Security
of Old Routine

Threat to
Discipline
Territoriality

Advantages of
the New System

Ability to
Learn System

No Knowledge
of System

Imposition of
Change on Staff

Staff

HEALTH CARE ORGANIZATION

Figure 19–4. Diagram of opposing change forces in computerized patient record example.

The nurse educator identified the following driving forces:

▷ Advantages of the new system.
▷ Administrative support for the change.
▷ Staff concern about quality care.
▷ Staff ability to learn the new system.

On the other hand, the nurse educator also found the following restraining forces.

▷ Lack of staff participation in the selection of the system.
▷ Little or no staff knowledge of the new system.
▷ Potential threats to staff feelings of security when giving up their old routine.
▷ Potential threats to territoriality of various disciplines because of equal access to the information in the new system.

These opposing forces are diagrammed in Figure 19–4. The diagram shows you what factors will help and hinder your efforts to bring about change. In some situations, you might also want to note which of the forces are especially strong by adding extra lines as was done in Figure 19–4 for illustrative purposes only.

UNFREEZING. Target systems usually need a push to get them moving toward change. Technically, open systems cannot be completely frozen, but they can be very resistant to change and so appear to be frozen to the leader-manager trying to introduce a change. Particular patterns of behavior can be so entrenched that it takes a great deal of energy to change them. You must then deliberately stir things up to unfreeze the situation.

There are three main tactics used to unfreeze the target system: creating disconfirmation, inducing guilt and anxiety, and providing psychologic safety. They can be used together to get the system ready to change.

Introducing disconfirmation is a confrontation with conflicting evidence. This confrontation makes the target system feel uncomfortable or dissatisfied with its present condition so that it will want to change. The disconfirming evidence may be information, examples, or experiences that challenge the status quo.

People often resist disconfirmation. They may try to ignore the evidence or to rationalize that the evidence is ambiguous or atypical. Or they may blame the problem on someone else. These responses may be defensive behaviors aimed at protecting security, esteem, or some other need.

Inducing guilt and anxiety will overcome resistance to disconfirmation. This is done by demonstrating that a goal or value that is important to the target system is not being met or upheld. This upsets the balance between the driving and restraining forces and raises the tension level within the target system.

Providing psychologic safety is the third tactic. Making a change requires some risk on the part of the target system, so the leader needs to provide sufficient security to minimize the risk. This would seem to be in conflict with the second tactic of inducing guilt and anxiety, but it is not really because the guilt or anxiety induced is specific to the planned change, while the feeling of security is developed as a general climate of trust and acceptance.

Many changes are resisted mainly because they present some kind of threat to the target system. If this threat is reduced or removed, people will feel comfortable enough to reduce their defensive behavior and attempt the change.

Much time and energy may be needed to unfreeze the target system enough to get it moving toward change. As a general rule, the most energy is needed to reduce or eliminate the strongest restraining forces and to strengthen the weaker driving forces. For a large-scale change, it may take weeks or even months to achieve unfreezing. Even the ordinary change situation described in the computerized record system example may require several weeks for unfreezing.

To unfreeze the staff, the nurse educator took the following actions:

Disconfirmation	Meet with every staff member in small groups to discuss the inadequacies of the current system.
	Present examples of problems found in the old system.
Inducing Guilt and Anxiety	Demonstrate ways in which the old system interferes with quality care.
	Indicate that the staff is not doing the best job possible in using the old system.
	Tell staff members how strongly administrators and board members support the new system. (This implies that they would be unhappy with the staff if the new system were not accepted.)
Providing Psychological Safety	Assure staff members that they will have ample time and opportunity to learn the new system.
	Indicate that staff will be involved in planning the implementation phase.
	Point out similarities between the old and new systems and that the new system will not change the routine too much.
	Express approval of staff's concern for the quality of the care given and confidence in their ability to learn the system.
	Ensure the continued identity of each discipline; use examples for each one; show how others will be better able to see and appreciate each discipline's contribution with the new system.

Each of the driving and restraining forces are dealt with in at least one of the three tactics. Many situations have more, or stronger, restraining forces than this example does and may require more emphasis on the disconfirmation and guilt-inducing tactics.

CHANGING. This is the implementation phase of the change process. Once the target system is unfrozen and moving toward change, the leader can begin putting the planned change into effect. The unfreezing process leaves people feeling unbalanced. A natural response to such change efforts is a state of high energy, called *hyper-energy* by Gillen (1986). This energy needs to be directed into productive actions. If it is not, it can provoke serious resistance to the proposed change (Gillen, 1986). The leader still plays a very active role in this phase.

The following is a list of the activities in which the leader will be engaged during the changing phase.

1. Introduce any new information that is needed to implement the change.
2. Encourage the new behavior so that it becomes part of the system's regular patterns of behavior. Allow practice and experimentation with the change behavior if possible.
3. Continue to provide a supportive climate to avoid an increase in defensive behavior and resistance to the change.
4. Provide opportunities to ventilate the guilt and anxiety deliberately aroused as well as other feelings, such as anger or hostility, that are aroused by the change process.
5. Provide feedback on progress and clarification of goals to reinforce the change process and to keep people from getting sidetracked.
6. Present yourself as a trustworthy person in order to keep communication open.
7. Act as an energizer to keep interest high and the change process moving forward.
8. Overcome resistance that may still arise by using the tactics of the unfreezing phase.

You probably noticed that most of the leader actions listed above are basic leadership skills derived from the components of effective leadership.

EXAMPLE. The following list shows how these change activities were translated into specific actions taken by the nurse educator:

Introduce New Information	Teach the staff how to use the new system.
Encourage the New Behavior	Begin with practice using examples from the real situations. Then, have the staff begin using the new system according to the plan they devised for implementation.
Continue the Supportive Climate	Allow adequate time for learning and practice before implementation. Point out how the staff is raising its standards of care.
Provide Opportunities for Ventilation	Ask staff how they feel about the new system; listen and respond to what they say about it.
Provide Feedback and Clarification of Goals	Check computerized records to evaluate progress.

	Ask staff how well the new system is working.
	Remind staff personally and through memos as needed about the use of the system and why it is being implemented.
Present Yourself as Trustworthy	Make sure that all staff were included in the implementation planning as promised.
	Follow through on other promises as well.
	Keep communications open and direct.
Overcome Resistance	Repeat, increase, and, if necessary, expand the tactics described in the unfreezing phase. If, for example, staff continue to use the old system, confront them with this evidence and with its consequences.
Act as an Energizer	Take every opportunity to promote the new system at meetings, mention it in newsletters, and so forth.
	Demonstrate interest in staff progress.

REFREEZING. The purpose of the refreezing phase is to stabilize and integrate the change so that it becomes a part of the regular functioning of the target system. It is similar to the institutionalization stage of the rational model.

At the beginning of this phase, the situation is still fluid. Because the target system is still in the process of changing and could still take a different course than planned change, the guidance of the leader is needed to ensure that the new pattern of behavior persists. However, the leader role does become a less active one in this phase than it was in the preceding phases.

To facilitate the integration of the planned change, the leader-manager continues to act as an energizer and to guide the new behavior but also increasingly delegates responsibility for the change behavior to other people in the target system.

Although high interest and even excitement about the change was more important in the previous phases, continued interest and support is still needed to keep the target system moving toward integration or refreezing. It is important to maintain the visibility and credibility of the change during this phase so that the integration process continues to proceed to completion (Lawless, 1987).

By the time this phase is reached, other interested and capable people should be ready to accept responsibility for continuing the new behavior. The leader-manager can gradually reduce participation as other people become increasingly involved.

The leader continues guiding new behavior only as long as necessary to ensure correct implementation. Because change continues to take place in an open system, some kind of continued supervision of the new behavior may also be needed. In some cases, the leader-manager relinquishes all responsibility for continued supervision at the end of this phase; in others, this supervision becomes a part of his or her regular functions.

Let's return to the patient information system example once more to see how the refreezing phase is accomplished.

EXAMPLE.   Having succeeded in implementing the new patient information system, the nurse educator took the following actions to ensure its continued use:

Continue Acting as Energizer	Keep the new system visible through memos, newsletters, frequent mention at meetings, and so forth. Continue to show interest in staff progress and feelings about the new system. Praise staff for genuine progress.
Continue Guiding New Behavior	Continue to check computerized records to see how well the new system is working and to intervene if problems arise. Help staff correct mistakes, and provide needed information. (Delegate both of these responsibilities as much and as soon as possible.)
Delegate Increased Responsibility to Others	Designate certain staff members as resources for staff to turn to for help. Turn over responsibility for checking implementation to supervisors.

The nurse educator continued to orient new staff members to the new patient information system and to act as a resource person when other staff people did not have the information needed to answer questions. The nurse educator also continued to show interest in the outcome of the new system but otherwise turned over all other responsibility for the system to staff members and their supervisors by the end of the last phase of Lewin's change model.

Havelock and Lippitt's Steps in the Change Process

This second normative change model is derived from Havelock (1973), Havelock & Havelock (1973) and Lippitt's (1973) work. It is oriented more directly toward the action of the leader rather than toward the evolution of the change as Lewin's phases were. This model is also more specific in its description of steps to follow when planning a change within a target system. You will see that it emphasizes the use of the democratic, participative leadership style in the planning and implementation of change.

ASSUMPTIONS OF THE CHANGE AGENT MODEL. These steps focus on the use of communication skills and the development of a good working relationship between the leader (or *change agent*) and the person or people of the target system. The target system is more involved in the initial planning of the change process in this model than in any of the other models. This emphasis on involvement is based on the assumptions similar to the motivational theories and the participative or democratic styles of leadership: that people will be more cooperative if they are included in decisions about things that will affect them and that most people will make appropriate decisions given sufficient time, information, and motivation.

This model begins with the development of a relationship with the target system and proceeds by engaging the target system in the problem-solving process. The last step deals with integration of the change into the regular behavior patterns of the target system and its environment.

Step 1. Build a Relationship. To work effectively with the target system, the leader must first earn that system's trust and respect. Several actions help to accomplish this task. The first way to earn trust and respect is by using good communication techniques, especially active listening. Offering some kind of help or assistance is another way to develop positive ties with the system. Openness and honesty are also needed to gain people's trust.

There are two commonly used ways to gain the target system's respect. The first is to provide people with information about your skills, credentials, and relevant experiences. The second is to demonstrate your ability to the group in some way.

Building an effective working relationship is fairly simple when the target system is a group of people who already know, trust, and respect you. Both clients and coworkers are frequently in this category. However, some of your colleagues in other professions may not be familiar with the full range of skills and knowledge possessed by a nurse, so your credibility and respectability would have to be further developed with them. Some clients' respect for the nurse may also have to be reinforced, but building trust is more frequently needed. Clients may lack trust because of negative experiences with health caregivers or because they see the leader as someone who does not have the same background or experience they have had. This lack of trust may also be found in coworkers for the same reasons.

EXAMPLE. A situation in which a new relationship had to be developed with a client system is described below:

> A nurse from a community service organization obtained permission to offer health services to the people held in a county jail. The nurse had never been inside the jail before except to meet with jail officials to get permission to work with the prisoners.
>
> Jail officials asked the nurse, Miss W., to begin by working with the women held in the jail, so she arranged to meet with the women and their guards (correction officers). In general, prisoners do not trust people easily. Miss W. knew that she could not pretend to understand how it feels to be arrested and imprisoned. She told the women honestly that she did not know what it was like to be in prison and that she needed to learn this from them before she could help them effectively. The nurse told the women about her nursing experience and credentials to gain credibility, but mostly she encouraged them to talk about their experiences and their health needs in order to begin developing a positive relationship with them.

In this situation, both trust and respect had to be developed to begin the change in the target system.

Step 2. Diagnose the Problem.   The purpose of this step is to identify a felt need for change. The people in the target system are actively involved in this process.

There are many ways to get the input of the people in the target system into the diagnosis of the problem. Individual and group meetings, conferences, informal discussion, surveys, questionnaires, telephone interviews, and casual conversation may all be used. Whatever method is used, the leader must ensure that people feel free to express their thoughts and feelings and that each person's input is in some way reflected in the final diagnosis of the problem.

Some face-to-face interaction should be included to allow for exchange and clarification of ideas leading to a consensus from the group (including the leader) regarding the situation in need of change.

This consensus among the people in the target system is an essential element of this change model. When the entire group has been involved in identification of the problem and has agreed that change is needed, resistance to change is decreased and motivation to change is increased. The planned change is perceived as coming from within the group rather than being imposed from the outside. It is a change that the group believes is needed. Through this approach, the group becomes committed to the change process, because the change belongs to the group and meets the needs of the group.

The leader's role in this process has several dimensions. The leader usually initiates the change process. Although this initiative could come from the group, the leader-manager is more often the initiator of the process because many people who have been working within a system for any extended period of time just move along with the currents of the daily routine and fail to recognize the need for change. They become so accustomed to the system's patterns that they do not think about ways to change or improve these patterns until stimulated to do so. Others simply fail to take the initiative to begin the change process or have given up trying to change the system.

The leader acts as an energizer in stimulating and continuing the exchange and guides the choice of methods for obtaining input from members of the target system. The leader provides input to the discussion and facilitates the exchange by engaging in open communication and promoting a climate of trust.

Finally, the leader encourages and guides movement toward the development of consensus on the problem. Generally speaking, the group should choose the problem of most concern or the one on which there is the greatest agreement in order to increase the motivation to change. However, when the group is immature, it is wise to start with a problem that has a good chance of being resolved. The success of the first attempt at planned change improves the group's function and increases the group's confidence in its ability to solve a harder problem next time.

EXAMPLE.   The group of women prisoners described above was not a highly functional group because of its high turnover rate and the fact that the women were very concerned about their individual problems and therefore unable to concentrate on group concerns. This limitation had to be taken into consideration in the process of diagnosing the problem.

> The nurse encouraged the women to talk about their health needs. Many problems arose in the discussion: needed diagnostic tests were not done, blankets were not cleaned between uses, no showers were allowed on Sundays, starchy high-calorie meals thwarted dieters, the women had fewer exercise times and television privileges than the men, they had difficulty contacting lawyers and families, there were interpersonal and racial conflicts among the women, and many women were concerned about young children left with friends or placed in foster care.
>
> When so many problems face a group, a decision must be made about where to begin. The problems could not all be dealt with at once, especially by an immature group, but several of them could be handled because they had a common source. The nurse encouraged them to choose one of the problems to work on first. The women decided that they would work on the inequity between the men and the women in the prison. They focused their attention on a particularly irritating but simple problem — they were not allowed to shower on Sunday, which was visiting day.

Step 3. Assess Resources. Once a consensus has been reached on the diagnosis of the problem, the resources available to the group are assessed. They can belong to the leader, to the target system, or they can come from the environment in which the change is to take place.

The particular resources needed to bring about change varies depending on the type of change the target system selects. In general, however, there are certain categories of resources to consider in making this assessment. These categories are the following:

▷ Motivation and commitment to change.
▷ Knowledge and skills needed to implement the actual change behavior.
▷ Sources of power and influence that support the change.
▷ Economic resources available.
▷ Time and energy available.
▷ Social norms, roles, and values that support the change.

This assessment of resources is somewhat like Lewin's analysis of the driving and restraining forces, except that it emphasizes the forces for change while neglecting the forces resisting change. In spite of this drawback, it does indicate when a group's resources are inadequate to bring about the change. More often, the assessment shows a group that it had more resources than it realized and encourages them to continue their movement toward change. Once you are familiar with these change models, you can combine their different strategies to suit a particular situation. You could, for example, use Lewin's analysis of the driving and restraining forces within this change-agent model.

EXAMPLE. It may seem that a realistic assessment of the resources available to a group of prisoners would be discouraging, but even this group had some resources they could draw on to bring about change:

▷ Knowledge of the informal system of the prison, especially what rules could be broken without punishment and the type of complaint prison officials were likely to respond to.
▷ Ability to gain the sympathy of the guards.
▷ Motivation of the women and the nurse to work for change.

▷ Potential support from the community because conditions in the jail could be publicized.

▷ Jail officials' recognition of the nurse's professional status and ability.

After assessing their resources, the group decided that their resources were adequate for the selected change.

Step 4. Set Goals and Select Strategies.   After diagnosing the problem and assessing the resources, the group is ready to set specific goals and decide how it will implement the change. The people in the target system are as actively involved as they were in diagnosing the problem. The leader continues to act as guide, resource person, supporter, and energizer in this step.

The goal set by the group should be *specific* to provide direction and *attainable* to avoid discouragement. When the goal has been specifically stated and agreed on, the group can decide how to implement its goal. Again, the group is actively involved in this decision-making process. The strategies selected need to be realistic in terms of the resources available to the group and appropriate both for the change desired and the setting in which it takes place.

Beginning with a *leverage point* is often a good idea. A leverage point is a point at which it is most easy to get movement toward change. A person or group that is likely to be receptive to the proposed change is one such leverage point.

EXAMPLE.   The women prisoners began with one strategy for change and shifted to another, more power-oriented, strategy when the first one failed to bring quick results. The goal they set and the two strategies they used were as follows.

> Goal. The immediate, specific goal set by the group was to get permission to shower on Sunday. In addition, they wanted TV and exercise privileges equal to those of the male prisoners.
>
> 1st STRATEGY. The women asked the nurse to speak to jail officials on their behalf. The nurse first spoke to the guard on duty with the women present. The guard said that showers were not allowed on Sundays because it was a visiting day and that the guard could not change the rule. The nurse then met with Warden L. who said he would think about the women's request.

At this point, the reader may note that the target system has actually been enlarged to include the guards and jail officials. However, these people were not included in the participative planning of the change and so were likely to resist the change.

> 2nd STRATEGY. The next day, Saturday, was very hot. The women asked the guard if they could take showers on Sunday. The guard responded, "No, the rule hasn't been changed." The women became more and more frustrated and angry. When they were put back in their cells after television privileges ended at 8 P.M., they set fire to their mattresses.
>
> The fires were quickly extinguished, but the incident frightened the guard and led to a meeting with the warden later that night during which the women presented their requests directly.
>
> On Sunday, the women were allowed showers before visiting hours, given equal television privileges, and promised equal outdoor exercise time.

The women had used a power tactic to take advantage of the warden's concern about public criticism of the way the jail was run.

Step 5. Stabilize, Consolidate, and Reinforce the Change.   This important last step is similar to Lewin's refreezing and Rogers' institutionalization. The leader's role in this step is to continue action to maintain the change, provide feedback on progress, and to support the change.

EXAMPLE.   Once the women succeeded in implementing the change they had been involved in planning, their motivation remained high enough to complete the change process and accomplish integration of the change.

> The women continued to remind their guards about their new privileges and took full advantage of the privileges. The nurse followed through on the change with prison officials until equal privileges became a written regulation of the prison.

You can see from this example that when you involve the target system in the whole process, both the process and the change can turn out to be quite different from what the leader originally had in mind. In this case, a normative change strategy evolved into a power-coercive strategy.

Discussion

The normative models for change are holistic, responsive, democratic, flexible, and adaptable. Their approach is responsive and democratic, particularly the change agent model in which the target system is actively involved in the planning of the change. Both models encourage responsiveness to the characteristics and needs of the target system. They are also far more holistic in their approach than the rational model is and applicable to a wider range of situations than the paradoxical model that will be discussed next. In fact, the normative models are so flexible that they can be applied to almost any change situation and are frequently used to challenge the status quo (Peters & Teng, 1984). In Research Example 19–1, you will see that the researcher attempted to determine what factors in a situation increase the likelihood of success for a planned change and came up with recommendations that parallel the strategies of the normative approach.

Although effective in a wide range of situations, the normative approaches do not always work. Normative change models work well when there is a low to moderate amount of resistance to change. They are basically persuasive, problem-solving methods. But there are individuals and even whole groups of people who are not easily persuaded, if at all, and there are situations that are not amenable to logical solution. In some of these cases, the paradoxical model may be effective.

At times, strong resistance to change is due to conflicting beliefs, norms, or values that simply cannot be made compatible with one another. The controversy over abortion is an example of conflicting values in which each side uses moral or ethical beliefs to support their arguments. Normative models will not work when people cannot eventually reach some kind of consensus.

In other situations, the resistance to change is very strong because the target system believes that the change will be detrimental to its position or well-being. There are, for example, many individuals and groups who value their positions of prestige, power, influence, or economic strength. A change that threatens any one of these elements will be strongly resisted.

RESEARCH EXAMPLE 19–1. Successful Planned Changes

What factors facilitate planned change? What factors increase resistance? Schermerhorn (1981) asked middle managers from hospitals of different types in New England to rate the effect of a number of different factors on a typical planned change. Most of these changes were common events such as altering admission procedures, asking lab employees to begin wearing lab coats, or trying to change the attitudes of uncooperative employees. A total of 70 actual successful and unsuccessful attempts to implement change were analyzed.

The factors rates by the managers as having increased success included the presence of a felt need, providing information about the change, using coercion and personal attraction to induce change, frequent communication, direct assistance, and top management support. Success in implementing change decreased when alternative actions were available. The perception that coercion was effective but that the use of special incentives (rewards) was not seemed to surprise the researcher.

The managers surveyed also thought that conflict increased when coercion or data gathering was done but decreased when a problem existed that created a felt need to change. The data gathering may be threatening to some people. Resistance was perceived to increase when information was provided or when alternatives to the change were available but decreased when there was a felt need, personal attraction to the person implementing the change, and top management support.

On the basis of these results, the researcher suggested the following guidelines for implementing change:

▷ Build the change around a felt need.
▷ Conduct data gathering in a nonthreatening manner.
▷ Use effective communication skills when presenting information and any alternatives.
▷ Maintain good interpersonal relations with staff to use the influence of personal attraction.
▷ Encourage free exchange of ideas to develop a sense of participation.
▷ Provide assistance and avoid overloading the group to facilitate the change process.
▷ Use the pressure of coercion to help unfreeze a situation.

When the restraining forces such as those mentioned above are too strong, the normative approach will not be effective. In these situations, a more powerful model — the power-coercive model — is needed to bring about planned change.

PARADOXICAL MODEL

The originators of the paradoxical model for change have a background in psychotherapy that is apparent in their perspectives on change (Watzlawick, Weakland, & Fisch, 1974). Their model is especially concerned with the way in which problems arise and why some persist while others are resolved. It grew out of their observation of a paradox: that logical, reasonable approaches to change often failed while illogical, backward-seeming approaches succeeded.

There are two different types or levels of change according to Watzlawick and associates, called *first-order* and *second-order* changes. The first-order changes are those that seem logical; the second-order changes are those that seem illogical.

First-Order Change

In a first-order change, the patterns of behavior and the nature of relationships between the systems involved remains virtually the same. A first-order change has far less impact on the function of a system than does a second-order change. The following example illustrates a first-order type of change.

> The professionals on an interdisciplinary child abuse evaluation team have had difficulty relating to one another as peers. Instead of a pattern of communication between equals, the communications have been superior to subordinate in nature.
>
> Whenever one member of the team approaches another team member as an equal, changing the pattern of communication, the other member retreats into a subordinate or superior position and so the overall pattern of interpersonal relationships remains the same. No permanent change in communication between equals has occurred.

The Paradoxes

Several different paradoxes affect the way change takes place.

NOTHING CHANGES.   From the example, you can see that first-order changes do not significantly alter old behavior patterns and may actually reinforce them, making them even more entrenched than ever. This is the paradox operating: some attempts to solve a problem by bringing about change can actually make the problem worse. If the old behavior pattern is not the most effective one (as in the example given of the child abuse team), first-order change is not adequate when you want to improve a system's function. Let's return to the child abuse team example to see how first-order changes can reinforce old behavior patterns.

> The child abuse team has become divided into two groups: the lower-status professionals (teacher, nurse, social worker) and the higher-status professionals (physician, psychiatrist). This division is reinforced by a superior to subordinate communication pattern.
>
> The lower-status members try to improve their position on the team by thoroughly preparing their reports on each child evaluated by the team and by asserting themselves at team conferences. The more they assert themselves, the more the higher-status professionals use a superior tone of voice and try to ignore their input in making decisions, even to the point of dictating the team's recommendations. The team is caught in this status struggle, and the valuable input of several team members is lost under these circumstances, which impairs the function of the team.

BE SPONTANEOUS.   Another kind of paradox is especially common on the individual level of change. This is the "be spontaneous" paradox. It occurs in the form of a demand, from yourself or others, to engage in some kind of natural behavior that can only occur spontaneously. In fact, the harder you try to perform the desired behavior, the harder it becomes to do so. For example, urging depressed patients to "Cheer up!" is asking them to do the impossible. Paradoxically, it can make them feel even worse because they are unable to please you by being cheerful. Another interesting example of the "be spontaneous" paradox is insomnia. Falling asleep is a natural behavior, but for insomniac patients, the harder they try to fall asleep, the wider awake they feel. The more conscious efforts they make to get to sleep on time, such as counting sheep or going to bed earlier, the less likely they are to succeed in falling asleep naturally.

Because of these paradoxes, first-order changes fail to break up old patterns of behavior and may actually result in reinforcing the unwanted pattern. A second-order change is needed to break up this pattern.

Second-Order Change

Shifting from an ineffective first-order change to a second-order change requires taking a new perspective on the problem. Watzlawick and associates (1974) use a familiar puzzle to illustrate this shift from first-order change (Fig. 19–5). If you have not seen the puzzle before, try doing it as directed.

The solution to the puzzle requires going outside of the square. While the directions do not prohibit your doing this, most people cannot solve the puzzle because the edge of the square becomes an imaginary boundary that keeps them from looking outside the square for a solution. This is an example of a first-order attempt to change. A second-order change, requiring that you go outside the logical boundaries of the square, is needed to solve this puzzle. Once you see the second-order solution, it becomes clear why you couldn't solve it with a first-order change.

REFRAMING. As you can see in the puzzle solution, second-order change requires a rethinking of a problem from a new perspective. This is called *reframing*. Before considering more second-order solutions to problems, the steps suggested by Watzlawick and associates for reframing the original problem will be considered. You may notice that they resemble the familiar problem-solving process somewhat at first, but they are *not* the same. These steps outlining the paradoxical model for change emphasize the need to reframe problems to eliminate the paradoxes that keep you from solving them. In fact, you might use this model when simple problem solving has failed to produce a lasting solution. The steps are as follows.

1. Define the problem in concrete terms.
2. List the solutions attempted so far.
3. Clearly define a realistic change.
4. Select and implement a second-order change strategy.

Step 1. Define the Problem in Concrete Terms. The purpose of this step is to help you to concentrate on the specific, solvable aspect of the situation and avoid trying to solve global or inevitable problems. Some problems are really inevitable and cannot be changed although you can change the way in which you cope with them. You cannot, for example, remove the threat of a hurricane or tornado, but you can either prepare for them or move out of their path. The storm itself is not amenable to change, but your response to the storm is amenable to change.

Example. In the same way, many social problems are amenable to change only over the long term and are not sufficiently concrete to tackle in order to gain relief from an immediate problem. To return to the child abuse team, here is a list of three possible ways to define the problem from the point of view of the nurse, teacher, and social worker:

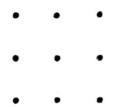

Puzzle: Connect the nine dots with four straight lines without lifting your pencil from the paper.

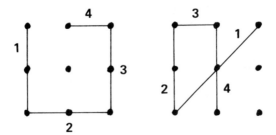

Wrong: First-order attempts to solve the puzzle.

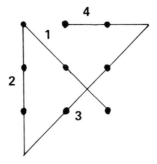

Solution: Second-order solution requires going outside the square.

Figure 19-5. An illustration of the difference between first- and second-order changes. (From Watzlawick, P, Weakland, J, and Fisch, R: Change: Principles of Problem Formation and Problem Resolution. WW Norton & Norton & Co, New York, 1974, with permission.)

▷ Our professional status is too low.
▷ Our value to the team is not recognized.
▷ Our input is ignored.

The first definition of the problem is too global to be amenable to immediate solution. It is a long-term problem that goes beyond the team and requires a change in social attitudes. The second definition of the problem is more specific, and the third one is the most specific and concrete. It also avoids analyzing the reasons behind the problem and defines the present dilemma of the lower status members of the team.

Step 2. List the Solutions Attempted So Far.   Once you have defined the problem in concrete terms, you are ready to look for solutions to the problem. Usually the previously attempted solutions were first-order changes that failed to bring about any lasting changes in behavior and, in fact, may have even made the problem worse than it was originally. The main purpose of this step is to help you avoid repeating previous unsuccessful attempts to change the situation.

Example. In the child abuse team example, the lower status professionals had made several attempts to change their position on the team. They repeatedly tried to do the following:

▷ Relate to other team members as equals.
▷ Prove their expertise by writing excellent evaluation reports.
▷ Demonstrate their worth by working harder than the rest of the team and by being more thorough in their assessments than the rest of the team.

None of these solutions worked. In fact, they made the situation worse. (These strategies frequently do succeed in bringing about change. The emphasis in this chapter, however, is on situations in which these simpler attempts to change have not succeeded and it is necessary to apply the strategies for planned change.)

Step 3. Clearly Define a Realistic Change.   In this step, you will define the goal of the planned change. Again, as in the first step, the emphasis is on the specific and concrete. To be avoided are goals that are too global or too vague, or attempts to solve a problem that is not amenable to change as stated (the inevitable storms, for example).

Example. The nurse, social worker, and teacher on the child abuse team wanted to achieve the following outcomes:

▷ Raise our status.
▷ Gain respect and recognition from the rest of the team.
▷ Increase use of our input in making recommendations.

The first goal is global; it defines an attempt to change social phenomenon and is a long-term goal. The second is more specific but still general in comparison with the third goal. The third goal, increased use of their input, is more specific and more amenable to immediate change than the first two. It would, therefore, be the most realistic of the three goals listed by the team members.

Step 4. Select and Implement a Second-Order Strategy.   The most distinctive aspect of the paradoxical model for change is the type of strategies recommended to bring about change. When first-order strategies have been tried without success, a second-order change is recommended. The previous steps were designed to help you to reframe the problem in need of solution so that you can shift into the second-order change perspective.

The key to designing a second-order change comes from the list of unsuccessful solutions rather than from usual approaches to the problem. The second-order change is usually the *opposite* of the original attempts to solve the problem. In fact, it more closely resembles the problem than the original solutions. The second-order change is frequently an imaginative solution that brings a smile to the face of the person who is to carry out the strategy. Here is an example of this:

Mr. D. had developed a fear that he would faint in hot, crowded stores. He could not shake this fear no matter how hard he tried to reason with himself that he was quite healthy and unlikely to faint (a first-order change strategy).

Finally, a second-order change strategy was prescribed for Mr. D. He was told to go into a crowded department store at the busy noon hour and lie down flat on the floor in the middle of the main aisle as if he had fainted. When he went to the store, he walked around looking for a place to pretend to faint, smiling to himself at the thought of deliberately stretching out on the floor, blocking traffic, and creating a hubbub.

He did not actually carry out the prescription; he had no need to do it because the unshakeable fear had been converted into a private joke he was tempted to play on the department store (Watzlawick, Weakland, & Fisch, 1974).

You can see how closely the solution resembled the problem and was almost the opposite of the original first-order change in which Mr. D. tried so hard to avoid feeling faint. The same strategy can be applied to the fear of speaking in public. Instead of trying to cover up your fear (which often makes people more nervous because they are sure their fear is showing), try telling the audience how scared you are of speaking to them. By announcing your fear, you not only eliminate its worst consequence but also win the support of the group to whom you are speaking.

The "be spontaneous" paradox can be dealt with in the same way. Insomnia was mentioned as an example of the paradox. The insomniac patients who cannot force themselves to go to sleep are told to go to bed but to be sure to keep their eyes open. With their efforts turned away from trying to fall asleep, they are able to fall asleep naturally. Their original solutions (counting sheep, going to bed earlier, trying harder to get to sleep) had become part of the problem and were dealt with by reframing the problem: by trying to stay awake, the insomniac patients were able to fall asleep spontaneously.

EXAMPLE. As you can see, every situation or problem calls for its own unique second-order strategy. Let's return once more to the child care evaluation team example to see what kind of second-order change strategy could be devised for this problem.

The nurse, teacher, and social worker had defined the desired change as "increased use of our input in making recommendations." But they also had found that their attempts to prove their worth on the team only provoked more resistance and resulted in less recognition for their work rather than more.

To implement a second-order change, the nurse, teacher, and social worker agreed with one another to use a second-order change strategy. Instead of working so hard to prove their ability, they started asking the physician and psychiatrist to do their work for them. They stopped trying to be recognized at the team conferences and began omitting important parts of their evaluations, asking the physician or psychiatrist to fill these parts in for them. Each one politely but insistently asked for time to meet with the physician and psychiatrist several times a week and telephoned them several times a day as well "just to check with you on this point."

Within 2 weeks, the physician and psychiatrist were telling the nurse, teacher, and social worker that they were quite capable of doing their own work. They also began to encourage them to contribute to the team conferences, saying, "You can't expect the two of us to do all the work!"

Comments on the Paradoxical Model

The paradoxical model seems particularly suited to those situations in which other solutions have failed. In fact, it was designed to deal with just this type of situation in which first-order change has not solved the problem.

While this model can be applied to larger systems, it does not include strategies for communicating the paradoxical message to large numbers of people. In this sense, the model is not complete in itself but can be used in conjunction with other change strategies.

There are some drawbacks to this model. First, the person who carries out the second-order change strategy must be highly motivated to be willing to carry out a seemingly absurd strategy. While it is true that often people do feel a desperate need to change a situation and are willing to do almost anything to resolve their problems, the model does not provide a way to increase this motivation. Because it does require motivation, however, it is classified here along with the other moderate-strength change strategies.

A second drawback to this model is that there is some risk that the strategy could backfire, although people faced with a persistent problem may see the risk as negligible in comparison with the problem. Finally, reframing requires imagination, the kind of creativity needed to be humorous and willing to alter your perspective (to step out of the nine-dot box of the puzzle). In a sense, this is the same kind of creativity Greene (1973) refers to when she talks about taking a stranger's point of view. In spite of these drawbacks, the creative leader will find the paradoxical model for change an effective approach for dealing with the persistent and seemingly unresolvable dilemmas that prevented the solution to the problem.

POWER-COERCIVE MODEL

The power-coercive model for change focuses on resistance to change and how to overcome that resistance. It is also concerned with the target system and the actions of the change agent. While it recognizes the influence of people's needs, feelings, attitudes, and values on change, the power-coercive model does not necessarily respect them.

Assumptions

The power-coercive model is located on the far end of the power continuum, at the opposite end from the rational model (see Fig. 19–1). A great deal of resistance is anticipated, so much that only an exercise of power is expected to be able to overcome this resistance. It is assumed that a consensus cannot be reached through the use of the softer, more persuasive approaches of the rational or normative models.

The power-coercive approach is neither democratic nor participative. The target system is truly a target in this model. The members of the target system are very resistant, sometimes actively resistant to the change and are not included in the decisions made during the change process. It is not responsive to the needs of the people of the target system except when this responsiveness would bring about the desired change.

Power-coercive strategies emphasize the use of some type of force that pushes the target system toward change. Their use are appropriate when the less powerful approaches fail. The leader who decides to use this approach is entering a win-lose situation and assumes the risk of losing the contest.

However, when you consider that the alternative is not to fight at all, the benefits often outweigh the risks of using the power-coercive model.

Power

Power is the ability to change people's behavior whether they want it changed or not. It has also been defined as the ability to impose your will on others even when they resist you (Hook, 1979). Power involves the use of some type of force, although it is not necessarily physical force. The force may be gentle or harsh, but it is used to overcome whatever resistance there is to the change.

Power tactics involve the use of coercion to bring about change (Zaltman & Duncan, 1972). The target system is not willing to change but is forced to by the use of power. Many also involve the use of threats to bring about change. For example, in collective bargaining, an employee group can threaten to strike if the employer does not agree to the group's demands.

Sources of Power

Although power is not evenly distributed among individuals or groups, everyone has some power and, therefore, some resources for using power tactics. These resources are multidimensional (Das, 1988). They include physical strength, ability to threaten harm, positional power, money, legal power, public recognition and support, expert power, the power of an idea, strength in numbers, and control of access to resources.

These power sources are interrelated, so the categories are not clear cut or exclusive. They do, however, provide a guide for assessing your actual and potential power and your opponent's actual and potential power.

PHYSICAL STRENGTH.   Physical force can be used to change behavior. For example, a parent will bodily remove a toddler from an immediate danger rather than try to persuade the child to move away from the danger. Police use physical force when necessary but usually try to use other powers (legal and positional) first. Nurses occasionally use force to restrain patients in danger of doing harm to themselves or others. A manager may step bodily between two arguing staff members to break up a fight.

With these few exceptions, physical force is rarely considered appropriate for use in leadership situations. A serious drawback to its use is that it can provoke return physical force and an escalation of hostility into violence. Its use also violates many social norms and values in most situations.

ABILITY TO HARM.   The ability to inflict some kind of harm on others is another source of power. For example, an employer can fire an employee, but employees can also quit, leaving the employer without anyone to do the work. Many other more subtle kinds of harm can be threatened, such as public embarrassment, loss of prestige, or loss of popularity.

The threat of harm does not have to be made directly to influence another's behavior. For example, an employer negotiating with a union knows that the union can call a strike and does not have to be told this directly. In fact, the veiled, ambiguous threat of harm is often more frightening and more effective than the direct threat in which the threatened person or group knows exactly what is risked by continuing to resist.

POSITIONAL POWER.   Some positions or offices, both public and private, have inherent power. The office of the president of the United States is an example of a very powerful position. On a less lofty level, the person who is the director of nursing or vice-president for nursing has some power over the entire nursing department. The director makes decisions that affect everyone working in the nursing department, and the director's requests or orders are usually obeyed because of the power in this individual's position as head of the department.

Positional power comes from the position itself rather than from the individual who holds that position. Part of this power is delegated. For example, an elected official is given power by the voters. A supervisor or nurse-manager has power delegated by the administration of the agency or institution. Another part of this power comes from the people who work under the direction of the person with positional power. They grant the person this power by respecting the position and being willing to carry out the requests made by the holder of this position. Another source of positional power comes from having a social position with high status. Two examples of this are being known as a community leader or being the spokesperson for a particular group.

Since positional power is delegated and granted by others, it is not too effective against very strong resistance, especially from those who have granted this power. However, it is often effective when used in combination with other sources of power.

MONEY.   Money is thought by some to be the greatest source of power and is certainly a very effective power source in many situations. The opportunity to gain monetarily or the fear of losing money affects much behavior. For example, money in the form of a salary influences the behavior of many workers. Since money is needed to purchase the basic necessities of food, clothing, and shelter, the loss of salary threatens these basic needs. As a result, people tend to behave in a way that they believe will keep that salary secure.

Economic motivation works at other levels too. For example, most organizations need money to survive; those that lose too much money will cease to exist. Accordingly, much behavior in organizations is aimed at bringing money into the organization or preventing the loss of money already earned.

People or groups who are able to control access to money have a tremendous source of power. There are indirect ways in which this source of power can be tapped. For example, information that leads the public to believe that an institution's services are inferior will indirectly lead to economic losses for that institution by reducing the number of people seeking and paying for its services. A poor evaluation that means a staff member will not receive a raise this year is another example of an indirect way to control economic resources. You can see that even if you do not have direct control over economic resources, you may be able to influence access to these resources and therefore gain power.

LEGAL POWER.   The legal system is a more specific source of power than some of the sources already mentioned. When the behavior you want to change is contrary to an existing law, you can use the law to force the target system to change. For example, nursing practice acts define the legal scope of the profession and may be used to support efforts to expand nursing functions. There are also laws regarding fair employment practices, health and safety standards for employees, legal precedents in malpractice cases, and regulations defining adequate health care for reimbursement purposes. These are just a few examples of ways in which laws can be used to support your efforts to bring about change. You can also challenge existing laws and regulations and/or work to get them changed at the local, state, or federal level of government.

Using legal power is not a simple thing to do. It requires knowledge of the law, of the way courts and legislatures operate, and money to support your effort. However, many important changes have been brought about through the legal system. The laws against discrimination in employment are just one example of these changes.

PUBLIC RECOGNITION AND SUPPORT. Although public recognition and support may seem to be a nebulous entity, it can be a very useful source of power. Most people want to avoid embarrassment or disapproval and will often change their behavior to do so.

Pressure from peers can be an effective way to change behavior. For example, aides who have gotten into the habit of coming in to work late will change their behavior if their coworkers begin to criticize their lateness.

Most people want recognition and approval. Letters of thanks from former patients or a favorable article in the newspaper about the high-quality care given on a particular unit strongly reinforce the care givers' desire to function at a high level. This public recognition not only raises morale but also keeps the administration from trying to make any unwanted changes on this popular unit.

Hospitals and other health care organizations find it very difficult to operate in a climate of unfavorable public opinion. Public recognition and support is so important that large health care organizations actually have public relations departments whose major purpose is to win this approval and recognition. Favorable public opinion about an organization brings increased numbers of clients and increased financial contributions to the organization.

Public sympathy can also be aroused and used to bring about change. For example, you can use public sympathy for abused children to support the expansion of family counseling and child protective services.

EXPERT POWER. Expert power is based on the education, skills, and experience of the individual or group. Patients often follow the nurse's directions simply because they believe the nurse is the expert on health matters. A well-known example of the use of expert power by a group is the American Dental Association's endorsement of fluoride toothpaste.

Expert power is gained by first preparing yourself as an expert, identifying yourself as an expert, and then seeking recognition as an expert. It is especially useful in influencing public opinion to support your side. By itself, expert power is not usually sufficient to overcome strong resistance, but it is useful in establishing the legitimacy of your claims to power and in combination with other sources of power.

POWER OF AN IDEA. Ideas by themselves have a certain amount of power. For example, a nursing home staff can be depressed and discouraged by the idea that they are only providing a place to warehouse old people until it is time to die. The idea that a nursing home is a rehabilitation center that aims to send some people home can completely change the feelings of the staff and the climate of the nursing home.

For an idea to have power, it must be heard. The idea that a nursing home means rehabilitation not warehousing would not have had any effect if it were not effectively communicated to the staff. The power of an idea is also enhanced when the idea can be stated simply, remembered easily and accepted by large numbers of people.

STRENGTH IN NUMBERS. The sheer number of people who support a change is an important source of power. It is so important that organizing a following is one of the basic steps in carrying out a power-coercive change strategy.

The larger the number of people who support a change, the harder it becomes for others to oppose the change. When other factors are equal, the side with the most supporters appears strong, and the side with fewer supporters appears weak. Gaining many supporters for your side increases the strength of the entire strategy for change.

CONTROL OF ACCESS TO RESOURCES. This last source of power overlaps several of the others already mentioned. The person or group who controls access to money, communications, or information has a potentially enormous source of power available, because very little can be accomplished without money, communication, or information.

Basic Steps of the Power-Coercive Model

The steps given here are derived primarily from the work of Alinsky (1972) and Haley (1969). Both Alinsky and Haley have concentrated on the use of power by people who are ''have-nots'' in contrast to the ''haves,'' to use Alinsky's term. In other words, these are the tactics used by people who do not have the advantage of holding high positions, great wealth, or other vast resources to support their desire to bring about change. The haves tend to be especially afraid of losing their power and react defensively to any challenges to their power.

The following tactics are designed to take advantage of the sources of power most available to the have-nots. The steps in this model are not as orderly as those of the previous models, but they do serve as an outline to guide you in the use of this powerful leadership strategy.

STEP 1. DEFINE THE ISSUE AND IDENTIFY THE OPPONENT. As with most strategies for change, you need to be clear about exactly what change is desired. In a power-coercive strategy, you also need to reduce the change to a single issue around which you can polarize (divide into groups for and against) people and rally support.

The issue must be specific enough that people can take sides for or against it. It also needs to be expressed in a few simple words that can be easily communicated to a large number of people and can serve as a slogan or battle cry. Finally, the issue should express a goal that is realistic and has the possibility of being achieved.

In a power strategy, the target system becomes the opponent. The opponent is the person or group that has the ability to bring about the desired change, not necessarily the person or group who will actually implement the change but whoever controls the behavior targeted to be changed. You need to identify the opponent as sharply as the issue to focus all the pressure on this point.

EXAMPLE. This example will illustrate how health caregivers can use the power-coercive model to fight restrictions on their professional roles:

> Several incidents had come to the attention of the chief of the medical staff in regard to patient teaching. Two very traditional obstetricians complained about the post-partum exercises their patients were taught. Then, an oncologist found a patient weeping and complained that the nurses had spoken to this patient about dying. Finally, one patient called the attending physician because the patient had discovered during routine preoperative teaching that the scheduled surgery would be much more extensive than the patient had expected.
>
> The chief of the medical staff brought these complaints to the hospital administrator and asked the administrator to do something about them. The administrator then asked the director of nursing to tell all nurses that they could do no patient teaching without a physician order. The director protested strongly and listed the reasons why nurses are expected to teach patients as needed and pointed out that other staff also did some patient teaching. The administrator was adamant and told the director, "If you do not take care of it, then I will." The director replied, "You are making a mistake."
>
> The next day, a memo from the administrator was distributed to every nursing unit. The memo stated that nurses in that hospital would do no patient teaching without a physician's order.
>
> A head nurse, Miss B., who had been planning an extensive new patient-teaching program with her staff, was infuriated by the memo. She decided to fight the new rule. The issue as she saw it was nurses' rights to teach their patients and her opponent was the administrator who signed the memo.

STEP 2. ORGANIZE A FOLLOWING. You may be completely alone when you begin to implement this strategy but you cannot succeed if you remain alone. You can remain the leader of the strategy, but you need to form a group to support you.

Actually, two kinds of groups are needed. The first is a small cadre of people who are just as strongly in favor of the change as you are and who are willing and able to help you plan and carry out the tactics needed. This cadre will be the core group, the key people on whom you can depend throughout the rest of the steps.

The second group is a larger following of people, as many as possible, who will support you and take part in some of the tactics. These people do not have to be as dedicated or skillful as the key people, but it will be important to keep up their interest and motivation (Griffin, 1987). This larger number of people is needed to provide the strength of numbers. The size of the group will be one demonstration of your side's power.

Some organizing tactics may be needed to develop a following. The issue and the identity of the opponent need to be clearly and simply communicated to anyone you want to recruit. The opponent is defined as the enemy of your following, an enemy who threatens harm to your group. Identification of a common enemy increases the cohesiveness of your following and appeals to the needs or interests of the people on your side. It is important to define your side as having the ability to bring about the desired change and as being right in demanding this change, while the other side is defined as wrong and as a threat to your group that can and must be overcome.

It may be difficult to attract a large following immediately. If this happens, Alinsky has a formula for dealing with this problem:

▷ If you have a vast number of people, "you can parade it visibly" and "openly show your power. . . ."

▷ If you have a small number of people, conceal them in the dark but make a lot of noise so its sounds like a lot of people. . . .

▷ If you have a tiny number, "too tiny even for noise, stink up the place" (Alinsky, 1972).

EXAMPLE. In the example so far, a head nurse has decided to fight the new rule limiting nurses' rights to teach their patients.

> Miss B. talked with two of her friends after the head nurse meeting about the memo. Both were angry about it but not sure what to do. Miss B. suggested that they meet after work to talk about it some more.
>
> After work, the three head nurses met. One had brought the evening supervisor, who was known to be in agreement, to join them. They discussed the problem for a while. They all thought that most of the nurses in the hospital were unhappy about the memo, so they decided to collect as many signatures as possible to send with a reasonable letter stating their position to the administrator.
>
> The first head nurse mentioned including the director of nursing, but the supervisor suggested that they wait until the signatures were collected. Each of the four nurses took a section of the hospital and planned to collect the signatures immediately so that the letter could be sent within 48 hours.

STEP 3. BUILD A POWER BASE. This step lays the groundwork for the implementation of specific tactics in the next step. The development of a following was the beginning of the power base that now needs to be expanded. The leader and key people need to assess carefully what types of power they have or can develop. As many as possible of the power sources listed earlier in this section should be used to build the power base from which pressure can be put on the opponent.

The power available to your opponent should also be assessed. Even more important is an assessment of the opponent's weak points, which will be the targets of the power tactics in the next step. For example, if your opponent is violating a law or regulation, this violation is an obvious weak point. Or your opponent may be particularly sensitive to public opinion, which would then be a logical target. No opponent has an unshakeable power base — there is always an Achilles heel to attack if you search hard enough for it.

EXAMPLE. The four nurses found that most of their colleagues supported their fight for nurses' rights:

> Several nurses offered to collect signatures and, within the 48 hours, they had signatures from more than half of the nurses working in the hospital. The first head nurse also prepared a letter to the administrator that gave a rationale for patient teaching and pointed out that it was an independent function mentioned specifically in their state's nurse practice act.
>
> The administrator, Mr C., was impressed with the number of signatures and began to wonder if he'd acted too hastily. However, he was concerned that if he gave in to this petition, the hospital staff would think they could always get him to change his mind by presenting a petition. So he decided to ignore the petition and did not respond to it at all. When Ms. B. called his office, his secretary told her that no action would be taken.
>
> Ms. B. called the key people together again to plan their next move. They reassessed their position. What could they do next? They had several sources of power available: many nurses on their side (numbers), the law supported but did not demand they be allowed to do patient teaching (some legal power), the patients wanted teaching (potential

public support), and they were good at it (expert power). Also, they could refuse to work (threat of harm) and paralyze the hospital, although they did not want to do this. The administrator had positional power, economic power, and the support of some physicians, but seemed susceptible to a change in public opinion or to pressure from others with positional power.

STEP 4. BEGIN ACTION PHASE. In the action phase of the power-coercive model for change, tactics that will push the opponent into accepting the desired change are selected and implemented. These tactics are designated to create fear, confusion, and anger in the opponent. Conflict and controversy are *encouraged* in this approach in contrast to other models for change.

Several factors should be considered in the selection of tactics. First, the tactic must suit your following. For example, health care professionals are likely to be more comfortable with petitions and even picket signs than with any tactic that is illegal or dangerous. The tactic should also be one that your group can enjoy carrying out. One that has drama or humor in it is more than fun and usually more effective. Paradoxical tactics have this element of humor in them.

Alinsky was a master at creating effective tactics that people enjoyed. For example, he developed a harmless way to tie up a busy airport completely: have your people go into the restrooms and keep them occupied — for hours. A bank can be paralyzed the same way by large numbers of people opening new accounts with small amounts of money.

Alinsky also used ridicule effectively. He found that it not only infuriates the opponent but is very hard to counterattack. When obeyed to the letter, most rules become absurd, and this can be an effective way to ridicule an opponent's rule.

Threats have already been mentioned as effective tactics. However, if you decide to use a threat, be sure that you can fulfill it, because your opponent may challenge you to carry it out. In other words, do not bluff.

Haley recommends that you set yourself up as an authority or expert on the issue and speak to the opponent as an equal or better, never as a subordinate. It is also important to respond to any attack on your side with either a question or another attack, not with a defensive reply because it will be perceived as a sign of weakness.

At the same time, you can paradoxically define yourself as not seeking power — this makes your opponent appear to be the power-hungry one. You can also say that you are not calling for a change and then call for a change — this confuses your opponent and makes it harder to attack your side. This is a pretended meekness that makes your opponent appear to be the bad guy and builds public sympathy for your side.

You cannot actually be meek when implementing a power-coercive strategy. An effective strategy demands strength. Each tactic either demonstrates your group's power or challenges the power of your opponent.

EXAMPLE. Based on their assessment of the power available to them and to their opponent, the four nurses planned a tactic that they believed their following would be willing to carry out:

> The four nurses decided to launch a campaign to publicize their fight and build more support. They distributed buttons saying "Nurses' Rights" to all nurses who would wear

them. Many patients, visitors, and staff members asked what the buttons meant and expressed support for the nurses' group.

The administrator began to wish he had just let the nurses keep on teaching, but he was still concerned about the physicians who had originally complained and about appearing weak (losing power) by giving in to the nurses. So he decided to live with both the buttons and his memo.

STEP 5. KEEP THE PRESSURE ON.   It may be necessary to continue the pressure on your opponent by carrying out several different tactics until your opponent agrees to the desired change. The pressure is continued by changing tactics. The changes serve two purposes. First, they keep your opponent off balance and unable to predict your next move. Second, they keep your following interested and excited. A single tactic used for a long time becomes predictable and boring. New tactics help to keep your group's motivation high.

EXAMPLE.   Although the administrator was definitely feeling the pressure, he had not agreed to change after both the petitions and/or the buttons with the ''Nurses' Rights'' slogan had won some public support for the nurses:

The four nurses decided that it was time to increase the pressure on the administrator by getting increased public support and by using ridicule. They asked the people in their group to encourage anyone who expressed support to call the administrator. The nurses also asked every physician who supported them to stop by the administrator's office to tell him what they thought, because the administrator seemed to be susceptible to physician influence.

In the meantime, the key people in the group began telling hospital staff members that the only reason the memo had been sent was because the administrator was afraid of one of the outspoken physicians. They started referring to the administrator as ''Chicken Charlie.'' They also decided to meet with the director of nursing.

Because the administrator originally issued the memo in response to physician complaints, the administrator assumed he had their support until they began to visit his office. The number of calls to his office increased that day to the point that his secretary threatened to resign. The administrator went home a little earlier than usual that day.

STEP 6. THE FINAL STRUGGLE.   Neither side can continue to give or take such pressure indefinitely. If the opponent has not yet agreed to the desired change despite several different tactics, it is time to increase the pressure enough to force a decision. Several new and stronger tactics are needed to do this.

EXAMPLE.   The four nurses thought that they were close to winning and wanted to force a decision.

The four nurses met with the director of nursing, who had closely followed their activities and quietly supported their efforts. They asked the director for more direct support. With the director, they planned the final attack.

The attack focused on two points: making the administrator look foolish by overly obeying his rules and bringing on pressure from outside the hospital for the first time. The four nurses went back to their group and asked each nurse to point out to the physicians every time there was an indication that a patient needed any information at all. At the same time, the director of nursing canceled all prenatal classes held at the hospital, declaring that they were in violation of the administrator's rule. To inform the people who attended the classes, the director asked the local newspaper and radio stations to announce the cancellations.

After it was all over, the administrator could not remember whether it was the chief of the medical staff or the president of the board of trustees who called him first. The president of the board demanded to know why they were going to be the only hospital in the city without those very popular prenatal classes. The chief of the medical staff told the administrator to stop being ridiculous and let the nurses get on with their work so that the physicians could get on with their work.

The four nurses celebrated their victory with their following. Along with several members of their group, they were asked to serve on a nursing advisory committee that made recommendations about any new policies affecting nurses. The director of nursing took advantage of the situation to strengthen the power of the director's position in relation to the administrator, so that any further policies affecting nursing would come only from the office of the director of nursing.

Not every power-coercive strategy will end in victory. Effective implementation of a power-coercive strategy demands a great deal of time and energy from the leader and from supporters. However, since it is used when other change strategies are ineffective, deciding not to use the strategy is actually an acceptance of defeat on that issue.

Power tactics are used frequently in work situations, so an effective leader must be able to recognize them and respond to them with equally strong tactics as well as to initiate their use to bring about change.

SUMMARY ⎯⎯⎯⎯⎯⎯⎯⎯⎯⎯⎯⎯⎯⎯⎯⎯⎯⎯⎯⎯⎯⎯⎯⎯⎯⎯⎯⎯⎯⎯⎯⎯⎯⎯⎯⎯

Planned change is the deliberate application of knowledge and skills by the leader to bring about change. Change is inherent in open systems. It may be positive or negative, welcome or resisted by the system. Many factors influence a system's response to change, including the perceived value of the change, the rate of change, and the needs, experiences, culture, values, and coping abilities of the system within a given environment.

The rational model is based on the assumption that people will respond in a logical fashion to change. It works best when there is little resistance to change. This model has three steps: invention, diffusion, and consequences. A change is more easily communicated or diffused if it has an advantage over the old way, is compatible, is not too complex, can be tried out on a limited basis, and has observable results. In the last phase, the change may be either accepted or rejected. If accepted, it will pass through three typical phases: trial, installation, and institutionalization.

Normative change models deal with people's needs, feelings, values, and potential resistance to change. The first model, derived primarily from Lewin, began with an analysis of the forces for (driving) and against (restraining) change. The leader then proceeds to work through the unfreezing, changing, and refreezing phases of change.

In the second normative model, derived from the work of Havelock (1973) and Lippitt (1973), the leader begins by developing a positive relationship with the target system. The target system itself is then actively involved in the rest of the change process: diagnosing the problem, assessing resources, choosing a goal and selecting strategies, and finally, reinforcing and integrating the change into the function of the target system.

The normative approach works best when the resistance to change is low to moderate and when some consensus on the planned change can eventually be reached.

The paradoxical model for change divides change strategies into two types: first-order and second-order changes. The logical solutions to problems of the first-order type often fail to break up old patterns of behavior and, paradoxically, may even make the problem worse. The second-order change strategy is usually the opposite of the logical first-order change. By reframing the problem, the second-order change resolves the paradox that prevented the solution to the problem.

Power is the ability to change people's behavior despite their often strong resistance. Everybody has some sources of power available to them that can be used to carry out a power-coercive strategy for change. These sources include physical strength, ability to threaten harm, positional power, money, legal power, public recognition and support, expert power, the power of an idea, strength in numbers, and control of access to resources. After defining the issue and identifying the opponent, the leader organizes a following, builds a power base, and then carries out the power tactics needed to pressure the opponent into the desired change in behavior.

REFERENCES*

*Alinsky, S.D. (1972). *Rules for Radicals: A Practical Primer for Realistic Radicals.* New York: Vintage Books.

*Bennis, W.G. et al. (1976). *The Planning of Change.* ed. 3. New York: Holt, Rinehart & Winston.

Das, H. (1988). Relevance of symbolic interactionist approach in understanding power: A preliminary analysis. *Journal of Management Studies,* 25 (3), 251–267.

Dutton, W.H., Rogers, E.M., & Jun, S-H. (1987). Diffusion and social impacts of personal computers. *Communication Research.* 14, 219–250.

Gillen, D.J. (1986). Harnessing the energy from change anxiety. *Supervisory Management.* 31 (3), 40–45.

Greene, M. (1973). *Teacher as Stranger.* Belmont, California: Wadsworth.

Griffin, (1987). Ralph Nader presents: More action for a change. New York: December Books.

*Haley, J. (1969). *The Power Tactics of Jesus Christ and Other Essays.* New York: Avon Books.

Havelock, R.G. (1973). *The Change Agent's Guide to Innovation in Education.* Englewood Cliffs, New Jersey: Educational Technology Publications.

Havelock, R.G., & Havelock, M.C. (1973). *Training for Change Agents: A Guide to the Design of Training Programs in Education and Other Fields.* Ann Arbor: University of Michigan Press.

Holmes, T.H. & Rahe, R. (1967). The social readjustment rating scale. *Journal of Psychosomatic Research,* 2 (4), 213.

Hook, S. The conceptual structure of power—An overview. In Harward DW: *Power: Its Nature, Its Use, and Its Limits.* Boston, Schenkman Publishing.

Lawless, M.W. (1987). Institutionalization of a management science innovation in police departments. *Management Science,* 33 (2), 244–252.

Lewin, K. (1951). *Field Theory in Social Science: Selected Theoretical Papers.* New York: Harper & Row.

*Lippitt, G.L. (1973). *Visualizing Change: Model Building and the Change Process.* La Jolla, California: University Associates.

Lounamaa, P.H. & March, J.G. (1987). Adaptive coordination of a learning team. *Management Science,* 33 (1), 107–123.

Mathwig, G. (nd). *The Nurse as a Change Agent.* (mimeographed) New York: New York University.

Peters, J.P. & Teng, S. (1984). Managing strategic change: Moving others from awareness to action. *Hospitals and Health Services Administration,* 29, 7–18.

Rogers, E.M. & Shoemaker, F.F. (1971). *Communication of Innovation.* ed 2. New York: The Free Press.

Schein, E.H. & Bennis, W. (1975). *Personal and Organizational Change Through Group Methods.* New York, John Wiley & Sons.

Schermerhorn, J.R. (1981). Guidelines for change in health care organizations. *Health Care Management Review,* 6 (3), 9.

*Watzlawick, P, Weakland, J, & Fisch, R. (1974). *Change: Principles of Problem Formation and Problem Resolution.* New York: W.W. Norton & Co.

Zaltman, G. & Duncan, R. (1972). *Strategies for Planned Change.* New York: Vintage Books.

*References marked with an asterisk are suggested for further reading.

Chapter 20 ━━━━━━━━

OUTLINE ─────────────────────────────────────

The Concept of Community
Definitions of Community
  Geographical Community
  Community of Interest
  Community of Solution
Functions of a Community
The Community as an Open System
  Wholeness
  Openness
  Pattern
  Energy
  Goals
Power Distribution in the Community

Community Action
Mutual Identification of Need
Prioritize Needs
Develop Motivation
Take Stock of Resources and Build
    Confidence
Develop a Plan of Action
Implement the Plan
Evaluate Results

**Political Action: Influencing the Flow
  of Power and Decision Making**
Entering the Decision-Making Channel
  The Proposal or Desired Change
  Identify the People For and Against
    the Change
  Barrier I. Community Values
  Barrier II. Blocking Procedures
  Barrier III. The Decision-Making Arena
  Barrier IV. Administrative Interpretation
    and Enforcements
Effective Community Leadership
  Goals
  Skills and Knowledge
  Self-Awareness
  Communication
  Energy
  Action

Summary

LEARNING OBJECTIVES ─────────────────────────

Upon completion of this chapter, the reader will be able to:

▷ Describe a community as an open system.

▷ Identify sources of power within a community.

▷ Use the community action approach to bring about change in a community.

▷ Participate in a political action to bring about change.

▷ Discuss the components of effective leadership in a community setting.

LEADERSHIP IN THE COMMUNITY

Communities are even larger and more complex than those open systems considered so far. They contain a larger number of subsystems within them. A community can be the setting in which the health professional works, or it can be the "client" of the health professional, or both. The tremendous size and complexity of some communities makes it even more difficult to see them as systems that have characteristics as a whole; but they do, in much the same way that organizations have these characteristics.

In this chapter, a simplified concept of community and its characteristics as an open system are considered. Then, leadership in the community is discussed including the basic power structures of a community, the process of community action, and strategies for influencing the flow of power and decision making in the community.

THE CONCEPT OF COMMUNITY

Definitions of Community

There are many definitions and uses of the term *community*. Most of these uses fall into one of two categories—those that emphasize geography or place and those that do not. Both emphasize the common bonds and interrelationships between people that are the basis of a community (Braden & Herban, 1976; Gottschalk, 1975; Hall & Weaver, 1985; Hanchett, 1979; Warren, 1963). With either type of definition, the basic elements of the concept of community are the people and whatever they share that makes them a community.

GEOGRAPHICAL COMMUNITY. Those definitions that emphasize *place* define a community as an open system comprised of a number of people who share a common place and common resources, interests, or needs. The community may be a neighborhood, parish, ghetto, village, town, city, metropolitan area, county, or other locale. Its boundaries may be defined geographically by rivers, mountains, streets, and fields, or politically by boundary lines such as those drawn between a city and its suburbs. A geographical community usually contains a number of different organizations within its boundaries and usually has a political and legal structure as well as the informal relationships that develop among people who share a common place.

COMMUNITY OF INTEREST. Those definitions that do not emphasize place define a community as an open system comprising a number of people who have common resources, interests, or needs, and a potential sense of belonging or identification with one another. This community of interest may be a religious community, a migrant population, people in the same occupation such as coal miners or asbestos workers, people with a physical disability such as blindness, people with a psychosocial problem such as alcoholism, or people with a common ethnic background. People who belong to any of these groups have a common need or interest and could (potentially, at least) identify with one another on the basis of that common need or interest.

COMMUNITY OF SOLUTION. The concept of a community of solution helps to bridge the gap between these two different definitions of community by combining them to some extent. It is a helpful way to look at a community for both health caregivers and health care planners. A community of solution is comprised of a number of people (a specific population) who have an identifiable need or problem and constitute the system *within which the solution to this problem can be implemented.* To be a viable community of solution, a system must have a sufficient number of people with the same problem or need, sufficient resources to meet this need or solve the problem, and the capability and authority to carry out the solution. The following is an example of a community of solution:

> A large number of migrant workers come through a small farming community every year to pick fruit. The migrant workers have some serious health needs, but this small farming community has neither the money nor the trained people to meet these needs. Several other farm communities in the area also have migrant workers coming through but no resources to provide for their health care needs. However, the county health department has access to the funds and the health care professionals required to meet these needs, so all the migrant workers who come through the entire county became the community of solution for this particular problem.

The community of solution was defined by both the need and the capability to meet the need.

Functions of a Community

Communities are formed and maintained because they fulfill important functions for the people who belong to them. These functions are generally broader than those of an organization. The basic functions of a community are to provide safety and security, mutual support, a network for the distribution of resources, shared meanings and values, and a place of belonging for its members. It is the ability of a community to meet these needs that makes most people willing to contribute in some way to the continuation of their communities.

Nongeographical communities of interest are more likely to emphasize the provision of mutual support, socialization, and significance than the provision of safety measures or distribution of resources.

The Community as an Open System

WHOLENESS. Some communities are highly integrated wholes in which there are active ties between most of the people and organizations within them. Others are poorly integrated with few ties between their various subsystems. There may be conflicts among these subsystems, for example, among different age groups, ethnic groups, or political organizations. In fact, conflict may characterize the interactions in some communities, while others may be characterized by friendly and cooperative interactions among subsystems.

OPENNESS. Communities are open systems that influence and are influenced by their environment. The political structure is an example of this influence moving in both directions. The people in the community elect representatives for the state legislature and for Congress. In turn, both the legislature and Congress will pass laws that the community and its members must obey. However, if the people are dissatisfied with the laws supported by their representatives, they can protest them, elect new representatives, and even have the current ones removed from office. So the influence flows both ways: the community decides who will represent them in the legislatures, and the legislatures decide what laws the community must obey.

PATTERN. Like organizations, many communities evidence differences in activity patterns between weekdays and weekends. Many health care services, for example, are available only on weekdays, often only during working hours. In communities where people commute long distances to work, a predictable flow of traffic in and out of the community can be observed.

The patterns of communication and decision making in the community are of particular interest to the leader. On careful observation, you will note in some communities that people interact most with those who live nearby or those with whom they share a common interest, and that communication between different neighborhoods and different interest groups within the community is minimal. This type of communication pattern has important implications for the leader attempting to communicate a message to everyone in the community.

There are also identifiable patterns to the way decisions are made. You may note, for example, that certain people and groups are influential in a large number of decisions, while others are only occasionally involved, and still others seem never to be involved in decision making. This information is valuable when you are attempting to influence a decision within the community. Another behavior pattern of interest to the leader who wants to bring about change is the way in which a community responds to change and the kinds of changes that seem to provoke resistance.

ENERGY. Because of the community's dependence on an adequate flow of energy, the ability to influence or control this flow is an important source of power in a community (Hanchett, 1979). People who are in a position to affect the flow of money (such as bankers and people in government) or the flow of goods (such as merchants and other businessmen) or the flow of information (such as professionals and people in the media) may be sources of considerable influence in the community.

GOALS. Like organizations, communities have both official and operative goals. However, people seem to be more aware of the fact that the official goals of communities have their unspoken, covert counterparts that are equally or even more influential.

One of the best ways to identify the community's operative goals is to observe what happens and where the community's energies are spent, especially its scarce resources. For example, does the community use its limited funds to improve its schools and health services, or is the money spent on a new municipal building? If the community's operative goal is to educate its children and keep its people healthy, the money will be spent on the schools and health services. If the community's operative goal is to be more attractive than its neighbor, the money will be spent on that municipal building.

Different socioeconomic or cultural groups within a community often have different and conflicting goals. The following is an example of such a conflict:

> A group representing several churches and temples from a mixed low-to-moderate income neighborhood requested permission from the town council to use an empty town-owned building for a youth drop-in center. The group was concerned about the delinquency rate in the neighborhood and wanted to find a positive solution that would help troubled adolescents and be of benefit to the community as well.
>
> A second private group, from a more affluent part of the community, offered to purchase the building from the town. They intended to renovate the building and convert it into meeting rooms that could be rented to a number of different social groups, primarily groups of adults with moderate to high incomes. They argued that the town would gain financially from the sale of an unused building, which would go back on the tax rolls when sold to this private group.

Both groups believed that they could make good use of the building and that their plans for the building would be of benefit to the community. However, their plans were not congruent and led to a long and bitter conflict between the two groups and dissension among town council members.

Such incongruence among the goals of different socioeconomic or cultural groups within a community can have serious consequences for the community. In an organization, every person *could* be consulted (as was described in the discussion of Theory Z), although it is rarely done. This is far more difficult to do in all but the smallest communities. Instead, community leaders frequently rely on their ability to identify and consult with groups and individuals who represent a cross section of community opinion and on their own intuitive sense of community feeling developed from their knowledge and interactions with the community.

Power Distribution in the Community

The questions of who has the most power and who has the ability to influence decisions within a community has been a difficult one to answer or even to study. A community is far too large and complex to re-create in a laboratory for careful study, which has been done with groups. The community can be observed in its natural setting, but power, authority, and influence relationships are multiple and interconnected and at the same time can be quite subtle and difficult to observe by an outsider.

One of the early solutions to the problem of identifying the power distribution in communities was to ask people to list the most influential leaders in their community. It was found that a small number of people were consistently named. These people, primarily from the top ranks of commerce, finance, and industry in the community, were considered the ruling elite, the group that made the decisions in the community (Hunter, 1970).

However, when additional methods (such as studying actual participation in decision making; memberships in community organizations; and positions within business, government, educational, labor, and religious organizations) were used, it was found that different people were influential in regard to different issues. Power and influence were found to vary according to the particular issue and the particular resources controlled by the individual or group. The power structure of a community is not a single hierarchy of the elite but a complex network of many actors, each with varying amounts of power and influence and diverse, often conflicting, interests (Coleman, 1977; Freeman & Laumann, 1970; Marsden et al, 1977; Polsby, 1970).

One useful, although simplified, way of visualizing the distribution of power in the community is to divide those who are powerful into three major groups, the influentials, the effectors, and the activists. The institutional leaders or *influentials* are the people who head the largest business, government, political, educational, and other types of organizations. They are the people mentioned earlier whose reputations for being influential are based on their positions within these organizations. It is interesting to note that most of the influentials are not particularly active in community affairs. Their influence is felt primarily by their prestige and support of one side or other on an issue but also through the next group, the effectors.

Effectors are very active in the community's decision-making processes. Although they are not heads of organizations as the influentials are, they are professionals, government officials, and employees of corporations. They often become involved in the community's decision-making processes through specific work assignments and are most influential in decisions that require technical or specialized knowledge.

Although a number of other sources of authority can be found in the community, one of the most influential is the hierarchy of government officials and organizations, from the local level through the county, state, and national levels. The influence of government in the community is of particular interest to the leader in the health care fields because the government has become increasingly involved in the planning, financing, delivery, and regulation of health care. The fact that we are reaching a point where nearly half the money spent on health care comes through government channels is just one indicator of the public sector's increasing influence on health care (Hanlon & Pickett, 1984; MacIntosh, 1978; Williams, 1980).

The *activists* are different. They come primarily from voluntary, civic, or service organizations. While they do not have the effectors' power bases of a government agency or large corporation behind them, they influence decisions by committing their time and energy to involvement in community affairs. The activists are less likely to be involved in economic decisions than are the influentials and effectors.

The people who participate regularly in decisions that affect the community are a diverse but powerful group. Some of their power is derived from their positions and is based on authority relationships; ability to control the flow of money, credit, and jobs; and expert technical knowledge unavailable to most people in the community. Another source of power is derived from their reputations as people who can mediate negotiations, respect for their ability to get things done in the community, connections with other influential people, and influence in community organizations such as political parties or volunteer organizations. Outside political and economic ties are also power sources. People who are influentials, effectors, or activists usually have a cluster of these characteristics, rather than just one or two of them.

For most purposes, the leader will find that the categories of influential, effector, and activist are sufficient for analysis and action. However, the power distribution in a community is actually more complex than these categories indicate, encompassing a large network of people and groups with different resources and links with the decision-making processes of the community. To complicate matters further, different issues are settled in different arenas within the community, so that certain people and groups will be close to one decision-making process but completely removed from, and not even interested in, other decisions.

Those people in the community who do not regularly participate in community decisions still have some potential for influence on decisions. When they do participate, they usually take one of two general patterns: the high-initiative, direct-action pattern, or the low-initiative pattern of participation (Litwack, Meyer, & Hollister, 1977).

The high-initiative pattern includes group actions such as consumer boycotts, picketing, agitation, and protest marches. It also includes such direct actions as hiring professional advocates (for example, lawyers) and using ombudsman organizations, consumer protection agencies, outside auditors, and investigative agencies to bring about desired change.

The low-initiative pattern includes group actions such as holding formal meetings and presenting formal requests for change. Individual actions include writing letters, telephoning, and meeting with those who will make the decision and presenting individual requests for change. Although these are low-pressure tactics, they can influence the outcome of community decision-making processes by providing information about community values and positions on particular issues that decision makers, especially politicians and public office holders, know they cannot completely ignore without risking community protest.

COMMUNITY ACTION

The intent of the *community action* or *community development* approach is to work with members of the community to help them initiate action to meet their own needs. It is a process based on the principles of democratic leadership and uses the same process as does Havelock and Lippitt's model for change (Chapter 19). Because it is a normative (moderate in strength) approach to change, it is most effective with minimal to moderate resistance. When there is strong, organized resistance to change, Bachrach and Baratz's (1970) power model (discussed later in this chapter) is more appropriate.

Leaders working in the community quickly learn that they must gain the support of the community one way or another to succeed with any project intended to improve the health of the community. If the members of the community do not want a particular service, they can ignore it, avoid it, and refuse to support it (Maxwell, 1986; Whyte, 1984).

For example, if you offer people health information for which they see no need, they may listen politely but not use it. If the offered service offends them, they might even ask you to remove it. The ability of a community to reject your offer of help is part of both the frustration and the challenge of working with communities, particularly when working in a community whose culture is different from your own.

Community action is a mutual problem-solving process. Its dual purposes are to help the community learn how to meet its own needs and to find ways to meet an immediate need. It also serves to develop more connections among people and increase their sense of belonging as they learn how to help themselves and others.

Ross developed a series of steps that provide a useful outline for the community action approach. They begin with the mutual identification of a community's needs, followed by prioritizing those needs, developing the community's motivation, taking stock of the resources available and building up the community's confidence, developing a plan of action, implementing that plan, and then evaluating the results (McDowell, 1977; Ross, with Lappin, 1967). You can easily see some parallels to the basic nursing process as it begins with assessment, proceeds through implementation, and ends with evaluation. You could say that it is the nursing process applied to the community with the community as the identified patient.

Mutual Identification of Need

Once you have identified the community with which you are going to work and established some kind of contact with that community, you are ready to find out from the people themselves what they consider their needs to be.

As a knowledgeable professional, you could probably generate your own list of the community's health needs and select several that are of top priority. But, however accurate your list might be, doing it without the input of the community fails to generate any interest or commitment from the community. You may also find that the people in the community have a very different idea of what their needs are.

It is important to *try* to reach everyone in the community with which you are working, although they may not all respond. If you plan to hold a community meeting, personal contacts before the meeting will help to make individual people believe that their attendance is needed and desired. A door-to-door survey is another way to meet with members of the community. It can be quite informative but is also very time consuming. When it is not possible to involve every member of the community (the size of the community is an important factor), you can try to reach a representational cross section of the population to assess accurately the needs and priorities of the community as a whole.

When you first approach them, the people of the community may have trouble identifying their needs, and you may have to offer some ideas to get the discussion started. Questions aimed at discovering areas of discontent and dissatisfaction usually lead to an identification of needs.

EXAMPLE.   A student was assigned to a clinic that served the three apartment buildings of a small senior retirement community in an urban area. The student tried to find out what health care needs of the community were not being met.

To find out what kind of project would be most use to the people who lived in the retirement community, the student distributed flyers that asked everyone living in the three buildings to meet with the student the next week. The student expected that these older people would have many physical problems and that they would want information about their problems.

Only 10 people came to the meeting. The student was disappointed but went ahead with the plan and began by explaining the purpose of the meeting. The student asked the people who came to suggest ways in which they thought their health care could be improved. Most of the people told the student that they had private physicians and were quite satisfied with the services provided by the clinic nurses. At that point, the student expressed disappointment at the small number who came, and the people told the student that this happened whenever they had a tenants' meeting or community function. They began talking about the problem of apathy in their community, and by the end of the meeting, they had decided to meet again to work on reducing the apathy of their community.

Prioritize Needs

The community's priorities may also be quite different from those of the leader. For example, you might expect that a group of parents would agree that having their children immunized would be a top priority and be surprised to find that their priority is to get an extra police officer stationed at a dangerous school crossing. Both, of course, are important, but you will find a community is much more cooperative and actively involved when you begin with their priorities.

EXAMPLE.   In the retirement community, the people had identified apathy as their primary concern, so a listing of priorities was not needed at that time.

Develop Motivation

The next step is to generate sufficient interest and motivation in the community to sustain action and involvement. To motivate people to take action, the project and its outcomes have to have some personal meaning to each individual community member. It is important to get people excited about the project and to believe in its importance. The effective leader will also encourage the development of good working relationships among the people involved in the project.

EXAMPLE.   One of the most effective ways to engage people in the process of improving their own community is to help them see the connection between the proposed action and a strongly felt personal need, as the student does in this example.

The same 10 people came to the second meeting and began to talk about the lack of interest of other members of their community. The student noticed that many were saying, "What's the use? They'll never come out of their apartments," and wanted to revive their sinking enthusiasm. So the student led them into talking about the effects of the prevailing apathy on each one of them personally—how it depressed them, how it discouraged them from suggesting any activities, and how it kept them from enjoying life in that community as much as they could. By the end of the discussion, the people were all angry about the way the apathy was cheating them and preventing them from deriving pleasure from their residence.

Take Stock of Resources and Build Confidence

Community groups frequently feel unable to do anything about their identified needs. A common sign of this is when people say, "What's the use? There's nothing we can do about this problem." The leader can help them take a more realistic and positive view of their own resources and the resources available to them. The leader can also encourage and support their efforts and offer assistance where necessary. Once people begin to evaluate their power and the help that is available, they usually begin to feel capable of carrying out the action needed to solve their own problems.

EXAMPLE.   The group from the retirement community thought at first that they could not handle the apathy problems alone.

> The group asked the student to offer some suggestions, but the student turned the question back to them and asked them what it is that gets them out of their apartments to attend meetings. After they gave several answers, the student pointed out that they might have some ideas about getting other people to meetings. They agreed, and began to discuss who else might be able to help them fight the apathy. They decided that they might want to call on the city recreation department and the agency on aging for some help in carrying out their plan.

Develop a Plan of Action

Although time consuming, it is important to involve the community in the development of a plan of action. In some cases, learning how to approach a problem and solve it may actually be more valuable for the future than the resolution of the present problem. Participation increases the community's commitment to the plan, and the result is more likely to be a plan that is congruent with the community's culture. The leader's willingness to let the community develop the plan communicates the leader's confidence in its ability to handle this responsible task.

Involving the community does not mean that the leader allows the group to formulate a completely inappropriate or unrealistic plan. The leader's role in planning is to offer information when no one else in the group has that information and to guide the group in developing an effective plan. Asking questions about the feasibility of suggested actions and encouraging consideration of alternative actions helps people to develop an effective, realistic plan.

EXAMPLE.   By this time, the group had begun to take some initiative:

> Most people in the group knew others in the apartment building who did not attend any meetings. They talked about some of the reasons why these friends and neighbors did not become involved. They came up with several common reasons: physical disabilities that made it difficult to go out; a life-long pattern of noninvolvement; a lack of any sense of belonging to the community, which was self-perpetuating; and lack of interest in the few activities available.
>
> They developed a three-stage plan: Stage 1: Personally contact all residents in the three buildings to find out what activities they would enjoy and to invite them to the next meeting. Stage 2: Begin a voluntary support service to help people with physical disabilities get out more often. Try to involve the new people who come to the next meeting in this project. Stage 3: Ask the city recreation department to help them establish a better activity program based on the results of their survey.

The student was impressed with the plan, especially with the residents' intent to get other community members involved. The student also realized that not even Stage 1 of the plan could have been carried out by the student alone before the assignment to the clinic was over.

Implement the Plan

The next step is to carry out the plan. Again, the members of the community should be involved as much as possible. For example, they can contact other agencies, write to their representatives, seek new funds, get involved in writing proposals, and assist in the delivery of health care services. The degree to which the community is involved has a great impact on both the success of the initial implementation and on the maintenance of the project after the leader withdraws or has to turn attention to another problem.

EXAMPLE.   The group immediately implemented Stage 1 of their plan.

The 10 residents and the student were excited about beginning the visits. They planned to keep in touch with one another to see how the visits were going and in case they ran into any problems.

The next community project meeting attracted 50 people. Most of the new people were interested in the original group's plans for reducing the apathy of their community and offered to help complete the visiting of each resident.

The next meeting attracted even more people, who formed committees to analyze the data collected about desired activities and to plan the operation of a support group.

Evaluate Results

It is always helpful to pause at intervals during a project to evaluate the progress made so far and to decide whether new strategies are needed to complete the project successfully. The dynamics of the group and the degree to which the members of the community are involved in the activities of the project should also be evaluated. An evaluation of the outcome should also be done at the end of the project.

EXAMPLE.   After the meeting in which the committees were formed, the student met informally with the 10 original group members.

These residents thought that they had successfully launched their project and had already reduced the apathy somewhat by getting more people to attend their project meetings. They decided that it would be important to continue to involve as many people in the project as possible and that they would have to take responsibility for keeping up the community's interest and enthusiasm after the student left.

The 10 original members were preparing themselves to assume the leadership of the project after the student left. Their leadership would be a very important factor in maintaining the success of the project.

POLITICAL ACTION: INFLUENCING THE FLOW OF POWER AND DECISION MAKING

The community action process just described cannot be used on every occasion. When there is strong resistance to a proposed change, an approach is needed that recognizes and deals with the ever-present politics and the relevant sources of power and influence.

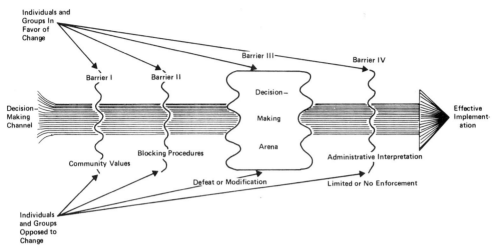

Figure 20 – 1. Flow of decision making in the community. (Adapted from Bachrach, P and Baratz, MS: Power and Poverty: Theory and Practice. Oxford University Press, London, 1970.)

Bachrach and Baratz (1970) developed a model that outlines the process of decision making in the community, the directions in which power and influence flow, and the major barriers encountered en route to implementing a change. This model (Fig. 20 – 1) is applicable to a wide range of decisions at either the local, state, or national level of decision making. It is an outline of the process; the content must be filled in from your knowledge of the particular community and the particular situation.

The model is especially useful as a guideline for analyzing a situation in which a large number of variables are involved in order to sort out the complexities of the situation. Once the situation has been analyzed using this model, you can see where it is possible to have an impact on the decision-making process.

According to this model, once the proposal or issue is clearly understood, the analysis begins with the identification of the individuals and groups who will support the change and those who will oppose it. Then it follows the proposed change through the decision-making channel past four major barriers (community values, blocking procedures, the decision-making arena itself, and administrative interpretation and enforcement) until it is finally implemented effectively. At any barrier, the proposed change can be defeated or delayed indefinitely by the opposing group. This model uses elements of Lewin's analysis of driving and restraining forces and some tactics of the power-coercive approach to change (see Chapter 19).

Entering the Decision-Making Channel

When entering the decision-making channel, it is important to identify clearly the basic elements involved in the process. These are the proposal or desired change and the way in which different individuals and groups in the community feel about the change.

THE PROPOSAL OR DESIRED CHANGE.   So many different types of decisions are made in a community that it is difficult to categorize all of them except in terms of the broad functions of a community listed earlier in this chapter. In the health care field alone, myriad decisions are made about the kind of services to offer, who will be eligible for them, how to support them, and how they will operate and by whom and so forth.

The proposal for change may come from any individual or group. They include health care organizations; government officials; civic, social, and religious groups; interest groups; professionals; concerned citizens; and individuals who are in need of the service. They may also come from individuals and groups outside the community.

EXAMPLE.   The proposal we will follow through the decision-making channels is one that came from concerned professionals who lived in a particular community:

> Two community mental health nurses who were employed outside the community become concerned about reports of inadequate health care in a correctional facility located in their community. News items about problems with the county jail included stories about serious incidents arising from the neglect of the prisoners' health needs. Two prisoners had committed suicide within the past month, and one died from a neglected perforated ulcer, although the prisoner had pleaded for medical attention.
>
> After confirming these reports and trying unsuccessfully to work with prison officials to improve the situation, the two nurses decided to become involved in a campaign to improve the health services at the jail.

IDENTIFY THE PEOPLE FOR AND AGAINST THE CHANGE.   Every proposal or desired change involves some kind of issue around which people can align themselves as being for or against the proposal. At this early stage of the process, many people will be potential rather than actual supporters or opponents. There will also be people who remain indifferent or uninformed about the issue.

The individuals and groups who are in favor of the proposed change will try to push it through the decision-making channel, while the opposing forces will try to keep it out of the channel or, once it gets into the channel, to slow or stop its progress. These people must be identified to estimate their strength and the sources of their power.

EXAMPLE.   In the example being used, the correctional facility was becoming a controversial issue in the community. Because of the many news stories, a number of individuals and groups were on each side of the issue:

> The two nurses found several groups in favor of improving conditions at the jail. A key citizens' organization in the community, the Civic Union, was considering doing a study of the situation and invited one of the nurses, who was a member of the organization, to head the study group. The Interfaith Council, which included representatives from every church and temple in the community, had been trying to begin some social services at the jail and was very much in support of the proposed change. The major political parties were divided on the issue, but a few in the majority party of the county legislature (which provided the funds to run the jail) supported the idea of making improvements but had not yet worked out the details of any improvement plan. A number of individuals also spoke out against the present conditions in the facility and called for reforms. Among them were several inmates and the parent of the young man who died in the jail.
>
> Opposing any changes were many individuals who believed that being in prison was supposed to be a punishment. Among them were several people who had been victims of

crimes committed by people in the jail. The county sheriff, who was responsible for operating the jail, opposed any changes at the jail except improvements of the building. The sheriff was supported by most members of the sheriff's political party, which was currently the minority party in the county legislature but had only two seats fewer than the majority party. Two active taxpayers' groups from different parts of the county opposed spending any more money on the jail at all if it would mean raising taxes.

At the time the nurses joined the movement to improve the jail, many people in the community were beginning to be concerned about what had happened at the jail. They were not sure what should be done about it, however.

BARRIER I. COMMUNITY VALUES. Those individuals and groups who are opposed to the change will try to keep it from being considered in any decision-making arena. To do this, they will reinforce any existing community values that support the status quo (present situation). These values are the first barrier to any proposed change in the community and are already in place when the change is proposed.

You can almost always find some community values that can be called on in support of the change, but there will usually be more or stronger prevailing values that support the status quo. The proponents of change will have to overcome the status quo.

EXAMPLE. Strong community values supported spending as little money as possible on the jail, but the recent reports of problems at the jail threatened to upset the status quo.

The county prison was constructed as a place to detain people accused but not convicted of crimes and to punish those found guilty of relatively minor offenses. Those who were given long sentences for serious crimes were not held at the county prison but sent to the state prison.

Most people in the community preferred to ignore the jail and leave it to the sheriff and the sheriff's administrators to operate in such a way that it didn't cost the taxpayer too much but did keep the inmates securely inside. The prevailing value, then, was to provide the minimum necessary for the jail and its inmates. There was also an undercurrent of feeling that the victim of a crime was more neglected than the person who committed the crime.

Values in support of improving the correctional facility were primarily based on a belief in humane treatment of any individual regardless of past behavior, and a belief that most people found in county jails would be more accurately described as troubled than as evil and dangerous.

When people in the community heard news reports of a series of escapes from the jail, they began to wonder if even the minimal necessities were presently taken care of at the jail, and they began to think about their own safety and feelings of security in a community that had frequent prison escapes.

The incidents at the facility (especially the deaths) sparked a grand jury investigation that uncovered numerous instances of inhumane treatment, including neglect of the most basic health needs, even emergency treatment. Dissemination of the grand jury findings through news stories and discussions at gathering places throughout the community upset the status quo — the community could no longer ignore the jail, and too many of its values were in conflict with conditions at the jail.

The proposed change passed Barrier I when it became apparent to the community that the jail was not well managed and that its inmates were treated far worse than they had imagined.

BARRIER II. BLOCKING PROCEDURES. Once the first barrier has been passed, the opponents of the change will try various maneuvers to block its movement into the decision-making arena. This is a stage at which a working knowledge of the community and its organizations and of the different levels and branches of government is particularly vital information. You will need this information to set up your own blocks or maneuver around those set up by opposing groups.

Those who oppose the change will try both *avoidance tactics* and *direct blocking tactics*. The specific tactics used vary somewhat according to the situation, but some common ones are used in many situations. The following is an example commonly found in health care organizations:

> If you were trying to get a change made in a particular social service, but the administrator, Mr. D., and his staff are opposed to your idea, the administrator will first try avoidance tactics, such as not returning your calls and not answering your letters. When you finally succeed in speaking with him (perhaps catching him at a public meeting), he will be politely evasive. If you persist, he may claim that you do not understand the situation and therefore cannot understand why your proposal cannot be implemented. If pressed further, he will probably say he cannot make the decision alone but will not tell you who can make the decision. When you try to approach others in the agency, you may find that they have been instructed to direct all inquiries back to the administrator. If you try to go around him to his supervisors, you will find that he has been there first and that they have issued a new policy that all requests for changes in the agency's services must come through the administrator.

When these so-called normal channels of communication are effectively blocked, it becomes necessary to circumvent them or to open them up.

The type of avoidance and blocking described above is very common. It succeeds in discouraging all but the most persistent agent for change. However, no person or group is completely immune to public pressure to change. If the channels are blocked, you *can* break down the barrier through the use of power tactics.

EXAMPLE. In the jail situation, it became necessary to use some power tactics to move the issue into the decision-making arena. For this issue, the arena was the county legislature:

> At first, the sheriff simply refused to comment on the news stories about the jail. When the grand jury report was released, the sheriff told reporters it was full of erroneous statements. These avoidance tactics succeeded for several months. Finally, the legislators thought that they had to do something about the rapidly deteriorating situation and placed the prison on the agenda of their next meeting. The sheriff came to the meeting and told the legislators that since a sheriff is a duly-elected official of the county, they could not tell a sheriff how to run the county jail. This direct block succeeded, and the issue was dropped for the time being.
>
> The groups supporting the proposal searched for a way around this block. The Civic Union study group, led by one of the nurses, met with several county legislators who were known to oppose the sheriff and support the proposed change. The legislators decided to bring the study group's data and the grand jury reports to the attention of the state investigation commission. At the same time, a group of former inmates decided to sue the sheriff for inadequate medical care. These two actions kept the jail on the front page of the county's newspaper and kept up the pressure on the county legislature.
>
> State investigators visited the jail and issued yet another critical report on prison conditions. Based on this new report, unidentified sources in the governor's office were quoted as saying that they were looking into ways to remove the sheriff from office. When this news story broke, county legislators were spurred back into action. They found a different way to deal with the prison situation—through control of the funds needed to operate the jail.

Supporters of the proposals to improve the jail finally had succeeded in moving the issue into the decision-making arena.

BARRIER III. THE DECISION-MAKING ARENA. Once an issue reaches this stage, both the supporters and opponents are likely to become more open about their viewpoints, and the lines between the groups become clearer. The decision-making arena often provides an opportunity for the groups or their representatives to face each other directly for the first time to debate the proposal. Evasion is more difficult at this point, but stalling and blocking tactics can still be used by opponents of the proposal.

The arena itself varies according to the particular issue. The legislatures at any level of government are frequent arenas, but the courts and administrative arms of government and regulatory appeals boards are also common arenas. In the jail issue discussed here, for example, the former inmates' lawsuits could have become the decision-making channel if the county legislators had failed to respond, and the courts could have ordered improvements at the jail if the inmates won their suit. The executive branch of government can also conduct investigations and hearings that become arenas for decision making. The election process is another arena for community decision making.

There are also arenas outside of government. Schools, colleges, and a wide range of community organizations can hold meetings and forums that have the potential to be decision-making arenas. Neighborhood gatherings and formal meetings of representatives from various organizations can also become arenas. The media—especially newspapers, radio, and television stations—disseminate information, encourage debates on issues, and sometimes support one side but are not usually decision-making arenas.

EXAMPLE.   The jail issue has finally been brought before the county legislature:

At the preliminary hearing of the legislature, a number of proposals were presented. The two nurses led a coalition between the Civic Union group and the Interfaith Council that presented a well-developed, comprehensive plan that called for changing the administrative structure of the jail, providing a wide range of health, social, and vocational services for the inmates and petitioning the state legislature to remove the county prison from the sheriff's control. One of the supporting legislators presented a similar but less expensive plan.

Another legislator who supported the sheriff presented a proposal that simply allocated more funds for the jail, which would be used at the sheriff's discretion. The sheriff had previously requested more money to renovate the prison building, and this request was read to the group. A representative of one of the taxpayers' groups cautioned the legislators against getting caught up in the emotionalism of the issue and against throwing money at problems instead of trying to solve them inexpensively.

Now the lines were clearly drawn. Both sides supported an increase in funds for the jail. However, one side wanted the money to be spent on services and to remove control of the prison from the sheriff; the other wanted the sheriff to retain control of the prison and to spend any additional funds on construction.

As often happens, the positions and proposals of the two sides were reduced to two-word descriptions and they became known as the anti-sheriff and pro-sheriff groups. The division also followed political lines, with most members of the sheriff's political party supporting the sheriff and many from the other party opposing the sheriff.

The sheriff was a well-known, popular figure in the community. At the legislative hearing, the sheriff spoke persuasively of a long fight to retain law and order in the community and implied that the other side wanted to coddle the prisoners and let them run loose in the community. One of the guards (correction officers) at the jail described the unruly behavior and abusive language guards had to deal with daily. The county engineer described the deteriorating condition of the prison building.

The anti-sheriff group, including the two nurses, described the inhumane treatment of the inmates in dramatic tones, implied that the sheriff was not capable of operating the prison properly and that the sheriff's methods would turn relatively harmless people into dangerous criminals by the time they were released back into the community. The parents of the young man who died described their pleas for help and the way their son was treated in the hours before he died. The hearing lasted 6 hours and received extensive news coverage.

The legislature adjourned at 2:00 AM and reconvened the next afternoon to vote on the proposals. The coalition's proposal to expand services was approved after cuts were made in the budget. However, the proposal to remove control of the jail from the sheriff was defeated by a small margin. Both groups claimed victory but neither side actually felt satisfied. The sheriff retained control of the prison but was now supposed to provide more services for the inmates.

BARRIER IV. ADMINISTRATIVE INTERPRETATION AND ENFORCE-MENTS.   It would seem that once a decision is made, especially if it is in the form of a law, that battle would be over. It is not that simple, however. As is done with the official goals of an organization, official laws can be ignored or only partially enforced, particularly if the community does not support the law and pressure a reluctant administrator to enforce the law firmly and fully. In addition, some laws are so vaguely worded that they can be interpreted in several ways.

The same is true of any decision. Any ruling, procedure, or decision can be ignored or evaded by its opponents if its enforcement is not closely followed by its supporters.

EXAMPLE.   The results of the county legislature's decisions left a situation in which limited enforcement was almost a predictable outcome:

The sheriff continued to control the prison. After the funds were appropriated, the sheriff quickly initiated renovation plans and publicized the physical improvements being made. However, the introduction of new services did not conform with the approved plan. A part-time social work student and licensed practical nurse were hired but given little direction or support. One community group was given permission to visit inmates once a week, but group members were treated so rudely by some of the guards that they did not want to return.

Although news items about the jail decreased considerably, both the coalition and supporting legislators continued to pay close attention to what was happening at the jail. When it became apparent that only token attempts to improve health, social, and vocational services were being made, they brought their data and complaints back to the state investigating commission, which renewed its pressure on the sheriff (the threat to remove the sheriff from office was a real possibility, although such action is a rare occurrence), and the sheriff finally hired an experienced and capable administrator for the jail. The new administrator appointed several community advisory boards to develop plans for improving conditions in the prison, and within a year, most of the services described in the coalition's original proposal were implemented.

The tremendous amount of time and energy required to implement the proposal described in the example was due not only to the strength of the opposing side but also to the community's fundamental lack of interest in what happened at the prison so long as members of the community did not feel that it affected them personally. The combination of strong opposition, initial community disinterest, and conflicting beliefs and values made it very difficult to move the issue through the channels of decision making to effective implementation.

You may have noticed that the nurses in the example were only a small part of the group that finally succeeded in improving prison conditions. A number of different individuals and groups within the community and outside the community were eventually involved and brought their collective power and influence to bear on the situation. Without this convergence of power and influence from many sources, the change would not have taken place. As an individual leader, you can act as a catalyst in bringing these forces together. As an energizer in helping to keep up interest and momentum, you can greatly extend your influence in the community.

Effective Community Leadership

To some readers, it may seem that this chapter has presented a very different perspective on leadership, one that is not closely tied to leadership and management *within* health care organizations. But the basic principles of leadership and management actually remain the same. To illustrate this, let's review the components of effective leadership to see how they were applied to this last example of leadership in the community.

GOALS. Although the goals of the various individuals and groups who supported the change were far from identical, they were sufficiently congruent for the people to work together. The two groups that formed the coalition identified and agreed upon mutual goals through the development of the written proposal for improving the county prison.

SKILLS AND KNOWLEDGE. A great deal of knowledge and skill was needed to implement this change. Knowledge of the conditions at the jail and what was needed to improve conditions was frequently used as data to support the desired change. Familiarity with the community's beliefs and values helped the group to overcome the first barrier by indicating how the community's values were in conflict with the status quo at the jail. Use of the legislators' knowledge of the way in which the state government could apply pressure was a turning point in bringing the issue to the legislature and enforcing full enforcement of the decision.

SELF-AWARENESS. The need for self-awareness was not as evident in this particular situation as it is in some others. However, it did enter into the development of effective working relationships within the groups forming the coalition and among all of the individuals and groups forming the supporting side. The people who led the movement for change also had to be aware of their own motives. If their desires for individual recognition or power had overridden their desire to bring about change, it could have destroyed the coalition.

COMMUNICATION. Communication between the individuals and groups forming the coalition was essential. It brought the people together at the beginning of this process and, later, helped them to coordinate their actions. Even more essential to the success of the entire project was the steady flow of communication with other people in the community through the media, meetings, and personal interaction. Without this communication, the supporting side could not have gained the support from the community and the pressure from the media needed to press the county legislature to act. It also involved as many people in the community as possible in the movement to bring about change.

ENERGY. As mentioned earlier, a great deal of energy was required to initiate and maintain interest in the issue, particularly at the barrier points where the opposition nearly succeeded in blocking the proposed change completely. Energy was also needed to keep the supporting group interested and excited about its work and to follow up on enforcement, a time when energies are likely to flag because the battle appears to be over.

ACTION. The initiative of the two nurses helped to bring the two community groups together into a coalition. This is a good example of the linking function. Other actions included the frequent use of the media, the number of meetings called, and the nurses' continuing presence and participation in the many meetings and hearings about the jail.

SUMMARY

A community may be defined as a geographical place, a number of people with shared interests and needs, or as a population within which a problem can be solved. The functions of a community are to provide safety and security, mutual support, socialization, significance, and a network for the distribution of goods and services.

A community is an open, living system that has unique characteristics as a whole that are different from those of its many subsystems. They have their own sets of goals, which may or may not be congruent. Like other living systems, communities have identifiable rhythms and patterns of activity. They also exchange energy in the form of information, materials, money, and services with their environment.

Power is unevenly distributed in the community. People who regularly influence decision making can be categorized as influentials, effectors, or activists. Others in the community participate at irregular intervals and can be categorized as having high- or low-initiative patterns.

The goal of the community action process is to involve members of the community in helping themselves and others. The leader's primary roles are to act as a catalyst, energizer, supporter, and source of information. The process begins with the mutual identification of needs and a prioritizing of those needs by the community. The next steps are to develop motivation, take stock of the resources available and build community members' confidence in their ability to help themselves, develop a plan of action, implement the plan, and evaluate the results.

The model for analyzing the flow of power and decision making in the community begins with the identification of the proposed change, its supporters, and its opponents. The four barriers in the way of effective implementation are prevailing community values, blocking procedures, the decision-making arena, and administrative interpretation and enforcement of the change. Using the components of effective leadership, the leader can act as a catalyst and energizer in bringing together the sources of power and influence in the community needed to move a proposal past the barriers and into effective implementation.

REFERENCES*

Bachrach, P. & Baratz, M.S. (1970). *Power and Poverty: Theory and Practice.* London: Oxford University Press.

*Braden, C.J. & Herban, N.L. (1976). *Community Health: A Systems Approach.* New York: Appleton-Century-Crofts.

Coleman, J.S. (1977). Notes on the study of power. In Liebert, R.J. & Imershein, A.W. (eds.): *Power, Paradigms, and Community Research.* Beverly Hills: Sage Publications.

Freeman, L.C. et al. (1970). Locating leaders in local communities: A comparison of some alternative approaches. In Aiken, M. & Mott, P.E. (eds.): *The Structure of Community Power.* New York: Random House.

*Gottschalk, S.S. (1975). *Communities and Alternatives: An Exploration of the Limits of Planning.* New York: Schenkman.

Griffin, K. (1987). *Ralph Nader Presents: More Action for a Change.* New York: Dembner Books.

*Hall, J.E. & Weaver, B.R. (1985). *A System Approach to Community Health.* Philadelphia: J.B. Lippincott.

*Hanchett, E. (1979). *Community Health Assessment: A Conceptual Tool Kit.* New York: John Wiley & Sons.

*Hanlon, J.J. & Pickett, G.E. (1984). *Public Health: Administration and Practice,* ed. 7. St. Louis: C.V. Mosby.

Hunter, F. (1970). Methods of study: Community power structure. In Aiken, M. & Mott, P.E. (eds): *The Structure of Community Power.* New York: Random House.

Klein, D.C. (1968). *Community Dynamics and Mental Health.* New York: John Wiley & Sons.

Litwack, E., Meyer, J.J., & Hollister, C.D. (1977). The role of linkage mechanisms between bureaucracies and families: Education and health as empirical cases in point. In Liebert, R.J. & Imershein, A.W. (eds): *Power, Paradigms, and Community Research.* Beverly Hills, California: Sage Publications.

MacIntosh, D.R. (1978). *Systems of Health Care.* Boulder, Colorado: Westview Press.

Marsden, P.V. & Laumann, E.O. (1977). Collective action in a community elite: Exchange, influence resources and issue resolution. In Liebert, R.J. & Imershein, A.W. (eds.): *Power, Paradigms, and Community Research.* Beverly Hills, California: Sage Publications.

Maxwell, R.J. (1986). Learning from the third world. *The Lancet,* January 25, 1986.

McDowell, D. (1977). *The New Older Citizen's Guide: Advocacy and Action.* Harrisburg, Pennsylvania: Office for the Aging, Pennsylvania Department of Public Welfare.

Polsby, N.W. (1970). How to study community power: The pluralist alternative. In Aiken, M. & Mott, P.E. (eds): *The Structure of Community Power.* New York: Random House.

*Ross, M.G. with Lappin, B.W. (1967). *Community Organization: Theory, Principles and Practice,* ed 2. New York: Harper & Row.

Solomon, S.B. & Roe, S.C. (1986). *Integrating Public Policy into the Curriculum.* New York: National League for Nursing.

*Warren, R. (1963). *The Community in America.* Chicago: Rand McNally.

Whyte, W.F. (1984). *Learning from the Field.* Beverly Hills: Sage.

Williams, S.J. & Torrens, P.R. (1980). *Introduction to Health Services.* New York: John Wiley & Sons.

*References marked with an asterisk are suggested for further reading.

UNIT IV LEARNING ACTIVITIES ─────────────

▷ Conduct a mock problem-solving conference using either a patient/client problem or typical nursing team problem as the focus. A volunteer leader and five or six team members is a good size for the group. Assign functional roles to half of the team and nonfunctional roles to the other half (not known to the leader) to play in the session. Analyze the outcomes as was done for the script, including a sociogram, seating arrangement, communication pattern, roles played, maturity of the group, course of discussion, decision making and the outcome, dominant synchronizers, and leadership style and effectiveness.

▷ With a colleague or classmate, role play a negotiation session with your immediate supervisor in which you are requesting a substantial salary increase based on merit.

▷ Using information about the patients or clients served by your assigned agency or unit, devise an ideal assignment plan. Be sure that assignments are both appropriate and fair and that their outcomes would promote both the efficiency and effectiveness of the care given.

▷ Select a particular change in health care that you would like to see occur. Work through the steps of phases of *each* change model from the rational to the power-coercive as they would be used to bring about your selected change. Evaluate the appropriateness and potential effectiveness of each model for the given situation.

▷ Using newspaper accounts and local informants, trace the progress (or lack of progress) of an important health-related issue in your community. Using the political action model, identify the forces for and against change, the decision-making channel, the barriers to change in the decision-making arena, and the degree to which the change was implemented. Analyze the outcome in terms of actions that could have taken place either to promote or prevent it.

Unit V

EVALUATION AND PROFESSIONAL DEVELOPMENT

Chapter 21.   Formal and Informal Evaluation Procedures
Chapter 22.   Accountability and Quality Assurance
Chapter 23.   Staff Development
Chapter 24.   Leading Information Conferences
Unit V Learning Activities

Chapter 21 ━━━━━━━━━━

OUTLINE ━━━━━━━━━━━━━━━━━━━━━━━━━━━━━━━━

Informal Evaluation
Informal Versus Formal Evaluation
Purpose of Providing Evaluative Feedback
Clarify Performance Expectations
Reinforce Constructive Behavior
Correct Unsatisfactory Behavior
Provide Recognition
Increase Self-awareness
Promote Growth and Change
Guidelines for Providing Constructive
Feedback
Both Positive and Negative
Immediate
Frequent
Private
Objective
Based on Observable Behavior
Appropriately Communicated
Include Suggestions for Change
Nonthreatening

Seeking Evaluative Feedback
When Is Evaluative Feedback Needed?
Responding to Evaluative Feedback

Formal Evaluation
Purpose of Formal Evaluation
Accountability
Administrative Intervention
Rewards
Identification of Educational Needs
Data Base
Performance Appraisals by Managers
and Supervisors
General Guidelines
Evaluating the Marginal Staff Member
Formal Review by Peers
Fundamentals of Peer Review
A Comprehensive Peer Review System

Summary

LEARNING OBJECTIVES ━━━━━━━━━━━━━━━━━━━━━━

Upon completion of this chapter, the reader will be able to:

▷ Distinguish formal from informal evaluation.

▷ Provide both positive and negative feedback in a constructive manner.

▷ Conduct a formal performance appraisal.

▷ Evaluate the objectivity and constructiveness of informal and formal evaluation procedures.

▷ Participate in the development and implementation of a formal peer review system.

FORMAL AND INFORMAL EVALUATION PROCEDURES*

Everyone needs to know how well they are doing. From the chief executive officer to the lowest-paid maintenance worker, people need to know where they stand and what impact they have on the organization. They need to know how valued they are, how others respond to them, how well they have solved a problem, whether they have been helpful to other people, and, in general, how effective their work is.

Informal evaluation provides this kind of information on a regular moment-by-moment basis. It is a continuous process of giving and receiving evaluative feedback that includes both positive and negative comments on people's effectiveness as caregivers, coworkers, team members, leaders, and managers. Although some of this feedback will be negative, it can still be constructive in the sense that it improves performance and promotes growth.

Formal evaluation is the planned process of giving and receiving feedback as part of the stated procedures of most organizations. Formal evaluations are much less frequent but usually more structured. Employee participation in these procedures is usually required by the organization.

Formal evaluation begins with the setting of standards against which the individual will be judged. These standards should be objective, in written form and communicated in advance to those who will be evaluated.

This chapter begins with the principles of seeking and providing evaluative feedback that apply to both formal and informal evaluation. Both the manager's and staff member's point of view will be considered in later sections of the chapter to provide a broader perspective on evaluation.

INFORMAL EVALUATION

Informal Versus Formal Evaluation

The term *informal evaluation* is used to distinguish it from the formal procedures such as peer review and performance appraisals that are mandated by organizations or by accrediting agencies. Informal evaluation occurs during the give and take of other work activities. It is a continuous process, an action that occurs often and whenever it is needed rather than according to schedule. It is also an integral part of the activities of a well-

---

*Co-authored by Ruth M. Tappen, R.N., Ed.D. and Phyllis George, R.N., M.A.

functioning team and is the responsibility of every member of the team, not just the team leader. The leader-manager has the extra responsibility of ensuring that it occurs and is done appropriately.

Formal evaluations usually have an explicit structure, including specific forms to fill out and timetables for carrying out the procedures.

Formal evaluation procedures may occur only once or twice a year. Alone, this method is inadequate to provide the continuous guidance and recognition that people need at work. Providing frequent informal feedback can meet these needs and is an important function of the leader-manager. You may recall that giving feedback was one of the actions listed in the components of effective leadership and that monitoring work was one of the components of effective management.

Purpose of Providing Evaluative Feedback

People function better when they receive constructive feedback about their performance. More specifically, providing evaluative feedback serves to clarify performance expectations, reinforce constructive behavior, correct negative behavior, provide recognition, increase self-awareness, and promote growth and change (Mager & Pipe, 1970).

CLARIFY PERFORMANCE EXPECTATIONS. No matter how clearly job descriptions are written (and sometimes they do not even exist), the details of a particular job cannot be fully described in writing. Informal feedback is an effective way to communicate these details as questions arise in the course of the work being done. Feedback also verifies for people either that they did understand what was expected of them or that they need to clarify these expectations.

REINFORCE CONSTRUCTIVE BEHAVIOR. Evaluative feedback can confirm that people are performing well. Providing positive feedback encourages constructive behavior, increases motivation, and promotes job satisfaction.

CORRECT UNSATISFACTORY BEHAVIOR. Correcting unsatisfactory behavior is often thought of as the only purpose for evaluation. Poor performance must be acknowledged and steps must be taken to correct it.

PROVIDE RECOGNITION. Recognition for work well done is a powerful and inexpensive reward for good performance. It meets those needs for esteem and recognition that all people have to varying degrees.

INCREASE SELF-AWARENESS. Feedback helps people identify their strengths and weaknesses so that their efforts can be directed toward reinforcing strengths and developing more skill in areas of weakness.

PROMOTE GROWTH AND CHANGE. Frequent feedback is one way to challenge caregivers to continually use the very best methods in providing health care. It also encourages people to use their best resources whenever they face a problem or difficult decision and to look for opportunities to upgrade their knowledge and skills. By serving these purposes, informal evaluation also improves the quality of the health care given.

Both positive and negative feedback are needed to fulfill these purposes. Neglect or avoidance of either will reduce your effectiveness as a leader-manager.

Guidelines for Providing Constructive Feedback

Evaluation involves making judgments and communicating these judgments to others. People make judgments all the time about all types of things. Many times these judgments are based on opinions, preferences, and dislikes rather than facts or on inaccurate or partial information.

Biased, hasty judgments offered as objective feedback have given evaluation a bad name for many. Poorly communicated feedback has an equally negative effect. In fact, you will find that many people who are threatened by evaluation have been the recipients of biased and/or poorly communicated evaluations in the past.

Evaluation can be destructive. When poorly done, it reinforces ineffective work habits, reduces self-esteem, and destroys motivation. On the other hand, when it is done well, it reinforces motivation, strengthens the team, and improves the quality of care given.

Evaluative feedback is most effective when it is given immediately, frequently, and privately. To be constructive, it must be objective, based on observed behavior, and skillfully communicated. The feedback message should include the reason why a behavior has been judged good or poor in order to promote growth and learning. If the message is negative, it should be nonthreatening and include suggestions and support for change and improvement. Each of these criteria is discussed below.

BOTH POSITIVE AND NEGATIVE.   Positive feedback may be easier to give, but leader-managers often neglect to do so. If questioned, people who do not give positive feedback will explain that, "If I don't say anything, that means everything is okay." Unfortunately, they don't realize that some people will assume that everything is *not* okay when they receive no feedback. Others assume that no one is aware of how much effort has gone into their work unless it is acknowledged with positive feedback.

Most people want to do their work well. They also want to know that their efforts are recognized and appreciated; it is a real pleasure to be able to share the satisfaction of a job well done with someone else. If you neglect to give positive feedback, you have failed to use a powerful and readily available motivator (Huntsman, 1987). Kron (1981) calls positive feedback a "psychological paycheck" and points out that it is almost as important to people as their actual paycheck.

It has been said that nurses do not do enough to support each other as colleagues. Whether that is true or not, giving positive feedback to one's colleagues is an important way to support them.

Negative feedback is just as necessary as positive feedback but probably more difficult to do well. Too often, negative feedback is critical rather than constructive. It is easier to just tell people that something has gone wrong or could have been done better than it is to make the feedback a learning experience for the receiver by suggesting ways to make the needed changes or working together to develop a strategy for improvement. It is also easier to make broad, critical comments such as, "You're too slow," than it is to describe very specifically the behavior that needs improvement such as saying, "Waiting in Mr. D.'s room while he finishes his breakfast takes up too much of your time," and then add a suggestion for change such as, "You could get your bath supplies together while he finishes eating."

Providing no negative feedback at all is the easiest but least effective solution to the problem of being too critical. Unsatisfactory work must be acknowledged and discussed with the people involved. The "gutless wonder" (Del Bueno, 1977) who silently tolerates poor work encourages it to continue and undermines the motivation of the whole team.

IMMEDIATE. The most helpful feedback is given as soon as possible after the behavior has occurred. There are several reasons for this. Immediate feedback is more meaningful to the person receiving it. If feedback is delayed too long, the person may have assumed that your silence indicated approval or may have forgotten the incident altogether.

Also, like other confrontation situations, problems that are ignored often get worse, and, in the meantime, a lot of frustration and anger can build up. When feedback is given as soon as possible, there is no time for this build-up and results can be seen immediately.

FREQUENT. Feedback should not only be immediate but frequent. Frequent constructive feedback keeps motivation and awareness levels high and avoids the possibility that problems will grow larger and more serious before they are confronted. It also becomes easier with practice. If giving and receiving feedback is a frequent and integral part of team functioning, it will be easier to do and less threatening to most people. It becomes an ordinary occurrence, one that happens spontaneously and is familiar to everyone to the team.

PRIVATE. Giving negative feedback privately rather than in front of others avoids embarrassment. It also avoids the possibility that those who overhear the discussion may misunderstand it and draw erroneous conclusions from it. As one writer has said, a manager should praise staff in public but punish (correct) them in private (Matejka, 1986).

OBJECTIVE. It can be very difficult to be objective when giving feedback to others. The use of critical analysis techniques discussed in Chapter 6 (such as avoiding emotional arguments or ensuring that data are adequate) can be helpful here. People should be evaluated on the basis of job expectations, not compared, whether favorably or unfavorably, with other staff members (Gellerman & Hodgson, 1988). Another way to increase objectivity is to always give a reason why you have judged a behavior as good or poor. Reasons should be given for both positive and negative messages. For example, if you tell a coworker, "That was a good interview," you have told that person nothing except that the interview pleased you. However, when you add to the message, "because you asked many open-ended questions that encouraged the client to explore personal feelings," you have identified the specific behavior that made your evaluation positive and reinforced this specific behavior.

Finally, use as broad and generally accepted a standard for judgments as possible to avoid basing evaluation on personal likes or dislikes. Formal evaluation should always be based on previously agreed-upon, written standards of what is acceptable behavior. Informal evaluation, however, is based on unwritten standards. If these standards are based on idiosyncratic personal preferences, the evaluation will be highly subjective. Objectivity can be increased by using standards that reflect the consensus of the team, the organization, the community, or the profession as a whole. Here are some examples:

A team leader who describes a female social worker as having a professional appearance because she wears dark suits instead of bright dresses to work is using a personal standard to evaluate that social worker.

A supervisor who asks an employee to stop wearing jewelry that could get caught in the equipment used at work is applying a more generally accepted standard of safety in making the evaluative statement.

The nursing home administrator who insists that staff include every resident in the weekly birthday party game is applying a narrower and more personal standard than the administrator who insists that staff members offer every resident the opportunity to participate in weekly activities.

BASED ON OBSERVABLE BEHAVIOR. An evaluative statement should describe directly observed behavior, not personality traits, attitudes, or interpretation of behavior. The observation is much more likely to be factual and accurate than the interpretation and less likely to evoke a defensive response. Here is an example:

Saying, "You were impatient with Mrs. G. today," is an interpretive comment. Saying, "You interrupted Mrs. G. before she finished explaining her problem," is based on observable behavior. It is more specific and may be more accurate because the caregiver may have been trying to redirect the conversation to more immediate concerns rather than simply being impatient. The second statement is more likely to evoke an explanation rather than a defensive response.

APPROPRIATELY COMMUNICATED. An evaluative statement is a form of confrontation. Any message that contains a statement about the behavior of a staff member is confronting that staff member with information. The guidelines given in Chapter 15 about the appropriate way to confront another person or group apply to giving evaluative feedback. It is, for example, particularly important to avoid sending put-down or blaming messages.

As with other confrontations, the leader who gives evaluative feedback needs to be prepared to receive feedback in return and to engage in active listening. Active listening is especially important when the person receiving the evaluation responds with disagreement and high emotion. Here is an example:

Let's say that you point out to Mr. S. that his patients need to be monitored more frequently. Mr. S. responds emotionally about doing everything possible for the patients and not having a free moment all day for one extra thing. In fact, Mr. S. tells you that he never even takes a lunch break and goes home exhausted. Active listening and problem solving with this coworker to relieve his overloaded time schedule are a must in this situation.

When you give negative feedback, it is often necessary to allow time for ventilation of feelings and then for problem solving with the individual to find ways to improve a situation. This is particularly true if the problem has been ignored long enough to become as serious as in the example given.

INCLUDE SUGGESTIONS FOR CHANGE. When you give feedback to someone that indicates some kind of change in behavior is needed, it is helpful to suggest alternative behaviors. This is easier to do when the change is a simple one.

When it is a complex change that is needed (as in the example given above), you may find that the person is aware of the problem but does not know how to solve it. In such a case, overly simple solutions are inappropriate, but an offer to engage in the search for a solution is appropriate. A demonstrated willingness to listen to the other person's side of the story and to assist in finding a solution also indicates that your purpose in providing the negative feedback was to help rather than to criticize or attack the individual.

NONTHREATENING. An appropriately communicated statement should not be threatening. Highly threatening messages divert people's energies into activities aimed specifically at reducing the threat. Although a small degree of anxiety may increase learning, too much fear immobilizes and reduces functional capacity to grow. The ultimate purpose for providing informal evaluation is, after all, to improve the function of the team and its individual members. When the feedback is negative, the focus of the message should be on the specific behavior, not on the person as a whole, which devalues the person and threatens self-esteem.

Negative feedback often contains veiled or even open threats and hints of dire consequences, probably in the mistaken belief that it will increase the person's motivation to change. The following are some common examples:

"You're not going to last long if you keep doing that."

"People who want to do well here make sure their assignments are done on time."

"Don't argue with the doctors, they'll report you to the nursing office."

When a person's behavior actually does threaten job security, a formal evaluation directly stating this fact and proposing needed changes is appropriate. The examples given above threaten job security, but other evaluative statements can threaten other types of safety and security needs, self-esteem, or the need for love and belonging.

You may have assumed that people in the ranks above you (manager, head nurse, supervisor, director, and so forth) could not be threatened by feedback from you. This is not true. They are all human and as susceptible to feeling threatened as your coworkers are. You need to follow these same guidelines in giving feedback to people above you in the organization.

Seeking Evaluative Feedback

Just as important as knowing how to give feedback is knowing when to look for it and how to take it. The purposes for seeking feedback are the same as those for giving it to others. The criteria for evaluating the feedback you receive are also the same.

WHEN IS EVALUATIVE FEEDBACK NEEDED? There are a number of different situations in which you need to seek feedback. For example, you could find yourself in a work situation where you receive very little feedback from any source except your own self-evaluation. Or you may be getting only positive and no negative comments, or vice versa.

Another time when you need to look for feedback is when you feel uncertain about how well you are doing or whether you have correctly interpreted the expectations of the job. The following are some examples of these situations:

You have been told that good patient care is the first consideration of your job but feel totally frustrated by never having enough staff to give good care.

You thought you were expected to do case finding and health teaching in your community but receive the most recognition for the number of home visits made and for the completeness of your records.

An additional instance in which you should request feedback is when you feel that your needs for recognition and job satisfaction have not been met adequately.

Requests for feedback should be made in form of "I" messages. If you have received only negative comments, ask, "In what ways have I done well?" If you receive only positive comments, you can ask, "In what areas do I need to improve?" Or, if you are seeking feedback from a patient, you could ask, "How can I be of more help to you?"

RESPONDING TO EVALUATIVE FEEDBACK. There are times when it is appropriate to critically analyze the feedback you are getting. If the feedback seems totally negative or you feel threatened when receiving it, ask for further explanation. You may have misunderstood what the person meant to say.

It is hard to avoid responding defensively to negative feedback that is subjective or laced with threats and blame. But if you are the recipient of such poorly done evaluation, it may help both of you to try to guide the discussion into more constructive areas. You can ask for reasons why the evaluation was negative, what standard it is based upon or what the person's expectations were, and what the person suggests as alternative behavior.

When the feedback is positive but nonspecific, you may also want to ask for some clarification so that you can find out what that person's expectations are. Do not hesitate to seek that psychological paycheck. Tell other people about your successes — most are happy to share the satisfaction of a successful outcome or positive development in a patient's care.

FORMAL EVALUATION _____

As a first-line manager, you will be expected to do formal evaluations and you may be involved in setting up evaluation procedures. To do this effectively, you need to know the purposes of formal evaluation, how to develop and use standards, and how to write objectives. Even more important is the ability to be objective in your evaluation and to use communication skills effectively in sharing the evaluation with the person or group that was evaluated. You can see that you need to have learned leadership and management well to be an effective evaluator. This is so important that many organizations hold workshops on evaluation and schedule skill-training sessions for people who do performance appraisals (employee evaluations).

As an employee, you will also be the *subject* of evaluation procedures. When this is the case, you still need to know what constitutes an objective evaluation and how to communicate effectively. You also need to know what you can reasonably expect from your employer.

Purpose of Formal Evaluation

The purposes of informal evaluation described earlier (providing recognition, increasing self-awareness, and so forth) also apply to formal evaluation. Formal evaluation has some additional purposes that are related to the function of the organization, to the regulatory agencies that mandate the procedures, and to the professions that are involved in the procedures. These purposes are discussed briefly below.

ACCOUNTABILITY. Evaluation is an important demonstration of both the individual's and the health care organization's acceptance of responsibility for the services provided. It is a demonstration to the public that efforts are being made to provide quality care.

Individual health care professionals are accountable for the care they give. Participation in evaluation procedures in which the caregiver is judged against an accepted standard is one way to achieve this accountability.

Entire health care organizations should also be accountable for the health care that they offer to consumers. The development and implementation of comprehensive evaluation programs is one way to achieve accountability. Not every organization has been willing to do this, but pressure from state and national levels of government and accrediting bodies has helped promote the development of organizational accountability.

ADMINISTRATIVE INTERVENTION. Evaluation that is taken seriously by the administrator of an organization can be a stimulus for change within that organization. In particular, evaluation documents success or failure in meeting objectives and identifies specific obstacles in the way of achieving these objectives.

Regular evaluation of the individual staff members can help to identify weaknesses and problems before they become major obstacles to achieving the desired objectives. If these evaluations are based on the goals and standards of the organization, they can answer such questions as the following:

▷ Are expected objectives being achieved?
▷ Are patients' needs being met?
▷ Are standards for quality being met?
▷ Is care being given efficiently as well as effectively?

Because the leadership and administration of a program can be crucial to its effectiveness, upper-level management people should also be evaluated.

REWARDS. Formal evaluations should serve as the basis upon which employees are given raises and promotions as rewards for satisfactory or better performance.

An objective, comprehensive evaluation of an employee's work can identify the person's potential for growth, point out deficiencies in a person's work, and help in the identification of ways to improve that person's performance and contribute to professional growth. Evaluations may also be the basis for termination of employment when consistently poor appraisals follow substantial efforts to remedy the problem.

IDENTIFICATION OF EDUCATIONAL NEEDS. The data resulting from formal evaluation procedures can be used to analyze the continuing educational needs of the people who work in that organization. For example, the analysis could point out a specific need such as inconsistency in diabetic teaching or more general educational needs of the staff such as exploring new approaches to practice or improving leadership skills.

DATA BASE.   Although it is not generally the main purpose for formal evaluation, the information collected and recorded during evaluation procedures can serve as a valuable data base for the evaluation of health care procedures.

There are many problems in health care for which solutions have not been found. For example, many diabetic patients do not follow their diets, many alcoholic patients are not sufficiently motivated to stop drinking, and too many hemiplegic patients are not restored to maximum function. The chances of finding a way to achieve better results are improved if we look for solutions in a number of places, including the data from evaluation procedures.

Performance Appraisals by Managers and Supervisors

GENERAL GUIDELINES.   *Performance appraisal* is the term generally used to describe the formal evaluation of an employee by a superior (usually a manager or supervisor). The employee's behavior is compared with a standard describing how the employee is expected to perform. Employees need to know *what* has to be done, *how much* has to be done, and *when* it has to be done (Hansen, 1986). The standards that provide this information are often written in the form of objectives. Actual performance is evaluated, not good intentions.

The Procedure.   In the ideal situation, the performance appraisal procedure begins when the employee is hired. Based on the written job description, the employee and manager or supervisor discuss the expected standard of performance and then write a set of objectives that they believe the employee can reasonably accomplish within a given period of time. The objectives should be written at a level of performance that demonstrates that some learning, attainment or refinement of skill, or advancement toward some long-range objective has taken place. The following are examples of objectives that could be set for a patient educator to accomplish in 6 months:

▷ Conduct a survey of patient use and response to the closed circuit television patient education programs.
▷ Include staff in development of a proposal for a neuropsychological rehabilitation program.
▷ Continue to conduct diet and exercise classes for the community.
▷ Implement developed series of Stop Smoking classes.

The 6-month objectives for a staff nurse would be quite different. They could include such items as the following:

▷ Assume charge duties on a 3:00-to-11:00 shift when the assistant head nurse is not on duty.
▷ Attend two appropriate continuing education seminars.
▷ Precept one new graduate nurse assigned to the unit.

Six months later, at a previously agreed upon time, the employee and supervisor meet again and evaluate the employee's performance in comparison with the previously set goals. The evaluation should be based on both the employee's self-assessment and the supervisor's observation of specific behaviors. New objectives and plans for achieving them may be agreed on at the time of the appraisal or at a separate meeting (Beer, 1981). A copy of the performance appraisal and the projected goals must be available to the employee so that he or she can refer back to them and check on progress toward the agreed-upon goals.

It is important to set aside adequate time for the feedback and goal-setting processes. Rushing through these important discussions is certainly not the best way to handle them (Hunter, 1988). Both the employee and the supervisor should come to this session with data for use at this session. The data should include a self-evaluation by the employee and observations by the evaluator of the employee's activities and outcomes. Data may also be obtained from peers and patients or clients. Some organizations use surveys for getting this information from patients.

The guidelines for providing informal evaluative feedback apply to the conduct of performance appraisals. While not as frequent or immediate as informal feedback, they should be just as objective, private, nonthreatening, skillfully communicated, and growth promoting.

Standards for Evaluation.   Many organizations, unfortunately, have employee evaluation procedures that are far from ideal. Their procedures may be inconsistent, subjective, and even unknown to the employee in some cases. The following is a list of standards for a fair and objective employee evaluation procedure that you may want to use to judge your own or your employer's procedures:

1. Standards are clear, objective, and known in advance.
2. Criteria for pay raises and promotions are clearly spelled out and uniformly applied.
3. Conditions under which employment may be terminated are known.
4. Appraisals are part of the employee's permanent record and have space for employee comments.
5. Employees may inspect their own personnel files.
6. Employees may request and be given a reasonable explanation of any rating and may appeal the rating if they do not agree with it.
7. Employees are given a reasonable amount of time to correct any serious deficiencies before other action is taken, unless the safety of self or others is immediately threatened.

In some organizations, collective bargaining agreements are used to enforce adherence to fair and objective performance appraisals. However, these agreements often emphasize seniority (length of service) over merit, a situation that does not promote growth and change.

EVALUATING THE MARGINAL STAFF MEMBER.   Conducting the performance appraisal of a highly motivated, competent staff member is usually a demanding but satisfying experience for the first-line manager. The appraisal meeting provides an opportunity to recognize and reward the individual for work well done and to plan for further growth and development. Generally, it reaches an agreeable conclusion even if it begins with some tension or apprehension on your part or that of the staff member being evaluated.

Evaluation of a staff member whose performance has not been satisfactory is an entirely different story. Very few people find it easy to sit down and discuss a person's shortcomings with him or her directly. It is usually an uncomfortable but necessary experience for both the evaluator and the evaluatee.

Excuses for Inaction.   It is quite easy to rationalize your failure to confront unsatisfactory performance. You may rationalize that the poor performance is just a temporary lapse that will soon disappear or that it is due to a personal problem at home. If these *are* legitimate reasons, you must set a time limit to your tolerance of poor performance.

Another common rationalization is that you want to give the employee a fair chance to improve on his or her own before intervening. Or, you may tell yourself that the employee really is trying hard and any negative feedback may discourage him or her. Both of these excuses imply that negative feedback cannot be helpful, that you are doing Employee X a favor by not telling Employee X that a problem exists.

Often, just the fact that Employee X is really a very nice person can inhibit a manager. Employee X may be the person who always has a cheerful smile early in the morning, the one who never complains, or the one who can lighten up a serious staff meeting with a funny story. The problem with these excuses is that you are confusing personality with performance (Hansen, 1986).

Finally, inaction is encouraged when the unsatisfactory employee is thought to be leaving, transferring out of the department, or retiring. The excuse is that there is no point in raising the issue because Employee X is leaving soon. In the meantime, however, Employee X is drawing a salary but not doing a fair share of the work.

Importance of Intervention.   The importance of intervening has probably already become clear to the reader. Like the failure to confront problems generally, failure to confront unsatisfactory performance is likely to result in the problem growing larger, not smaller. The longer unsatisfactory behavior is tolerated, the more difficult it is to change it.

The unsatisfactory performer, Employee X, is still being paid as if performance were satisfactory. This fact alone makes Employee X a liability to the organization. Unless another staff member is doing Employee X's work (which obviously is not fair), there is work that is not being done. Can your unit afford to allow Employee X to continue performing poorly? Isn't it affecting patient care? Or morale within the team?

Excessive tolerance of poor performance also affects your image as a leader-manager. The leader-manager who fails to confront problems affecting the group may be seen as laissez-faire, uncaring, ineffective, powerless, cowardly, or simply lazy. Some of these interpretations may be true. Failure to confront poor performance results in increased cost to the organization, an unfair work burden on other staff members, work bottlenecks within the team, lower quality of care to the clients being served, and the potential for reduced morale among the employees whose performance is satisfactory (Pulick, 1986).

Factors Leading to Marginal Performance.   The cause of poor performance is not necessarily found in the employee. An open systems perspective makes this very clear. Consider the elements of a management situation: the leader-manager, the employee, the work to be done, and the environment in which they interact.

The problem may have begun all the way back at the selection and hiring process. The employee may not have been carefully screened and interviewed, or the requirements for the position may not have been clear at the time. The employee may not have had enough *prior experience and/or education* to be ready for the responsibilities of this position. The orientation and training provided may also have been inadequate.

Sometimes the manager's or organization's *expectations are vague or unrealistic.* Vagueness is especially a problem in a newly created position unless deliberate efforts are made to clarify expectations through initial discussion, written job descriptions, and frequent feedback. Other times, the expectations for a single person or person with limited preparation are far too high. A new graduate should not be placed in charge of a unit on the evening or night shift, yet this is still done when there are staff shortages (which is the worst time!). One nurse cannot provide good primary care for 10 or 15 patients on most acute care units, and yet this unrealistic standard is often used. The employee may also have had unrealistic expectations and may have tried to take on too many responsibilities too quickly.

A *lack of communication regarding priorities and expectations* may be another factor in poor performance. Leader-managers often do not realize that their attention to such details as a clean utility area or tidy patient units can inadvertently communicate to employees that appearance rather than substance is a priority. They may also assume that an experienced nurse needs little orientation to a new unit. Poor management can certainly be a factor in poor employee performance.

Poor work habits often contribute to poor performance. Time management skills may be undeveloped: procrastination and delay are a source of much poor performance. Other problems may include defensiveness, frequent absenteeism or lateness, frequent complaints (which may be legitimate), lack of confidence, or failure to take the initiative. Each one requires investigation to determine how the problem can be resolved.

Resolution of the Problem. The first step in resolving a problem of poor performance is to observe and objectively document the problem. Documentation should be of the behavior itself, not your interpretation. Remember also that your concern is with the employee's performance not personality traits that you might find unattractive. Behavior that actually disrupts team or department function, however, is a legitimate management concern.

Once the problem behavior is carefully documented, it is time for a counseling session with the employee. Both positive and negative feedback should be given, but the emphasis should be on the behavior that is cause for concern. The purpose of the session is to communicate the problem and to develop a plan for resolution of the problem. It is very important that the employee's point of view be heard and that the employee is treated with respect and concern. During the session, your support in resolving the problem should be offered, but the employee must also be clearly informed of the consequences of continued poor performance (no raise, no promotion, a cut in pay, a demotion, or termination of employment). Before the session is done, guidelines for re-evaluation should be agreed upon. Some of the actions to be taken before that time could be further orientation or education, reassignment of the employee, a change in either or both parties' expectations, and/or a change in the work environment. A transfer to another team or unit may be a solution, but too often it is used as an escape from confrontation, leaving the fundamental problem unresolved. The counseling session should, of course, be carefully and thoroughly documented.

Minor problems can usually be resolved through discussion between the first-line manager and the employee. However, any serious or long-standing difficulty should be discussed with your second-line manager or supervisor before you conduct a counseling session. For most first-line managers, especially new ones, it is a relief to have someone to turn to for guidance and support in handling these situations. Furthermore, upper-level management may have to make a decision regarding demotion or termination if the problem is sufficiently serious and cannot be resolved.

Every employee should be given at least a second and third opportunity to improve. This means that several recounseling sessions may be necessary and that your support and guidance may be needed for a long time. However, if all efforts to resolve the problem and improve performance have failed, demotion or termination of the employee, however difficult and painful it may be to all concerned, may be the only solution to the problem.

Formal Review by Peers

FUNDAMENTALS OF PEER REVIEW.   Peer review is the evaluation of an individual's practice by colleagues (peers) who have similar education, experience, and occupational status. Its purpose is to provide the individual with feedback from those who are best acquainted with the requirements and demands of that particular position. It is usually concerned with both process and outcomes of practice.

Whenever staff members meet to audit records or otherwise evaluate the quality of care they have given, they are actually engaging in a kind of peer review. However, formal peer review programs are often one of the last formal evaluation procedures to be implemented in a health care organization.

On an informal basis, professionals frequently observe and judge their colleagues' performance. But many people feel uncomfortable about telling others what they think of their performance, so the evaluations made are not shared with the individual practitioner as often as they could be unless a formal system is established.

Formal peer review begins with precisely defining the scope of professional practice and setting standards for quality care. Observations of performance are made by one or more peers, compared with previously set standards, and then shared with the person being reviewed. The reviewer is expected to look for those behaviors indicated by the standards and to avoid making judgments based on personal standards or subjective feelings.

Peer review reinforces good performance and stimulates health care professionals to scrutinize their own practice and continue their learning in order to maintain or improve their level of practice. Although it is often perceived as threatening when it is introduced, it can be a rewarding experience when it is conducted according to the guidelines for providing objective, nonthreatening, evaluative feedback.

There are a number of possible variations in the peer review process. For example, the observations may be shared only with the person being reviewed or with the person's supervisor or with a review committee. The evaluation report may be written by the reviewer or it may come from the review committee. However, the use of a committee defeats the purpose of peer review if the committee members are not truly peers of the individual being reviewed.

A COMPREHENSIVE PEER REVIEW SYSTEM. Peer review systems can consist of simple, informal feedback shared among colleagues, or they can be developed into comprehensive systems that are fully integrated into the formal evaluation structure of a health care organization. When a peer review system is fully integrated, the evaluative feedback from one's peers is joined with the performance appraisals done by the nurse manager and is used to determine pay raises and promotions for individual staff nurses. Using peer review in this way is a far more collegial style of formal evaluation that the hierarchical one generally used.

A comprehensive peer review system begins with the development of job descriptions (Fig. 21–1) and performance standards (Fig. 21–2) for each level within the nursing staff. You probably have noticed from comparing Figures 21–1 and 21–2 that the job description is a very general statement while the standards are quite specific behaviors that can be observed and recorded.

In some organizations, the standards may be considered the *minimum* qualifications for each level. In this case, additional activities and professional development are expected before promotion to the next level. Evidence of this development can include such things as documented participation in the quality assurance program, evaluating a new product or procedure, serving as a translator or disaster volunteer, or making postdischarge visits to patients from the unit.

In a truly participative environment, the work of developing these standards would be done by committees having representatives of different units and of each staff level, from the beginning staff nurse to representatives of top-level management. Writing useful job descriptions and objective, measurable standards of performance is an arduous but rewarding task. It requires a clarification and explication of the work nurses actually do that goes beyond our usual generalizations about what nursing is and what nurses do. Under effective group leadership and with strong administrative support for this process, it can be a challenging and stimulating experience. Without it, the committee work can be frustrating and discouraging when the group gets bogged down in details and disagreements.

Once the job descriptions and performance standards for each level have been developed and agreed upon, a procedure for their use must also be worked out. There are several ways in which this can be done. An evaluation form listing the performance standards can be completed by one or two colleagues selected by the individual staff member. The information from these forms is then used, along with the nurse manager's evaluation, to determine pay raises and promotions. In some organizations, the evaluation

Responsibility To Patient	CN I	CN II	CN III	CN IV
1. Plans care for duration of stay on clinical unit.	a. Family/social concerns are addressed in the assessment process, as evidenced by nursing care documentation. b. All admission documentation on assigned patients is recorded. c. History reflects information relevant to current hospitalization. d. Patient problem/outcome statements are current and/or designated as achieved. e. Patient teaching, transfer, and/or discharge preparation is documented.	a. through e. f. Uses nursing history for care planning as evidenced by auditing charts for integration of problem statements. g. Assesses supplies/equipment and has them readily available for patient use. h. Initiates discharge summary sheet prior to discharge.	a. through h. i. Identifies need for and/or initiates appropriate family/social referrals with documentation. j. Assesses and documents cultural differences, patient support systems, and expectations for hospitalization. k. Documents patient's response to teaching as identified in nursing care documentation.	a. through k. l. Collaborates with the Department of Patient Education in designing and revising patient teaching materials.
Responsibility to Peers				
1. Avails him/herself to coworkers at all times.	a. Notifies peers when required to leave the clinical area. b. Assumes responsibility for IVs and orders of LPN on assigned patients. c. Responds promptly to all emergency situations that arise in the district.	a. through c. d. Takes initiative to offer assistance to other nurses and with assigned patients. e. Serves as preceptor to students/orientees.	a. through e. f. Acts as senior resource coordinator in absence of nurse manager.	a. through f. g. Coordinates/teaches two programs in conjunction with the Department of Nursing Education annually. h. Conducts staff conferences to evaluate clinical competencies of personnel with documentation.

Figure 21–1. Sample job descriptions. (Adapted with permission from Baptist Hospital of Miami, Florida, Professional Nursing Advancement Programs.)

Clinical Nurse I (CN I)

The CN I supports the philosophy of primary nursing by planning and coordinating nursing care for a group of patients within his/her district. It is the CN I's responsibility to direct auxillary personnel for full implementation of the plan of care. The CN I supports the management of the unit and uses resource persons and/or materials when the need arises. He/she has satisfactorily mastered the basic skills required to work on the assigned unit. The CN I's scope of nursing practice is focused on his/her assigned group of patients and does not extend into the administrative aspects of the unit at large.

Clinical Nurse IV (CN IV)—Unit Clinician

The CN IV is an advanced clinical nurse who supports the practice of primary nursing on the unit, as well as hospital-wide. He/she is recognized within the specialty area, as well as throughout the hospital, as being proficient in the delivery of complex nursing care. The CN IV has mastered the many facets of nursing care required at the CN II and CN III levels. This qualification is validated through the acquisition of national certification in the appropriate specialty area.

The CN IV coordinates and directs emergency situations, seeks out learning opportunities for the unit staff, and serves as a resource for all aspects of nursing care delivery.

The CN IV collaborates closely with physicians on the unit for the implementation of the plan of care. This may be facilitated through assessing special equipment needs and planning multidisciplinary programs.

The CN IV works closely with the nurse manager in planning unit goals and objectives and unit specific orientation programs, as well as assisting with staff performance evaluations.

The CN IV acts as a liaison between his/her unit and the Departments of Nursing Education and Patient Education.

Figure 21–2. Sample performance standards. (Adapted with permission from Baptist Hospital of Miami, Florida, Professional Nursing Advancement Program.)

from one's peers is used for counseling purposes only and is not taken into consideration in determining pay raises or promotions, an approach that provides useful feedback but weakens the impact of peer review on the individual or on the system as a whole.

A third approach uses a peer review committee. This committee, composed of colleagues selected by the nursing staff, reviews the evaluation forms and makes its recommendations to the director of nursing (or vice-president for patient care services) who then makes the final decision regarding the appropriate rewards (raises, promotions, commendations) or punishment (demotion, transfer, termination of employment). It may surprise the reader who has not participated in such a peer review process that the recommendations of one's peers may be harsher than the recommendations made by management (Dison, 1986).

A comprehensive peer review system can be an effective mechanism for both evaluation and staff development. Done well, a comprehensive system can provide many opportunities for increased professionalism and learning and ensure appropriate rewards for high performance levels and professionalism on the job.

SUMMARY

Informal evaluation is a continuing process of seeking and providing feedback that should be an integral part of team function. The purposes of this type of evaluation are to provide recognition, increase self-awareness, clarify expectations, promote change and growth on the job, facilitate team function, and challenge staff members to improve their performances.

People need both positive and negative feedback. Constructive feedback is immediate, frequent, private, objective, based on observable behavior, appropriately communicated, nonthreatening, and includes suggestions for change. Seeking feedback is as important as providing feedback and uses the same guidelines. Responding to feedback is also important and may help to clarify both positive and negative feedback.

Formal evaluation procedures in organizations serve as a source of data, a demonstration of accountability, an identification of educational needs, and the basis for the reward system and for administrative intervention.

A performance appraisal begins with setting goals to be accomplished within a specified period of time. The degree to which these goals were met is evaluated at the end of this time, reasons for success or failure are discussed, and new goals are set. This process becomes more difficult when the staff member to be evaluated has been a marginal or poor performer. In this case, counseling sessions may be scheduled more frequently, more support and guidance from the manager is needed, and the consequences of failing to meet the objectives must be clearly spelled out.

Peer review is another potentially effective mechanism for formal evaluation and staff development. It is done by one's equals or peers rather than by one's manager and supports a collegial relationship between evaluator and evaluatee. Peer review should be based on clear and measurable written standards for a particular position. The result of peer review may be used for counseling purposes only or for determining appropriate rewards (pay raises, promotions, or commendations) or punishments (reassignment, demotion, termination of employment) within the organization.

REFERENCES*

Beer, M. (1981). Performance appraisal: Dilemmas and possibilities. *Organizational Dynamics*, (Winter 1981) 24.

*Del Bueno, D. (1977). Performance evaluation: When all is said and done, more is said than done. *Journal of Nursing Administration*, 7 (10).

Dison, C. (1986). Professional Nursing Advancement in the Work Place. Annual Nursing Research Conference, Sigma Theta Tau, Beta Tau Chapter, Miami, Florida.

Gellerman, S.W. & Hodgson, W.G. (1988). Gyanamid's new table on performance appraisal. *Harvard Business Review*, 88 (3), 36–41.

*Hansen, M.R. (1986). To-do lists for managers. *Supervisory Management*, 31 (5), 37–39.

*Hunter, W.L. (1988). Relieving the pain of performance appraisals. *Management World*, 17 (3), 7–9.

*Huntsman, A.J. (1987). A model for employee development. *Nursing Management*, 18 (2), 51–54.

Kron, T. (1981). *The Management of Patient Care: Putting Leadership Skills to Work*. Philadelphia: W.B. Saunders.

Lynch, E.A. (1978). Evaluation Principles. NLN Publication # 23-1721. New York: National League for Nursing.

Mager, R.F. & Pipe, P. (1970). *Analyzing Performance Problems*. Belmont, California: Lear Sigler/Fearon.

*Matejka, J.K., Ashworth, D.N. & Dodd-McCue, D. (1986). Discipline without guilt. *Supervisory Management*, 31 (5), 34–36.

*Pulick, M.A. (1986). What to do with incompetent employees. *Supervisory Management*, 31 (3), 10–16.

*References marked with an asterisk are suggested for further reading.

Chapter 22 ▬▬▬▬▬▬▬▬

OUTLINE ────────────────────────────────────

Accountability

Quality Assurance
  Purposes of Quality Assurance
  Comprehensive Evaluation
    Structure
    Process
    Outcome
  Evaluation Standards
  Procedures
    Record Audit
    Observation
    Interviewing

Quality Circles
Incentive Programs
Policies, Regulations, and Laws
Utilization Review

Implementing Quality-Assurance
  Programs
  A Participative Approach
  Example of a Chart Audit for Quality
    Assurance

Summary

LEARNING OBJECTIVES ──────────────────────────

Upon completion of this chapter, the reader will be able to:

▷ Discuss accountability from the perspective of the practicing health professional.

▷ Distinguish structure, process, and outcome in formal evaluation procedures.

▷ Describe the various approaches to quality assurance.

▷ Participate in the development and implementation of a comprehensive quality assurance program.

ACCOUNTABILITY AND QUALITY ASSURANCE*

To achieve excellence in health care, we must strive for both quality and productivity. The need to ensure that high standards of care are maintained has received increasing attention in health care, and the methods for evaluating and improving the quality of nursing care have become increasingly sophisticated. We can no longer call evaluation the "stepchild" of the nursing process, the forgotten final phase.

In this chapter, we will continue our consideration of formal evaluation procedures. Those discussed in the previous chapter were concerned mostly with evaluation of the individual employee. The formal evaluation procedures discussed in this chapter have a wider scope and broader purposes. They are used for evaluating and improving the quality of care given by particular units or departments and by the organization as a whole. Many of the procedures are applicable to other health care professions as well.

Involvement in quality-assurance programs begins at the staff nurse level and extends to the top of the management hierarchy. It is an increasingly important and interesting process, one that demands clarification and articulation of what nurses do and what impact their actions should have on the outcomes of care.

The chapter begins with a discussion of the concepts of accountability and quality assurance. Then we will look at the three aspects of care that should be evaluated, some specific procedures for carrying out the evaluation, and implementation of quality-assurance programs.

ACCOUNTABILITY

Accountability is one of the identifying characteristics of a profession. It is the ability and willingness to take responsibility for one's behavior while engaged in the practice of one's profession. The accountable person is expected to be able to distinguish between right and wrong and to think and act rationally. The educational and licensing processes required of professionals are meant to ensure that they possess the skills and understanding necessary to make correct decisions and to apply their unique knowledge appropriately.

If someone were to explain to you what the word *quality* means to him, he would probably say he expects a high-quality product to be the best it can

---

*Co-authored by Ruth M. Tappen, R.N., Ed.D. and Phyllis George, R.N., M.A.

be, that it will perform as well or better than other products of its kind, and that there will be some guarantee on the part of the person selling the product that it will not break down, or, if it does, that it will be fixed. Implied in those expectations are the concepts of excellence, conformance with a standard of performance, and reliability (Gross, 1986). People have similar expectations about quality in health care. The service provider is expected to perform in accordance with standard rules for providing the service, to be adequately trained, and to take due care to reduce the likelihood of mistakes.

The methods for evaluating the practice of professionals and assuring consumers of the quality of their services are generally known as the process of *quality assurance*. Health care institutions are developing quality-assurance programs as part of their routine operation, and nurses are very much involved in the processes of quality assurance.

There is an increasing demand for an accounting of the quality of the health care services being given. There are a number of reasons for this increased public concern. Three major factors are the increasing costs of providing services, the increasing sophistication of consumers, and the determination of consumers to hold health care professionals and institutions responsible for providing the best possible care. One approach is to take them to court when the outcomes of the services are less than satisfactory. Another is to demand stricter legal restrictions. A third is simply to take one's business elsewhere, that is, to seek a better source of care (an option available to many but not all consumers).

QUALITY ASSURANCE

A quality-assurance program is a system of procedures used to evaluate a service and to give feedback to the providers of the service so that it can be improved (Brown, 1983). Ideally, it involves the entire institution. It should be done in conjunction with other departments in the institution that are supportive or complementary to nursing services. Although the discussion here will focus primarily on evaluation of the nursing component, it actually occurs within the context of the entire organization. Whatever the evaluation of the nursing program reveals is, of course, relevant to the quality of the entire institution's services.

Comprehensive quality assurance programs are more than simply auditing records or evaluating policies and procedures and staffing patterns. They can be *retrospective* (evaluate past performance), *concurrent* (current performance), or *prospective* (future oriented) and should incorporate the problem-identification and problem-solving elements that are also part of a performance appraisal. The perspective is unit- and system-wide, not just at the level of the individual practitioner. For example, there may be a study to find out what the patient care outcomes are on a particular unit, whether care planning is occurring appropriately, whether nursing intervention includes patient and family teaching, and whether these activities are affecting the length of stay of the patients on the unit. Depending on the method used to gather the information, it may also be possible to identify the individual staff member's performance in relation to the rest of the unit and to compare the performance of the entire unit with an institutional standard (Gross, 1986).

Quality-assurance programs are also being asked to evaluate how long it took and how much it cost to deliver the service:

> Medicare's DRG system of reimbursing for hospital care is based on the development of a standard of what is "reasonable and necessary" to achieve the desired result. The care of a patient whose length of stay exceeds the DRG limit will not be reimbursed beyond the DRG limit. In home care, it may be possible for a patient to recover full use of the lower extremities following an auto accident, but if it takes a year of physical therapy at home, that is unlikely to be considered a reasonable and necessary investment of resources to be reimbursed by Medicare. (The patient and family may have a very different opinion on how reasonable and necessary an investment this is.)

Another reason that quality-assurance programs have become an integral part of the institution's functions is to identify the areas in which cost savings can occur without adversely affecting the processes and outcomes of care.

Purposes of Quality Assurance

Improving the efficiency and effectiveness of the services rendered are the fundamental purpose of the quality-assurance program. You can see that it is beneficial to have staff involved in the process, and that the nursing quality-assurance program needs to be compatible with the institution's overall quality assurance program. Quality assurance does not end with the collection of data and the determination that standards either are or are not being met. There is little point in this unless the information is used to identify and resolve the problems that keep care from happening as desired.

Building into the data collection process some means of identifying the nature and causes of a problem can be helpful in beginning to determine the solutions. There may be a need to improve the orientation of new employees, for example, or for an inservice program on a new procedure or on how to include the family in a patient assessment. There may be some problem with the environment (overcrowding or a poorly planned transport system, for example) or policies or procedures that interfere with the desired performance. It may be necessary to collect further information about why the desired performance is not occurring (Meisenheimer, 1983).

The quality-assurance program can also stimulate research efforts to learn more about the relationship between interventions and expected outcomes. Perhaps, for example, the standard procedures are no longer efficient and can be improved with the assistance of computers. Quality-assurance procedures may provide the documentation needed to demonstrate the need for new equipment or a new procedure.

The cost of the evaluation process must be considered in relationship to its outcomes. The time required of a number of people in the organization to engage in these investigations must be counted as part of the cost of providing that service. The time needed to develop tools, select methods, collect and interpret data, identify problems, and solve them must all be considered. Several questions should be asked about the quality-assurance program itself: "Is it accomplishing what we want it to accomplish? What are the outcomes? Are they the ones we want?" If subsequent data collection shows increased cost-effectiveness—for example, reductions in lengths of stay, improvements in patients' self-care ability after discharge, reduced wound infection rate—and these changes occur because problems previously identified have been addressed and improved procedures or outcomes of care have resulted, then it can be said that the quality assurance program itself is cost-effective.

Some methods may ultimately be too time-consuming for the results obtained. On the other hand, failure to invest adequate time in the process of quality assurance may result in great waste in the long run if the care is poor and/or costly in terms of resources.

Comprehensive Evaluation

Three different aspects of health care can be evaluated: the structure in which the care is given, the process of giving that care, and the outcome of that care. To be comprehensive, an evaluation program must include all three aspects of health care (Donabedian, 1969; Donabedian, 1977; Brook, 1980).

STRUCTURE. Structure refers to the *setting* in which the care is given and the *resources* that are available. It is the easiest of the three aspects to measure and yet is still overlooked in some evaluation procedures. The following is a list of some of the structural aspects of a health care organization that can be included in a formal evaluation:

1. **Facilities:** adequate space, comfort, convenience of layout, accessibility of support services, safety.
2. **Equipment:** adequate supply, state-of-the-art equipment, staff ability to use it.
3. **Staff:** credentials, absenteeism, turnover rate, staff-patient ratios.
4. **Finances:** salary levels, adequacy, sources.

None of these structural factors alone can guarantee that good care will be given, but they are factors that make good care more likely to occur. High nurse-patient ratios and low staff absenteeism rates, for example, are structural factors that are associated with quality nursing care (Chance, 1980).

The most common pitfall in evaluating structural factors, however, is to neglect the other two aspects (process and outcome). The following is an example that illustrates the problems that occur when evaluating only structure:

> One hospital measured the quality of nursing care given in its eight-bed critical care unit by comparing its staffing ratio with the standard ratio of one nurse to two patients. The inadequacy of this structural measure became apparent during a period when the unit had six (out of a total of eight) patients who each required the care of one nurse. Under the standard that was set, four nurses were on duty, which created a severe staff shortage because seven nurses were actually needed to provide adequate care.

PROCESS. Process refers to the *actual activities* carried out by caregivers. It includes psychosocial interventions, such as teaching and counseling, as well as physical care measures and can include leadership skills and writing care plans as well as actual patient/client interventions.

There are several ways to collect process data. The most direct is by observation of caregiving activities. Another is self-report of the caregiver. A third source of data is the chart or record that is kept, called an *audit*.

Whatever source of data is used, some set of objectives is needed as a standard against which to compare the activities. This set of objectives can be very specific, such as listing all the steps in a catheterization procedure, or it can be a very general list of objectives, such as "offer information on breastfeeding to all expectant parents" or "conduct weekly staff meetings." The example at the end of this chapter describes the collection of process data through use of a chart audit based on very general objectives.

OUTCOME.   Outcome refers to the *results* of the activities or process in which the health care givers have been involved. Outcome measures evaluate the effectiveness of these activities by answering such questions as "Did the patient recover? Is the family more independent now? Has team functioning improved?"

These questions are very general and reflect overall goals of the caregivers and the organizations in which they work. The outcome questions asked during an actual evaluation should be far more specific and should measure observable behavior such as the following:

Patient: Well hydrated.
          No elevated temperature.
          Absence of infections.
Family: Increased time between visits to the emergency room.
          Applied for food stamps.
Team: Decisions reached by consensus.
          Attendance at meetings by all team members.

Some of these outcomes—such as temperature, attendance, or time between visits—are easier to measure than other equally important outcomes, such as increased satisfaction or changes in attitude. While these less tangible outcomes cannot be measured as precisely, it is still important to include them because omitting them may imply that they are not important outcomes (Lynch, 1978).

A major problem in using outcome measures in evaluation is that they are influenced by many factors, not by just one factor or by just one person. Here is an example:

> The outcome of patient teaching done by a nurse on a home visit is affected by the patient's interest and ability to learn, the quality of the teaching materials, the presence or absence of family support, the information given by other care givers (which may conflict), and by the environment in which the teaching is done. If the teaching is successful, can the nurse be given full credit for the success? It it is not successful, who has failed?

It would be necessary to evaluate at least the process as well as the outcome to determine why an intervention such as patient teaching succeeds or fails. A comprehensive evaluation would include all three aspects: structure, process, and outcome.

Evaluation Standards

An evaluation standard is a criterion for judging the work of an individual, team, or organization. It supplies a basis for comparison. The following are examples of standards that have been mentioned before in this chapter:

Structural Standard: A ratio of one nurse to two patients in the critical care unit is maintained at all times.

Process Standard: Every expectant parent is offered information on breastfeeding.

Outcome Standard: All families who qualify will have applied for food stamps before discharge.

The major reason for setting standards is to increase objectivity by defining as clearly as possible what is acceptable and what is not acceptable. Without these standards, the judgments that take place in the evaluation process can be very variable, subjective, and susceptible to the whims and biases of the evaluator.

A second function of these standards is to communicate clearly to everyone involved with the organization (including staff, administrators, consumers, accreditors, and regulators), what level of service is expected in that organization. This can be done only if the standards are available to all these people. In the past, such standards have not been made available to the consumer, but there is some evidence to indicate that this will change in the future.

The standards and measurements used for evaluating performance may vary with the institution, the purpose of the evaluation, and the evaluator. They can rapidly become outdated and should be reviewed regularly. Outdated standards perpetuate the use of ineffective practices and make the evaluation results useless at best.

Procedures

The different procedures used in a quality-assurance program will depend on the purposes of the program. A variety of methods is usually employed in order to be comprehensive.

RECORD AUDIT. Record audits are one of the most commonly used procedures. Using standards developed by the nursing staff, patient records are evaluated to determine whether care plans are being developed for patients, if implementation is occurring as planned, and if the outcomes occur as expected. Audits may be done *concurrently*, while the patient is receiving care, or *retrospectively*, some time after the patient has been discharged (Phaneuf, 1976). Actually, record audits can provide only a limited amount of information, because they reveal only what has been *documented*, not necessarily what has occurred. Other methods are needed to supplement the record audit. Ideally, the record audit would take place *while* the care is being rendered rather than afterward, because it is impossible to develop solutions for a particular patient after he or she has been discharged.

In hospitals, retrospective audits are often done by people in the Medical Records Department who have ready access to patient records. They may also develop a coding and filing system that makes it easier to pull out records for the patients who are on a particular service unit, have a particular diagnosis, or were discharged within a certain time period.

The standards of care and expected outcomes for a nursing audit, however, should be prepared by the nursing staff. The data recorded by the auditors are then examined by a nursing audit committee or by the staff of a particular service area so that the information can be evaluated and the results can be communicated to the entire staff involved. Sometimes nurses themselves conduct the entire audit.

No matter who retrieves the information from the chart, the audit of the record is based on previously developed standards of care for particular health care problems. For example, the standards of care (evaluating process) for a diabetic patient at home might include the following:

1. Teach and observe patient drawing up insulin accurately and self-administering it correctly.
2. Teach patient importance of skin and foot care and what constitutes such care.
3. Teach patient to recognize and respond appropriately to episodes of hypoglycemia and hyperglycemia.

A concurrent or retrospective audit would look for documentation of these nursing behaviors in the chart.

Recorded outcomes are compared to the expected (standard) outcomes of care. The following list gives some examples of the outcomes of teaching a diabetic patient, which could be found in a chart audit:

1. Patient was observed on three occasions drawing up insulin accurately and injecting correctly, rotating sites.
2. Patient states importance of good foot and skin care, but refused to inspect feet daily, answered the door barefoot, and stated it was too much trouble to put shoes on all the time.
3. Patient states signs of hypoglycemia and hyperglycemia and appropriate intervention. Keeps orange juice on hand.

The outcomes listed above are typical in the sense that 100-percent compliance is not always achieved: while two standards were met, the third was only partially met.

One of the problems with the record audit, especially in the early stages of its use in quality assurance, is that it only gives information about what is actually documented in the record. For example, if the auditor is looking for evidence of patient teaching, the failure to find evidence of that care and its outcome *could* mean that what actually happened was not documented. If so, the audit may point up a need for staff inservice training about documentation.

Feedback to the staff about the results of an audit is a crucial part of the audit process because it reinforces both group and individual accountability for the care given, the outcomes achieved, and proper documentation of both of these. The results also give each care giver information that may be useful in self-evaluation. Information from audits can be used in appraising an employee's performance.

The effectiveness of inservice education programs can also be evaluated through a chart audit. For example, an audit of the self-care abilities of diabetic patients would look for an increase in the number of patients who are able to give their own insulin at discharge after an inservice program on diabetic teaching was given.

OBSERVATION. Observation, actually watching the care that is being given, is probably the most reliable, albeit the most difficult, way to evaluate care. You can observe that complete assessments are being done, that care is actually being given as planned and includes the patient's goals and expectations, that interventions are occurring as planned, and that desired outcomes are actually resulting. This method of gathering information about the quality of care being rendered by an individual practitioner or on a nursing unit is probably the most time-consuming and requires very clear categories or standards that should be tested for reliability (consistency among observers).

INTERVIEWING. Interviewing or distributing questionnaires to patients, families, and those rendering care can provide information about the care provided and the outcomes that result. This method is most helpful when used in conjunction with other methods, because the subjective elements of memory, anxiety, and individual interpretation are likely to enter into people's responses. The quality of the questionnaire is also an important factor in determining the value of the data.

QUALITY CIRCLES. The origin of quality circles is uncertain but they began to receive attention when Theory Z was introduced (Chapter 2). They are usually formed by administration in an attempt to involve workers in the identification of problems and their solutions. They are organized by work area, so that employees involved in the same tasks can work on solving mutual problems. Employees form a group that meets regularly to identify problems (or potential problems) and brainstorm about their origin, suggest solutions, and show how solution can contribute to the improvement of service. Quality circles have been introduced in human service settings with some degree of success (Wassaic Developmental Disabilities Office, 1986):

> In a state institution for the care of the developmentally disabled, the staff in one of the group homes identified the use of toothpaste tubes as presenting a problem. They saw that a lot of toothpaste was wasted because of residents' carelessness or lack of dexterity, and this caused problems in keeping bathrooms clean. Furthermore, the tube posed a danger at times because the cap of the toothpaste tube got lost, sometimes down the drain where it might clog the plumbing, sometimes on the floor where it might cause someone to fall. The further possibility existed that a resident might swallow the cap. The quality circle decided to do a study to determine whether toothpaste pumps might be more economical and reduce some of the inconveniences and dangers of the tubes. They very methodically tested the two containers and documented the number of "brushes" that could be obtained from each, then brainstormed all the advantages and disadvantages of the toothpaste pump and compared them to those of the tube. They were able to calculate the costs of the two containers and concluded that the pump was more cost-efficient and had fewer disadvantages than the tube. (The cost savings, when projected for the entire state, were quite impressive.)

Quality circles are perceived as "enriching the work life" of the employees (Wassaic Developmental Disabilities Office, 1986) because they involve them in the process of being accountable in a visible way for the quality of their care. Yet, the cost in time and commitment to the process on the part of both employees and their managers is considerable. Goddard (1988) claims that 75 percent of all quality circles fail because the work culture (environment) and management were not supportive. Resistance may come from first-line managers threatened by the involvement of staff in identifying and solving management problems. If not carefully administered, quality circles may be seen as still another task imposed with no more time in the day to get the additional work done. The manager who watches a group searching for a suitable problem for brainstorming may have qualms about the cost-effectiveness of the process even though it is enhancing the group process and the effectiveness of the work group. Some believe that the increase in self-esteem and job satisfaction that comes to the group that successfully masters a problem makes it worthwhile (Cornell, 1984), while others believe that it is worthwhile only if it results in demonstrable cost savings.

INCENTIVE PROGRAMS. In an attempt to upgrade the quality of care provided by employees, some organizations develop incentive programs that encourage and reward behaviors that are not normally expected of the average worker. The most common involves awards for the best cost-saving suggestion offered by a staff member or by an entire unit. More extensive incentive programs may provide a career ladder or reward system in a setting where the opportunities for such advancement or recognition are otherwise few or nonexistent. There may also be incentives for doing special projects that will contribute to the institution in some meaningful way, such as a patient or staff education program or a research project (Woldum et al., 1983). Incentive programs should not, however, become a substitute for adequate financial compensation.

An institution offering such incentives is perceived as being committed to improving the quality of care. Employees are expected to be serious about the quality of the care they provide because there are specific rewards for going beyond what is expected, pushing the boundaries of the ordinary to provide even extraordinary care.

Policies, Regulations, and Laws. Quality assurance is often mandated as part of a group of policies, regulations, or laws. The institution itself may, as a result of its quality-assurance investigations, develop certain rules or policies that are designed to ensure that uniform procedures are followed and that they assure the practice of certain interventions or reduce wasteful practices. These policies may include directions about who will be responsible for the distribution of drug education materials, for completing incident reports, or for initiating discharge planning.

The state or federal government also sets up laws and regulations containing specific standards which the institution must meet in order to be certified to provide care. The Health Care Finance Administration (HCFA), a division of the Social Security Administration responsible for the administration of the Medicare program, has developed certain regulations that define the circumstances under which care will or will not be reimbursed. The prospective payment system (described in Chapter 5) is one such set of regulations. Another set regulates the way home care services will be reimbursed. The institution or agency that does not follow the regulations will not be paid for its services. Most institutions cannot afford to operate that way for very long.

UTILIZATION REVIEW. Utilization review was originally mandated by the federal government as a quality-control measure tied to Medicare reimbursement. Basically, a utilization review asks the question, "Does the patient have to be here?" and then, if the physician has shown in the record why the patient does have to be here, the utilization review answers, "Okay, but only for this many days." Utilization review is done in any health care agency where care is reimbursed by Medicare, including hospitals, health departments, and home health care agencies.

The utilization review process has become increasingly restrictive over the years in order to ensure that reimbursements are not being made for trivial or unjustified expenses. For example, patients must have acceptable diagnoses and the length of their hospital stays must conform to the guidelines set for that particular diagnosis. The following is an example of how these guidelines operate:

> A 65-year-old man who is admitted to the hospital with a diagnosis of appendicitis and has an appendectomy would be expected to be discharged by the sixth postoperative day.
> Complications that require further treatment and a longer stay must be justified. For example, if the 65-year-old man could not be discharged by the sixth day, the physician would have to record the development and treatment of the new problem such as atelectasis, wound infection, thrombophlebitis, or urinary tract infection. It would not be acceptable simply to say that the patient cannot go home yet because he is too weak or there is nobody at home to take care of him.

The utilization review process has generated a new department within the hospital for documenting patients' legitimate needs for hospital care and treatment. The person who performs the mechanics of the utilization review is paid by federal money if the hospital is in compliance with the regulations. If not, that money goes to pay the regional surveyor, who not only does surveillance but also assists organizations in setting up their own procedures according to guidelines. The findings are reviewed on a regular basis by a committee of physicians, nurses, and other care givers called the Professional Review Organization (known as PROs). This review provides an opportunity for health care professionals to evaluate care not only for conformity to utilization review standards but also to acceptable practice standards.

Health care organizations that do not do utilization review or do it poorly risk losing reimbursement (payments) for the care they give to Medicare patients. By requiring hospitals to set standards to receive reimbursement, utilization review is a potential force for the improvement of care.

In most cases, these regulations or laws are set up to ensure a minimum standard of care that can be expected by consumers. Home care has recently been identified by some consumer advocate groups as one area where insufficient guarantees exist to protect the consumer (ABA report, 1986; AARP, 1986). The response has been to introduce legislation controlling the home health care industry (Home Health Journal).

IMPLEMENTING QUALITY-ASSURANCE PROGRAMS ⎯⎯⎯

A Participative Approach

Quality-assurance programs need to include consideration of those being evaluated as well as those receiving the care. People often feel uncomfortable when they know that someone else is going to be looking at their work, judging it for quality and completeness, and making these findings known publicly. This is why it is a good idea to involve these same people in the development of the process, from planning to the evaluation of the information collected. There is likely to be more investment in the quality-assurance program when staff sees the results—evidence of true excellence in care or the identification of problems that interfere with providing quality care. Staff can also provide insight into the problems they encounter in providing care and will be more willing to participate in the problem-solving process when they are part of a joint effort.

Many institutions implement their quality-assurance program through a quality-assurance committee. For nursing, this may consist of nurse managers, clinical specialists, and staff representatives. For the entire institution, the committee will have representation from all departments, so that the quality of the services provided by the institution as a whole may be evaluated in an integrated and coordinated fashion. The methods used and information gathered by the nursing quality-assurance committee contribute to the information-gathering system developed by the institution-wide committee. Involvement of employees from all departments in the institution's quality-assurance program can be very useful in giving them a real sense of the importance of the department's contribution to the overall mission of the institution.

Example of a Chart Audit for Quality Assurance

A typical chart audit routine is illustrated in the following example:

A large home health agency has four district offices located within the county it serves. The quality-assurance committee of this agency has developed a set of general standards for home health care record review that can be applied to the record of any of the agency's clients, whether the client is in the terminal stages of AIDS, needs instruction in the care of a new colostomy, or is receiving rehabilitative therapy to improve ambulation after a stroke.

Once a month, representatives from each of the four district offices bring three randomly selected records from his or her current caseload for audit. At the meeting, the records are exchanged and audited by the representatives from the other district offices. Each record is audited according to the system developed by the agency's quality assurance committee. This particular system consists of 44 separate standards divided into seven categories designed to reflect the functions of the home health nurse:

1. Assessment of the client.
2. Assessment of those participating in care.
3. Planning and execution of nursing procedures and techniques.
4. Execution of physician's orders.
5. Observation of client symptoms and responses.
6. Management and coordination of total plan of care.
7. Reporting and recording. (Dutchess County Health Department, n.d.).

Examples of the individual standards within some of these categories are given in Figure 22–1.

Fully documented compliance with each individual standard is given a score of 7, partial evidence of compliance is given a score of 3, and no evidence of compliance is scored 0. The total score is meant to reflect the level of service as defined by this agency and its quality-assurance committee from *excellent*, for a score over 210, to *unsafe*, for a score under 63. Reviewers are also asked to comment on the results of the audit and make

Category: Assessment of those participating in care
  Examples:
    Care procedures are taught to patient, family, and others participating in his or her care.
    Ability and readiness of those to be taught was taken into account.
    Results of initial and additional teaching are assessed with appropriate follow-up.

Category: Planning and execution of nursing procedures and techniques
  Examples:
    The patient's patterns of sleep and rest are taken into account when planning his or her care.
    Patient has been instructed on what to do in an emergency situation.
    Efforts are made to reconcile actual physical activity and independence in self-care with
      clinically estimated tolerance level.

Category: Reporting and recording
  Examples:
    Results and evaluation thereof are recorded for every nursing procedure.
    Significant clinical observations are reported to the appropriate professional.
    Flow sheets are complete.

Figure 22–1. Sample standards for a home health chart audit.

recommendations for improvements in policies, procedures, practices, and the audit form itself.

This audit procedure is designed to provide objective feedback to the home health agency nurses and their supervisors. The feedback concerns both the individual practitioner and the care given by the agency as a whole. Both strengths and deficiencies are discussed and recorded. The process has resulted in the identification of some problems that have been resolved by the agency. For example, they found that some parts of the record could be improved to more readily and more accurately report some of the care given, including patient teaching, emotional support, and efforts to involve the client and family in the care. Improvements in the record followed directly from recommendations made by the quality-assurance committee.

You can see from this example that the results of a quality-assurance evaluation procedure such as a chart audit can and do lead directly to recommendations for change and improvement in the organization's procedures. Future audits should then evaluate the extent to which the changes made have resulted in improved performance.

The involvement of both staff and management was also evident in the example. For quality-assurance programs to have maximum impact, they should have the wholehearted support of management and should involve as many staff nurses as possible. Ideally, all staff members should have input into both the setting of the standards and the use of the standards in implementing the quality-assurance program.

SUMMARY

Quality assurance is a broadly defined means of acknowledging the responsibility of the institution and the professional to be accountable for the care provided. Comprehensive quality assurance includes evaluation of structure, process, and outcome based upon clearly written standards. Its purpose is to focus on specific problems that interfere with the provision of quality care, and develop solutions that allow more efficient procedures and desired outcomes to occur.

Quality assurance is important as a means of ensuring consumers of a minimum standard of care that can be expected, as a means of controlling costs, as a means of maintaining and even improving the standard of professionalism, and as a necessary means of monitoring providers' practice to minimize the risk of malpractice.

Quality assurance is also important to the individual practitioner as a means of developing skills and growing in stature in the practice of the profession. It helps to identify strengths and weaknesses and can provide a supportive milieu for improving skills and recognizing high-quality performance. It is integral to professional practice.

Attempts to ensure quality of care and even promote higher standards of care can be seen in such forms as institutional policies and procedures, government regulations and laws, quality circles, and professional incentive programs. Implementation of quality-assurance programs is usually done through quality-assurance committees, which should represent all of the organization's health care professionals and would, ideally, involve every staff members in some way in the process.

REFERENCES*

ABA Report. (1986). Homecare Quality Assurance—the "Black Box" Home Health Journal, 7 (9), 1ff.

AARP (1986). Seriously deficient claims report. Home Health Journal, 7 (9), 3.

*Beyers, M. (1986). Cost and quality: Balancing the issues through management. Journal of Nursing Quality Assurance, 1 (1), 47–54.

Brook, R.H., Davis, A.R. & Kamberg, C. (1980). Selected reflections on quality of medical care evaluations in the 1980s. Nursing Research, 29 (2), 127.

Brown, B.J. (1983). From the editor. Nursing Administration Quarterly, 7 (3), viii–ix.

*Chance, K.S. (1980). The quest for quality: an exploration of attempts to define and measure quality nursing care. Image, 12 (2), 41.

Cornell, L. (1984). Quality circles: A new cure for hospital dysfunction? Hospitals and Health Services Administration, 29, 88–93.

*Crisham, P. (1986). Ethics, economics, and quality. Journal of Nursing Quality Assurance, 1 (1), 26–35.

*Curtis, B.J. & Simpson, L.J. (1985). Auditing: A method for evaluating quality of care. Journal of Nursing Administration, 15 (10), 14–21.

Donabedian, A. (1969). A guide to medical care administration. vol II. Medical Care Appraisal—Quality and Utilization. New York: American Public Health Association.

Donabedian, A. (1977). Evaluating the quality of medical care. Milbank Memorial Fund Quarterly, 44 (part 2), 166.

Dutchess County Health Department (n.d.). Nursing audit chart review schedule. Poughkeepsie, New York: Nursing Division, Dutchess County Health Department.

Edwardson, S.R. & Anderson, D.I. (1978). Hospital nurses' valuation of quality assurance. Journal of Nursing Administration, 8 (7,8), 33–39.

*Goddard, R.W. (1988). Gathering a great team. Management World, 17 (4), 20–23.

*Greaves, P.E. & Sloquist, R.S. (1983). Impact evaluation: A competency-based approach. Nursing Administration Quarterly, 7 (3), 81–86.

Gross, K.F. (1986). A quality and cost control model for managing nursing utilization. Journal of Nursing Quality Assurance, 1 (1), 36–46.

Larson, E.L. & Peters, D.A. (1986). Integrating cost analyses in quality assurance. Journal of Nursing Quality Assurance, 1 (1), 1–7.

Lewis, E.M., Nitta, D.E., Biczi, T. & Robinson, M. (1986). Downsizing: Measuring its effects on quality of care. Journal of Nursing Quality Assurance, 1 (1), 17–25.

*Lillesand, K.M. & Korff, S. (1983). Nursing process evaluation: A quality assurance tool. Nursing Administration Quarterly, 7 (3), 9–14.

Lynch, E.A. (1978). Evaluation: principles and processes. NLN Publication, No. 23-1721, 32 pp.

Maciorowski, L., Larson, E. & Keane, A. (1985). Quality assurance: Evaluate thyself. Journal of Nursing Administration, 15 (6), 38–42.

Meisenheimer, C.G. (1983). Incorporating JCAH standards into a quality assurance program. *Nursing Administration Quarterly, 7* (3), 1–8.

Pelle, D. (1986). An integrative approach to quality assurance. *Journal of Nursing Quality Assurance, 1* (1), 8–16.

Phaneuf, M. (1976). *The Nursing Audit: Self-Regulation in Nursing Practice.* New York: Appleton-Century-Crofts.

"Quality Circles in Human Services" (1986) presented by Wassaic Developmental Disabilities Services Office. August 6.

"Reaction–NAHC Counters ABA" *Home Health Journal, 7* (9), 1ff.

"Roybal Introduces Major QA Bill" *Home Health Journal, 7* (9), 5.

Wilson, C.K. (1986). Strategies for monitoring the cost and quality of care. *Journal of Nursing Quality Assurance, 1* (1) 55–65.

*Woldum, K.M., Halsey, S., Murray, M. & Solovieff, N. (1983). The professional development program: an alternative to clinical ladders. *Nursing Administration Quarterly, 7* (3), 87–93.

*References marked with an asterisk are suggested for further reading.

Chapter 23

STAFF DEVELOPMENT

Chapter 23

OUTLINE

A Climate for Growth
Encourage Critical Thinking
Provide Educational Opportunities
Encourage New Ideas
Involve Staff in Decision Making
Reward Professional Growth

Prevention of Reality Shock and Burn-out
Reality Shock
The Honeymoon
The Conflicts

Additional Pressures on the New Graduate
Unsuccessful Coping Efforts
Resolving the Conflicts — Leader-Manager Actions
New Graduate Actions
Burn-out
Factors Contributing to Burn-out
Counteracting Burn-out
Impaired-Nurse Programs

Summary

LEARNING OBJECTIVES

Upon completion of this chapter, the reader will be able to:

▷ Describe the factors that promote staff growth and development.

▷ Contribute to staff development in the role of leader-manager.

▷ Recognize reality shock and take steps to prevent and/or counteract it.

▷ Recognize staff burn-out and impairment and take steps to prevent and/or counteract it.

STAFF DEVELOPMENT

Staff development is an important component of effective management. It is an area that is neglected to a surprising extent in some health care organizations because of budget restraints and priorities placed on other areas. It is neglected by some administrators who would never think to allow peeling paint or poorly maintained equipment and yet allow their most costly and valuable resource, the staff, to be unmaintained and unrefreshed by new ideas or new challenges.

Much of the responsibility for promoting staff development rests with upper-level management people who have the authority and available resources to do such things as plan seminars, conduct organization-wide workshops, institute education policies, develop clinical ladders for promotions, and encourage organization-wide growth and change. However, there is still quite a lot that the first-line nurse manager can do at the team or department level to foster staff development. We will concentrate on these possibilities in this chapter. Two aspects of staff development are considered: the creation of an environment that fosters professional growth and learning and the prevention of such negative outcomes as reality shock and burn-out. Staff development is a long-term building strategy (Bernhard & Ingals, 1988). Training, on the other hand, is shorter term and focused on a more specific need. Sharing new knowledge through the format of information conferences is considered in the next chapter.

A CLIMATE FOR GROWTH

The difference between a climate that encourages staff development and one that does not can be quite subtle. In fact, many people are only partly aware, if at all, of whether they work in an environment that fosters professional growth and learning or not. Yet the effect on the quality of the work done is pervasive, and it is an important factor in distinguishing the merely good health care facility from the excellent one.

Some of the ways in which the leader-manager can develop and support a climate of professional growth are to encourage critical thinking, provide opportunities for educational programs, encourage new ideas and projects, involve staff in decision making, and reward those who take advantage of these opportunities. We will briefly consider examples of each positive approach and then examine prevention of some serious problems that can occur within nursing staff: reality shock, burn-out, and impairment of function.

Encourage Critical Thinking

If you ever find yourself or other staff saying to a colleague something like, "Don't ask me why, just go ahead and do it," you need to evaluate carefully the type of climate in which your staff is functioning. An inquisitive frame of mind is relatively easy to suppress in a work environment. Staff members quickly perceive a team leader's or manager's tendency to become impatient or defensive when too many questions are raised. Their response will be simply to give up asking these questions.

On the other hand, if you encourage the critical thinker and act as a role model who adopts a questioning attitude, you can encourage others to do the same. Like motivation in general, interest and curiosity are intrinsic; the leader-manager's responsibility is to stimulate and reward their occurrence.

Provide Educational Opportunities

In most organizations, first-line managers do not have discretionary funds that can be allocated for educational purposes. However, they can usually support a staff member's request for educational leave or for financial support and often have a small budgeted amount that can be used for seminars or workshops.

Perhaps even more important, team leaders and first-line managers can either make it easy or difficult for staff members to further their education. They can make it easier by being flexible in scheduling and allowing an occasional day off to finish a paper or study for an exam. They can be generally encouraging and include the pursuit of further education in performance appraisal reports. Or, they can make things difficult for the staff member who is trying to balance work, home, and school responsibilities. Unsupportive supervisors have even attacked staff members who pursue further education, criticizing every minor error and blocking their advancement. Obviously, such behavior should be dealt with quickly by upper-level management.

Encourage New Ideas

Every move up the professional ladder should bring new challenges and job enrichment (Roedel & Nystrom 1987). The leader-manager can do a great deal to foster an environment in which every staff member is challenged and rewarded for meeting these challenges. Informal or formal brainstorming, nominal group technique, synectics, problem solving conferences, and problem discussions all encourage the generation of new ideas. New ideas need to be nurtured; the leader-manager can ensure that they at least get a fair amount of consideration and that many are implemented. The success of one new idea can have a synergistic effect, encouraging the generation and testing of many more ideas. In addition, the leader-manager can encourage staff to develop and implement new projects to improve or expand patient services or unit management. Job enhancement in general makes work more satisfying (Hurston, 1988).

Involve Staff in Decision Making

Staff development has two major facets: a focus on enhancing leadership and a focus on improving patient care. Although staff involvement in decision making is primarily aimed at enhancing each member's leadership capability, its ultimate result should be a better functioning unit that provides better patient care. The benefits of participative leadership and management have been discussed in great detail earlier.

Reward Professional Growth

Both tangible and intangible rewards for professional growth should be considered. Specific mention of active involvement in continuing education should be a part of every professional employee's performance appraisal. Contributions to the smooth functioning of the unit or to improved patient care should also be rewarded. Some organizations have special incentive programs in which they reward innovative or cost-saving suggestions.

The intangible rewards of positive feedback and widespread recognition of a staff member's contribution are very effective in encouraging pursuit of professional growth. These pursuits also have their own intrinsic rewards of course, but they are not under the direct influence of the leader-manager (Knowles, 1984).

PREVENTION OF REALITY SHOCK AND BURN-OUT _____

Reality shock and burn-out are related conflicts experienced by a number of people in helping professions. They severely deplete motivation and inhibit staff development. Both of these terms refer to conflicts between a person's professional ideals and the realities of the work situation. Reality shock refers specifically to the occurrence of this conflict when nurses first leave school (Kramer, 1974, 1981; Kramer & Schmalenberg, 1977; Schmalenberg & Kramer, 1979). Burn-out is a broader term describing the way this conflict is experienced by people at any time in any of the human service professions who become chronically disillusioned and apathetic about their work (Edelwich & Brodsky, 1980; Freudenberger, 1974).

Reality Shock

Reality shock occurs when the new graduate suddenly becomes aware of the discrepancy between the real world and the ideals of the nursing profession. The shock stems from the realization that the way the graduate was taught to do things in school and believes is the right way to do things is not necessarily the way things are actually done on the job.

THE HONEYMOON.   The first few weeks on a new job are the honeymoon phase. During the honeymoon phase, the new employee is excited and enthusiastic about the new position and everything seems rosy. Coworkers usually go out of their way to make the new person feel welcome and overlook any problems that arise.

Honeymoons do not last forever. The new graduate is soon expected to behave just like everyone else and discovers that expectations for a professional employed in an organization are quite different than expectations for a student in school. Those behaviors that brought rewards in school are not necessarily valued by the organization. In fact, some of them are criticized. The new graduate who is not prepared for this change feels confused, angry, disillusioned, and shocked. The tension and stress of the situation can become almost unbearable if not resolved.

THE CONFLICTS.   What are these differences in expectations? Kramer, who has studied reality shock for many years, found some substantial differences between organizational and professional goals and expectations. These discrepancies include a mechanistic versus holistic organization, the priority of efficiency over effectiveness, the way expectations are communicated, and the way feedback is given.

Ideally, health care should be comprehensive. Not only should it meet all of the patient's needs, but it should be delivered in a way that considers the client as a whole person, as a member of a particular family that has certain unique characteristics and needs, and as a member of a particular community. Most health care professionals, however, are not employed to provide comprehensive, holistic care. Instead, they are asked to give medications, to provide counseling, to make home visits, or to prepare someone for surgery, but rarely to do all these things. These tasks are divided among different people, each a specialist, for the sake of efficiency rather than continuity or effectiveness.

When efficiency is the goal, the speed and amount of work done is rewarded rather than the quality of the work. This also creates a conflict for the new graduate who was allowed to take as much time as needed to provide good care while in school.

Expectations are communicated in different ways. In school, an effort is made to provide explicit directions so that students know what they are expected to accomplish. In many work settings, however, instructions are brief and many expectations are left unspoken. New graduates who are not aware of these unspoken expectations (part of the informal level of operations) may find that they have unknowingly left tasks undone or are considered inept by co-workers who believe they know the "right" way to do things. The following is an example:

> A new graduate was assigned to give medications to all the patients cared for by the team. Because this was a fairly light assignment, the graduate spent some time looking up the medications and explaining their actions to the patients receiving them. The graduate also straightened up the medicine room and filled out the order forms, which the graduate thought would please the task-oriented team leader.
>
> At the end of the day, the graduate reported these activities with some satisfaction to the team leader. The graduate expected the team leader to be pleased with the way the time had been used. Instead, the team leader looked annoyed and told the graduate that whoever passes meds always does the blood pressures too and that the other nurse on the team who had a heavier assignment had to do them. Also, since supplies were always ordered on Fridays for the weekend, it would have to be done again tomorrow so the graduate had, in fact, wasted time.

If this new graduate had been more aware of the existence of the informal level of operations, the graduate would have discussed the plans with the team leader earlier in the day. Of course, an effective leader would have communicated the expectations much more clearly, but many people in leadership positions are not particularly effective leaders.

The example of the new graduate also illustrates some differences in the way feedback is given. The feedback given was all negative and it was given too late. Other common problems are messages that are too vague or global such as, "You're doing fine"; very indirect messages such as grumbling under the breath or redoing something that has just been done; or a complete lack of feedback until something goes wrong.

ADDITIONAL PRESSURES ON THE NEW GRADUATE. The first job a person takes after finishing school is often thought of as a proving-ground for testing newly gained knowledge and skills. People often set up mental tests for themselves that they believe must be passed before they can be confident of their ability to function. Passing these mental tests also confirms achievement of identity as a practitioner rather than a student.

It is important to take a positive, assertive approach to your abilities at this time and to avoid minimizing them. For example, when you need to ask for assistance or information, you can make a point of first telling your co-worker what you do know and then indicate where you need help rather than presenting yourself as a helpless person or saying you have never done something before, which is damaging to your confidence.

A feeling of uncertainty about your competency can also come from the ambiguities of a situation. Many clinical situations demand professional judgment because there is no single right way to handle them. It also has been suggested that nurses are socialized into being very concerned about not making a mistake or harming the patient rather than into feeling confident of their abilities.

At the same time the new graduates are undergoing testing by their co-workers. The co-workers are also interested in finding out whether the new graduates can handle the job. This testing is somewhat like hazing of freshmen entering high school or college. The new graduate is entering a new group, and the group will decide whether to accept this new member. This testing is usually reasonable, but sometimes new graduates will be given tasks they are not ready to handle. If this happens, Kramer (1981) recommends that you refuse to take the test rather than fail it. Another opportunity for proving yourself will soon come along.

The discrepancies in role expectations and the need for a feeling of competency are the top two concerns of new graduates, according to most surveys. Next in order of concern are the system that must be dealt with, self-concept, and the type of feedback that is given (or not given). Some other problems (which have already been discussed), such as dealing with resistant staff members, cultural differences, and age differences, are of concern here as well. Before considering positive ways to resolve these problems, we will look at some less successful ways of coping with these problems.

UNSUCCESSFUL COPING EFFORTS. When faced with reality shock, some new graduates give up their professional goals and ideals completely, adopting the organization's operative goals as their own. By doing this, they eliminate their conflict but become less effective caregivers. This coping strategy results in putting the needs of the organization before your own needs or the needs of the client and reinforces operative goals that might better be challenged and changed.

Other people give up their professional ideals but do not adopt any others to replace them. This concession has a deadening effect: they become automatons believing in nothing relating to their work except in doing what is necessary to earn a day's pay.

Of those who do not give up their professional goals and ideals, many try to find an organization that will support them. Some will succeed and thrive in these organizations, but others will find themselves switching from one job to another until they find what they seek. Unfortunately, a significant percentage escape these conflicts by leaving their jobs and not returning to their profession.

RESOLVING THE CONFLICTS—LEADER-MANAGER ACTIONS. Some of the shock experienced by the graduate can be prevented. Prevention of reality shock should begin with the interview process. An honest description of the organization's work environment and employee policies is the first step in preparing the new employee. This is also important during orientation. Together, the interview and orientation make a lasting impression (George, 1986) that is difficult to reverse.

Once the classroom portion of orientation is done, follow-ups over the next 3 months should be at frequent intervals and then continue but gradually decrease over the next year. Regular meetings with groups of new staff are helpful because a sharing of concerns prevents the feeling that one is alone in having difficulty adjusting. Probably the worst way to handle new employees, especially new graduates, is to let them "sink or swim."

There are several other things that the leader-manager can do to ease the transition from school to work. First, of course, you must recognize that these conflicts do occur and be willing to listen to the person's criticisms or suggestions for change without becoming defensive. Second, it may be possible to implement some of these suggestions. Third, you need to adjust your high expectations of staff members somewhat to allow time for adjustment. This should not create any difficulty with other staff members if they understand what is being done and had been accorded the same kind of consideration when they were new to the organization. Finally, the new employee needs more frequent informal feedback and closer supervision until he or she is functioning well within the new environment. Assigning new staff members to work with experienced staff in a preceptor-preceptee relationship is an effective way of facilitating adjustment and providing extra feedback. It is important, however, to select staff who provide excellent role models, who function well within the organization, and who have maintained their professional ideals.

NEW GRADUATE ACTIONS. The new graduate who understands the difference between the formal and informal levels of operation in an organization, knows how to identify its operative goals, and recognizes the games that organizations play will not be as shocked as the naïve individual.

Experience also helps. Opportunities to challenge your competence and develop your identity as a professional can begin in school. Success in meeting these challenges can immunize you against the loss of confidence that accompanies reality shock.

When you begin a new job, it is important to learn as much as you can about the organization's formal and informal levels and operative goals. This not only saves you from some nasty surprises but also gives you some ideas about how to work within the system and how to make the system work for you. The following is an example of how one team leader figured out how to use the system:

> A new team leader realized that patient care conferences were never held in the home health agency but were needed to improve the care given. When the team leader

approached team members (who were all long-term employees of the agency) about this, they expressed no interest in having conferences. The supervisor's response was also negative.

The agency was an extremely rigid and bureaucratic one that allowed team leaders very little authority, so the team leader could not begin the conferences without the supervisor's approval. (The team members would not attend the meetings unless they were approved anyway.) However, the agency did have strong bias in favor of education, held many classes for its employees, and rewarded employees for accumulating large numbers of education credits or contact hours.

The new team leader took advantage of the value placed on education. The team leader adopted the patient care conference format to focus on the teaching and learning aspects of it and presented the idea to the supervisor as twice-weekly seminars for staff. The supervisor recognized the seminars' similarity to patient care conferences but felt a need to approve the plan because of the strong emphasis on education in the agency. The staff agreed to attend because it was a good way to accumulate continuing education credits on work time. The patient care conference/seminars became an accepted part of the team's operation, and the team leader was later praised for interest in meeting the educational needs of the team.

The team leader in the example did not abandon or even compromise the goal to improve care but adapted it to the realities of the work situation.

Keep in mind that a great deal of energy goes into learning a new job. Attempting to implement change also takes time and energy on your part so you need to make some choices regarding any changes and improvements that you see are needed. It is also a good idea to make a list of these things so that you do not forget them later when you have become socialized into the system.

Three other actions can help to reduce the shock effects of these conflicts. The first is to *seek feedback* often and persistently. This tactic not only provides you with needed information but also pushes the people you work with to be more specific about their expectations of you. A second is to *use confronting communications* to deal with the problems that can arise with coworkers. The third action is at least as important and helpful: *develop a support network* for yourself. Identifying colleagues who have held onto their professional goals and sharing with them not only your problems but the work of improving the organization is a very helpful cushion against reality shock. The mutual support of colleagues reinforces your self-confidence if it wavers. Their praise of your work can keep you going while rewards from the organization are meager. A support network is a source of strength when resisting pressure to give up professional ideals and a source of power when attempting to bring about change. Work on developing your potential in each of the components of effective leadership can also help to prevent the problems of reality shock.

Reality shock may occur whenever you begin a new position, even if you are not a new graduate (see Research Example 1–1). Because reality shock and burn-out are related conflicts, you may also find some of the suggestions for counteracting burn-out helpful in coping with reality shock.

Burn-out

The term *burn-out* refers to a state of exhaustion, a depletion of energies that seems to be a particular problem for people in helping professions. It begins with frustration, disillusionment, or doubts about your work and leads to the loss of ideals, purpose, and energy.

The burned-out individual may feel apathetic, alienated, or exhausted. Stress-related physical symptoms such as headaches, backaches, indigestion, and lowered resistance to infection may be experienced. Family difficulties and social problems may also occur. Like reality shock, the cost of burn-out to individuals, their families, employing organizations, and clients is enormous.

People who enter helping professions usually do so with a lot of enthusiasm and idealism. They want to help people and expect that their interventions will have a great deal of impact. The system needs changing, and they frequently intend to do something about it. Support and success can nourish their high hopes. But nursing environments often lack the support and nurturing of creativity that people in the helping professions need (Moch & Diemert, 1987), and when they meet continuous resistance and disinterest, many begin to burn out.

FACTORS CONTRIBUTING TO BURN-OUT. Burn-out is the result of the negative interaction between the expectations and behavior of the health care professional and the systems with which the professional is working. The following is a list of the factors most commonly involved in this negative interaction.

Low Pay. In comparison with professionals in other fields, many health care professionals are poorly paid for the amount of education they have and the degree of responsibility they are given. In some communities, nurses are still paid less than sanitation workers or grocery store cashiers.

Long Hours. Not only is the work demanding, but many find themselves working well beyond the typical 40-hour week. For example, nurses are frequently asked to work rotating shifts or 16-hour days, both of which are a considerable stress.

Too Much Paper Work. People who enter helping professions derive their satisfaction from interacting with people, not with paper. When much of their time is spent on filling out forms, charts, and reports, they become frustrated by the loss of time that could be spent with their clients.

Lack of Success with Clients. When you commit yourself to helping people, their failure to recover can be a personal disappointment. Health care professionals find that the people they counsel often return to destructive behavior and that many they care for do not recover but die. This happens to intensive care nurses, oncology unit staff, counselors, rehabilitation workers, hospice nurses, and many others. The continual loss of patients alone can result in burn-out.

Lack of Appreciation and Understanding. Getting intangible rewards (that psychological paycheck) meets an important need for esteem and recognition. Patients or clients do express their appreciation many times, but supervisors frequently fail to comment favorably on a job well done. Also, the public does not fully understand what many nurses do and does not appreciate how demanding some of these jobs are. Many people still think of nurses as bedpan carriers and doctors' helpers until they require the services of a nurse and find out what nurses really do.

Lack of Support. Many health care professionals find themselves working in organizations that do not support their efforts to improve the quality of the services offered. Continually fighting for the right to practice in a professional manner has left many burned out.

Unresponsiveness to Client Needs. The health care system's lack of responsiveness to clients needs (impersonal, fragmented care; restrictive eligibility requirements; lack of respect for the dignity of the individual) conflicts with the professional ideals of a helping person. Finding out that the operative goals of a health care organization emphasize efficiency and monetary gain over the needs of the people served leads to much frustration and disillusionment.

Powerlessness. A feeling of powerlessness can contribute to burn-out. This stems from a failure to recognize and use the potential power available to any large group that performs a vital function. Many people in the helping professions feel it inappropriate to use their power and react with dismay when they find themselves the target of a power play.

Discrimination. Although progress has been made in reducing discrimination, you will still find more women and minorities in the lower-status, lower-paid positions in health care. Most physicians are still men; most nurses are still women and they still find themselves resisting physician dominance and the myths that women and nurses are weaker, less dependable, or less intelligent than men. This problem is quite evident in the health care field but not unique to it.

Inadequate Advancement Opportunities. People at the lower levels in the helping professions are often discouraged by the educational prerequisites for moving up the career ladder. Those who are higher up on the ladder find that further advancement means moving into management or teaching and further away from the people they want to help. This frustration also is not unique to the helping professions.

COUNTERACTING BURN-OUT. It is difficult to devote much energy to counteracting burn-out when your energies are seriously depleted. For this reason, it is a good idea to intervene for yourself and others before burn-out becomes too severe.

Some of the suggestions given previously for dealing with reality shock are also helpful in counteracting burn-out. The suggestions offered here focus on long-term interventions.

You may have noticed when reading the list of factors contributing to burn-out that several of them were based on unrealistic expectations. People who define success in terms of having all their patients recover or all their clients rehabilitated have set themselves up for failure. In contrast, if you are able to define success as having made *some* contribution to the health and welfare of *some* of the people you care for, then you have set yourself up for success.

You can also divide overall goals into partial goals that are more likely to be successfully met. For example, if your staff's goal is to rehabilitate a stroke patient completely, they may fail, especially if the patient has another stroke. But if they set several partial goals or separate steps leading to the patient's full recovery, such as finding a new means of transportation or being able to prepare meals, they have a much greater probability of meeting at least some of these goals. In general, a focus on one's successes rather than on one's failures helps to reduce feelings of discouragement and disappointment.

You can also redefine the extent of your responsibility and your team's responsibility to your clients. If you recall the victim-rescuer-persecutor roles of the Karpman Triangle (from Chapter 15), you'll see that helping persons who take on full responsibility for what happens to a client are acting in the role of rescuer. In contrast, caregivers who recognize that their clients have some responsibility too and who allow clients to exercise that responsibility have taken a burden off their shoulders and at the same time become more effective helping persons. This strategy has more utility in some settings than in others, but even in intensive care units, caregivers can learn to recognize their own limits and can focus their thoughts on the people who would not have survived without their care.

The use of effective leadership actions was mentioned as a way to cope with reality shock. They are equally helpful in dealing with burn-out. It is especially important to learn how to use change strategies to fight back when work situations are unsatisfactory. In particular, it is important to overcome the idea that the use of change strategies, especially power tactics, is unprofessional. Power tactics can and will be used on you by other people (including other professionals) so you will need to know how to use them in return or at least recognize when they are occurring. Many people in the helping professions are reluctant to let go of the myth that rewards somehow come automatically to those who do their work well. While this happens occasionally, more often the rewards go to those who know how to ask for and even demand them.

Stress reduction, relaxation techniques, exercise, and good nutrition are all helpful in keeping energy levels high. However, they are not solutions to the conflicts that lead to reality shock and burn-out and are supplements rather than substitutes for the other strategies discussed here.

When work takes up too much of a person's time and energy, little time is left for other important activities and relationships. Your job can become the center of your world and your world can become very small. When your interests and satisfactions are limited to your work, you are more susceptible to burn-out; trouble at work becomes trouble with your whole life. Two ways out of this are: set limits on your commitment to work and expand the number of satisfying activities and relationships you have outside of work.

Many people in the helping professions have difficulty setting such limits on their commitment. It is fine if they enjoy working extra hours and taking calls at night and on weekends; but if it exhausts them, they need to stop doing it or risk serious burn-out. When you are asked to work another double shift or the third weekend in a row, you can say no. At the same time that you are setting limits at work, you can expand your outside activities so that you live in a large world in which a blow to one part can be cushioned by support from other parts. If you are the team leader or nurse manager, you need to recognize and accept staff members' need to do this as well.

IMPAIRED-NURSE PROGRAMS. Mention should also be made of a specific problem that has been receiving increasing attention: the impaired nurse. Generally speaking, this term applies to the nurse who is having personal difficulty with substance abuse, although, of course, impairment of function can be the result of other problems as well. While impairment is not as directly related to the work environment as are reality shock and burn-out, a stressful, conflicted work environment can certainly contribute to the problem.

Nurse managers and administrators can choose to offer support and help (treatment) to the impaired. Or they can punish them, most often by terminating their employment (O'Connor & Robinson, 1985). Sometimes this is done by contributing to their arrest and legal proceedings against them. An offer of support is in keeping with the attitude that a staff member is a colleague and valued resource.

It is most important that the problem of impairment be confronted rather than hidden or ignored until it is so bad that a serious incident occurs, one that could harm staff or client. Often, the impaired individual is relieved that he or she no longer has to hide the problem and that support and understanding are offered. The staff member's colleagues may be relieved that they no longer have to cover for the impaired person. Many states have developed impaired-nurse programs that offer specific treatment to the impaired person and guidelines for employer intervention.

SUMMARY

Leader-manager actions that contribute to a climate that fosters staff growth development include encouraging critical thinking, supporting educational pursuits, encouraging new ideas and projects, involving staff in decision making, and rewarding these activities.

Prevention of reality shock and burn-out and effective intervention with impaired employees also foster staff development by reducing common inhibitors of it.

Reality shock and burn-out are related conflicts between a person's professional goals and ideals and the realities of the work situation. Reality shock occurs when nurses leave school and discover the discrepancies between professional and organizational goals: a holistic versus mechanistic orientation, the priority of efficiency over effectiveness, the way expectations are communicated, and the way feedback is given. Burn-out stems from the frustration and disillusionment of unsatisfactory working conditions and unrealistic expectations. Strategies for counteracting these problems include a realistic and supportive orientation for new employees; flexibility in management style to allow staff to resolve these conflicts in a positive manner; obtaining adequate knowledge, confidence, and skills to do the job; giving and receiving frequent feedback; using confrontation; developing a support network; improving and using leadership skills; redefining success; setting realistic goals; setting limits on one's work responsibilities; and expanding one's world outside of work.

Employees who evidence such impairments of function such as substance abuse should be offered rehabilitation rather than immediate termination.

REFERENCES*

*Bernhard, H.B. & Ingals, C.A. (1988). Six lessons for the corporate classroom. *Harvard Business Review,* 88 (5), 40–48.

*Edelwick, J. & Brodsky, A. (1980). *Burn-Out: Stages of Disillusionment in the Helping Professions.* New York: Human Science Press.

Freudenberger, H.J. (1974). Staff burn-out. *Journal of Social Issues,* 30 (1), 159.

George, R.T. (1986). First impressions: How they affect long-term performance. *Supervisory Management, 31* (3), 2–8.

Hurston, C.J. (1988). Job reconstruction in progress. *Management World, 17* (2), 19–21.

Knowles, M. (1984). *The Adult Learner: A Neglected Species.* Houston: Gulf Publishing.

*Kramer, M. (1974). *Reality Shock: Why Nurses Leave Nursing.* St. Louis: C.V. Mosby.

Kramer, M. (1981). Coping with Reality Shock. Workshop presented at Jackson Memorial Hospital, Miami, Florida. January 27–28.

Kramer, M. & Schmalenberg, C. (1977). *Path to Bicul-*turalism. Wakefield, Massachusetts: Contemporary Publishing.

*Moch, S.D. & Diemert, C.A. (1987). Health promotion within the nursing work environment. *Nursing Administration Quarterly, 11* (3), 9–12.

*O'Connor, P. & Robinson, R.S. (1985). Managing impaired nurses. *Nursing Administration Quarterly, 9* (12), 1–9.

Roedel, R.S. & Nsytrom, P.C. (1987). Clinical ladders and job enrichment. *Hospital Topics, 65* (2), 22–24.

Schmalenberg, C. & Kramer, M. (1979). *Coping with Reality Shock: Voices of Experience.* Wakefield, Massachusetts: Nursing Resources.

*References marked with an asterisk are suggested for further reading.

Chapter 24

LEADING INFORMATION CONFERENCES

Chapter 24

OUTLINE

Information Conferences

Design Phases
State the General Purpose Within a
    Conceptual Framework
    Conceptual Framework
Identify Relevant Characteristics of
    Learners and Environment
    Adult Learners
    The Setting
Write Specific Behavioral Objectives
    Common Mistakes
    Categories of Objectives
    Sharing Objectives
List Content Areas for Each Objective
    Need to Know
    Sequencing

Assess Learners' Preinstructional Level of
    Achievement for Each Objective
Select Appropriate Teaching/Learning
    Activities
    Basic Principles of Learning
    Presentation of Content
Provide a Facilitative Environment
Implement Teaching Plan
Evaluate Outcomes, Revise as Needed
    Identify the Behaviors to Be Measured
    Evoke the Identified Behaviors
    Record the Behavior
    Analyze the Results
    Use the Results

Summary

LEARNING OBJECTIVES

Upon completion of this chapter, the reader will be able to:

▷ List the steps in planning and conducting an information conference for staff or clients.

▷ Use the principles of adult learning in conducting an information conference.

▷ Write appropriate objectives for a learning situation.

▷ Lead an information conference effectively.

▷ Evaluate the outcomes of an information conference.

LEADING INFORMATION CONFERENCES

This chapter continues the subject of staff development from the previous chapter. Leader-managers are frequently called on to present information to both small and large groups of staff or clients. It is often assumed that this can be done effectively by anyone. Such an assumption ignores the fact that, like other areas of leadership and management, there are certain principles and processes which, if followed, will make the presentation of the information more effective.

In this chapter, we will first consider some of the important characteristics of both the learning environment and the adult employee as a learner. Then we will proceed through the process of planning, implementing, and evaluating an information conference in a work setting.

INFORMATION CONFERENCES

The information conference is essentially a short-term, teaching–learning situation that can be implemented on the team or unit level by the leader-manager. Even though it is brief, the design still needs to be based on an understanding of the teaching-learning process. Although our major interest here is in staff development, the basic principles can be adapted to almost any group of adults (including clients) so long as you keep their special characteristics and needs in mind.

An information conference is the sharing of knowledge, skills, and experience with others. The conference can be on almost any subject: a lecture on an aspect of nursing care; a report about a new nursing service; a class for patients preparing for discharge; or a miniworkshop in health promotion strategies for the community. The information conference usually has a more general application than the problem-solving conference, which focuses on a specific situation. It is an excellent vehicle for staff development.

DESIGN PHASES

The design of an information conference has nine important phases according to Kemp (1977). These phases are summarized in Figure 24–1. The leader-manager begins with an idea of the general purpose of the conference. You will also need to assess the characteristics and needs of the people attending the conference and the setting or environment in which the

> ▷ State the general purpose within a conceptual framework.
> ▷ Identify relevant characteristics of learners and environment.
> ▷ Write specific behavioral objectives.
> ▷ List content areas for each objective.
> ▷ Assess learner's preinstructional level of achievement for each objective.
> ▷ Select appropriate teaching/learning activities.
> ▷ Provide a facilitative environment.
> ▷ Implement a teaching plan.
> ▷ Evaluate outcomes and revise as needed.

Figure 24 – 1. Phases in the development of an information conference.

conference will take place. Once you have decided on these general conditions, you can write specific objectives for the conference and assess some more specific characteristics of the learner. The content of the conference and the way in which it is presented are based on your assessment and your objectives. You also need to provide a comfortable, facilitative setting for the conference. Finally, the outcomes of the conference need to be evaluated.

The planning of information conferences is often haphazard and incomplete. These phases of instructional design provide a clear guide for systematic planning and implementation that will increase the effectiveness of your information conferences by directing your attention to the many aspects of the situation that need careful consideration. Each of these phases will be discussed in the following sections. The environmental aspect of planning an information conference (selecting a convenient time and place, creating a climate of trust, and so forth) are virtually the same as for the problem-solving conference (discussed in Chapter 17) and will be mentioned only briefly here.

State the General Purpose within a Conceptual Framework

Begin your planning of an information conference by stating the purpose in broad terms. The purpose is the reason for the conference. It should be a simple general statement. For example:

▷ Make sure other agencies understand our new pilot program for families of developmentally disabled children.
▷ Improvement of our crisis intervention techniques.
▷ Increase staff understanding of the new hyperalimentation procedure.

Writing specific objectives or using the correct form is not necessary at this point. In fact, being so specific may be premature because you have not yet found out the needs of the group.

You also need to decide whether an information conference is the most appropriate approach. For example, do you want the staff to figure out why a patient is suddenly confused or do you want to improve the staff's ability to intervene with confused patients? In the first case, which involves an individual patient, a problem-solving conference would be more appropriate; in the second case, which has a more general perspective, an information conference is appropriate. Your choice should be based upon an adequate assessment of needs (Bernhard & Ingals, 1988).

CONCEPTUAL FRAMEWORK.   A concept is a statement describing a common property of several facts or pieces of information (Gagne, 1975). It is a classification of things, ideas, or relations. A conceptual framework serves the purpose of organizing or unifying the information you plan to present. It organizes the content to make it more meaningful and easier for people to remember. (Higher-level principles and theories that predict or prescribe may also be used as a framework, of course.)

The following is a sampling of some commonly used concepts in nursing:

Crisis Intervention	Nursing Process	Body Image
Sensory Deprivation	Grief Work	Self-Actualization
Developmental Tasks	Hope	Support Systems
Regulatory Mechanisms	Mobility	Isolation
Autoimmunity	Self-Efficacy	Pain

Example.   To illustrate how these phases can be applied to the planning of an actual information conference, a pilot program for families of developmentally disabled children will be followed through each phase.

For the Family Project pilot program, the conceptual framework could be networking (increasing the network or number of supports available to a person or family) to increase support systems for families with developmentally disabled children.

Identify Relevant Characteristics of Learners and Environment

For whom are you planning this conference? Who needs this information? To write appropriate objectives for your conference, you need to know several things about the group and the environment.

ADULT LEARNERS.   Although it varies somewhat according to the purposes of the conference, the following list includes the characteristics and needs of adult learners that most often influence the outcome of an information conference.

Goals: What does the group want to accomplish? What does it need to know? Are its goals congruent with yours?

Motivation: What incentives are there for the group? Does the group have a need for the information? Does it recognize this need? Other sources of motivation include expectation of some kind of reward, career achievement goals, general desire to improve skills and upgrade knowledge and the satisfaction inherent in mastering new skills or acquiring more knowledge (Gagne, 1975).

Abilities: People differ in academic ability, knowledge, and skill already gained from other learning situations and on the job. For some groups, it is important to find out if everyone in the group is able to read because people rarely volunteer this information.

Learning Style: Individuals and groups learn at different rates and approach learning in different ways. For example, some prefer a step-by-step explanation, while others prefer open-ended discussions and use of general principles (Biehler & Snowran, 1978).

Maturation: Adult learners tend to prefer self-directed activities and are able to assume responsibility for their own learning. As with any authoritarian style, a "teacher-knows-best" attitude is likely to elicit resentment and resistance (Vacca & Walke, 1980).

Example.   To illustrate the characteristics listed above, let us continue the Family Project example:

> Based on your contacts with the agency personnel involved, you can conclude that they are able to understand the relatively basic level of information you plan to present (ability). However, you will need to find out if they are familiar with similar programs and the services they offer because more details are necessary if they are not. On the other hand, if the agency personnel is familiar with a similar service, you can compare and contrast the two.
>
> If the group is not interested, members may not even come to your meeting unless you build up their interest, perhaps by indicating how the new service can be of use to them (motivation). Finally, what do these people from other professions think about your agency beginning such a program? Do they, perhaps, see it as an invasion of their turf (goals and sociocultural factors)?

THE SETTING.   The setting in which you hold your conference can either facilitate learning or be a barrier. As with any group, an open climate facilitates group process and learning. People need to feel free to make comments and ask questions. For some, an informal arrangement is much more comfortable than a classroom setting, especially for people who have had negative school experiences or who think that classrooms are only for the young. The beliefs that education ends in the early twenties and that the ability to learn declines with age still influence the way some adults feel about learning something new.

A comfortable physical setting facilitates learning. When you are too hot, too cold, or sitting on a hard chair, your discomfort can distract your attention from the conference. Outside noises can also be very distracting. An inconvenient time and place can often keep people from attending even a worthwhile conference.

The environment within which you are working must also be considered. Will people be rewarded for attending your conference and using what they have learned? Or, will they be penalized for "taking time off from their work" or for bringing back new ideas? You need to know what is rewarded in your organization and how to tap into these sources of power in gaining support for staff development activities (Willey, 1987). Resistant coworkers can also have a deleterious effect on staff. Potential conflicts with sociocultural values are of special concern with patient or health education but need to be considered with staff as well. For example, home health agency staff who are accustomed to working with the elderly may have some difficulty adjusting to an increased caseload of AIDS patients whose lifestyles are quite different from theirs.

Write Specific Behavioral Objectives

Now that you have a clear idea of the purpose, participants, and environment, it is time to be more specific about what you hope to accomplish. A discussion of objective writing can be found in Chapter 3. To summarize, the objectives should begin with an action verb and include a description of the behavior you expect of the group members at the end of the conference. Your purpose, conceptual framework, assessment of the group and environment, and knowledge of the subject are your guides in selecting appropriate objectives for your information conference. Two examples of objectives that could be used in a leadership course for staff members are, "Compare the primary and team methods of delivering nurse care," and, "Plan an information conference based on principles of teaching and learning."

Many people find it difficult to write objectives because they are concerned about the correct form and because it demands a very clear idea of what outcomes you expect from your teaching. However, it is this demanding nature of correctly written objectives that makes them worth writing down. Clearly stated objectives reduce much of the vagueness of purpose that plagues formal learning situations.

COMMON MISTAKES. There are several common mistakes people make when writing objectives. One is to write the objectives in terms of the teacher or group leader rather than outcomes for the group. For example:

TEACHER-ORIENTED OBJECTIVE: Show a film about insulin injections.

LEARNER OBJECTIVE: Select appropriate site for insulin injection.

There are times when you will write objectives for yourself, such as in a job description or in an independent learning situation. For information conferences, however, objectives are written as specific behaviors you expect the group to be able to carry out at the end of the conference.

Objectives should also be specific. Notice in the above example that the second objective is more specific than the first. Another common mistake is to begin the objective with a vague verb such as *understands*, which is difficult to define in terms of how you will observe that the group has actually accomplished the objective.

As much as possible, use observable behavior in your objectives. However, many important objectives related to attitudes and expression of feelings are difficult to measure directly. In this case, observable behavior may provide you with some indirect indications of a change in attitude. For example, acceptance of AIDS patients might be measured indirectly by a person's willingness to accept an assignment to care for an AIDs patient. It is preferable to include a hard-to-measure objective rather than omit it because measurement of the outcome will be difficult.

There is also a tendency to write more objectives for the simpler kind of learning (such as *knows, defines, names, recognizes*) than for the more complex kinds (such as *use, apply, analyze, compare, design, plan, appraise, evaluate*) (Bloom, 1956), which are often important goals of a conference. For example, in a class for people with diabetes, you would want the people to know not only what the symptoms of impending hypoglycemia are, but also how to differentiate these from hyperglycemic symptoms and to be able to take appropriate measures:

LOW-LEVEL OBJECTIVE: Defines hypoglycemia.

HIGHER-LEVEL OBJECTIVE: Distinguishes between symptoms of hypoglycemia and hyperglycemia.

CATEGORIES OF OBJECTIVES.   There are three different categories of objectives: cognitive, affective, and psychomotor. *Cognitive* refers to the knowledge type of objective; *affective* refers to attitudes (such as *accepts, defends, challenges, supports*); and *psychomotor* refers to skills (such as *injects, bathes, communicates*). The names of each of these types of objectives is probably not as important as is the fact that these categories help to remind you to consider using objectives from all three areas as appropriate.

SHARING OBJECTIVES.   Educators usually recommend sharing your objectives with the group. From a leadership point of view, this does not go far enough. Objectives are essentially statements of a group's goals. You will recall from the components of effective leadership that congruence between group and leader goals influences the leader's effectiveness with a group.

The effective leader includes group members in the planning of an information conference. Writing the objectives may be a too demanding and time-consuming task, but group members can participate in setting goals for the conference. Involvement of group members will both increase goal congruence and increase group motivation to participate in the conference and to support the objectives of the conference.

A set of objectives for an information conference about the Family Project pilot program could be stated as follows:

At the end of the conference, participants will be able to:

▷ Describe the goals of the Family Project.

▷ Explain the services of the Family Project to their clients.

▷ Make appropriate referrals to the Family Project.

▷ Support the Family Project's goals.

List Content Areas for Each Objective

The objectives you wrote with the input of the group can now serve as your guide in selecting content and, later, in planning and evaluating the actual activities of the conference. The content includes whatever information the group needs to accomplish the objectives. It should include the concepts that provide the framework for the conference. If you have psychomotor objectives, you may include demonstration and practice of some skills. To achieve affective (feeling or attitude) objectives, you can include discussion of common myths, of positive and negative experiences, and of people's reactions to or feelings about the subject.

NEED TO KNOW.   Probably the most common mistake in selecting content for any kind of learning experience is to confuse what is "nice to know" with what people "need to know." It is very tempting to throw in some interesting facts about the subject or a few anecdotes that are amusing but not really pertinent. This occurs in patient education, for example, where patients are told the intricate details of their surgery or how a new valve replacement was invented, but not how they are going to feel during the procedure or what they will need to know to care for themselves when they get home. Relating the content to each specific objectives will help you to avoid this mistake.

SEQUENCING.   It is usually helpful to begin with content that is familiar to the people in the group and then proceed to the unknown. Another useful sequence is to begin with the simple or concrete and proceed to what is complex or abstract. Some content has an inherent logical order, such as a procedure that you would probably want to demonstrate step by step from beginning to end.

EXAMPLE.   Let us look now at what kind of content would be appropriate for the information conference about the Family Project. To see how the content flows from the objectives, they are repeated with the related content listed alongside.

Objective	Content
1. Describe the goals of the Family Project.	1. The assessed needs of the families and how the Family Project is designed to meet these needs.
2. Explain the services of the Family Project to its clients.	2. List and describe each service offered: family support groups, telephone networks, counseling, legal consultation, financial assistance, health guidance, respite care.
3. Make appropriate referrals to the Family Project.	3. Specific procedure for referral; whom to contact; eligibility requirements (need, financial, residence).
4. Support the Family Project's goals.	4. How the agencies represented plan to use the service; what the group thinks of the project; how the project can meet the needs of the agencies.

Assess Learners' Preinstructional Level of Achievement for Each Objective

The main reason for doing this specific assessment in regard to each objective is to ensure that you will begin at a level that is comprehensible to your audience but not waste their time by repeating what they already know. There are two aspects to this assessment. The first is the *prerequisite knowledge and skills* that are needed to begin the learning experience. These prerequisites could include background knowledge in math, psychology, or nursing, or previous practice and experience. If the group members have this background, they are ready for your conference.

The second aspect of this assessment, *specific achievement*, is the extent to which members of the group have already achieved specific objectives. You can determine this by using a pretest or questionnaire, or by informal questioning and discussion before the conference. This specific assessment will also help you to apply another important leadership principle: begin where the group is. The pretest may have a useful side effect — it can arouse interest and awareness of the need to learn if presented in an effective manner.

In the Family Project example, you would need to assess the following:

Prerequisites:
   Ability to assess clients' needs.
   Experience in making referrals.
   Familiarity with networking.

Specific Achievement:
   Experience using the agency's referral procedures.
   Extent of information already received about the Family Project's goals and services.
   Attitudes toward the Family Project.

The emphasis on a thorough assessment may seem excessive for planning an information conference. A thorough assessment can save time for the group as a whole, however. A saying, often related in patient education, may be appropriate here: *Assume nothing* (Gulko & Butherus, 1977). Failure to do an assessment has led to many poor conferences where information is presented that the group already knew or that the group could not comprehend because it was assumed that they had the prerequisite knowledge or skills.

Every person and every group has different characteristics, needs, and experiences, so assessment is always important. For example, caregivers frequently assume that their well-educated clients understand what is happening to them. The community nurse might be surprised to find that even a well-educated client thinks it is okay to share an insulin syringe with another family member. An inservice educator might find that many nursing assistants do not know the location of many vital organs in the body or that they confuse similar-sounding terms such as *gall bladder* and *urinary bladder*.

Select Appropriate Teaching/Learning Activities

Some guidelines and factors should be considered in making your choice from the almost infinite variety of ways in which you can structure a learning experience. A list of some basic, generally accepted principles of learning is presented next, and then, the most common ways of presenting content are described.

BASIC PRINCIPLES OF LEARNING. The following list is not exhaustive, but it includes some of the most commonly agreed-upon principles for facilitating learning. The first four have been mentioned already, others may already be familiar to you.

1. Begin where the learner is.
2. Stimulate motivation to learn.
3. Make a thorough assessment: assume nothing.

4. Allow for individual differences in abilities, style, and sociocultural background.
5. Vary the rate of presentation according to the abilities of the learners and the difficulty of the material.
6. Provide opportunities for success.
7. Present challenging materials and activities to stimulate interest.
8. Provide sufficient repetition and emphasis of main points to promote remembering.
9. Provide opportunities for practice and for application of learning to new situations to promote transfer of learning.
10. Provide feedback as close to the event as possible.

Some principles of learning apply specifically to adult learners, which are your target group. These are derived from Knowles' (1984) principles of adult learning.

1. Adults want to know *why* they should learn something and will put a lot of energy into it if they recognize their need to know.
2. Motivation is stimulated when adults see that what they are learning will help them perform a task or solve a problem.
3. All adults have intrinsic motivation to continue learning, but it can be blocked by a negative self-concept, the pressure of other responsibilities, lack of opportunity, and poorly designed educational programs (Knowles, 1984).
4. Adults believe that they are responsible for themselves and can make their own decisions, that is, they can be self-directed (Mooney, 1987). Past experiences in authoritarian classrooms may lead them to resist a return to the classroom or, paradoxically, to become passive when they first re-enter a formal learning situation.
5. Adults bring more life experience with them than younger learners, experiences that can be a rich resource if they are encouraged to share them.

While these principles are easily understood, it takes thorough preparation and often some ingenuity and creativity to apply them to a specific conference.

PRESENTATION OF CONTENT. The many ways to present content are divided into three broad categories: autotutorial, presentation to the group, and active interaction (Kemp, 1977; Green et al., 1983).

Autotutorial. *Autotutorial* literally means *self-teaching.* Most adults can assume much of the responsibility for their own learning. They can make decisions about what they need to learn and can seek opportunities to fulfill these needs. This does not mean, however, that guidance and feedback are unnecessary; both are helpful to even the most skilled and autonomous people.

People can learn on their own in many ways. Television, films, books, modules, and programmed instructions are all forms of autotutorial learning. The content can be fed into a computer, printed in a book, put on film or tape, put into a notebook format, or a combination of these. Preplanned autotutorial programs usually include objectives, pretests, exercises and other learning activities, and then a posttest.

One particular advantage of autotutorial learning is that it can be highly individualized. It allows as many opportunities for repetition and review as are needed by each learner, and each learner can proceed at his or her own pace. It is also efficient in terms of the leader's time, once the materials have been prepared. For example, an inservice instructor can put together a learning module explaining the use of a new crash cart. Then, staff members can work on the module whenever they have the time, and the instructor only needs to be available to answer questions that may come up and to administer the posttest.

In completely autotutorial learning, the person interacts with the material but not with other people. No opportunities are provided for sharing ideas with others. Such opportunities not only are stimulating but also reinforce learning. Discussion is also particularly helpful in bringing out feelings and attitudes. Some programmed materials become monotonous after a while. Unless sophisticated equipment is available, learners cannot get frequent feedback on the quality of their work nor can they get a question answered readily, which can be frustrating.

Presentation to the Group.   Probably the first method you thought of in this category is the lecture, one of the most popular and yet most maligned of all teaching strategies. A lecture can be virtually one-way communication (but not *completely* because you cannot not communicate) from a speaker to a passive listening group. But it can also be made more interactive through the use of question-and-answer sessions and discussion.

A lecture is particularly useful when you want to introduce a subject, to clarify and explain a complex subject, or to share your experiences with a group. You can present a large amount of information quickly. When giving a lecture, it is important to pay attention to feedback from the group because it is likely to be more subtle (unless they fall asleep or protest loudly). Audiovisuals of all types, from the blackboard to videotapes, can be used for visual stimulation, but they are also relatively passive modes of learning.

A second popular form of presentation is the demonstration. Here, the group leader shows a group how to carry out a skill, which could be anything from an aseptic technique to a client interview. Although usually interesting to watch, the group is still relatively passive unless you provide opportunities for practice and return demonstrations.

Active Interaction.   In this mode, the learner interacts more actively with both the learning materials and with other members of the group. The leader's role in active interaction is to facilitate learning, focus attention on the objectives, challenge assumptions, provide feedback, and summarize learning. The role is still an active one, but it is less controlling than in the presentation to the group.

Open discussion is one of the most common ways to encourage active interaction. It is useful in encouraging expression of feelings and attitudes, for stimulating creative and divergent thinking, and for group problem solving.

There are many other ways to provide active interaction even when equipment and facilities are limited. Role playing, games, and group exercises are some of these. An example would be to hold a mock conference, with learners taking the roles of different staff members, and then analyzing the group dynamics and outcome.

In simulations, learners try out their skills in an imitation-of-life setting. The almost life-like simulators called *Annies* used in CPR instruction are a well-known example. Another increasingly popular one is computer simulation of patient care problems. Simulations are an effective way to promote active participation and transfer of learning, especially for complex psychomotor skills. They tend to require more equipment than other modes but can accelerate learning (De Geus, 1988).

A combination of two or all three modes is sometimes the most effective way to allow for different learning styles and to accomplish all the objectives of an information conference.

EXAMPLE. To return to the Family Project example, the following teaching strategies could be chosen from the three modes.

▷ Distribute written materials to participants before the conference (autotutorial).
▷ Briefly tell the group about the project's services and referral procedures (presentation to the group).
▷ Give participants case study examples and ask them to determine eligibility and to fill out actual referral forms (active interaction).
▷ Discuss the group's reactions to the program and how they think it will be of use to them (active interaction).

Provide a Facilitative Environment

Adequate, well-prepared materials and functional equipment are important for learning situations. Inadequate or broken equipment creates frustration, wastes time, and reduces learning. The well-prepared leader checks all these things ahead of time to ensure a smooth-running conference.

Provision of comfort, psychological security, and sometimes privacy make group members feel at ease. Setting a convenient time and place makes it easier for people to attend the conference and shows the leader's consideration for group members. Stimulation of motivation, including a supportive organizational or community climate, will also encourage people to attend the conference.

Implement Teaching Plan

The leadership skills required to implement an information conference are similar to those needed for other conferences. Among the most important points to consider in conducting an information conference are the following, drawn from the components of effective leadership.

GOALS: Be sure that the leader's and group's objectives are congruent.

KNOWLEDGE: Know your subject well.

SELF-AWARENESS: Be yourself; do not try to mold yourself into a teacher role (especially the role of authoritarian expert) that does not suit your personal style or the style of the group.

COMMUNICATION: Use language that people can understand; watch the

	use of jargon or technical terms. Encourage feedback from the group; provide frequent feedback to the group.
ENERGY:	Share your interest and excitement about the subject with the group.
ACTION:	Start the conference on time. Engage the group in the purpose of the conference by stimulating motivation. Guide the learning process; keep group members on the track. Keep the pace lively but not so fast that you lose people. Encourage the active participation of *all* group members. Summarize at the end of the conference.

Evaluate Outcomes, Revise as Needed

Evaluation serves several purposes: it is a measure of your effectiveness as the conference leader; it measures the extent to which the group achieved its objectives; and it provides some direction for improvements for your next conference. The objectives you wrote in the planning stage are now your guidelines in evaluating the conference. The outcomes of the conference should be measured in terms of observable behaviors defined by the objectives.

A careful analysis of the objectives will tell you what behaviors need to be evaluated. Then, you need to decide how you are going to evoke the identified behaviors, record them in some way, and analyze the results (Gronlund, 1976). Each of the steps will be discussed briefly.

IDENTIFY THE BEHAVIORS TO BE MEASURED. The more specific your objectives were, the easier this step will be. If, for example, the objective was concerned with selecting the appropriate site for insulin injection, it is clear that asking the client for a return demonstration of an insulin injection is one way to meet the objective.

More general objectives like the one in the Family Project example about making appropriate referrals are harder to evaluate. To evaluate this objective, it is necessary to observe a cluster of behaviors, including the ability to determine need and eligibility and the ability to fill out the referral form correctly.

EVOKE THE IDENTIFIED BEHAVIORS. Paper-and-pencil tests are the most common ways to evoke the identified behaviors. The tendency with these tests, however, is to measure more lower-level objectives such as defining terms or recalling information.

> An example of this would be to ask a person to list the appropriate sites for insulin injection. Asking instead to point out appropriate sites on a diagram or on oneself would test a higher-level objective and an important ability for a person with diabetes to have.

Tests are usually more relevant when case studies or other ways to apply knowledge are used rather than simply asking for definitions or recall of facts.

Often you also need to find our whether or not a person can actually perform in a given situation (Gronlund, 1976). Simulations of various kinds can be set up to measure the degree to which this type of objective was met.

You can, for example, ask people to react to a problem situation, select the correct procedure, perform in a laboratory simulation, or evaluate a videotape performance.

Two other strategies are often used to evaluate learning. The first is to ask for a *final product* such as a project report, a case study, or a videotape. The second is to test people in real-life situations. The latter has the advantage of high relevance, but errors in performance can be more serious.

Affective objectives, those looking for changes in feelings or attitudes, are usually measured indirectly. Some ways to do this include the use of opinion surveys, questionnaires, and interviews. Another way is to keep anecdotal records of comments or observed behavior.

> For example, one way to judge whether or not patients have accepted their diagnoses is to note whether or not they ever talk about their diagnoses. Another way, also indirect, is to observe the degree to which patients are following the prescribed treatment plan.

RECORD THE BEHAVIOR. Some kind of permanent record is needed to share the results of the evaluation with others. A written test or final product provides its own record. Other ways to record behavior include videotapes, audiotapes, behavior checklists, and anecdotal notes. The last two methods (checklists and notes) are harder to keep objective.

ANALYZE THE RESULTS. Grades are neither necessary nor relevant for information conferences. A clear idea of what behaviors would indicate to you that the objectives have been met is needed.

Several approaches exist for defining an acceptable outcome. You can write out the correct answers to the test questions, write a model answer to a case study question, or produce a tape of an acceptable performance for comparison. Another approach is to draw up checklists that provide detailed descriptions of acceptable performance. For example, you can list each step in giving an insulin injection (draws up correct dose, cleans site before injection, and so forth) and then check that each step is done correctly.

When the outcomes defined by the objectives are more general, you can describe the behavior, and, if possible, specify a frequency. For example:

> You may decide that hearing a patient mention the diagnosis only once is not adequate evidence of acceptance of that diagnosis, but that the patient is mentioning it on three occasions to three different people would be acceptable evidence.

USE THE RESULTS. The evaluation will tell you how much has been learned and whether you need to hold another conference on the same subject. It will also tell you where your instructional design was done well and where it was weak and needs improvement. You can see that being involved in the evaluation process can contribute to your development as a leader-manager.

Evaluation has a use for the people attending the conference, too. It provides them with feedback about their behavior. By asking for some kind of return performance, it also reinforces learning.

Example. One of the objectives of the Family Project was to enable people from other agencies to make appropriate referrals to the project. This includes the ability to determine need, to determine eligibility, and to fill out the forms correctly.

> Presenting a case study of a client applying to the project for assistance would be an

appropriate way to evoke most of these behaviors (except the ability to elicit the necessary information from a client during an actual interview). Group members could be asked to evaluate the hypothetical client's need and eligibility and to fill out a referral form.

The answers could be compared to a model evaluation and referral form you prepared before the conference. Any discrepancies between the model and the group's answers could be discussed with the group to determine what people had learned and what further information was still needed. The discussion should also give you some indications of the strengths and weaknesses of your design of the conference as well as the degree to which you fulfilled the original objectives for the conference.

SUMMARY

When planning an information conference, the leader begins with an idea of the general purpose of the conference and then identifies an appropriate conceptual framework within which to organize the information to be shared. An assessment of the characteristics of the group members and the environment is the next step. Then, the leader is ready to write specific objectives for the conference.

Once the objectives have been determined, the content for the conference can be outlined and a more specific assessment of the learners can be done. Selection of appropriate activities completes the planning process. The leader then implements the conference, keeping in mind the factors that facilitate the learning and applying the components of effective leadership. An evaluation based on the degree to which the specific objectives were met provides useful feedback to both the leader and the other members of the group.

REFERENCES*

Albanetti, J. & Carroll, D. (1984). In-service nursing education through clinical units. In Knowles, M. (ed) *Andragogy in Action.* San Francisco: Jossey-Bass.

*Bernhard, H.B. & Ingals, C.A. (1988). Six lessons for the corporate classroom. *Harvard Business Review,* 88 (5), 40–48.

*Biehler, R.F. & Snowran, J. (1982). *Psychology Applied to Teaching.* Boston: Houghton Mifflin.

Bloom, B.S., et al. (1956). *Taxonomy of Educational Objectives. Handbook I. Cognitive Domain.* New York, David McKay.

De Geus, A.P. (1988). Planning as learning. *Harvard Business Review,* 88 (2), 70–74.

Gagne, R.M. (1975). *Essentials of Learning for Instruction.* Hinsdale, Illinois: Dryden Press.

*Green, L.W., Kreuter, M.W., Deeds, S.G. & Partridge, K.B. (1980). *Health Education Planning: A Diagnostic Approach.* Palo Alto: Mayfield.

Gronlund, N.E. (1976). *Measurement and Evaluation in Teaching.* New York: Macmillan.

Gulko, C.S. & Butherus, C. (1977). Toward better patient teaching. *Nurses' Drug Alert.* Vol. I, No. 8, p. 52.

*Kemp, J.E. (1977). *Instructional Design: A Plan for Unit and Course Development.* Belmont, California: Feron-Pitman.

*Knowles, M. (1984). *The Adult Learner: A Neglected Species.* Houston: Gulf Publishing.

Mooney, M.A. (1987). Use of adult education principles in medication instruction. *Journal of Continuing Education in Nursing,* 18 (3), 89–92.

Vacca, R. & Walke, J.E. (1980). Andragogy: The missing link in college reading programs. *Lifelong Learning: The Adult Years,* Vol. III, No. 6, p. 16.

Willey, E. (1987). Acquiring and using power effectively. *Journal of Continuing Education in Nursing,* 18 (1), 25–27.

*References marked with an asterisk are suggested for further reading.

UNIT V LEARNING ACTIVITIES _____

▷ Evaluate the extent to which your assigned unit or agency promotes staff development. Suggest ways in which staff development could be promoted and estimate the relative costs and benefits of your suggestions.

▷ With another colleague or classmate, role play a performance appraisal session in which the staff member has failed to achieve all but one of the objectives that had been mutually agreed upon 6 months ago. Evaluate the nurse-manager's actions in terms of effective communication, the components of effective management, and adherence to the guidelines for providing feedback. Then evaluate the staff member in terms of effective communication skills, the components of effective leadership, and guidelines for receiving feedback. You may have to refer to earlier chapters for some of these guidelines. If time permits, switch roles and repeat the session.

▷ Investigate the laws and regulations concerning impaired nurses in your state. Interview several employers and staff nurses to determine their knowledge of these rules and opinions regarding their fairness and effectiveness, particularly the degree to which they provide safeguards for the patient, the employee, and the employer.

▷ Plan a 10-minute information conference. Work through all phases of the design from a statement of purpose through evaluation and revision as outlined in Chapter 24. If possible, implement your plan and evaluate both your effectiveness and the degree to which following the phases in development did or did not help you plan and implement an effective information conference.

INDEX

A page number in *italics* indicates a figure. A "*t*" following a page number indicates a table.

Accountability, 464, 475–476
Action, 57, 75
  in effective leadership in community, 452
  to increase motivation, 371, 372
  initiating, 75–76
  leadership and, 82
  of new graduates, 496–497
  selecting course of, 158–161
  types of, 76–79
Action orientation, 21
Active listening, 69
Activists, 439–440
Activities, categorization of, 244
Acuity index, 223
  staff mix and, 226
Administration
  as barrier to change, 450–451
  computer systems for, 254–255
  formal evaluation and, 464
  representation of, 101
Administrator, 207
  cost monitoring of, 113
Adult learners, 507–508
Advocate role, 100
Affection needs, 17–18
Aggression, as coping mechanism, 14
Aggressor role, 329
Ambiguity, of roles, 25
American Nurses' Association, in collective
  bargaining, 264
Antibiotics, introduction of, 108
Application, theory and, 4
Assertiveness, 70
Assignments
  communication of, 388
  criteria for, 385–388
  relation factors of, 387–388
  task-related factors of, 385–387
  undesirable, 391
Attending, 288–290
Authoritarian leader, 34–37
Authority, 22
  budget and, 173–174
  in organizational relationships, 206–209
Automation, 245
Autonomy, 21–22

"Be spontaneous" paradox, 418, 422
Bear trap, 211–212
Becoming orientation, 21
Behavior
  assumptions about, 11–12
  coping patterns of, 12–14
  cultural differences and, 24
  factors influencing, 11
  human needs hierarchy and, 14–20
  of leaders, 37–38
  meaning of, 11–12
  roles and, 24–28
Behavioral management, 46–47
Behavioral theories, 33–40, 53
Being orientation, 21
Belonging needs, 17–18, 370
Biased arguments, 129–130
Billing, computerized, 254
Binding arbitration, 270–271, 273–274
Biorhythms, 10
Blocker role, 329, 359
Blocking procedures, 447–449
Board
  financial management and, 174–175
  function of, 207–208
Body stance, 287
Brainstorming, 156
Budget. *See also* Budgeting
  blaming, 171–172
  operating, components of, 172*t*
  planning of, 172–173
  power and authority of, 173–174
  for staffing, 228
  types of, 176–178
  types of calculations for, 179–180
Budget committee, 175
Budgeting
  computer systems for, 254
  incremental, 176, 178, 183
  process of
    modification and approval of, 181
    monitoring of, 181–182
    planning phase of, 178–179
    preparation phase of, 179–181
  zero-base, 177–178, 183
Bureaucracy, 195–198

Bureaucracy—*Continued*
diffusion of responsibility in, 197
division of labor in, 197–198
elements of, 196
Burn-out, 497–498
counteracting, 499–500
factors contributing to, 498–499
programs for, 500–501

Care. *See* Health care costs; Health care
organizations; Health care system;
Nursing care
Case method, 217–218
Chain of command, in bureaucracy, 196–197
Change, 107–119
anticipated response to, 154–155
barriers to, 447–451
dynamics of, 396–399
first-order, 418, 422
identification of people for and against,
446–447
implementation phase of, 408–410
multifactorial influences on, 397–398
myths about, 397
normative model of, 404–417
paradoxical model of, 417–423
planned, 395–396, 432, 433
potential for, 396
power-coercive model of, 423–432
proposal of, 446
psychological safety and, 407–408
rate of, 398–399
rational model of, 400–404
reinforcing and stabilizing, 416
second-order, 419–422, 423
strategies for, 395–433
system response to, 397–399
Change agent model, 416–417
assumptions of, 412–416
Chaotic communication, 332–333
Chart audits, 96
for quality assurance, 485–486
Chief executive officer, 194
financial management and, 174
Clarifying perceptions, 292
Clerical computer support, 251–252
Clichés, 129
Collective bargaining, 280
definition of, 263–264
employee and, 268–274
issues arising from, 266–268
management and, 274–279
purposes of, 264–266
stalemates in, 270–271
Collective decision making, 45–46
Comfort, seeking, 13
Common bonds, 311–312
Communication
basic skills of, 288–294
channels of, 203–204

checking perceptions and, 71
confrontation techniques in, 294–303
control of in preventing unionization, 277
effective, 57
in effective leadership, 69–73
in community, 451–452
as an exchange, 285–288
feedback and, 71
interpretation of, 287–288
leadership and, 82
negotiation and, 303–308, 309
nonverbal, 286–289
open, in teams, 382–383
patterns of in groups, 330–333
patterns of in meeting, 358
Communication networks, 50
Community. *See also* Community action
concept of, 435–440
definitions of, 435–436
functions of, 436
of interest, 435–436
as open system, 436–438
power distribution in, 438–440
of solution, 436
values of, 447
Community action, 440–441
developing motivation for, 442
developing plan for, 443–444
evaluation of, 444
implementation of, 444
mutual identification of need for, 441–442
prioritization of need for, 442
resources and building confidence for, 443
Compatibility, in making assignments, 388
Compensation, 12
Complex man, 51
Comptroller, 175
Computer printer, 250
Computer systems
adequacy of, 258
applications
for clerical and secretarial support,
251–252
for education and information resources,
253–254
for nursing administration, 254–255
for patient assessment and monitoring,
253
for patient records, 252–253
for research, 255–256
compatibility and coordination of, 257
comprehensive plan for, 257
consultants for, 257
cost vs. benefits of, 260
depersonalization with, 258–259
equipment, 249–250
expectations for, 256–257
overdependence on, 259–260
personnel training for, 258
privacy and security with, 259
programs for, 250–251

finding right, 258
simulation, 159
purpose of, 256
Computerized records, privacy and security
of, 259
Conferences. *See* Information conferences;
Problem-solving conferences
Conflicts
of interest, 303
resolving with leader-manager actions,
496–497
in staff, 494–495
in teams, 383–384
Confrontation, 76
avoidance of, 294–296
by calling the other's game, 298–300
definition of, 294
inappropriate, 297, 298
indirect vs. direct, 301
through information, 296–298
meeting, 301–303
processing of, 300–301
in resolving conflicts, 497
tape recordings in, 300
Connections, making, 126–127
Consensus taker, 329
Consideration, 38
Contingency plans, 90
Contingency theory, 47–49, 54
Contributor role, 358–359
Control need, 369
Cooperative orientation, 307
Coordinator role, 100, 101, 329
Coping behavior patterns, 12–14
unsuccessful, 495–496
Crises
planning for, 90
recurrent, 243–244
Critical analysis, 127
of group's work, 244
questions for, 128–133
uses of, 127–128
Critical path method, 166
Critical thinking, 64–66
critical analysis and, 127–133
encouragement of, 492
problem solving and, 77
purpose of, 125–127
Criticism
avoidance of, 201–202
premature, 158
Crosscultural research, 23
Crossroads approach, 162
Cultural awareness, 23–24
Cultural beliefs, 24
Culture, 20, 28
differences in and shared meaning,
20–23
working with differences in, 23–24
Current work planning, 90–91
Customer behavior analysis, 115

Data
relevant, 131
verifiable, 130
Data base, from formal evaluation, 465
Deadlines, 91
Decision making
arena of, 449–450
collective, 45–46
critical thinking and, 125–126
entering channel of, 445–451
influencing of, 444–452
in problem discussion meeting, 360–361
staff involvement in, 492–493
in teams, 379–380, 381
Decision package, 177
Decision to act, 78–79
Delegation, 241–242. *See also* Responsibility,
delegation of
criteria of, 392
difficulty with, 388–389
issues and problems in, 388–391
Deliberative coping mechanisms, 13–14
Democratic leadership, 34–36, 37
Denial, 13
Dependence, 21–22
Dependency needs, 17
Depersonalization, computers and, 258–259
Depression, 108
Designated leader, 373
Development, 98–99
Diagnoser, 329
Diagnosis-related groups (DRGs), 112, 477
Differential marketing, 115
Direct role bargaining, 26
Direction, effective management and, 92–94
Directness, 70
Disagreer, 329
Disconfirmation, 407, 408
Discussion of problems, 14
Displacement, 13
Division of labor, 196, 197–198
Dominator/usurper role, 329
DRGs, 112, 477
Driving forces, 405–407, 445

Eating, as coping mechanism, 14
Economic issues, 264
Economic security, 369
Education
computer-assisted, 253–254
identification of needs for, 464–465
opportunities for, 492
Effectors, 439
Efficiency, goal of, 201
Elaborator, 329, 358–359
Emergent leader, 373
Emotional arguments, 129–130
Emotional energy, 73
Emotional issues, 304
Employee attitudes, 42

Encounter groups, 341
Encourager role, 329, 359
Energizer, 329
  in change, 410, 411, 413
Energy
  in effective leadership in community, 452
  flow and reserves of, 74–75
  flow of in community, 437
  inventory, 75
  leadership effectiveness and, 73–74, 82
  mobilization of, 57
  neural and emotional, 73
Energy fields, 8–9
Environment, 6
  changing, 107–119
  people's interaction with, 5–11
Esprit de corps, 378–379
Esteem needs, 18, 19
Evaluation
  formal procedures of, 463–473
  informal procedures of, 457–463, 472–473
Evil, innate, 20–21
Exchange, 285–286
  elements of, 286
Exercise, as coping mechanism, 14
Experience, drawing on, 14
Expert power, 426
Explanation, theory and, 4
Expresser, 329, 358–359
Expressiveness, 22
Eye contact, 22, 289

Fact finding, 270
Fair play, appeal to, 307
Fairness, in making assignments, 387
Federal Mediation and Conciliation Service, 270
Feedback, 52, 97. See also Negative feedback; Positive feedback
  constructive, 473
  evaluative, 458
    guidelines for, 459–462
    responding to, 463
    seeking, 462–463
  immediate, 460
  loop, 8, 285
  marketing, 115
  nonthreatening, 462
  providing, 71
  on record audit, 481
  in resolving conflicts, 497
  as reward, 97
  seeking, 462–463
  self-awareness and, 68
  in teamwork, 375
Filing systems, 239
Financial gain, 200–201
Financial management
  budget process in, 178–183
  effects of on nursing, 171
  importance of, 171–174
  responsibility for, 174–175
  types of budgets in, 176–178
First-line manager
  tasks of, 88
  under union contract, 278–279
Fiscal officer, chief, 175
Flextime, 227
Focusing, 291–292
Follower role, 329, 358–359, 360
Formal evaluation, 463, 473
  vs. informal, 457–458
  purpose of, 464–465
  types of, 465–473
Functional group-building roles, 329
Functional health care delivery method, 218–219
Functional task roles, 328–329
Functional theories. See Behavioral theories
Future work planning, 91–92

Game, breaking up, 298–300
Gantt charts, 165
Gatekeeper, 329, 359
Genuineness, 290
Geographical community, 435
Goal setting
  advantages and disadvantages of, 144–145, 146
  in change agent model, 415–416
  personal and career, 234–236
  time management and, 234–236
Goal-based motivation model, 370–372
Goals, 52. See also Goal setting
  actions needed to meet, 236
  clear, 61–62
  of community, 437–438
  congruent, meaningful, 60
  environmental, 59–60
  group, 59
  individual, 59
  keeping reasonable, 241
  levels of, 58–60
  of organization, formal and informal, 199–202
  setting of, 57. See also Goal setting
Goodness, 20–21
Great man theory, 32, 53
Great Society, 109
  unfulfilled promises of, 110
Grievances, 271–273
  handling under collective bargaining, 278–279
  procedure for handling, 265, 276
Group adjourning stage, 326–327
Group dynamics, 335–337
Group formation stage, 313–317
Group norming stage, 321–323
Group performing stage, 323–326
Group size, 50

Group storming stage, 317–321
Group-leader interaction, 51–52
Groups. *See also* Meetings; Problem-solving
    conferences
  clarification of goals of, 316
  communication patterns in, 330–333
  dominant synchronizers of, 335–337
  mature and immature, 325*t*
  maturity of, 360
  norms of, 380–382
  as open system, 312–313
  patterns of communication in, 10
  patterns of interaction in, 328–337
  position in, 50
  public and hidden agendas in, 333–335
  roles in, 328–330
    in meetings, 358–360
  small, 311–313
  social interactions in, 328–337
  stage of development of, 313–327
  understanding of, 311–338
Growth, 9
Guidance, 76

Hard copy, 250
Harm, ability to, 424
Hawthorne Effect, 42
Hawthorne studies, 41–42, 43
Health care costs. *See also* Financial
    Management
  with computerization, 260
  payment plans for, 111–114
  rising, 110–111
Health care organizations, 187, 213. *See also*
    Health maintenance organizations
    (HMOs); Hospitals
  as complex, open systems, 189–194
  for-profit vs. not-for-profit, 188
  function of, 199–206
  patterns of relationships in, 206–212
  structures of, 194–199
  types of, 187–189
Health care system, *See also* Health care costs
  business-orientation of, 113–114
  early evolution of, 107–108
  evolution of, 119
  finances in, 111–114
  growth and prosperity and, 109
  marketing of, 114–117
  nursing image and, 117–119
  outcome of, 479
  process of, 478–479
  scientific, technologic, and social
    expansion of, 108–109
  skepticism and disillusionment in,
    109–111
  structure of, 478
Health insurance. *See also* Medicaid; Medicare
  commercial, 108
  comprehensive, 109

  private, 111
Health maintenance organizations (HMOs),
    110
  advertising and marketing of, 115
Hidden agendas, 333–335
  dominant synchronizers and, 337
Hierarchy. *See also* Needs hierarchy
  authority and power in, 206–209
  in bureaucracy, 196
  of organizations, 191–192, *193*, 194–195
Hill-Burton Program, 109
Hill-Harris amendment, 109
HMOs. *See* Health maintenance
    organizations (HMOs)
Holistic management, 46
Honeymoon, 493–494
Horizontal health care systems, 112–113
Hospitals
  advertising and marketing of, 115–117
  diversification of, 113
  establishment of first, 107–108
  merging of, 112–113
Human behavior. *See* Behavior
Human needs, 15. *See also* Needs hierarchy
Human relations, 41–42, 43
Hygiene factors, 44–45

"I" messages, 463
"I told you so" game, 211
Ideas
  encouraging new, 492
  power of, 426–427
Identification, 13
Immunization programs, 108
Impaired-nurse programs, 500–501
Incentive programs, 483
Incompetence, in role, 26
Incongruity, of roles, 25–26
Indirect role bargaining, 26–27
Individual characteristics, 32–33
Individual needs, meeting, 202
Individuality, 10, 189–190
Influentials, 439
Informal evaluation, 472–473
  feedback in, 458
  vs. formal evaluation, 457–458
  guidelines for constructive feedback in,
    459–462
  seeking feedback in, 462–463
Information. *See also* Data; Data base
  computer access to, 253–254
  confrontation through, 296–298
  encouraging flow of, 69–70
  giving, 293
  means of sharing, 94
  supplying, 307
Information conferences, 505
  behavioral objectives of, 509–510
  content areas for objectives of, 510–511
  design phases of, 505–518

Information conferences—*Continued*
evaluating and revising outcomes of,
516–518
facilitative environment in, 515
implementing teaching plan of, 515–516
learner's preinstructional levels in,
511–512
relevant learner and environment
characteristics of, 507–508
statement of purpose of, 506–507
teaching/learning activities of, 512–515
Information giver, 328, 358–359
Information seeker, 328
Initiating action, 75–76
Initiating structure, 38
Initiator/contributor role, 328
Insecurity, 70
Inservice education programs, effectiveness
of, 481
Integrated market planning, 115
Interactional theories, 50–53
Interdisciplinary team, 372
Interpersonal relationships, patterns of, 10
Interpersonal stress, 50
Interpretation, 287–288
Interruptions, reduction of, 242–243
Interviewing, 482

Job descriptions, 93
sample, *471*
Job enrichment, 492
Job satisfaction, leadership style and, 39
Job security, 267–268
Judgments, complex, 125–126

Karpman Triangle, 210–211, 278
in calling other's game, 299
Knowledge
leadership and, 62–63, 82
nursing, 63–64

Labor contract
administration of, 271–274
negotiation of, 269–271
ratification of, 271
Labor relations, 263. *See also* Collective
bargaining; Unionization
Labor union, formation of, 268–269
Laissez-faire leader, 35, 37, 53
in team, 373
Language, 22
Lawsuits, avoidance of, 202
Leader situation, elements of, 51
Leader-group interaction, 51–52
Leader-manager theories, 42–54. *See also*
Leadership, early theories of;
Management, early theories of

Leaders
assertiveness of, 365
behavior descriptions of, 37–38
competence of, 65
factors affecting effectiveness of, 54
feedback loop and, 8
least preferred coworker (LPC), 49
task-relationship orientation of, 38–40
types of, 373
Leadership. *See also* Leaders; Management
in community, 435–452
concept of wholeness and, 7
conceptual base for, 3–28
designation of, 50
early theories of, 31–40
in effective management, 89
effectiveness of, 57
action and, 75–79
checklist for, 79–82
communication in, 69–73
in community, 451–452
components of, 82
energy and, 73–75
leader situation and, 51
in problem discussion meeting, 361
self-awareness and, 66–69
enhancing productivity through, 245
goals of, 58–62
innate capacity of, 53
knowledge, 62–63
participative, 47
self-awareness and, 66–69
skills, 63–66
styles of, 34–37, 53
and nursing staff job satisfaction, 39
in problem discussion meeting, 361
of team, 373–374
Leadership ability, 32–33
Leadership event, elements of, 8
Least preferred coworker (LPC) leader, 49
Legal counsel, 279
Legal power, 425–426
Lewin's phase of change, 405–411
Limit setting, 239–242
Limited·communication, 332
Line authority, 196
Linker, 329
Linking, 72
List making, 237
Listening
active, 69
attentive, 289
supportive, 293–294
Long-term employment, 46
Love, need for, 17–18
LPC leader, 49

Mainframe computer, 249
Management. *See also* Leadership; Managers
behavioral, 46–47

collective bargaining and, 274–280
conceptual base for, 3–28
defining, 86–87
early theories of, 31, 40–42, 53–54
effectiveness of, 85–88, 104
  checklist for, 101, 102–103
  components of, 85–104, *86*
  development and, 98–99
  direction and, 92–94
  leadership and, 89
  monitoring staff and, 94–96
  planning and, 89–92
  recognition and rewards in, 97–98
  representation and, 99–101
opposition to unionization of, 274–277
participative, 93–94
practicing of, 87–88
scientific, 40–41
successful, 48
tasks of, 88
Management by objectives
  advantages and disadvantages of, 144–145
  essentials of, 141–144
  evaluating outcomes in, 144
  misuse of, 145
Management situation, 86, *87*
Managerial skills, 41–42
Managers
  as advocate, 100
  as coordinator, 100
  financial management and, 175
  problem in defining role of, 389–390
Marginal performance, 466–469
Marketing, 114
  definition of, 114–115, 119
  importance of to nurses, 117
  techniques of, 115–117
Maslow's hierarchy of needs, 3, 14–20, 28,
  44, 47, 54
Mass media, in diffusion of change, 401–402
Matrix organizations, 198–199
Mediation, 270
Medicaid, 109
Medical staff, structure of, 207–208
Medicare, 109, 111
  DRG system of, 112, 477
Meetings, 76. *See also* Groups
  choosing date for, 343–344
  communication pattern in, 358
  coverage for, 344–345
  follow-up on, 366
  guiding of, 346, 364–365
  opening of, 345–346, 364
  outcomes of, 366
  place for, 344
  problem discussion, 341, 367
    implementation of, 345–347
    preparation for, 341–345
    scripts for, 347–361
  publicize, 344
  reduce threats of, 345

refreshments for, 345
roles played by members of, 358–360
seating arrangements in, 358
summarizing of, 347, 366
time for, 344
Mintzberg's model, 195
Mission, 52
Misunderstandings, avoiding confrontation
  and, 295
Modem, 249
Money, as power, 425
Monitor (computer), 249
Monitoring
  effective management and, 94–96
  methods of, 96
Monopolizer, 329
Motivation, 391
  goal-based model of, 370–372
  of individual employee, 369–372
  needs hierarchy and, 14–20
Motivation factors, 44–45
Motivational theories, 42–47, 54
Motivators, five basic needs as, 369–370
Multi-hospital systems, 112–113
Multiple marketing tools, 115

National Health Planning and Resources
  Development Act, 109, 110
National Labor Relations Act, 263–264
National Labor Relations Board (NLRB),
  263–264
National prosperity, 109
Nature, relationship with, 21
Needs hierarchy, 3, 14–20, 28
  as motivators, 369–370
Negative feedback, 71, 97, 459–460, 473
Negotiation, 303
  continuing process of, 305–307
  opening move in, 304–305
  setting stage for, 303–304
  simulated, 306
  strategies to influence, 307–308
Networking, 72–73
Neural energy, 73
New Frontier, 109
NLRB, 263–264
No, saying, 239–240
Nominal group technique, 157
Nonconformity, 26–27
Nondeliberative coping mechanisms, 12–13
Nonfunctional roles, 329–330
Nonproductive time, 226
Nonverbal communication, 286–287
  attending, 289
  interpretation of, 287–288
Normative change model, 404, 416–417, 432
  assumptions of, 405
  Havelock and Lippitt's steps in, 411–417
  Lewin's phases of change in, 405–411
  types of, 405

Not-for-profit organizations, 188, 189
Numbers, strength in, 427
Nurse, interpreting role of, 78
Nurse administrators, 208
Nursing
  image of, 117–119
  marketing and, 117
  primary, 220–222
  team, 219–220
Nursing care
  acuity index and, 222–223
  determining staffing needs for, 222–226
  developing a system of, 228–230
  monitoring of, 94–95
  organization of, 217–230
  organizing delivery of, 217–222
  staffing and scheduling issues in, 227–228
Nursing knowledge, 63–64
Nursing skills, 82
Nursing staff, 208
Nursing team, 372
Nursing unit, monitoring of, 96

Objective. *See also* Goals; Management by
  objectives
  implementing of, 143–144
  individual, 141–143
  work-group, 143
  writing of, 141–143, 146
Observation, 482
  in monitoring, 96
One-way communication, 330–331
Open communication, 332
Open systems
  characteristics of, 5–11
  community as, 436–438
  complex man and, 51
  defined, 5
  factors influencing behavior in, 11
  health care organizations as, 189–194
  response of to change, 397–399
  small groups as, 312–313
Open-ended questions, 290–291
Openness, 7–8, 437
  to self, 66–67
Operating core, 194
Operation, levels of, 202–206
Opinion giver, 328, 358–359
Opinion seeker, 328
Organizational structure, 50
Organizations. *See also* Health care
  organizations
  bureaucratic, 195–198
  complexity of, 192
  formal and informal levels of operation
    in, 202–206, 213
  fully developed, 194–196
  function of, 199–206
  goals of, 91, 199–202, 212
  growth patterns of, 192–194

hierarchy of, 191–192, *193*
  individuality of, 190
  matrix, 198–199
  openness of, 192. *See also* Open systems
  proprietary, 188
  relationship patterns in, 206–212
  structures of, 194–199
  theory and, 3
  voluntary, 188
  of work, 236–239
Organizing, 77
Overload, of roles, 26
Overqualification, 26

Paperwork, unnecessary, 240
Paradoxical change model, 417–418, 423, 433
  first-order change and, 418
  paradoxes in, 418–419
  second-order change in, 419–422
Passive behavior, as coping mechanism, 14
Paternalism, 209–210
Path-goal theory, 49, 54
Patient assessment, computerized, 253
Patient census, 222
Patient classification systems, 223–225,
  229–230
Patient monitoring, computerized, 253
Patient records
  computer programs for, 252–523
  computerized, privacy and security of, 259
Patterns, 9–10
  long- and short-interval, 10
Peace Corps, 109
Peer review, 96, 473
  comprehensive, 470–472
  fundamentals of, 469–470
People-environment interaction, 5–11
Perceptions, checking out, 71, 292
Performance appraisals, 96, 473
  guidelines for, 465–466
  of marginal staff member, 466–469
Performance gap, 150–151, 155
Performance standards, 472
Personal computer, 249. *See also* Computer
  systems
Personal self-worth, 369
Personalizing, 292–293
Perspective, theory and, 3–4
PERT charts, 165, *166*
Physical strength, 424
Physiological needs, 15–16
Pilot projects, 160–161
Plan
  analysis of options and course of action
    in, 158–161
  analysis of situation in, 151–155
  establishing purpose of, 150–151
  evaluating outcome of, 167
  formulating objectives to, 155

generating alternative solutions to, 156–158
implementing and monitoring of, 164–167
obtaining approval for, 161
presentation of, 161–164
revising and updating of, 167
Planned change. *See* Change
Planning, 77, 168
computer systems for, 254–255
of current work, 90–91
development phase of, 150–161
in effective management, 89–92, 104
financial, 172–173
of future work, 91–92
implementing and monitoring phase of, 164–167
presentation phase of, 161–164
types of, 149–150
Playboy role, 329
Political action, 444–445
barriers to, 447–451
decision-making channels of, 445–451
effective community leadership and, 451–452
Positional power, 425
Positioning, in communication, 287–289
Positive feedback, 459–460, 473
Posture, communication and, 289
Power, 424, 433
budget and, 173–174
distribution of in community, 438–440
in organizational relationships, 206–209
sources of, 424–427
Power base, building, 429–430
Power-coercive change model, 423
assumptions of, 423–424
basic steps of, 427–432
power in, 424
sources of power in, 424–427
Prediction, theory and, 4
Presentations, 161–164
planning of, 342–343, 363
Primary nursing, 220–222
Priorities, 90
Prioritization, 237
Privacy, 259
Proactive planning, 151
Problem analysis, 152
Problem discussion meetings. *See* Meetings, problem discussion
Problem discussion script, 347–356
analysis of, 356–357
Problem solving, 26
critical thinking and, 77
individual approaches to, 140
purpose of, 135–136
steps in, 136–140
Problem-solving conferences, 362
analysis of, 366–367
implementation of, 364–366
preparation for, 362–364

Procedural technician, 329
Product definition, 115
Productive time, 226
Productivity, enhancing through leadership, 245
Product-line management system, 116
Professional activities, 77–78
Professional practice, promotion of, 265–266
Profits, 188
Project planning, 149–168
Projection, 13
Promoter role, 100
Promotions, slow, 46
Proprietary organizations, 188
Prospective payment, impact of, 111–114
Psychological safety, 407–408
Public agenda, 333
Public health agencies, 189
Public image, 201
Public Law 98–21. *See* Social Security Amendments of 1983
Public recognition, 426
Public support, 426
Punishments, 44
motivation and, 371–372

Quality, 475–476
Quality assurance, 476–477
chart audit for, 485–486
comprehensive, 476
comprehensive evaluation of, 478–479
evaluation standards in, 479–480
implementation of, 484–487
participative approach to, 484–485
procedures in, 480–488
purposes of, 477–478
Quality circles, 482–483
Quantity, priority of, 201

Rational change model, 400, 432
assumptions of, 400
consequences of, 403–404
diffusion of, 401–403
invention of, 400–401
Rationalization, 13
Reactive planning, 151
Reality shock, 27, 493–497, 501
Reassurance, 293–294
seeking, 13
Recognition, 104
need for, 369
seeking, 78
in teams, 374
Recognition seeker, 329, 358–359
Record audit, 480–481
Recorder, 329
Reflex actions, 12
Reframing, 419–422

Refreezing, 410–411
Regulations, in bureaucracy, 196
Relationship games, 209–212, 213
Relationship orientation, 38–40
Relationships, 21–22
Relaxation techniques, 14
Repetitive activity, as coping mechanism, 14
Repetitive tasks, automation of, 245
Repression, 12
Research, computer systems for, 255–256
Resources
    control of access to, 427
    taking stock of, 14
Responding, 290
Responsibility. *See also* Delegation
    delegation of, 385–391, 392
    diffusion of, 376
Restraining forces, 405–407, 445
Retrospective payment, 111
Rewards, 44, 52
    determining, 97–98
    formal evaluation and, 464
    in negotiation, 307
    for professional growth, 493
    types of, 97
Rhythm, as coping mechanism, 14
Rigidity, as coping mechanism, 14
Risk taking, 78–79
Role bargaining, 26–27
Role stress
    reduction of, 26–28
    sources of, 25–26
Roles. *See also* Groups, roles in; Social roles
    conflict of, 25, 27
    in groups, 328–330
    informal, expectations of, 205
Rules, in bureaucracy, 196

Safety needs, 16
Salaries, 276, 277
Scenarios, 159–160
Schedules
    for implementation, 164–165
    in time management, 238
Scheduling, 93–94
    computer systems for, 255
    issues of, 227–228
Scientific advances, 108–109
Scientific management, 40–41
Seasonal variations, 10
Secretarial computer support, 251–252
Security needs, 16–17
Selective attention, 126
Self-actualization, 19–20
Self-awareness, 57, 66
    effective leadership and, 245
    in effective leadership in community, 451
    hidden agendas and, 334
    importance of, 67–68
    increasing of, 68

openness and, 66–67
    stages of, 68–69
Self-esteem, 18–19
Sensitivity, 82
Sensitivity groups, 341
Sentience, 10–11
Sequence, 90
Shadow organization, 207–208
Shared meaning, 20–23
Silence, 289
Simulation, 158–159
Situational determinants, 49–50, 54
Situational leader, 373
Situational theories, 47–50, 54
Situational variables, 152–154
Sleeping, as coping mechanism, 14
Smoking, as coping mechanism, 14
Social relationships, 21–22
Social roles
    influence of, 24–28
    reduction of stress of, 26–28
    sources of stress in, 25–26
Social Security Act, 108
Social Security Amendments of 1983, 112
Social Security payroll deductions, 109
Social status, 50
Social welfare programs, 107
    government involvement in, 108
Socialization, 25
Sociocultural influences, 20–28
Sociogram, 357–358
Software, 250–251
    finding right, 258
    for nursing practice and management,
        251–256
Sound, as coping mechanism, 14
Spatial relationship, 22
Specialization, 227–228
SSI program, 108
Stability needs, 17
Staff
    budget for, 180
    computer training of, 258
    continuing education for, 98–99
    delegating responsibility in, 385–391
    development of, 98–99, 491–501
        climate for, 491–493
    direction for, 92–94
    effective management of, 104
    inadequate, 390–393
    monitoring of, 94–96
    pressures of, 495
    prevention of reality shock and burn-out
        in, 493–501
    representation of, 99–101
    specialization of, 227–228
    support, 195
    technical, 195
    temporary, 228
Staff mix, 225–226
Staff surveys, 277

Staffing, 93–94
    determining needs for, 222–226
    developing system for, 228–229
    issues of, 227–228
Standard setter, 329
Stereotypes, 129
Stilted communication, 331–332
Stimulants, as coping mechanism, 14
Stranger's viewpoint, 127
Strategic planning, 149–150
Streamlining work, 242–245
Stress, interpersonal, 50
Stress rating scale, 399
Substantive issues, 304
Substitution, 13
Subsystems, 6
Summarizer, 329
Supervision. *See also* Management
    under collective bargaining agreement,
        277–279
    indirect, 46
Supplemental Security Income (SSI)
        program, 108
Support, 293–294
    of work-unit culture, 52–53
Support network, 497
Support staff, 195
Support systems, mobilization of, 76–77
Suppression, 13
Suprasystems, 6, 187
    complexity of, 212
Synchronizers, 335
    dominant, 335–337
        in problem discussion meeting, 361
    types of, 336–337
Synectics, 157–158
Synergistic power, 74
Synergy, in teams, 374
Systems. *See also* Organizations
    hierarchy of, 6
    open. *See* Open systems

Target group, definition of, 115
Task orientation, 38–40, 49
Team nursing, 219–220
Teams, 372, 391
    building of, 376–384, 391–392
    composition of, 372
    defining roles in, 377
    flexibility of, 374–375
    function of, 373–374
    group norms in, 380–382
    guiding decision making in, 379–380
    leadership of, 373
    managing conflicts in, 383–384
    maturity of, 373
    open communication in, 382–383
    participative decision making in, 381
    purpose of, 373
    relationships in, 374

    selecting members of, 376
    setting goals of, 376–377
    team identity and cohesiveness in,
        377–379
Teamwork
    advantages and disadvantages of, 374–376
    facilitation of, 372–384
Technical competence, 196
Technical direction, 94
Technical staff, 195
Technological advances, 108–109
Temporary personnel, 228
Tension reliever, 329
Theory. *See also* Leader-manager theories;
        Leadership, early theories of;
        Management, early theories of
    empirical testing of, 5
    internal consistency of, 5
    selection of, 4–5
    uses of, 3–4
Theory X, 44–45, 48, 54
Theory Y, 44, 47, 48, 54
Theory Z, 45, 46, 54
Thinking, modes of, 22–23. *See also* Critical
        thinking
Threats, 308
    reduction of, 363–364
Tickler files, 237
Time
    blocks of, 238
    blocks to effective use of, 245
    tyranny of, 233–234, 246
Time lines, 238–239
Time log, 242, *243*
Time management, 90, 233–246
    enhancing productivity through, 245
    goal setting for, 234–236
    limit setting and, 239–242
    organizing work and, 236–239
    streamlining work in, 242–245
Time orientation, 21
Timing, 90
Trait studies, 33
Trait theories, 31–33, 53
Turnover, 93

Unfair labor practices, 264, 265
Unfreezing, 407–408
Unionization. *See also* Collective bargaining
    contract negotiations in, 269–271
    elections in, 269
    organizing council for, 268–269
    prevention of, 274–277
Unnecessary work, elimination of, 240–241
Utilization review, 483–484

Vagueness, as coping mechanism, 14
Value conflicts, 132–133
Value-adding partnerships (VAPs), 113

Values, 24
VAPs, 113
Ventilating feelings, 14
Vertical health care systems, 112
Vietnam era, 109–110
Vitamins, discovery of, 108
Voluntary organizations, 188

Weber, Max, 195–196
Wholeness, 6–7, 189–190, 436–437
    implications of, 7

Withdrawal, 13, 27–28
Work assignment, 92–93
Work stoppages, 271
Workaholics, 239
Worker groupings, 42
Worker relations, 41–43
Working with others, 76–77
Work-unit culture, 52–53

Zipper-mouth role, 329, 359

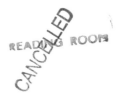
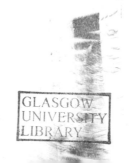